# CSA Symptom Solver

*Clinical frameworks for the MRCGP CSA exam*

**Muhammed Akunjee**

GP Principal

**Nazmul Akunjee**

GP Principal

*Clinical Prep* Publishing

London, UK

**Clinical Prep (Publishing), 2014**
339/341 West Green Road
London N15 3PB


**www.csaprep.co.uk**


**First published in 2014**

**Important Note from the Publisher**
The information contained within this book was obtained by Clinical Prep from sources believed to be reliable. Whilst every effort has been made to ensure the accuracy of the material contained herewith, no responsibility for loss, injury or exam failure whatsoever occasioned to any person acting or refraining from action as a result of information contained herein can be accepted by the authors or publishers.

Although every effort has been made to ensure that all owners of copyright material have been acknowledged where relevant in this publication, we would naturally be pleased to acknowledge in subsequent reprints or editions any omissions brought to our attention.

All readers should be aware that medical sciences are constantly evolving and whilst the publishers and authors have checked all dosages and guidance are based upon current indications, there may be specific practices and procedures that differ between countries and nations. You should always follow up-to-date guidelines laid down by the manufacturers of specific products and the relevant authorities in the country in which you are residing and/or practicing.

**ISBN-13: 978-0-9927661-1-5**
Typeset and designed by Clinical Prep, UK

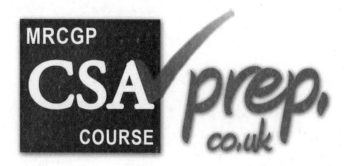

# Table of Contents

# 0.1 Preface

General practice can throw up an eclectic mix of patients presenting with a range of confounding and complex symptoms. Once qualified as a GP, you would be expected to deal with the majority of such patients; in fact, given the huge cutbacks and caps on NHS investment that the present economic climate has imposed upon us, GPs are expected more than ever to diagnose and managing a greater number of patients to reduce the ever burgeoning secondary care bill.

On this background, the RCGP created the CSA exam which now contains a bank of 600+ cases that have been tried and tested on 1000's of students since its inception. The RCGP curriculum is wide ranging and covers the plethora of medical specialties and subspecialties that GPs need to have some knowledge about. Of the cases, the vast majority are common and straightforward diagnosing and management stations. The remainder, are considerably more tricky, dealing with complex communication or ethical issues and are usually the ones that discriminate between a passing and failing candidate.

In an already busy GP registrar year with e-Portfolio updates, tutorials, VTS away days, home visits, and the daily rigmarole of clinics, there is perhaps not enough time to revise the whole of medicine, surgery and the specialities (ENT, Ophthalmology, gynaecology, paeds etc.) that would give you confidence to face the exams. With this in mind, we have written this book to try and lessen the load. It includes over 120 common symptoms that patients present with and those that often come up in the RCGP CSA exams. For each symptom a comprehensive consultation framework has been included to guide you through the best approach in dealing with the complaint.

This CSA book includes guidance such as what questions to ask, eliciting relevant past medical history, social history, family history and system review; the CSA framework then guides you to which examinations are relevant and what investigations should be requested in your exam. The final part of each chapter advises about possible differential diagnoses and evidence based ways of managing these. We have also included in this book simple explanation briefs that you can use to explain the pertinent diagnoses to the patient in a jargon free manner. This book has been specifically written to save you hours of time researching before your examinations and hopefully will become your core companion to ease you through the CSA exams and into your future as a fully fledged General Practitioner.

We hope that you find this book a useful aid to excel in the CSA exams and continue to use it well into your independent GP years!

**Muhammed & Nazmul Akunjee**
August 2014

# 0.2 About the Authors

### Muhammed Akunjee MBBS, MRCGP, PgCert (Diabetes), PgCert (MedEd)

Muhammed Akunjee has been a GP Principal in London since 2007. He is the mental health lead for Haringey CCG and is a Board Member. He is also the GP Director for the SE Haringey federation and has undertaken consultancy work for primary care procurement projects. He qualified from Guy's, King's and St. Thomas's Medical School in 2002 and completed his MRCGP gaining a distinction in 2006. During this time he was also awarded first prize for the Roche / RCGP Registrar award for a paper on miscommunication between secondary and primary care. He is a GP Appraiser for the NCL cluster as well as a BMA Book Award Appraiser.

He completed a Postgraduate Certificate in Medical Education at the University of Dundee and more recently, a Certificate in Diabetes at Warwick University. He has attended the London Deanery's, *Introduction to Teaching in Primary care course* and has taught and examined clinical skills at Imperial College, London. He is an avid medical book writer and has published a number of articles in peer reviewed journals.

### Nazmul Akunjee  MBBS, MRCGP

Nazmul Akunjee recently completed his GP vocational training and is currently a GP Principal in a large North London practice. He qualified from GKT medical school in 2005 and is currently actively engaged in teaching medical students and preparing them for their exams. He has published a number of articles related to examination skills in peer-reviewed journals and recently was appointed as a GP Appraiser by NHS England (London).

Nazmul Akunjee passed and excelled at his CSA exam in February 2011 passing all 13 stations at the first attempt. Since then, he has been involved in 1-2-1 private CSA coaching as well as group tuition with GP registrars. He completed the London Deanery's, *Introduction to Teaching in Primary care course* in June 2011 and has taught and examined medical students at University College London Medical School.

Nazmul is currently a GP lead for implementing the Primary Care Strategy as well as the IT lead for Haringey CCG. He is also the clinical lead for both the Haringey Primary Care Intelligence Group and CCG Access and Productivity Task Force looking to help improve quality in general practice across the borough. He is the Medical Director for Tottenham Primary Care Services LTD. In 2014, Nazmul was shortlisted for the GP Enterprise RCGP First5 award for his work in primary care.

### BMA Book Awards

Nazmul Akunjee and Muhammed Akunjee are both authors of *'The Easy Guide to OSCEs'* series published by Radcliffe. In 2008 their book the *'Easy Guide to OSCEs for Final Year medical students'* was Commended in the BMA book awards. Their second publication, *'The Easy Guide to OSCEs for Specialties'* was Highly Commended in the BMA book awards the following year in 2009. Their most recent work *'Clinical Skills Explained'* was Highly Commended at the BMA book awards in 2013. Radcliffe Publishing nominated the authors for the BMA Young Author of the Year in 2010.

# 0.3 The CSA Prep Course

The CSA Prep course commenced in the winter of 2011 providing an intense one-day coaching experience for GP registrars to help pass the RCGP CSA exit exams. It was the brainchild of Dr Nazmul Akunjee who sat and successfully passed the CSA examination at his first attempt. After he attended a number of courses, he felt that there was no course that accurately reflected the examination experience. Hence, he went about devising and creating a course that was, *'as close to the exam as possible.'*

The CSA Prep course is unique in that it solely utilizes MRCGP trained actors who have all acted out in the MRCGP CSA exams and appreciate the nuances of how to act out medical cases and when to drop cues. The full day course uses four different CSA actors who act out 18 different cases in total.

The course employs 2 course facilitators, both of whom are GP partners, each in charge of a group of 3 registrars so that each candidate gets at least 6 goes on the day and sees 12 further cases. The facilitators give honest and personalized feedback with a view to helping you through the CSA examination hurdle.

The cases used on the day have been written to be equivalent to the harder end of the CSA exam spectrum and focus on difficult consultations such as dealing with angry patients, breaking bad news, underage consent and negotiating shared management plan, areas that many GP registrars find challenging.

We pride ourselves in trying to give you an experience, *'as close to the exam as possible'* and in this vein we have created our own MRCGP course app that is similar in functionality and structure to that of the RCGP exam. Thus giving you plenty of practice with the Ipad before having to do so in the real examination.

*2-For-2 Course*
For those who have completed the full-day CSA course and want further personalised feedback and more challenging cases covering other areas of the RCGP curriculum, is a half-day mini-CSA exam. This course uses 2 CSA actors, but has 10 further challenging cases and each candidate is allocated a single GP facilitator to coach them on their communication and consulting skills.

*Free Cases*
The CSAPrep experience does not end there, but through the website, www.csaprep.co.uk you can gain access to free CSA cases as well as free communication skills material with quick reference tools on how to succeed in the examination. You can also download an exam-like free app onto your iOS device and practice cases in a similar format to that of the examination. The website also contains numerous articles on how to pass the CSA exam and how to interpret the RCGP feedback following the examination.

*MRCGP CSA Case Book*
The authors have also written a 366 page book entitled, *'Practice CSA Cases and Communication Skills for the MRCGP CSA Exam'*. The CSA Case book has been written with 26 cases to emulate two full circuits of the RCGP CSA exam. Each case has been written to a similar standard to the examination and includes nuances arounds cues, communication skills and complex negotiation stations. The book includes an introductory chapter that explains all the key skills one would need to employ during a doctor - patient consultation. The clinical cases have been written containing a doctor consultation brief as well as an actor brief so that you can practice with friends. At the end of each case is a full explanation walk-through that has been thoroughly researched according to recent guidance and gives you the relevant history, examination and management plans needed to excel in the exams.

# 0.4 Abbreviations

| | | | |
|---|---|---|---|
| ABG | Arterial blood gas | ABPI | Arterial brachial pressure index |
| ACS | Acute coronary syndrome | ACR | Albumin : creatinine ratio |
| AF | Atrial Fibrillation | AFP | Alpha-fetoprotein |
| ADPKD | Autosomal dominant polycystic kidney disease | ASD | Atrial septal defect |
| AXR | Abdominal X-ray | BD | Bis in die (twice a day) |
| BDZ | Benzodiazepine | BMI | Body Mass Index |
| BNF | British National Formulary | BP | Blood Pressure |
| BPH | Benign prostatic hypertrophy | BPM | Beats per minute |
| BTS | British Thoracic Society | Ca | Cancer |
| CABG | Coronary artery bypass graft | CBT | Cognitive behaviour therapy |
| CF | Cystic fibrosis | CFS | Chronic fatigue syndrome |
| CKD | Chronic kidney disease | CI | Contraindication |
| COPD | Chronic obstructive pulmonary disease | COCP | Combined  Oral Contraceptive Pill |
| CP | Chest Pain | CSA | Child support agency |
| CT | Computerised tomography | CVA | Cardiovascular Accident |
| CVD | Cardiovascular disease | CVS | Chorionic villus sampling |
| CXR | Chest X-ray | D | Daily |
| DEET | N,N-Diethyl-meta-toluamide (insect repellant) | DM | Diabetes Mellitus |
| DMD | Duchenne Muscular Dystrophy | DPT | Diphtheria, pertussis & tetanus |
| DVT | Deep Vein Thrombosis | ECG | Echocardiogram |
| ERCP | Endoscopic retrograde cholangiopancreatography | FB | Foreign body |
| FBC | Full blood count | FEV1 | Forced expiratory volume |
| FH | Family history | FOB | Faecal occult blood |
| GA | General anaesthetic | GAD | Generalised anxiety disorder |
| GORD | Gastro Oesophageal Reflux Disease | GP | General practitioner |
| GTN | Glyceryl Trinitrate | HF | Heart failure |
| HNPCC | Hereditary non-polyposis colorectal carcinoma | HIV | Human immunodeficiency virus |
| HRT | Hormone Replacement Therapy | HTN | Hypertension |
| HVS | High vaginal swab | Hx | History |
| IBD | Inflammatory bowel disease | IBS | Irritable bowel syndrome |
| IFG | Impaired fasting glucose | IGT | Impaired glucose tolerance |
| IHD | Ischaemic heart disease | IOP | Intraocular pressure |
| IV | Intravenous therapy | LA | Local anaesthetic |
| LBBB | Left bundle branch block | LOS | Lower oesophageal sphincter |
| LN | Lymph nodes | LRTI | Lower respiratory tract infection |
| LUQ | Left upper quadrant | MAOI | Monoamine oxidase inhibitor |
| MCS | Microscopy, culture and sensitivity | MG | Milligrams |
| MRCP | Magnetic resonance cholangiopancreatography | MI | Myocardial infarction |
| MRI | Magnetic resonance imaging | MS | Multiple sclerosis |
| MSK | Musculoskeletal | MSU | Midstream urine |
| Mx | Management | N&V | Nausea and vomiting |
| NICE | National Institute for Health & Care Excellence | NHS | National health service |
| NSAIDs | Non-steroidal anti-inflammatory drugs | OAB | Overactive bladder |
| OCP | Oral contraceptive pill | OD | Omni die (daily) |
| OE | On examination | OGD | Oesophago-gastro duodenoscopy |

| | | | |
|---|---|---|---|
| ON | Omne nocte (every night) | OT | Occupational therapist |
| PAD | Peripheral arterial disease | PCOS | Polycystic ovarian syndrome |
| PDA | Patent ductus arteriosa | PE | Pulmonary embolism |
| PEFR | Peak expiratory flow rate | PF | Peak flow |
| PHQ | Patient health questionnaire | PID | Pelvic inflammatory disease |
| PMHx | Past medical history | PMS | Premenstrual syndrome |
| POP | Progesterone only pill | PPI | Proton-pump inhibitors |
| PR | Per rectal | PRN | Pro re nata (as needed) |
| PSA | Prostate specific antigen | PVD | Peripheral vascular disease |
| QDS | Quater in die (four times a day) | RBBB | Right bundle branch block |
| RF | Renal failure | Ref | Reference |
| RUQ | Right upper quadrant | ROM | Range of movements |
| SIGN | Scottish Intercollegiate Guidelines Network | SLE | Systemic lupus erythematosus |
| SSRIs | Selective serotonin reuptake | SOB | Shortness of breath inhibitors |
| STI | Sexually transmitted infection | TB | Tuberculosis |
| TCA | Tricyclic antidepressants | TDS | Ter die sumendum (three times a day) |
| TIA | Transient ischaemic attack | TMJ | Temporomandibular joint |
| TURP | Transurethral resection of the prostate | U | Units |
| URTI | Upper respiratory tract infection | US | Ultrasound scan |
| UTI | Urinary tract infection | VF | Ventricular fibrillation |
| VQ scan | Ventilation perfusion scan | VT | Ventricular tachycardia |
| Wk | Week | WPW | Wolff Parkinson White |
| ZN stain | Ziehl–Neelsen stain | | |

# 1.1 Home Visits

Despite the rates of home visit requests declining in recent times, possibly due to improved transport access and the existence of alternative providers of medical care (A&E, OOH, pharmacy, matrons, DN), visiting a patient at home is still an important and necessary feature of the GP's work. Usually the most vulnerable or unwell patients make request for a visit having exhausted alternative treatment options.

When visiting a patient, the dynamics of the consultation change as no longer is the GP in the comfort of their consulting room, with easy access to medical equipment or colleagues for support and advise. Family members or carers may also be present, and their concerns, or fears may affect and tip the balance of the consultation. The doctors themselves are exposed to potential risk, injury or violence and it is essential that they inform other staff members before journeying out.

---

**Preparing for a Home Visit**

| | |
|---|---|
| *Telephone* | Confirm patient's address, phone no. and triage the call to ensure the HV is necessary |
| *Map* | Ensure you know how to get to the patient's house and have the correct address |
| *Bag* | Take with you a thermometer, BP, stethoscope, prescription pad, otoscope, ophthalmoscope, headed paper, swabs, gloves, lubricant, sample bottle, blood request forms, urine dipsticks and relevant emergency medications |
| *Inform* | Inform staff when and where you are going and when to expect you back |

---

**HISTORY**

***Principles***

| | |
|---|---|
| *Home visit request* | Establish the reason for the home visit and what the main issue of concern is |
| *Surroundings* | Observe the house / room. Is it clean and well looked after? Is it disordered or poorly kept? Does it smell of urine or faeces? Does the patient hoard items? Are there any worries about health and safety? |
| *Rapport* | Greet the patient as well as any carers when you enter the room. Maintain good eye contact when engaging with them |
| *Interaction* | Observe the interaction between the patient and the carer (if present) |
| Positive | Is the carer concerned and appropriately caring for the patient? |
| Negative | Does the carer have the patient's best interests at heart? |

**Focused history**

| | |
|---|---|
| *Detailed* | Establish in a chronological order how their symptoms developed |
| Onset | How did it begin/start? |
| Last well | When were they last well? |
| Triggers | Does anything make it better or worse? |
| Similar episodes | Any similar episodes/illnesses in the past? |
| Contact | Have they been in contact with anyone with similar symptoms i.e. at a home/day centre |

### General
| | |
|---|---|
| Bowels | How are their bowel movements? |
| Urine | Any problems with passing urine? Any accidents? |
| Weight | Have they lost or gained any weight recently? |
| Eating | How often do they eat? Has it changed? Are they refusing food? |
| Drink | Are they taking plenty of fluids? |
| Swallowing | Do they have problems swallowing? Is this for solid or liquids? |

### Functional history
| | |
|---|---|
| *Mobility* | How do they get around (stick, frame, wheelchair)? |
| *ADLs* | Are you having problems with looking after yourself? Are you able to cook? Can you feed yourself? Are you washing yourself regularly? |

### IDEA, CONCERNS, EXPECTATIONS
| | |
|---|---|
| *Ideas* | Did you have any thoughts as to what is causing your illness? |
| *Concerns* | Did you have any specific worries about your problems? |
| *Expectations* | How were you hoping we could address this problem? |
| *Impact on life* | How has the illness affected the patient and the carer? |

### PAST HISTORY
| | |
|---|---|
| *Medical* | Enquire whether they suffer from any medical conditions |

### DRUG HISTORY
| | |
|---|---|
| *Medication* | Are they taking any medications? Have they been reviewed? |

### FAMILY HISTORY
| | |
|---|---|
| *Genetic* | Establish if there are any conditions that run in the family? |

### SOCIAL HISTORY
| | |
|---|---|
| *Relationships* | Are they currently in a relationship? How are things? Do you have any children? |
| *Home* | Where do they live (residential, nursing home, own house)? Who lives with them? |
| Relatives | Are there any relatives close by? Do they help out? What do they do (cook, shop)? |
| Social services | Do they have any full-time carers or key-workers? |
| *Centre* | Do they attend a day centre? |
| *Occupation* | Are they working at the moment or unemployed? Are they on benefits? |
| *Smoker* | Do they smoke? How many cigarettes per day? |
| *Alcohol* | Do they drink alcohol? How much and how often? |

### EXAMINATION
| | |
|---|---|
| *Vitals* | BMI, weight, pulse, temp, BP, O2 sats |
| *Inspect* | Look at the general appearance |
| *Examination* | Examine the appropriate system for the relevant physical complaint |
| Resp | Signs of chest infection |
| CVS | Listen for murmurs |
| Abdomen | Palpate for masses or constipation |
| MSK | Check gait and mobility |
| ENT | Examine ear for wax. Screen for hearing disorders |

## INVESTIGATIONS

| | |
|---|---|
| *Bloods* | BM as needed. Refer for further tests depending on the condition |
| *Urine* | Dipstick and send for MC&S if symptomatic |
| *Phlebotomy* | Consider sending community phlebotomy to undertake any requested blood tests |

**RED FLAGS**        Deteriorating medically, unable to care for self

## CSA TIPS

Home visit cases in the CSA exam may at first appear to be quite daunting, as it involves a consultation that is away from the safety of your consultation room. Cases that crop up, usually deal with elderly patients with complicated chronic diseases or are around issues of palliative care and death planning. You will be led out of your room to another examination room where the case is assessed with the patient and examiner already present. The room is usually more sterile than your CSA consulting room with only a sofa or bed present where the patient may be resting.

## MANAGEMENT PLAN

| | |
|---|---|
| *Explaining* | When explaining the condition to the patient, incorporate vocabulary that they used to describe their own illness |

| | |
|---|---|
| **Medical** | Treat the condition as needed. Try and arrange for a carer or the pharmacy to deliver the medications if the patient is unable to leave the house |
| *Palliative* | Refer to the palliative care chapter for more details |
| *Admit* | Refer to hospital or call an ambulance via 999 if the patient is unwell and deteriorating or requires urgent assessment |

### Referral

| | |
|---|---|
| *OT / Physio* | If having difficulties with ADLs or mobility for consideration of home adaption or mobility aids |
| *Continence* | Refer to District Nurses or continence clinic for assessment and prescription of pads |
| *Social Services* | Consider referral for assessment of benefits or an assignment of carer. Consider referral for assessment for residential or nursing home placement |
| *Matron* | Can refer to a chronic disease matron who can also follow up the patient as needed |

## SAFETY NETTING

| | |
|---|---|
| *Follow up* | Offer the patient a convenient follow-up appointment if relevant. Consider ringing the patient the following day to check if things have improved |

# 1.2 Telephone consultations

Problems with GP access frequently make the press with successive governments pressing to increase access to primary care services. A key technology to improve access is the usage of telephone consultations. In the UK around 25% of GP consultations and over 50% of OOH are now conducted via the telephone. In some areas, surgeries triage all patients either using a nurse practitioner or a GP to ensure that patients are seen and assessed by the correct medical practitioner.

Tele-consulting allows patients better access, and on average, the consultation is shorter, allowing for more patients to be assessed. Although such consultations may be of a great advantage to patients as they are more convenient, timely and quicker than face-to-face consultations, the doctor conducting them must be aware of the key skills and communication necessary to ensure that they remain safe and provide an efficient and quality service for patients.

## Pitfalls of Telephone Consultations

| | |
|---|---|
| *Communication* | One relies entirely on verbal communication (what is being said) as opposed to non-verbal. Patient cues, body language and facial expression are lost |
| *Doctor Centred* | Consultations tend to be more Dr-centred and less psychosocial lines of questioning are usually employed |
| *Shorter* | Consultations tend to be shorter and less patient education as well as rapport building is undertaken by the doctor |
| *Miss information* | Occasionally, Drs miss out key areas of enquiry such as allergies. Doctors tend to underestimate symptom severity and tend to think patients are healthier than they may be |
| *Signs* | It is impossible to perform a physical examination and so valuable clinical signs may be missed when making an assessment |

## PRINCIPLES

| | |
|---|---|
| *Communication* | Ensure that you use your verbal communication skills to gather as much history as possible. Use active listening skills to obtain information. Try to clarify and repeat back to the patient to ensure there is no miscommunication or misunderstanding |
| Cues | Listen out for any verbal cues such as change of tone of voice, pace and pauses that may indicate fear, anxiety, pain or depression |
| Active listening | Allow the patient to speak without interruption for as long as they require |
| Repetition | Consider advising the caller to repeat back to you any medical advice (treatments, red flags) you have given to check understanding |
| *Telephone request* | Establish why the telephone call-back request was made from your staff and what the main issue of concern is |
| *Medical Records* | Read the medical records and candidate brief thoroughly. Is there anything there to give you a clue as to what the telephone consultation may be about? |

## HISTORY

| | |
|---|---|
| *Introduce yourself* | Clearly state your name and designation |
| *Establish caller* | Obtain the patient's name and telephone number (incase the line is cut). Enquire whether they are ringing about themselves or about another person |

| *Rapport* | Greet the patient and ask them to tell you what their problem is |
|---|---|

## Focused history

| *Detailed* | Establish in a chronological order how their symptoms have developed |
|---|---|
| Onset | How did it begin/start? |
| Last well | When were they last well? |
| Triggers | Does anything make it better or worse? |
| Similar episodes | Any similar episodes/illnesses in the past? |
| Contact | Have they been in contact with anyone with similar symptoms i.e. home/day centre |

## IDEA, CONCERNS, EXPECTATIONS

| *Ideas* | Did you have any thoughts as to what is causing it? |
|---|---|
| *Concerns* | Did you have any specific worries about your problems? |
| *Expectations* | How were you hoping we could address this problem? |
| *Impact on life* | How has the illness affected the patient and the carer? |

## PAST HISTORY

| *Medical* | Enquire whether they suffer from any medical conditions |
|---|---|

## DRUG HISTORY

| *Medication* | Are they taking any medications? |
|---|---|

## FAMILY HISTORY

| *Genetic* | Establish if there are any conditions that run in the family? |
|---|---|

## SOCIAL HISTORY

| *Relationships* | Are they currently in a relationship? How are things? Do you have any children? |
|---|---|
| *Home* | Where do they live (care home, own house)? Who lives with them? |
| *Occupation* | Are they working at the moment or unemployed? Are they on benefits? |
| *Smoker* | Do they smoke? How many cigarettes per day? |
| *Alcohol* | Do they drink alcohol? How much and how often? |

| **EXAMINATION** | Request the patient to attend the surgery if you need to examine them. Consider using community nursing services (as available) to check height, weight, urine and BP |
|---|---|
| **INVESTIGATIONS** | Request the patient to attend the surgery to pick up any investigation forms as relevant. Consider sending community phlebotomy to undertake any requested blood tests if housebound |

| **RED FLAGS** | As appropriate for the presenting complaint |
|---|---|

## CSA TIPS

Telephone consultations can be a quite daunting prospect for the trainee GP since it is a new skill to be learnt and one that, perhaps, has not been taught well during your medical training. As with most things, a good comprehensive and systematic approach will avoid you falling into any potential pitfalls. A key point to remember is that if you are in doubt or unhappy then either request the patient to attend in person or perform a home visit if they are incapacitated from doing so.

Be careful when taking a call and a patient is demanding results for a partner or relative. It is paramount that you confirm who you are talking with and gain explicit consent from the patient to discuss the case with any other parties. In the case of children, it is also important to ensure you are discussing with the carer who has the parenting responsibilities. If you are unsure with whom you are speaking or whether it is actually the patient or not, you should offer to ring them back using the telephone number recorded on the clinical system.

## MANAGEMENT PLAN

*Explaining*

Explain the condition using the patient's own description and terms as relevant. Ensure you break the information into small chunks and repeat to ensure clarity and to reduce the chance of miscommunication

***Management***

Treat the condition as necessary. Consider lifestyle changes, self-management and medical options

Script

Try and arrange for a carer or the pharmacy to deliver the medications if the patient is unable to attend the surgery

Refer

If the patient requires referral, consider whether this can be done without having to see or examine the patient

*Face-to-Face*

If at any point you are unhappy with the consultation, request the patient to attend the surgery. It they are unable to do so, consider whether a home visit is appropriate

*Signpost*

Signpost the patient to alternative ways of treatment such as self care, buying OTC medications from a pharmacist, attending UCC/WIC or A&E depending on the severity and appropriateness of their ailments

## SAFETY NETTING

*Red Flags*

Explain to the patient the natural course of the disease. Also clearly explain the red flag signs and symptoms when they should seek urgent medical help, either via another telephone consultation or by physically attending the surgery / A&E

*Follow up*

Offer the patient a convenient follow-up appointment if relevant. Consider ringing back the patient the following day to check if things have improved

*Closing-up*

Thank the patient and check if they are happy with the advice. End the consultation

*# 1.3 Angry patient*

Anger is one of the most intense of human emotions. All people get angry from time to time as it is a natural response to feeling threatened or attacked. Occasionally, the display of anger may be directed by patients towards doctors and/or health professionals, particularly when their own illnesses and sense of well-being is affected. Patients may get angry for a variety of reasons, such as receiving bad news, having to wait to see a Dr for a long time, however, anger may be also a sign of mental health illness, personality disorder or substance abuse. The key to responding to an angry patient is to remain calm and not to face anger with anger. Most situations can be easily diffused by apologising and giving the patient time to explain their predicament.

## HISTORY

Approach the topic sensitively in a non-threatening, non-judgemental manner. Adopt a relaxed open posture that is calm and inviting. Use the speed and tone of your voice to relax the patient and help appease them.

| | |
|---|---|
| **Open questions** | Good day Mr Smith. I am Dr Jones, one of the GPs here. How can I help? Can you please tell me what the problem is? |
| *Safety* | Ensure that the consultation is conducted in a safe, open place. If not, make sure that your colleagues know where you are. Try and be seated closer to an exit in the event that the patient becomes physically violent for a quick escape |
| *Cues* | Pick up any cues that the patient is getting angry such as changes in body posture (standing from seated), raising voice, clenched fists or becoming fidgety. *I can see that you are unhappy, please do tell me about it so I can help you* |
| *Avoid* | Do not be defensive or deny responsibility. It is important not to blame anyone without establishing all the facts. Do not be evasive when the patient asks you any questions as this may appear as if you are trying to cover up or whitewash their problem |
| **Open questions** | Tell me more about why you attended today? |
| **Establishing Events** | |
| *Establish Reason* | Try and establish why the patient is in the state they are in. What caused them to become angry and why? *Tell me exactly what happened* |
| *Listen* | Allow the patient time and space to express their story. Be empathic. *Thank you for telling me. I know it must have been difficult to do so* |
| *Acknowledge* | Recognise why the patient is angry and acknowledge their response if it is reasonable. Show appreciation to the patient for raising the complaint especially if it is of a serious nature. *I can see why that made you upset... I can imagine that it must have been quite difficult for you* |
| *Apologise* | Apologise even if you feel the complaint was not warranted and this should be offered as early as possible. *I am sorry for the experience you have had* |

## IDEA, CONCERNS, EXPECTATIONS

| | |
|---|---|
| *Ideas* | Why do you think this happened? |
| *Expectations* | Clarify with the patient what they were hoping for from the complaint. *How were you hoping we could address this problem?* |
| *Impact* | How has this affected you? |

## RED FLAGS

| | |
|---|---|
| *Abusive / Violent* | If the patient is not responding to your efforts or is increasingly getting more abusive or threatens violence, then you should explain to them that you are feeling uncomfortable and may terminate the consultation if they continue |

## PAST HISTORY

| | |
|---|---|
| *Mental Health* | Have you suffered with low mood or anxiety? |

## SOCIAL HISTORY

| | |
|---|---|
| *Home* | Who lives with you at home? |
| *Support networks* | Have you spoken to anyone about this? (friends, police) |
| *Occupation* | Are you working or studying at the moment? |
| *Alcohol* | Do you drink alcohol? How much do you drink and how often? |
| *Smoking* | Do you smoke? How many a day and for how long? |

## CSA TIPS

Patients may attend a consultation angry or may become angry during the course of a consultation as they are not getting the outcome they expected. You should pay attention to nonverbal cues that the patient is unhappy and try your best to deal with these as early as possible. Expect to have to deal with a second problem once the patient has been appeased (time permitting). Failure to allow them to discuss this may result in them becoming angry again!

## MANAGEMENT PLAN

### Explanation

| | |
|---|---|
| *Offer Reason* | Provide an honest explanation summarising the series of events. If a mistake happened then inform the patient as to how and why it occurred. If there are some mitigating circumstances surrounding the mishap then these can be stated without justifying the mistake |
| *Preventing* | State what immediate measures you have taken to rectify things and minimise the distress i.e. preventing the mistake from happening again. *We can try to prevent this from happening again by...* significant event analysis (SEA), practice audit, practice protocol, education event/retraining for the clinician, adding alerts to notes |
| *Complaints* | If they are still angry explain the practice's complaints procedure. Do not simply tell the patient to speak to the Practice Manager. Offer to ensure that their complaint is seen through and offer to take personal responsibility if appropriate. *If you still feel upset by it, I am happy to run through the complaints procedure with you* |

## SAFETY NETTING

| | |
|---|---|
| *Follow up* | Offer the patient a convenient follow-up appointment if relevant. If a complaint is being made, explain when the patient will expect to get a response |

# 1.4 Complaints

Complaints are rising in the consumer driving society that we live in. Patients' expectation are increasing and they are expecting higher standards of care than ever before. When their expectation is not met by service provision, a complaint is likely to be generated. People incorrectly assume that most complaints are around neglect, poor care or clinical negligence. However, research shows that most complaints centre around poor communication or attitude between patient and doctor.

The key to responding to a complaint is to allow the patient to vocalise and vent their concerns and then respond to them according to local policies and protocols. Most situations can be diffused by apologising and explaining to the patient what steps you will take to ensure that similar mistakes will not happen again.

## HISTORY

Approach the topic sensitively in a non-threatening, non-judgemental manner. Adopt a relaxed, open posture that is calm and inviting. Use the speed and tone of your voice to relax the patient and help appease them. Ensure that you read any patient notes fully before the patient enters the room to see if there is any indication that something has gone wrong or that a mistake has been made.

| | |
|---|---|
| **Open questions** | Good day Mr Smith. I am Dr Jones, one of the GPs here. How can I help? Can you please tell me what the problem is? |
| *Cues* | Pick up any cues that the patient is getting angry such as changes in body posture (standing from seated), raising voice, clenched fists, becoming fidgety. *I can see that you are unhappy, please do tell me about it so I can help you* |
| *Avoid* | Do not be defensive or deny responsibility. It is important not to blame anyone without establishing all the facts. Do not be evasive when the patient asks you any questions as this may appear as if you are trying to cover up or whitewash their problem |

## Establishing Events

| | |
|---|---|
| *Establish Reason* | Try and establish why the patient wants to complain. What happened and what went wrong? *Tell me exactly what happened* |
| *Listen* | Allow the patient time and space to express their story. Be empathic. *Thank you for telling me* |
| *Acknowledge* | Recognise why the patient is unhappy and acknowledge their response. Show appreciation to the patient for raising the complaint. *I am grateful that you have brought this to my attention* |
| *Apologise* | Apologise even if you feel the complaint was not warranted and this should be offered as early as possible. *I am sorry that happened* |

## IDEA, CONCERNS, EXPECTATIONS

| | |
|---|---|
| *Ideas* | Why do you think this happened? |
| *Expectations* | Clarify with the patient what they were hoping for from the complaint. *How were you hoping we could address this problem?* |
| *Impact* | How has this affected you? |

## RED FLAGS

*Abusive / Violent*    If the patient is not responding to your efforts or is getting abusive or threatens, violence then you should explain to them that you are feeling uncomfortable and may terminate the consultation if they continue

## SOCIAL HISTORY

| | |
|---|---|
| *Home* | Who lives with you at home? |
| *Support networks* | Have you spoken to anyone about this? (friends, police) |
| *Occupation* | Are you working or studying at the moment? |
| *Alcohol* | Do you drink alcohol? How much do you drink and how often? |
| *Smoking* | Do you smoke? How many a day and for how long? |

## CSA TIPS

Patients may wish to lodge a complaint for a wide number of reasons. It is important to be confident when dealing with a patient who wishes to complain and be able to advise them clearly regarding what will happen next. Many registrars simply advise the patient to go the Practice Manager to make a complaint, having spent the last 5 minutes explaining their complaint to you. This invariable will irk the patient, and possibly may turn them angry and aggressive! A better course of action would be to inform the patient about the procedure and tell them that you will record the complaint and escalate it to the PM on their behalf.

## MANAGEMENT PLAN

### Explanation

*Offer Reason*    Provide an honest explanation summarising the series of events. If a mistake happened then inform the patient as to how and why it occurred. If there are some mitigating circumstances surrounding the mishap, then these can be stated without justifying the mistake

*Complaints*    Explain to the patient the practice's complaints procedure. Do not simply tell the patient to speak to the Practice Manager. Offer to ensure that the patient's complaint is seen through and offer to take personal responsibility if appropriate. *I am sorry that you are still unhappy. Did you want to make a formal complaint?*

### Complaints Procedure

Explain to the patient the complaints procedure and protocol
- All complaints should be dated
- Verbal complaints should be recorded in writing
- Acknowledge all complaints in writing within 48hr of receipt
- A full investigation will take place within 10 working days
- May organise a practice meeting to establish all facts; patient can attend if they so wish
- A written response will be given within 2 weeks

*Preventing*    State what immediate measures you have taken to rectify things and minimise the risk of recurrence. *We can try to prevent this from happening again by...* significant event analysis, practice protocol, education event/retraining for the clinician, adding alerts to notes

*Escalation*    If the patient is still unhappy then you should advise them how to escalate. If local complaints resolution fails, the patient may be directed to the local CCG complaints officer, NHS England or to CQC directly. Alternatively, the patient may refer their complaint to an independent review panel (ICAS) or the patient's ombudsman. Patients may be guided to PALS (Patient Advice & Liaison Service), ICAS (NHS Complaints Independent Complaints Advocacy Service) at any time

## SAFETY NETTING

*Follow up*          Offer the patient a convenient follow-up appointment if relevant. If a complaint is being made, explain when the patient will expect to get a response

## EXPLANATIONS

*Complaints procedure*  I am sorry that this has happened and you want to make a complaint. We have a practice policy around complaints which I will guide you through. As you have told me your complaint, I will record it down and the practice manager, who is responsible for dealing with complaints, will write to you acknowledging that you have made a complaint. Within 10 working days, we will investigate what happened. This may be through a practice meeting; which you can come to if you so wish. Once we have investigated the matter, we will then write to you informing you of our findings. We expect this to happen within 2 weeks but sometimes it may take up to 1 month.

*Prevent reoccurrence*  Thank you for bringing the mistake to my attention. In order to prevent this mistake from happening again, there are a number of things we as a practice will do.

SEA          Firstly, we will convene a meeting known as a significant event audit and we will discuss this issue with all the key staff present, (Drs, PM, admin). In that meeting we will investigate what happened, what went wrong and what we can do to prevent this from happening again.

Protocols          If relevant, we will amend our protocols to ensure that this does not recur.

Retraining          We will also send all relevant staff to training to ensure that they are up-to-date with knowledge and procedures.

Alerts          Another thing we can do is to attach an alert message to all patients who have taken that drug. This will highlight to the Dr or staff that they need to be careful and hopefully reduce the chances of the same mistake happening.

Audits          We can also do a search of patients who have similar problems (medications, conditions) and ensure their medical records are updated to prevent this from happening again.

*Escalation*          I am sorry that despite my explanation you want to take the complaint further. I can assure you that you are within your rights to do this. You can complain to the local PALs service or CCG who has a dedicated officer who will explain to you what will happen next. If you so wish, you can also complain to NHS England who make decisions about our services. If you are still unhappy with their response, I can give you a leaflet which explains how to contact the ICAS (Independent Complaints Advocacy Service) or the patient's ombudsman.

# 1.5 Breaking Bad News

Breaking bad news is an important skill that doctors must be able to do well. It is a difficult skill to master, particularly if one has not been trained to do it proficiently or one is not exposed to doing it on a regular basis (oncology, palliative care). With patients having longer life expectancies, they are more likely to suffer from cancers and/or chronic illnesses than ever before.

Bad news is any news that may seriously or adversely affect the patient's well-being and view about their future. Invariably it is not about telling a patient that their death is imminent, but more commonly may be around communicating diagnoses of cancer, HIV, dementia, blindness or that a couple are infertile and cannot have children. If delivered incorrectly, it may increase anxiety in patients, make them misunderstand prognosis and lead to increased complaints and patient dissatisfaction.

## HISTORY

Approach the topic sensitively in a non-threatening, non-judgemental manner. Adopt an open posture that is calm and inviting. Use the speed and tone of your voice to relax the patient and help appease them. Ensure that you read the patient's notes fully before they enter the room to see if there is any documentation that may indicate there might be some difficult news to break (abnormal bloods, scan, smear results or letter from hospital). Consider possible differentials based on the results and what next steps will be necessary.

| | |
|---|---|
| **Open questions** | Good day I am Dr Jones, one of the GPs here. How are you today? |
| *Cues* | Pick up any cues that the patient is expecting any bad news. Try and establish why they have attended today and what they were expecting |
| *Tips* | Do not avoid breaking the news. You should try and inform the patient about what the results mean and not hide any information. It is best to be honest and open. Try and use non-medical jargon as much as possible. If you have to resort to medical terms, then explain what they mean in common language |

| | |
|---|---|
| **Setting Scene** | |
| *Establish Problem* | Thanks for coming in today. As we have not met before, can I just ask you a few questions before we speak about the test results today? |
| *Summarise* | Summarise what information you have to hand from previous consultations and check with the patient, if anything has changed in the meantime. If there has been change, find out more about what has happened |
| *Understanding* | What have you already been told about what is going on? |
| *Concerns* | With your symptoms going on for such a long time, did you think what may be causing it? Do you have any particular concerns you would like to raise with me today? |
| *Information* | How would you like me to give the information about the test results? Would you like to know everything about them? Or just the main points? |

| | |
|---|---|
| **SOCIAL HISTORY** | |
| *Home* | Who lives with you at home? |
| *Support networks* | Have you spoken to anyone about this? (friends, family) |
| *Occupation* | Are you currently working or studying? |

| **BREAKING NEWS** | Ensure that when you break the bad news you do not do it all in one go, but rather perform it in stages and fire a warning shot suggesting that some unpleasant news may follow |
|---|---|

*Warning Shot*

| Accompanied | Ask the patient whether they came alone or attended with someone. Do they want anyone else present in the consultation today? |
|---|---|
| | Before we begin can I just check if you came with someone or came alone? |
| Difficult | I'm afraid I have some difficult news to tell you. The results are a little more serious that we had hoped |

| *News* | Provide an honest and clear explanation about what the results show |
|---|---|
| | The results show some changes in your scan results. Although this may be caused by infection or inflammation, sadly at this stage we cannot exclude cancer as a possible cause |

| **Response** | Having broken the news, pause and await the patient's response |
|---|---|
| *Crying* | I am really sorry that I have to give you this news. I can see that it has really affected you; this is completely normal. Would you like some tissues? |
| *Anger* | You seem quite upset at the moment. That is perfectly understandable. However, I want you to know that I am here to help |
| *Silence* | I know this was totally unexpected. Do you want me to carry on? I can understand that it is a lot to take in, please take your time and tell me when you are ready to carry on |

---

**SPIKES - 6 step protocol for delivering bad news**

Consider using the SPIKES protocol to deliver the news to the patient;

- **S**etting up - Check the notes and rehearse how you want to break the news. Ensure privacy and sit close to the patient. Ensure you are not rushed or interrupted (calls, bleeps)
- **P**erception - Check what the patient knows so far and what their understanding is
- Patient's **I**nvitation - Find out how much the patient wants to know
- Giving **K**nowledge - Fire a warning shot. Give medical facts and avoid jargon
- Address **E**motions - Respond to their emotions
- **S**trategy & Summary - Explain the different options available. Share responsibility for decision making

*Ref: Adapted from Buckman, R. Breaking bad news: the S-P-I-K-E-S strategy. Community Oncology 2005*

---

**CSA TIPS**

In general practice, there is often little opportunity to infrom patients that they definitely have a cancer as we rarely take biopsies. Patients who have had biopsies are likely to be already under secondary care and would usually be pre-warned about the possible malignant nature of their lesion. In primary care, you will more likely have to explain to a patient an abnormal smear result or scan that shows something more serious may be amiss. In such cases, it is important to inform the patient about the possible sinister pathology, but also to convey to them the alternative benign diagnoses as well.

**MANAGEMENT PLAN**

**Explanation**

| *Referral* | Consider referring to specialist services via a 2WW if suspecting cancer. May require same day admission if worsening of a chronic condition or end-stage organ failure. Explain why you need to refer them and what the hospital may do in terms of treatments and investigations |
|---|---|

| | |
|---|---|
| Investigations | If relevant, consider referring for further investigations to help confirm or negate differential diagnoses |
| Treatment | Consider explaining what some of the possible treatment options will be i.e. radiotherapy, chemotherapy, surgery |
| *Prognosis* | Be honest if you know the seriousness of the condition. Do not pluck figures from the air, but if you are aware of the prognosis of the condition then you can communicate this to the patient |
| | Thankfully you have been diagnosed very early on and the lesion is very small. These days we have excellent treatments that can control the cells and prevent them from causing any permanent harm |

**SAFETY NETTING**

| | |
|---|---|
| *Support* | If the patient does not have any family or local friends, consider referring to a counsellor, bereavement service or patient support group |
| *Departing* | Offer to call in the receptionist or nurse to take the patient to a quiet room and have a cup of tea until they are well enough to go home. If the patient is due to go home alone, advise if they would like to contact a friend or family member to pick them up |
| *Follow up* | Offer the patient an early follow-up to address any new questions or concerns the patient may have following the news. Allow them telephone access or emergency consultations during this difficult early period |

# 1.6 Domestic violence

Domestic violence (DV) refers to abuse or violence that takes place between adults who are partners or who are close relations. Although violence conjures up thoughts of physicality, the definition also encompasses verbal abuse, intimidation, sexual assault and even rape. Sadly, DV is a common phenomenon affecting 1 in 4 women with 2 women a week killed by current or former partners.

---

### The Definition of Domestic Violence
Domestic violence has been defined by the Department of Health to refer to, *'Any incident of threatening behaviour, violence or abuse (psychological, physical, sexual, financial or emotional) between adults who are, or have been intimate partners or family members, regardless of gender or sexuality.'*

---

### HISTORY
Approach the topic sensitively in a non-threatening, non-judgemental manner. It can be quite difficult to broach the subject initially, so begin by making your first few questions designed to put the patient at ease. Avoid focusing only on injuries without addressing the underlying cause.

| | |
|---|---|
| **Open questions** | You look upset? Is everything alright at home? Is your partner taking care of you? Do you get on well with your partner? |
| *Confidentiality* | Reaffirm and emphasize that everything discussed is confidential |
| *Cues* | Pick up any cues such as multiple minor injuries, fractures |
| | I noticed that you have a number of bruises/cuts/burns, is everything alright? |
| | |
| **Leading questions** | Ask more direct and leading questions enquiring about possible injuries |
| | How does your partner treat you, are you having any problems? |
| | Do you ever feel frightened by your partner? Do you feel safe at home? |
| | Has your partner ever hurt you in any way? |
| | |
| *Partner* | Has your partner ever physically hurt or threatened you? |
| | Has your partner ever broken or destroyed things that were personal to you? Has your partner ever prevented you from doing things that you wanted to do, such as leaving the house or going to see friends? |
| | Does your partner have any criminal convictions? |
| | |
| *Listen* | Allow the patient time and space to express their story. Be empathic |
| | Thank you for telling me. I know it must have been difficult to do so. |
| | It's not your fault... you are not to blame... |
| | |
| *Frequency* | Enquire whether the violence has increased in frequency and severity |
| *Alcohol* | Is the abuser intoxicated? |

---

### Mnemonic 'HARK' for questions to ask in Domestic Violence
*Have you ever been ...*
- **H**umiliated (emotionally and verbally abused including put-downs)
- **A**fraid
- **R**aped (made to have non-consensual sex)

- **K**icked (physically assaulted)

*... by your partner?*

*Ref: Sohal H, Eldridge S, Feder G. The sensitivity and specificity of four questions (HARK) to identify intimate partner violence: a diagnostic accuracy study in general practice. BMC Fam Pract 2007; 8(49)*

## RED FLAGS

| | |
|---|---|
| *Self harm* | Have you ever felt so low that you wanted to end it all? Have you ever tried to take your own life? |
| *Children* | Enquire if there are any children in the home and establish if they are at risk. Has your partner ever threatened or abused your children? |
| *Rape* | Ask if their partner has ever sexually abused or raped them. Has your partner ever forced themselves on you even when you did not want to have sex? |

## Subtle Clues to Domestic Violence

Domestic violence is still considered a taboo subject with woman experiencing around 35 episodes of DV before seeking help. Patients delay presentation for a number of reasons, the most common of which include feeling shame or embarrassment, worry about reprisals from partners, or fear that their children will be taken away.

Patients may present with subtle signs and symptoms that may be a clue that DV is taking place. It is important to be aware of these such as delayed presentation, multiple injuries – abdominal, face & hands, fractures, unexplained bruising, burns and injuries at different stages of healing, history of loss of consciousness and miscarriages.

## PAST HISTORY

| | |
|---|---|
| *Obstetric* | Have you had any terminations or miscarriages? |
| *Mental* | Have you suffered with low mood or anxiety? |

## SOCIAL HISTORY

| | |
|---|---|
| *Home* | Who lives with you at home? |
| *Support networks* | Have you spoken to anyone about this (friends, police)? |
| *Occupation* | Are you currently working or studying at the moment? |
| *Alcohol* | Do you drink alcohol? How much do you drink and how often? |
| *Drugs* | Have you ever used illegal drugs? |

## Consequences for Victims of Domestic Violence - *Ref: Stark and Flitcraft (1996)*

Victims of domestic violence are:

- 15 times more likely to abuse alcohol
- 9 times more likely to abuse drugs
- 3 times more likely to be diagnosed as depressed or psychotic
- 5 times more likely to attempt suicide

## CSA TIPS

Domestic violence is extremely common and is not solely committed by men to women. It is important to broach the subject in an empathic way as many partners may find it difficult to talk about the subject for fear of retribution. The patient records may give an indication that they are undergoing domestic violence due to unexplained falls or injuries in an otherwise fit and well patient. However, when opening the subject remember that the patient is an adult and cannot be forced into making a disclosure or taking further action. Always ask whether there are children at home, and consider making a referral to the local child protection team if you are concerned that they are risk of abuse or neglect.

**MANAGEMENT PLAN**

| | |
|---|---|
| *Illegal* | Stress to the patient that domestic violence is illegal, unacceptable and should not be tolerated. Offer to contact the police if the patient consents. Respect autonomy if they do not wish to do so |
| *Children Safety* | If there are children involved, seek advice from your child protection lead. The child may require transfer to safe location if at risk. Refer to Multi-Agency Risk Assessment Conference (MARAC) |
| *VISA* | Reassure the patient that the government supports victims of domestic violence in their immigration applications |

---

**Government immigration policy towards domestic violence** - *Ref: UK Home Office 2013*
Domestic violence victims can apply for indefinite leave to remain in their own right, if they have been victims of DV during the first 2 years of that relationship

---

**Safety plan**

| | |
|---|---|
| *Escape route* | Plan an escape route (stairs, doors, windows) if you need to leave quickly |
| *Escape bag* | Pack an emergency bag that contains money, phone, keys, important documents i.e. passport. Can leave this at a friend's house |
| *Numbers* | Have a range of emergency numbers – e.g. friends, 999, refuge |
| *Neighbour* | Advise neighbour to contact police if they hear shouting or suspicious noises |
| *Safe house* | Have a safe house (friend, family, refuge) that you can reside in an emergency |
| *Services* | Contact National Domestic Violence Helpline, local services - Women's Aid groups, Refuge, Relate, local police domestic violence safety unit; housing association |
| *Follow up* | Offer open same-day emergency appointments taking into account that the patient may not be able to attend a routine due to circumstances. Add alert to notes – not to inform family (confidentiality) and highlighting that the patient is at risk of domestic violence |

---

**Principles of approaching domestic violence**

- Support, empathise and listen to the patient appreciating their capacity to act while respecting their autonomy – *Whatever you decide we are here to support you*
- Document any injuries and take photographs if indicated
- If there are children involved then a referral to child protection may be necessary. Inform them of the referral and need to breach of confidentiality before doing so

---

# 1.7 Child Protection

In 2012 over 600,000 children were referred to the local authority and social services due to concerns about their health and welfare, with just over 50,000 being subject to a child protection plan. Child protection is the process and system by which children are identified as being sufferers of, or at risk of, harm as a result of abuse or neglect.

---

**The Types of Child Maltreatment** - *Ref: Working together to safeguard children, DoH, 2013*
There are 4 types of child abuse as defined by the Department of Health
- *Physical Abuse:* May involve hitting, kicking, poisoning, burning or any method that causes a child harm or failing to prevent harm befalling a child
- *Emotional Abuse:* This is the persistent emotional mistreatment of a child that results in stunting of the child's emotional development. It may involve, swearing, shouting, making them feel worthless or unloved
- *Sexual Abuse:* This is forcing a child to take part in sexual activities that they do not understand the meaning of. This may include penetrative (anal, vaginal) or non-penetrative (kissing, fondling) acts
- *Neglect:* This is the failure to cater for a child's basic physical and psychological needs leading to impairment of the child's development. It may include failure to provide adequate food, clothing or shelter, or failure to ensure appropriate medical treatment

---

As professionals, we are often at the forefront when dealing with patients and their children and it is of exceptional importance that we are able to pick up the tell-tale signs of abuse or neglect early, to help safeguard and prevent suffering of children and young people.

---

**Professional duty towards Child Abuse** - *Ref: Working together to safeguard children, DoH, 2013*
- Safeguarding is everyone's responsibility: for services to be effective each professional and organisation should play their full part
- The child's needs are paramount, and the needs and wishes of each child, be they a baby or infant, or an older child, should be put first, so that every child receives the support they need before a problem escalates
- All professionals who come into contact with children and families are alerted to their needs and any risks of harm that individual abusers, or potential abusers, may pose to children
- All professionals share appropriate information in a timely way and can discuss any concerns about an individual child with colleagues and the local authority's children's social care services

---

### HISTORY
Approach the topic sensitively in a non-threatening, non-judgemental manner. It can be quite difficult to approach the subject initially, so begin by making your first few questions designed to put the patient at ease. Ensure that you read the patient's notes available to you fully before the patient or their carer enters the room to see if there is any documentation that may signify that there is evidence of abuse i.e. repeated A&E attendances, minor injuries, fractures or a third party disclosure (SW, school).

**Open questions**     You look upset? Is everything alright at home? Are your parents or carers taking care of you? Do you get on well with your family?

| | |
|---|---|
| *Confidentiality* | Reaffirm and emphasise that everything discussed is confidential as long as there is no risk to the child or others |
| *Attendance* | If the child is <16yr and attends alone, check if there is anyone with parental responsibility who can attend with them. Do not request this if the alleged abuse is being perpetrated from them. Have you spoken to your parents about it? Is there a reason why you have not? |
| *Cues* | Pick up any cues such as multiple minor injuries, fractures, multiple A&E attendances, poor growth and dentition, change in emotional state, underaged sexual activity. I noticed that you have been in and out of hospital a few times with bruises/cuts/burns, is everything at home alright? |
| **Leading questions** | Ask more direct and leading questions enquiring about possible child abuse. Do you feel safe at home? How do your carer / parents treat you? Are you having any problems? Do you ever feel frightened by them? Have they ever hurt you in any way? |
| *Physical* | Has your carer or parents ever physically hurt or threatened you? Have they ever kicked or punched you? Have you ever been burnt by hot water, the radiator or by cigarettes? |
| *Emotional* | Do they shout at you? What do they say? Do they always say that? How did that make you feel? |
| *Neglect* | Do you eat well or do you feel hungry? How often do you have a bath? How often do you change your clothes? When you are unwell does your carer take you to see a Dr or give you medicine? Are you up-to-date with your injections? |
| *Sexual* | Have you ever had sex? Who was it with? Did you want to have sex or were you pressurised into doing so? Have you ever been pregnant? Do you have an itch down below on your front or back passage? Have you had any discharge? |

**Associated History**

| | |
|---|---|
| *Mood* | How is your mood? Do you feel low or down? |
| *Sleep* | How is your sleep? Do you have recurrent nightmares? |
| *Self esteem* | How do you feel about yourself? Do you feel shy or worthless? |
| *Angry* | Do you feel angry all the time? Do you shout at your friends or siblings? |
| *Self-harm* | Have you ever felt that you wanted to harm or cut yourself? Have you ever felt so low that you wanted to end it all? Have you ever acted upon these thoughts? |
| *Urine* | Do you wet yourself at night? Do you have any pain when you pass urine? |

**HOME CIRCUMSTANCES**

| | |
|---|---|
| *Home* | Who is at home? Do you have any lodgers? Do you move a lot (traveller)? Have you ever been homeless? Have you ever run away from home? |
| *Carer / Parents* | Who looks after you - your own parents, foster carers or a relative? |
| Separate | Are your parents together or separate? How long has this been? |
| Illness | Does any of your parents suffer with depression, schizophrenia or other mental health illness? |
| Drugs | Do they use illegal drugs or drink alcohol? How often? |

# 1.8 End of life / Palliative care

Palliative care relates to the branch of medicine that deals with a patient's symptom management once there are no curative treatment options for a terminal illness. The ultimate aim is to improve the quality of life for both the patient and the family and to make the patient's life comfortable in the final stages of their illness. Palliative care usually involves a multidisciplinary approach with hospital specialists, GPs, community nurses, matrons, Macmillan nurses and pain specialists involved in delivering the care.

Common symptoms that present in palliative care patients include chronic pain, shortness of breath, nausea, vomiting and constipation. Such symptoms may be extreme or constant, affecting the patient's quality of life and causing distress and mental anguish. Good care planning and multi-disciplinary working can help patients and carers prepare them through this turbulent time.

## HISTORY

**Open questions**    Can you tell me more about the symptoms you have been experiencing? Can you tell me what has been troubling you?

**Focused questions**

| | |
|---|---|
| *Pain* | When did your pain first start? How long has it been going on for? |
| Frequency | Is it always there (continuous) or does it come and go (episodic)? |
| Site | Where exactly is the pain? (bone, viscera) |
| Severity | How severe is the pain? (score) |
| Character | How would you describe the pain? (sharp, dull, throbbing, burning, cramping) |
| Radiation | Does the pain go anywhere? |
| Triggers | Does anything make it better or worse? (respiration) |
| Breakthrough | Is this pain different to your regular level of pain? |

---

**Character of the Pain in Relation to Cause**

| | |
|---|---|
| *Bone pain* | Pain triggered by weight bearing, pressure on bone (mets/fracture) |
| *Nerve pain* | Shooting, burning, altered sensation, dermatological distribution (nerve compression) |
| *Increased ICP* | Headache with nausea & vomiting, worse in morning or coughing/sneezing |
| *Intestinal colic* | Colicky crampy pain that comes in waves (bowel obstruction) |
| *Liver pain* | RUQ tenderness with hepatomegaly |
| *Muscle spasm* | Pain over muscle (trigger points) with tenderness |

---

| | |
|---|---|
| *Dyspnoea* | When did your shortness of breath start? How long has it been going on for? Has it worsened recently? |
| Frequency | Is it always there (continuous) or does it come and go (episodic)? |
| Triggers | Does anything make it better or worse? (lying flat, sleep, dressing) |
| Noisy | Have you noticed increased noisy secretions in the throat or below? |
| Impact | Does it affect your sleep? Are you able to talk with it? How far can you walk before you have to stop to catch your breath? |

| | |
|---|---|
| *Cough* | When did your cough begin? How long has it been going on for? Has it worsened recently? |
| Frequency | Is it always there (continuous) or does it come come and go (episodic)? |

| Character | Describe the cough? (dry, barking, harsh, brassy) |
| Phlegm | Any phlegm? What colour is it? Is there any blood? |
| Associated | Any noisy secretions in the throat or below? Have you had any chest pain with it? Any shortness of breath? |

*Constipation*

| Frequency | How often do you open your bowels? Has it changed? |
| Absolute | Have you failed to open your bowels or pass wind? Have you been vomiting recently? Do you have any pain in your tummy? |
| Bloody stools | Any blood in your stools? Any dark stools? |

*Nausea & vomiting*

| | Do you feel sick or have you vomited? When did it start? How long has it been going on for? Has it worsened recently? What colour is it? |
| Frequency | Is it always there (continuous) or does it come come and go (episodic)? |
| Triggers | Did it start after taking any medications? Is it worse when you move your head? Do you have any headaches? |
| Associated | Any blood in your vomit? Have you had any heartburn? |

*Mental health*

| | Have you been feeling low recently? Do you feel disinterested in life or worthless inside? |
| Suicide | Have you ever felt so low that you wanted to end it all? |

**Associated history**

| *Appetite* | How is your appetite? |
| *Weight* | Have you lost any weight? |
| *Fatigue* | Do you feel tired or weak all the time? |

**RED FLAGS** — Dyspnoea at rest, intractable pain, bowel obstruction

**PAST HISTORY**

| *Medical* | Do you suffer from any medical conditions? |
| *Cancer* | Have you been diagnosed with cancer? When was it made? What treatment have you had (radio / chemotherapy, operation)? |
| *Place of death* | Has the patient decided where they would like to spend their remaining days (hospice, hospital, home)? |
| *Advanced directives* | Does the patient have an advanced directive? |
| *Care co-ordinator* | Establish who the care coordinator is and what input they have had |

**DRUG HISTORY**

| *Medication* | Are you taking any medications? What medicines have worked? How are you taking them (buccal, PO, IM, driver)? Are you using any OTC medications or herbal remedies? |
| Analgesia | Do you take any painkillers (opioids)? How often do you take them (overuse)? |

**SOCIAL HISTORY**

| *Spiritual* | Does the patient ascribe to any religion? Have they spoken to a priest or chaplain? |
| *Home* | Who is at home with you? |
| Relationships | Are you currently in a relationship? |
| Carers | Do you have any carers? How often do they attend? Are they coping? |
| QOL | What things can you do independently? (cook, bathe, dress, feed, continence) |

| Smoker | Do you smoke? How many cigarettes do you smoke per day? |
| Alcohol | Do you drink alcohol? How much do you drink and how often? |

## IDEA, CONCERNS, EXPECTATIONS

| Idea | Do you have any idea about what may be causing your symptoms? |
| Concerns | Do you have any worries about it? |
| Expectations | How were you hoping I could help you? (admission, hospice) |
| Impact | How have your symptoms affected your life? |

## CSA TIPS

Patients on the palliative care register should be reviewed regularly. They usually suffer with common complaints including pain, vomiting and shortness of breath. However, when Drs are called out to visit, this usually means that there has been some deterioration in symptoms. Drs should know how to manage such symptoms including being able to write them on a medication chart for DN administration. Always try and get access to any shared care plans that may have been created as this would give you good background about advanced directives and the patient's choice around treatment options.

## PHYSICAL EXAMINATION

| Vitals | BP, pulse, temp, O2 sats |
| Examination | Perform examination of appropriate system |

## INVESTIGATIONS

| Bloods | FBC, ferritin, calcium, U&Es |
| X-Ray | Abdominal X-ray if obstruction suspected, CXR if SOB |
| CT/MRI | Brain / spine scan if suggestive of pathology (raised ICP, spinal compression) |
| Specialist | LP |

## MANAGEMENT  *treat symptoms*

| **Care pathway** | Consider using a care pathway such as the Liverpool Care Pathway / or develop an individual end of life care package to help manage the patient's symptoms |
| Finance | If terminally ill (expectation will not live for >6mth) issue a DS1500. Disability living allowance and attendance allowance can be fast tracked. Discuss having living will |
| Dying | Discuss with the patient about DNR status, advanced directive, lasting power of attorney (see dementia chapter) |

## *Pain*

*Analgesic ladder*

| Mild | Use non-opioid such as paracetamol +/- NSAIDs |
| Moderate | Use weak opioid i.e. codeine, dihydrocodeine or tramadol in addition to non-opioid if necessary (co-codamol) |
| Laxative | Offer stimulant laxative (senna, bisacodyl) or softener (sodium docusate) |
| Severe | Consider strong opioid i.e. morphine. Start immediate release (rapid onset - 20min) oramorph 5mg 4hrly (2mg in elderly). Titrate dose in 30-50% increments until pain free. Offer laxative |
| Breakthrough | Consider 2hrly additional oramorph for breakthrough pain |
| Modified release | Morphine MR (onset in 1-2hrs with slow peak 4hr) offered for continuous pain or once pain control on immediate release. Calculate total 24hr morphine dose and divide by 2. Give as 12hrly dose. Offer oramorph (2hrly) for breakthrough pain |

| | |
|---|---|
| Side effects | Advise and treat side effect of drowsiness (often settles), N&V (metoclopramide, haloperidol), constipation (senna, bisacodyl, docusate) or dry mouth (sip cold water, ice cubes or lollies, chew gum/boiled sweet, have unsweetened drinks) |
| *Other pain* | |
| Intestinal colic | Try hyoscine hydrobromide |
| Muscle spasm | Suggest heat pad, massage, TENS or consider diazepam, baclofen |
| Neuropathic | Try amitriptyline, pregabalin or gabapentin |
| **Nausea & vomiting** | Treat underlying cause (medication, raised ICP, obstruction, hypercalcaemia, renal failure). Consider alternative route (syringe driver) |
| *Conservative* | Easy access to bowl, water. If sight or smell provokes nausea suggest someone else do cooking. Eat small meals/snacks with cool fizzy drinks, consider acupuncture |
| *Medical* | Treat with cyclizine (most), metoclopramide (gastric stasis), domperidone (gastric distension), ondansetron (post-radiotherapy), haloperidol (opioid induced) |
| **Cough** | Treat underlying cause (chest infection - abx, effusion - drainage, mass - radiotherapy) |
| *Conservative* | Recommend to sit upright, breathing exercises, stream inhalation, fan, open windows |
| *Medical* | Try simple or codeine linctus. If persistent, try codeine phosphate or MST. Nebulised saline can help secretions, bronchodilators for bronchospasm |
| **Constipation** | Treat underlying cause (opioids, dehydration, immobility, obstruction, hypercalcaemia). Stress good fluid intake |
| *Medical* | Offer stimulant laxative (senna, bisacodyl), softener (sodium docusate) or suppositories (bisacodyl, glycerol) for hard stools. Co-danthramer in terminally ill patients |
| **Dyspneoa** | Treat underlying cause (COPD, anxiety, asthma, chest infection) |
| *Conservative* | Use fans to help cool the patient. Advise relaxation techniques. Consider pursed lip breathing, sit upright |
| *Medical* | Offer oral strong opioids (morphine 2-2.5mg 4hrly). If they are unable to swallow use a SC syringe driver. BDZ (lorazepam, diazepam) may have a role for anxiety induced dyspnoea. Home oxygen if SOB worsens. Consider (nebulised) bronchodilators for partial airway obstruction |
| **QoF** | Maintain a register of palliative care patients. Ensure 3 monthly multidisciplinary discussions with allied health professionals around all patients on the register |
| **Referral** | |
| *Macmillan nurse* | Offer support and advice regarding medication for symptom control (pain, N&V) |
| *Marie Curie nurse* | Care for terminally ill, offers hands on care at home |
| *Pain Clinic* | Refer if despite maximal doses, ongoing pain |
| *Dietician* | Consider referral to dietician for advice on feeding and thickeners if problems swallowing |
| *Chaplain* | Consider referring to an appropriate NHS chaplain for advice around spiritual needs |
| *OOH* | Ensure that an appropriate handover form is sent to the OOH |
| *Other* | Physiotherapist, OT, social worker, benefits adviser |

**SAFETY NETTING**

*Follow up*                  Review 1-2 days if symptoms not improving. Offer home visits if deteriorating or bed bound

**EXPLANATIONS**

*Worsening prognosis*   I'm afraid I have some difficult news to tell you. Unfortunately it appears the cancer has spread to other parts of the body. This makes it harder to treat with medication (chemotherapy, radiotherapy) or surgery. Our priority now is to keep you as comfortable as possible. If you have any symptoms please inform me and I can try and offer you medications to keep you discomfort to a minimum.

# *1.9 Genetics Counselling*

At least 10% of GP-patient consultations is believed to be related to a disorder that may have a genetic basis. GPs play a pivotal role in diagnosing and screening patients for inherited disorders; but they also have an important role in communicating genetic information and educating the patient around their risks and the potential risks to as yet, unborn offspring. Decisions regarding when to refer to a specialist genetic counsellor need to be considered with the patient and the potential impact results may have on life or health insurance premiums.

With the increasing prominence of the genome project, more and more conditions can be detected at a genetic level to identify the presence of a mutation, and subsequently provide advice, warning and potentially intervention to prevent serious or debilitating disorders from developing. However, once a gene has been found, it is important to consider the implications this has, not only to the patient who has requested the test, but to the immediate and extended family.

---

**Genetic Counselling**

This is the process by which, patients who are at an increased risk of a disorder are counselled, being advised about the nature of the condition and its long-term sequelae. Consideration is made to their chances of developing it and their potential to subsequently pass it on to the next generation. Options are offered pertaining to management of the condition as well as family planning. The following issues should usually be discussed as part of a consent process during clinical consultations where medical and family history information is sought and/or where genetic investigations are initiated:

- Knowledge of a FHx of a condition, or test results, has a potential benefit to other family members
- Communication of certain aspects of information to family members may be recommended
- The means of contacting those at-risk family members where relevant
- The fact that a summary of relevant clinical and genetic information will usually be sent to other appropriate health professionals involved in their care
- The likely timescales for availability of test results
- The possibility of unexpected or incidental findings from testing and how these might be managed
- The predictive nature of certain genetic tests (e.g. indicating future risks rather than current risks)
- The routine practice of long-term storage of samples for possible future analysis and the patient's preferences regarding further testing if it becomes available

*Ref: Consent & confidentiality in clinical GP: A report of the Joint Committee on Medical Genetics 2011*

**HISTORY**

Approach the topic sensitively in a non-threatening, non-judgemental manner. Adopt an open posture that is calm and inviting. Use the speed and tone of your voice to relax the patient and help appease them. Ensure that you read the patient's notes available to you fully before they enter the room to see if there is any documentation that may indicate that this is a possible genetic case i.e. recently pregnant, letter from geneticist etc.

**Open questions**      Good day. I am Dr Jones, one of the GPs here. How are you today? Could you tell me about what has been troubling you?

## Focused history

| | |
|---|---|
| *Sufferer* | If the patient already suffers from an inherited condition, take a fuller history around it. Establish their ideas, concerns and expectations about their disorder |
| Onset | How did it begin/start? |
| Severity | How unwell are they? Is it worsening? |
| Coping | How have they been coping up until this time? |
| Treatment | Have they had any treatment for their condition? |
| FHx | Does anyone else in the family have this condition? |
| | |
| *At Risk* | If the patient has a family history of a condition and is worried about their own risk, take a fuller history around it. Establish their ideas, concerns and expectations about their disorder |
| FHx | Who has the condition? |
| Severity | How unwell are they? Is it worsening? |
| Coping | How have they been coping up until this time? |
| Treatment | Have they had any treatment for their condition? |
| | |
| *Pregnant* | If the patient is pregnant, congratulate them. Find out how the pregnancy is going and if there has been any problems |
| Scan | Have you had your dating (10-14wks) or anomaly (18-21wks) scans yet? |
| Down's Blood | Have you had your blood tests? What did the results show? |
| Children | Do you have any children? Are they well? Do they have any genetic conditions? |
| Outcome | If you found out that your baby had this condition, how would it change things? Would it change whether you wanted to keep this pregnancy or not? |

## IDEA, CONCERNS, EXPECTATIONS

| | |
|---|---|
| *Understanding* | Establish the patient's own understanding about the condition. What does it mean to them? |
| *Ideas* | Elicit their ideas about the genetic condition. How do you think you got the condition? |
| *Concerns* | Establish any concerns they have. Did you have any specific worries about your problems (becoming unwell in old age, passing on to children)? Do you have any concerns about conditions that appear to run in your or your partner's family? |
| *Expectations* | Clarify with the patient what they were hoping for today. How were you hoping we could address this problem (screening, referral to geneticist)? |
| *Impact on life* | How has the knowledge of this disorder affected the patient and immediate family members? |

## PAST HISTORY

| | |
|---|---|
| *Medical* | Enquire whether they suffer from any medical conditions |
| *Obstetric* | Have you been pregnant before? Did you have any miscarriages or stillbirths in the past? |

## FAMILY HISTORY

| | |
|---|---|
| *Genetic* | Establish if there are any conditions that run in the family? For each sufferer, establish when they were diagnosed and how severe the condition was |
| *Family Tree* | Draw out a family tree mapping the disease and inheritance |

## Compiling a Family Tree

A family tree is a useful way to depict inherited conditions and to map out their mode of inheritance. Usually, three generations (patient, children, parents) are enough to gain the information you need

| | |
|---|---|
| *Patient* | Begin by obtaining information about the health of the patient in front of you. Are they well? Do they have any inherited conditions? |
| *Partner* | Does their partner have any conditions or illnesses? Is the patient and their current partner related (consanguineous)? |
| *Children* | Do they have any children together? If so, how many and are they well too? Do they have any children from other relationships? How are they? Did they have any miscarriages or stillbirths? Did any children die prematurely due to ill-health? |
| *Parents* | Ask about both partners parents. Are they still alive? |
| *Siblings* | Enquire about the health of their respective siblings. Do they have any children? Are they well or do they have any conditions? |

## DRUG HISTORY

| | |
|---|---|
| *Medication* | Are they taking any medications? (Genetic malformations in pregnancy: tetracyclines, ACEI, warfarin, retinoids, NSAIDS - 3rd trimester, lithium, methotrexate, hydroxyzine) |

## SOCIAL HISTORY

| | |
|---|---|
| *Ethnicity* | Confirm the ethnicity of the patient (african caribbean, asian, ashkenazi) |
| *Partner* | Check ethnicity of partner and if consanguineous |
| *Home* | Who lives with them? |
| *Occupation* | Are they working at the moment or unemployed? |
| *Smoker* | Do they smoke? How many cigarettes per day? |
| *Alcohol* | Do they drink alcohol? How much and how often? |

## Ethnicity and Genetic disorders

Whilst many genetic disorders may run in families, some conditions are more common in people of a specific ethnicity. Conditions are also more common in consanguineous marriages.

| | |
|---|---|
| *African-Caribbean* | Beta-thalassaemia, Sickle cell anaemia |
| *Asian* | Alpha-thalassaemia, Beta-thalassaemia |
| *Ashkenazi Jews* | Tay-sachs disease, Maple Syrup urine disease, Gaucher disease |
| *European* | Cystic fibrosis, Hereditary haemochromatosis |
| *Mediterranean* | Sickle-cell anaemia, thalassaemia |

| | |
|---|---|
| **EXAMINATION** | Not usually indicated |
| **RED FLAGS** | Not usually indicated |

## INVESTIGATIONS

| | |
|---|---|
| *Bloods* | Haemoglobin electrophoresis (sickle cell, thalassaemia), CK (DMD), clotting (Haemophilia) |
| *Downs* | Blood test nuchal translucency US scan, quadruple blood test |
| *US Scan* | Ultrasound scan (ADPKD) |
| *Specialist* | Amniocentesis, CVS, Sweat test (CF) |

## CSA TIPS

More often than not, cases involving genetic counselling in the CSA will present with information pertaining to the condition written on a piece of paper or in the consultation notes. It is paramount that you check the patient's understanding and ask where they obtained the information about the disorder from. If explored correctly, invariably, the actor will hand you a piece of paper that explains their condition and it's inheritance patterns.

You will not be expected to know all the intricacies regarding diagnosis or management of the wide genetic disease populace, rather your job in the CSA will be to facilitate the patient's own understanding, and explore their concerns, fears and expectations. If a mother is presenting for antenatal screening, you should explain in simple terms the different procedures that can be used to check if the foetus has an inherited condition. Ensure that you explain the risks i.e. miscarriage and also the sensitivity or specificity of the results.

Always ensure that you check the patient's concerns. The concerns may not always be about the genetic condition and its consequences, but may be more generic such as pertaining to worries about the procedure itself i.e. causing miscarriage, or taking blood in a patient with needle phobia.

## MANAGEMENT PLAN

| | |
|---|---|
| *Explaining* | Explain the condition using the patient's own descriptions and terms as relevant. Ensure you break the information into small chunks and repeat to ensure clarity |
| Screening | Explain the difference between diagnostic and predictive genetic testing |
| *Leaflet* | Offer a leaflet explaining conditions and the genetic counselling process |
| *Refer* | Refer patient for genetic counselling if appropriate |

## Safety Netting

| | |
|---|---|
| *Follow up* | Offer the patient a convenient follow-up appointment i.e. after screening or diagnostic test |

## EXPLANATIONS

| | |
|---|---|
| *Genes* | A gene contains all the information or code that determines your characteristics, such as your eye, hair and face colour; very much like computer code to make up a game or software. They are the basic building blocks of life and are passed on from parent to children. |
| Chromosome | The many thousands of genes each of us have, are held on a spaghetti-like structure called a chromosome. Each person has 23 pairs of chromosomes; one pair that comes from your dad and the other pair from your mother to give 46 chromosomes in total. |
| *Genetic testing* | This is a special test that allows us to find out whether a person is carrying a specific faulty gene that may give rise to an inherited condition. It usually involves taking a sample of blood, or an inner cheek swab and then sending it to the lab to check for the faulty gene. |
| *Autosomal Dominant* | A person suffering from an autosomal dominant condition inherits one copy of the defective (bad) gene from the parent who is also a sufferer. If a person inherits a single defective gene then this means that they too have the disease and that this means they can pass on the gene to their children. |

| | |
|---|---|
| Inherit. (1 gene) | In your case, since you have only one copy of the faulty gene and your partner does not; there is a 1 in 2 (50%) chance that your baby will have the disorder. In other words, if you were to have 2 children with your partner we would expect 1 child completely well without any defective gene but the other will be a sufferer. |
| Inherit. (2 gene) | In your case, you have two copies of the faulty gene and your partner does not; sadly, there is a 100% chance that your baby will inherit and suffer from the disorder. |
| ADPKD | Autosomal Dominant Polycystic Kidney Disease is the most commonly inherited kidney problem. It is a problem with the kidneys where fluid filled collections or cysts develop in both kidneys and slowly increase over time. Initially you may not have any symptoms, but as the cysts get bigger you may start getting back pain, urinary infections, raised blood pressure and kidney stones. Eventually, the kidneys may no longer function well and you will need to go on to dialysis or even need a transplant. |
| Neurofibromatosis | Neurofibromatosis (NF) is a rare AD inherited condition that causes swellings or benign tumours to grow on the nerves of the body. It may also give rise to bending and bowing of the bones and the spine. Patients with NF may have a mild condition with no real impact on life. However, some may be seriously affected also suffering with learning disabilities. Not all NF is inherited, around half of cases just happen spontaneously (without cause) and in these sufferers, their children are not at an increased risk of inheriting it. Currently, there is no treatment for the condition and sufferers are watched closely to try and prevent any complications. |
| Huntington's | This is an AD inherited condition that affects the cells of the brain. Over time, the brain cells are attacked and start to get damaged. As more and more brain cells are affected, the functioning of the brain begins to deteriorate causing problems such as uncontrollable movements, loss of memory, change in behaviour and problems communicating and eating. Currently, there is no cure for the condition, however there are treatments that can help reduce some of the suffering. |
| Autosomal Recessive | A person who is a carrier of an autosomal recessive condition inherits one copy of the sleeping defective gene from the parent. This means they can pass on the gene to their children, but will not be affected with the disease themselves. |
| Inherit. (1 partner) | In your case, since you have only one copy of the sleeping faulty gene and your partner does not; there is a 1 in 2 (50%) chance that your baby will be a carrier. In other words if you were to have 4 children with your partner we would expect all children to be well with no disease, but 2 of them would be carriers in the same way you are. |
| Inherit. (2 partner) | In your case, since both your partner and yourself are carriers there is a 1 in 4 (25%) chance that your baby will have the disorder. In other words, if you were to have 4 children with your partner we would expect 1 child completely well without any defective gene, 2 children who are well and healthy but are carriers of the defective gene, and 1 child who will be a sufferer of the genetic disorder. |
| Cystic Fibrosis | This is an AR inherited condition that affects how the cells of the lung and pancreas work. Normally, the cells in these areas make sticky secretions that allow those organs |

to work well. In CF, there is a problem with the wateriness of the secretions and they become thicker. As a result of the lungs nor working well, the sufferer may experience a chronic cough, shortness of breath and repeated chest infections. If the pancreas is affected, then the sufferer with get problems breaking down food and may suffer from poor growth, bloating and constipation. Although there is no cure for the condition, there are a number of treatments that can help reduce some of the suffering and prolong the life and improve the quality of life of the sufferer.

*Sickle Cell*  This is an AR inherited condition that affects the blood cells of the body. Usually the red blood cells are circular and squishy, but in people with sickle cell they are more rigid and hard. As a result they can block or clog vessels in the body, stopping oxygen from going to the tissues, causing pain like a cramp. When this happens this is called a sickle cell crisis and you need to see a Dr. The condition also causes the blood cells not to last as long as they should and leaves the patient suffering with low blood levels as well. Unfortunately, the condition is life-long, but can be treated by reducing the number and severity of attacks and preventing complications.

Trait  This is when you have only one of the sleeping defective sickle cell gene. Usually you will not experience any symptoms but may pass the defective gene to your children. If both parents have the trait, then your child has a 1 in 4 chance of having full blown disease, 2 in 4 chance of being a carrier and a 1 in 4 chance of being completely normal.

*Thalassaemias*  This is a group of AR inherited conditions that affect the blood cells of the body. They make them weaker and more likely to breakdown. As a result, sufferers may experience low blood counts (anaemia), bone thickening and problems with growth. In the severe form, sufferers may get enlarged spleen and heart problems. There are 2 main types, alpha and beta, so-named depending on the genes affected. Unfortunately, the condition is life-long, but can be treated by having regular blood transfusions or a bone-marrow transplant.

*X-linked recessive*  This is when the inherited defective gene is linked to the 'X' chromosome and usually causes problems in children who are male. Males only have one 'X' chromosome whereas females have 2 'X' chromosomes. This means that if a man has a faulty 'X' chromosome they will suffer from the disease. On the other hand, if a female has one faulty 'X' gene, they normally do not have the condition but are carriers.

Inherit. (male)  In your case, since you have the copy of the faulty gene and your female partner does not; there is a 100% chance that if you have a female baby they will be a carrier but will not suffer from the disease. However, if you have a baby boy, they will be completely normal and neither be carriers nor sufferers of the illness.

Inherit. (female)  In your case, since you are well, but your female partner is carrying the sleeping defective gene, there is a 1 in 2 (50%) chance that if you have a female baby they will be a carrier but will not suffer from the disease. However, if you have a baby boy, then there is a a 1 in 2 (50%) chance that they will be completely normal and neither be carriers nor suffer from the illness. However, there is a 50% chance that a baby boy will suffer from the disease.

| | |
|---|---|
| *Duchenne's* | Duchenne's muscular dystrophy is an X-linked chromosomal disorder that affects the muscles. Initially it causes weakness of the muscles of the shoulder and the hip; and you may notice your child having problems with walking, running or when climbing the stairs. Over time, the disease progresses, and may leave the sufferer wheelchair bound and begin to affect their breathing. Not all duchenne's is inherited; around half of cases just happen spontaneously (without cause). Although there is no cure for the condition, there are a number of treatments such as steroids, that can help reduce some of the muscle weakness. |
| *Haemophilia* | This is an X-linked chromosomal disorder that affects the body's ability to clot. Normally, when we cut or hurt ourselves, the body sends special substances known as clotting factor to make the blood more sticky and helps plug the injury to stop bleeding. In haemophiliacs, patients do not have enough clotting factor and this can lead to bleeding longer than normal. Over time, this can cause joint and muscle damage and stiffness. Although there is no cure, there are treatments like artificial clotting factors that can reduce the bleeding time and prevent long term damage. |
| *Down's* | This is a fairly common condition affecting 1 in 1000 births. It is not inherited, but is due to the presence of a third copy of the 21st chromosome that occurs spontaneously. The extra genetic information gives rise to a number of problems including low intellect, short height and a characteristic facial and body appearance. Although there is no cure for it, there are a number of tests that can help during pregnancy to assess the risk of having a child with Down's. If the calculation states that the mother is high risk, they can have genetic tests (amniocentesis, CVS) to confirm or negate the likelihood of the condition in your child. |

# 1.10 Paternity test

The paternity test is a form of genetic testing to help determine as to whether a supposed father is in fact the actual biological father. Whilst it may appear an easy and quick test, it is riddled with ethical complexities and complications including the potential breakdown of the family unit. Patients often consult their GP assuming that the test is readily available on the NHS. Whilst it is not, it is still the GP's duty to counsel the individual and discuss the implications of having the test.

### HISTORY

| | |
|---|---|
| **Open questions** | Can you tell me more about why you would like to have a paternity test? |
| *Understanding* | Can you tell me what you already know about it? |
| *Preparation* | Before we go on to speak about the test I just need to ask you some sensitive questions about your current and previous relationships? Is that alright? |

| | |
|---|---|
| **Open questions** | Good day. I am Dr Jones, one of the GPs here. How are you today? Could you tell me about what has been troubling you? |

### Focused history

| | |
|---|---|
| *Partner* | How is your relationship with your current partner (boyfriend, husband)? Are there any stresses in the relationship? Why do you think he is not the father? |
| *UPSI* | When did you have unprotected sex with your casual partner? Do they know that they could be the father? Were you in a committed relationship with your long term partner at the time? |
| *Child* | How old is your child? Do you have any other children? How is their relationship with your long term partner/their dad? |
| Counselling | Have you discussed having the test with your partner? If you have not, is there any particular reason why you have not (relationship problems)? |
| Implications | How would he feel if he found out that he was not the biological father? Would that affect his relationship with you or your child (separation/divorce)? Would the biological father want to be involved with your child? How will that relationship work? |

### Legal Position Regarding the Paternity Test
- The Human Tissue Act 2004 state that consent is necessary for the storage or testing of DNA material. The paternity test falls under such regulation
- Declared fathers (on birth certificate) are permitted to consent for the test for the minor if the parental DNA being tested is their own
- In the case of mature minor who have the ability to understand and comprehend the issues, their explicit consent should be sought
- Whilst it is good practice to have consent of both parties (mother and father) it is not a legal requirement. The BMA advises: *'Legally, where the putative father has parental responsibility for the child, such testing could be undertaken without the knowledge of the mother. The BMA believes that this could be very harmful to the child, as well as to the family unit as a whole, and would prefer to see a situation in which the consent of all parties is required for paternity testing. In the absence of such a legal requirement, where doctors are consulted, they should encourage those seeking testing to discuss their plans with the child's mother and the BMA advises doctors not to become involved if that advice is rejected.'*

*Ref: Paternity testing, Guidance from the BMA Medical Ethics Department, August 2009*

| | |
|---|---|
| *Concerns* | Is there anything worrying you about having the test (who the father may be, 100% accurate)? |
| *Impact on life* | How will the results affect you (relationships/parenting)? |

**SOCIAL HISTORY**

| | |
|---|---|
| *Occupation* | Are you working at the moment? What do you work as? |
| *Stress* | Has your mind been preoccupied with having the test? Has this stressed you at all? |

**CSA TIPS**

Paternity testing is a complicated and often ethical request. Patients do not always consider what the potential ramifications would be for the results and it is important that you try and work through these with the patient. You must clarify the need for consent from one or both potential fathers and refuse to carry out the procedure if this is not explicitly sought correctly. A request for a paternity test may actually be a sign or a cue for more deep rooted relationship problems and these should be explored.

**MANAGEMENT**

| | |
|---|---|
| *Counselling* | Suggest to have an appointment with both partners to discuss the issues. Consider referring to couple's therapy if there are relationship stresses |
| *Consent* | Written consent is recommended for both partners before having the test |
| *Test* | Inform that the test is not available on the NHS. Recommend alternatives – possibly private providers or for the patient to contact the hospital labs directly. State it requires either blood or swab samples from both partners |

**EXPLANATIONS**

| | |
|---|---|
| *Paternity test* | It is a test that compares the DNA of the child with that of the parents. This may help you find out if your current partner is in fact the biological father. |
| *How to do* | A blood test or a simple swab of the inner lining of the mouth is needed from everyone (dad, mum, child) to get the most accurate results. |
| *Impact on life* | If the results are not what you expected or were hoping for, it can have a dramatic impact on your relationships with everyone involved including your child. Have you thought about what your partner would do if he found out that the child is not his? |

# 2.1 Chest pain

Chest pain is a common presentation in primary care. It may arise from a variety of pathological causes ranging from musculoskeletal to an acute coronary event. It is important to take a thorough history and conduct an examination to arrive at a diagnosis. Patients with cardiac sounding chest pain should be risk stratified for their cardiovascular risk factors. Take into consideration the patient's age, gender and lifestyle when considering potential differentials.

**HISTORY**

**Open questions**     Tell me more about the chest pain you have experienced? Talk me through how the chest pain started?

**Focused questions**

*Chest pain*      Where exactly is the pain? When did you first notice it? How long does it last for?

*Radiation*      Does the pain move anywhere, such as to your arms, jaw or back?

*Severity*      How severe is the pain on a scale of 1 to 10, ten being the most severe?

*Triggers*      Does anything make it better (analgesia, rest) or worse (exercise, movement, lying flat)?

*Character*      How would you describe it? Is it sharp, dull or a burning feeling? Does it feel like a pressure - like someone is sitting on your chest?

**Associated history**

*SOB*      Do you feel breathless with the chest pain? Did it come on suddenly?

*Cough*      Had you had a cough with it?

**Differentials**

*Angina*      Does the pain move down your arm or neck? Does it come on when exercising? How far can you walk before you feel it? Does it improve with rest or with a GTN spray?

*ACS*      Does it occur at rest? Did you feel sweaty and short of breath? Did you feel sick or vomited? Is it a crushing pain?

*GORD*      Does it feel like heartburn? Is it worse when you lie flat? Do you ever get excessive saliva (water brash) or an acidic taste in your mouth (acid brash)? Have you had any undue stress lately?

*MSK*      Is it worse with movement? Can you pinpoint it? Does it hurt when you press it?

*PE*      Did it come on suddenly? Is it a sharp pain? Were you coughing up any blood? Is it worse on breathing in? Do you have any leg pain?

*Pericarditis*      Does it improve with sitting up or leaning forwards? Is it worse on lying down?

*Aortic dissection*      Is it a tearing pain? Does it go to your back?

**RED FLAGS**      Haemoptysis, shortness of breath, severe crushing pain at rest. Angina pain that has become acutely more severe, increase in frequency or reduced walking distance

**PAST HISTORY**

*Previous*      Have you ever experienced these symptoms before?

*CVD*      Have you ever had a heart attack, high blood pressure, cholesterol or diabetes?

*PE*      Have you ever had a blood clot in the chest (PE) or leg (DVT)?

## DRUG HISTORY

| | |
|---|---|
| *Medication* | Are you taking any medications? |
| GORD | NSAIDs, steroids, bisphosphonates, nitrates, calcium channel antagonists |
| PE | OCP, HRT |

## SOCIAL HISTORY

| | |
|---|---|
| *Occupation* | Are you working at the moment? (builder, deliveries) |
| *Smoker* | Do you smoke? How many cigarettes do you smoke per day? |
| *Alcohol* | Do you drink alcohol? How much and how often? |
| *Drive* | Are you driving at the moment? |

## FAMILY HISTORY

| | |
|---|---|
| *IHD* | Anyone in the family suffer from heart problems? |
| *PE* | Does anyone else suffer from a blood clot in the leg/lung or blood disorders? |

---

### Risk factors for Ischaemic Heart Disease (IHD) or PEs

| | |
|---|---|
| *IHD* | Diabetes, smoking, hypertension, cholesterol, smoking, FHx of IHD, strokes/TIA, PVD |
| *PE* | Previous DVT/PE. Recent travel, trauma or surgery, prolonged bed rest, immobility, OCP, childbirth, cancer, recent fractures (hip or femur) |

---

## IDEA, CONCERNS, EXPECTATIONS

| | |
|---|---|
| *Idea* | What did you think was causing the chest pain? |
| *Concerns* | Do you have any worries about it (heart attack)? |
| *Expectations* | How were you hoping I could help you? |
| *Impact* | How have your symptoms affected your life? |

## CSA TIPS

Chest pain can cause much anxiety in patients with most worrying about suffering an acute cardiac event. Such patients may appear anxious or panicky, particularly if you do not address their concerns. Conversely, others may wish to play down their symptoms and attribute their chest pain to other less serious conditions such as GORD inspite of a clear ACS history.

## PHYSICAL EXAMINATION

| | |
|---|---|
| *Vitals* | BP, pulse (irregular- AF), temperature, respiratory rate (PE) |
| *Cardiovascular* | Listen for heart sounds, reproducible chest wall tenderness (MSK). Palpate legs for DVT |
| *Respiratory* | Listen to chest (reduced air entry & dullness to percussion – pneumothorax, pleural rub – PE) |
| *Abdominal* | Check for tenderness (gallstones, gastric ulcer, pancreatitis) |

## INVESTIGATIONS

| | |
|---|---|
| *Bloods* | FBC, U&E, lipids, fasting glucose, CRP, Troponin (if chest pain <72hrs), D-dimer (PE) |
| Other | LFTs, amylase (pancreatitis), CRP & ESR (infection) |
| *ECG* | IHD (ST elevation/depression, new LBBB, T wave inversion), PE (AF, RBBB, S1Q3T3) |
| *Exercise test* | No longer part of criteria to diagnose angina |
| *CXR* | Exclude chest infection, pneumothorax |
| *Other (specialist)* | Cardiac MRI/CT (calcium score), thallium scan, myocardial perfusion scintigraphy, angiogram |

| MANAGEMENT | treat underlying cause |
|---|---|

**IHD**

| | |
|---|---|
| *Conservative* | Stop smoking and exercise at least 30mins, 5x a week. Try and reduce stress. Improve diet (5x veg/fruit, less fat) and reduce alcohol intake to DoH levels |
| *Medical* | |
|   Unstable angina | Offer GTN spray, give 300mg aspirin stat and immediately refer to hospital. Perform ECG as soon as possible. Offer O2 if sats <94%. Avoid clopidogrel outside hospital |
|   Angina | Initiate treatment if history suggestive of stable angina and refer to chest pain clinic (within 2wks) for confirmation of diagnosis |

**Dyspepsia**

| | |
|---|---|
| *Conservative* | Avoid chilli and spicy food. Cut down on caffeine and alcohol. Stop smoking. Eat small, regular meals and ensure that the last meal is several hours before bedtime |
| *Medical* | Alginates – Gaviscon, H2 Antagonist - Ranitidine, PPI – Omeprazole |

| | |
|---|---|
| **Pulmon. Embolism** | If suspected, start on low molecular weight heparin (LMWH). If confirmed, start warfarin targeting an INR between 2-3. PE with transient risk factors (surgery, trauma, temporary immobility) commence warfarin for at least 3 months whilst permanent risk factors at least 6 months |
| **MSK/pericarditis** | Treat with NSAIDS and reassure. Steroids for pericarditis in resistant cases |
| **Aortic dissection** | Refer for urgent admission and intervention |
| **Pancreatitis** | Offer analgesia (paracetamol/NSAIDs or weak opioid) and refer to hospital for ERCP. Advise to stop smoking and alcohol |

**SAFETY NETTING**

| | |
|---|---|
| *Follow up* | Advise patient to seek medical advice if any red flags symptoms or if angina persists for 10-20min after resting or not relieved by GTN spray. Offer a follow-up appointment for 2-4 wks if stable |
| *Referral* | Refer if unsure of diagnosis. Admit if haemodynamically unstable (tachycardia, tachypnoea, BP <90/60, reduced O2 sats or altered consciousness) |

**DIFFERENTIAL DIAGNOSIS**

| Conditions | Characteristic exam feature |
|---|---|
| **Angina** | Cardiac pain (radiating to left arm/jaw). Worse on exercise, heavy meal or triggered by cold weather. Relieved by GTN and rest. Check for worsening of symptoms (change in character or decreasing walking distance). OE: nil may be found |
| **ACS/unstable angina** | Central, crushing cardiac pain (DM and elderly may have no chest pain). Pain at rest associated with nausea, vomiting, sweating and SOB. May or may not be relieved by GTN spray. OE: patient may be short of breath, sweaty with tachycardia |

| | |
|---|---|
| **GORD** | Burning sensation over epigastrium moving up to the neck. Worsened by lying down or bending over. Acid brash and water brash may be present. Can cause painful swallowing or nocturnal asthma. Relieved by antacids but related to spicy food, alcohol or hot caffeine drinks. OE: epigastric pain |
| **Pulmonary embolism** | Sudden shortness of breath with pleuritic chest pain. May also have haemoptysis and tachycardia. Risk factors: DVT, travel, trauma, OCP, malignancy. OE: tachypnea with calf tenderness |
| **Pneumothorax** | Sudden onset of pleuritic chest pain with shortness of breath. Can occur with existing lung disease. OE: reduced breath sounds, increased resonance and percussion note over affected area |
| **Pneumonia** | Pleuritic chest pain associated with fever, productive cough and dyspnoea. OE: coarse crackles with dull percussion note with fever |
| **Pericarditis** | Sharp stabbing retrosternal chest pain (can radiate to the jaw, back or to the left side of the chest). Pain made worse on deep inspiration (pleuritic) and lying flat, or left side or on inspiration. Relieved by sitting forwards. OE: pericardial friction rub noted |
| **Aortic Dissection** | Sudden severe retrosternal chest pain tearing in character. Radiates to back. OE: unequal pulses and blood pressures in both arms |
| **Pancreatitis** | Acute onset of boring epigastric pain associated with nausea and vomiting. Relieved on sitting up or leaning forward but worse on lying flat. Comes in waves. Risk factors include gallstones, alcohol excess, raised calcium and triglyceride levels |
| **Musculoskeletal** | Sharp pain at a specific point. No radiation. Reproducible on palpation and passive movements. History of colds, coughing or excessive physical activity may be elicited. OE: focal chest tenderness worse on movement |

**EXPLANATIONS**

*Angina*  In angina there is narrowing or furring of the vessels that provide your heart food and oxygen to function. This is usually caused by fat or cholesterol build up. When you exercise, the heart needs more blood that cannot reach it and so it feels a cramping pain much like you get when you experience a stitch when running.

*GORD*  The stomach contains acid that helps break down food that you eat. In GORD, there is a weakness of the trap-door (sphincter) that prevents the acid from entering your food pipe. As a result, some of the stomach's acid leaks back into your food pipe causing acid reflux. This can give you a burning feeling that starts from your stomach and moves up to your throat.

*PE*  A pulmonary embolism refers to a blockage of the vessels that carry blood to the lungs from the heart. This sometimes can happen because of a blood clot that has formed in your legs. There are things that can make this more likely such as not moving after a serious operation, being seated for long periods in a long-haul flight or because of a blood defect.

| | |
|---|---|
| *Pancreatitis* | This is where an organ called the pancreas is inflamed (swollen) and causes abdominal pain. The pancreas is important in producing chemicals (enzymes) that help digest and break down food so that our body can absorb them. |
| *Pneumonia* | This is simply a chest infection. It is very common and affects all ages of people. Usually a bacterial infection enters the lungs and causes the small sacs at the end of the breathing tubes called bronchioles to get inflamed and fill up with fluid. Most pneumonias can be treated quite comfortably with antibiotics. |
| *Pneumothorax* | A pneumothorax describes when air is trapped between the outer part of the lung and the chest wall. In some people who are tall and thin, it may happen out of the blue but in others it may be due to a chest injury, following an operation or be caused by illnesses such as TB or a chest infection. If the pneumothorax is small, it may simply go away itself. However, in some cases the trapped air may get larger and cause the lung to shrink a little. In some extreme cases, the lung may even collapse, making it difficult to breathe. |
| *Pericarditis* | This is when the sac that covers and holds the heart becomes inflamed and irritated. In most cases we do not know why this happens, but sometimes it is due to an infection and may even happen after certain types of treatment (chemo or radiotherapy). Although it sounds serious, usually with rest and simple pain relief the problem passes on its own. |
| *Aortic dissection* | An aortic dissection is when a tear develops inside the inner wall of the main blood vessel (artery) that carries blood away from the heart (aorta). As a result, blood can pool inside the tear creating a false channel (lumen) which may extend all the way down to your tummy. This means less blood goes to the rest of your organs. It is quite serious and you would need to see a specialist Dr today to deal with it. |

Ischaemic heart disease refers to a number of conditions including angina, unstable angina, and myocardial infarction. It is an extremely common condition affecting men and women alike with around 2 million sufferers in the UK. Symptoms classically include crushing central chest pain or pressure located behind the lower left sternal edge radiating to the left arm or jaw. In stable angina, the pain is brought on by exercise, a heavy meal or cold weather and abates once one rests. In unstable angina and MI (acute coronary syndromes), the pain comes on at rest, is severe and may be associated with a feeling of nausea, sweating and breathlessness. The pain is typically relieved or partially relieved by the use of sublingual nitrates (GTN spray). A strong FHx of heart disease (atherosclerosis) is normally present and risk factors such as hypercholesterolaemia, hypertension, smoking, male gender, diabetes, obesity, raised stress levels and lack of regular exercise are important to be elicited for risk stratification.

---

**Diagnosing Angina by History**

Patients with all 3 features can be diagnosed with typical angina. Atypical angina is 2 of these features. Patients with 1 or none of the features have non-anginal chest pain.

- Constricting discomfort in the front of the chest, neck, shoulders, jaw or arms
- Precipitated by physical exertion
- Relieved by rest or GTN within 5mins
- Factors making stable angina more likely include, increasing age, male, presence of risk factors, PMHx
- Stable angina is unlikely if the pain is prolonged, unrelated to activity, brought on by breathing or associated with dizziness, palpitations, tingling or difficulty swallowing

*Ref: NICE (2010): Chest pain of recent onset, Assessment and diagnosis … suspected cardiac origin*

---

**HISTORY**

**Open questions**

Tell me more about the chest pain you have experienced? Talk me through how the chest pain started?

**Focused questions**

*Angina pain*   Where exactly is the pain? When did you first notice it? What were you doing at the time? How long does it last for?

Radiation   Does the pain move to your arms, jaw or back?

Character   How would you describe it? Does it feel like a weight or pressure on your chest?

Severity   How severe is the pain on a scale of 1 to 10, ten being the most severe?

Aggr. / relieve   Does anything make it better (rest, GTN) or worse (stress)? Does the pain come on when you exercise (stable) or at rest (ACS)?

Exercise   If the pain comes on when walking, how far do you have to walk before you feel the pain? Has this distance changed recently?

**Associated history**

*SOB*   Do you feel sweaty, clammy or breathless with the chest pain?

*Nausea & vomiting*   Did you feel sick or have you vomited?

**Differentials**

*MI*   Is it a crushing chest pain? Does it occur at rest? Any shortness of breath?

*Pericarditis*   Does it improve with sitting up or leaning forwards? Is it worse on lying down?

| | |
|---|---|
| *Aortic dissection* | Is it a tearing pain? Does it go to your back? |
| **RED FLAGS** | Severe crushing pain at rest (MI) with shortness of breath. Angina pain that has become acutely more severe, increase in frequency or reduced walking distance |

**PAST HISTORY**

| | |
|---|---|
| *Previous* | Have you ever experienced these symptoms before? |
| *CVD* | Have you ever had a heart attack, high blood pressure, cholesterol or diabetes? Have you ever had a stroke or suffered from poor circulation to your feet (PVD)? |

**DRUG HISTORY**

| | |
|---|---|
| *Medication* | Are you taking any medications? |

---

**Anti-Anginal Medication and their side-effects**

| | |
|---|---|
| *Beta blocker* | Bronchospasm, cold peripheries, sleep disturbances (nightmares), fatigue, erectile dysfunction |
| CI | Asthma, COPD, bradycardia, heart block, PVD |
| *Ca2+ ch blocker* | Headache, flushing, ankle oedema |
| CI | Heart failure, heart block, do not combine rate limiting with B-blocker |
| *Nitrates* | Headache, postural hypotension, dizziness, tachycardia |
| Tolerance | Can develop tolerance with reduced effect. Avoid by having nitrate free period overnight i.e. giving 2nd doses of ISMN after 8hrs rather than 12hrs. Tolerance not noted in ISMN MR (modified release) |
| CI | AS, HOCM, MS, closed angle glaucoma |
| *K-ch activator* | (e.g. Nicorandil) Headaches (transitional), flushing, dizziness, anal ulceration |
| CI | left ventricular failure, hypotension |

---

**SOCIAL HISTORY**

| | |
|---|---|
| *Occupation* | Are you currently working at the moment? |
| *Smoker* | Do you smoke? How many cigarettes do you smoke per day? How long have you been smoking? |
| *Alcohol* | Do you drink alcohol? How much and how often? |
| *Drive* | Are you driving at the moment? |

**FAMILY HISTORY**

| | |
|---|---|
| *IHD* | Anyone in the family suffer from heart problems? |
| *Cholesterol* | Does anyone in your immediate family have raised cholesterol? |

---

**Risk factors for Ischaemic Heart Disease (IHD) or PEs**

| | |
|---|---|
| *IHD* | Diabetes, smoking, hypertension, cholesterol, smoking, family history of IHD, strokes/TIA, PVD |
| *PE* | Previous DVT/PE. Recent travel, trauma or surgery, prolonged bed rest, immobility, OCP, childbirth, cancer, recent fractures (hip or femur) |

---

**IDEA, CONCERNS, EXPECTATIONS**

| | |
|---|---|
| *Idea* | What did you think was causing the chest pain? |
| *Concerns* | Do you have any worries about it (heart attack)? |
| *Expectations* | How were you hoping I could help you? |

| Impact | How have your symptoms affected your life? |
|---|---|

## CSA TIPS

Patients who present within 72 hours with possible unstable angina require a same day hospital assessment to ensure that there is not an unstable plaque. However, it may require some negotiating to convince the patient to attend the hospital, particularly if they have a more pressing engagement such as attending a job interview, funeral or social event. In patients who drive Group 2 vehicles (i.e. bus/lorry) they may wish to downplay their symptoms to avoid losing their licence.

## PHYSICAL EXAMINATION

| *Vitals* | BP, pulse, O2 sats |
|---|---|
| *Cardiovascular* | Listen for heart sounds |

## INVESTIGATIONS

| *Bloods* | FBC, U&E, fasting cholesterol and glucose, Troponin (if chest pain <72hrs) |
|---|---|
| *ECG* | ST elevation/depression, new LBBB, T wave inversion |
| *Exercise test* | No longer part of criteria to diagnose angina |
| *CXR* | Exclude chest infection, cardiomegaly (HTN/cardiomyopathy) |
| *Other (specialist)* | Cardiac MRI/CT (calcium score), thallium scan, myocardial perfusion scintigraphy, angiogram |

## MANAGEMENT

### Conservative

| *Lifestyle* | Stop smoking, exercise (30min 5x/wk), stress reduction, recommend mediterranean diet (5x veg/fruit, less fat, 2 portions of fish /wk, low salt), reduced alcohol consumption. Try and lose weight to attain a BMI <25 kg/m2 |
|---|---|

### Post MI advice

| *Employment* | Patients in employment should try and return to work depending on the type of employment they are in. Sedentary workers can return within 1 month, light manual workers within 2 months and heavy manual workers within 3 months |
|---|---|
| *Exercise* | Advise to exercise lightly but regularly. Consider a stroll in the park after 2 wks. By 4-6 wks should aim to do 0.5 mile /day increasing to 2 miles a day |
| *Sexual intercourse* | Can resume 4 weeks post MI. If able to briskly climb 2 flights of stairs pain free then sexual activity should not be a problem |
| *Travel* | Should avoid driving for 4 weeks and avoid flying for up to 7-14 days uncomplicated MI and 4-6 weeks if complicated |

| *Immunisations* | Offer yearly influenza vaccination and one-off pneumococcal vaccination |
|---|---|
| *Driving* | Should inform the DVLA and not to drive if symptoms occur at rest or at the wheel, or with emotion for angina. Patients should be recommended to inform their insurance company about their diagnosis |

### Advice regarding travel and driving

| *Flying* | | |
|---|---|---|
| | Unstable angina | Cannot fly |
| | Stable Angina | if can climb a flight of stairs or walk 100 metres without pain or SOB can fly |
| | ACS/MI | 1-2wk (uncomplicated) or 4-6wk (complicated) |

| Angioplasty | 5-7 days |
| CABG | 14 days |

*Driving (group 1)*

| Unstable angina | Stop driving if pain occurs at the wheel or at rest |
| ACS/MI | No driving for 1 month or 1 week if treated successfully with angioplasty |
| CABG | No driving for 1 month |

## Medical

| *Unstable angina* | Offer GTN spray, give 300mg aspirin stat and immediately refer to hospital. Perform ECG as soon as possible. Offer O2 if sats <94%. Avoid clopidogrel outside hospital |
| *Angina* | Initiate treatment if history suggestive of angina and refer to chest pain clinic for confirmation |
| 2nd Prevention | All patients should be offered aspirin (75mg), statin (target: chol <4mmol/L, LDL <2mmol/L) and ACE inhibitor (if diabetic) |
| GTN | Glyceryl trinitrate spray (1-2 puffs) used as required when pain starts |
| 1st line | Consider B-blocker or Ca2+ channel blocker as first line |
| Beta blocker | If B-blocker (bisoprolol) not tolerated or contraindicated consider Ca2+ ch. blocker |
| Ca2+ ch block | Rate limiting calcium channel blocker (e.g. verapamil / diltiazem) however contraindicated in HF and heart block. Long-acting (e.g. amlodipine) best used in HF |
| Combination | If symptoms not controlled, try and combine therapy i.e. calcium channel blocker (amlodipine) with beta blocker or ISMN with B-blocker or Ca2+ ch. blocker. Avoid combining beta blocker with rate limiting Ca2+ ch. blocker |
| Nitrates | Start low dose nitrate and titrate up (Isosorbide mononitrate) |
| Nicorandil | Controls symptoms with similar efficacy to other anti-anginals (K-ch activator) |
| *QoF* | Maintain a register of patients with CHD. Monitor BP and cholesterol yearly. Ensure patient is on aspirin (and/or clopidogrel), ACE-I, beta-blocker and statin |

## SAFETY NETTING

| *Follow-up* | Review 2-4wk after initiating or changing medication. Seek medical advice if any red flags symptoms or if angina persists for more than 15 minutes after resting or not relieved by GTN spray |
| *Referral* | Consider referring to cardiologist if symptoms not controlled with combination therapy. Discuss with patient the possible need for CABG or angiogram |

## Referring Patient with Angina to Hospital

- If patient presents with chest pain or within 12 hours with abnormal ECG, consider urgent admission
- If patient had chest pain 12 - 72 hours ago then refer to hospital for same-day assessment
- If patient had chest pain more than 72 hours ago, perform risk assessment, take an ECG and troponin level before deciding next course of action

*Ref: NICE 2010: Chest pain of recent onset, Assessment and Dx... discomfort of suspected cardiac origin*

## EXPLANATIONS

| *Angina* | Your heart is a muscle that helps pump blood around the body. Like any other muscle, it has its own blood supply and needs oxygen and food to keep it working properly. In angina there is a narrowing or furring of these vessels (arteries) caused by cholesterol |

build up. So when you are exercising, the heart feels a cramping pain as less blood can reach it and supply the valuable oxygen it needs.

| | |
|---|---|
| GTN | GTN is a medication that works by relaxing the vessels in the body making it easier for the heart to pump blood round. It also allows more blood to flow to the heart muscle reducing the strain on it. Use it before any planned exercise or exertion. Be aware of side-effects as it can cause flushing, headaches and light-headedness. If after using it your chest pain does not improve, then repeat again after 5mins. Call 999 if the pain still continues after a further 5mins. |
| Beta blocker | Beta blockers work by reducing the heart rate and also the force of each heart beat. This means that the heart works less hard and need less oxygen to work and thus reduces strain. |
| MI | When the blood vessel has been completely blocked either by a cholesterol plaque or blood clot, the heart muscle is starved of oxygen causing severe chest pain. If this persists for a period of time, the heart muscle may begin to die and this is known as a heart attack. |
| Angiogram | This is an investigation that helps us see the blood vessels of the heart. A small wire is passed through a vessel in your groin or above the elbow, that tracks back to heart. A dye is injected which allows the doctor to see a narrowing or blockage in the arteries. |
| Angioplasty | A balloon at the end of the wire is slowly inflated in the narrowing of the artery and a wire mesh (stent) is left to keep the artery open. |
| CABG | This is a surgical operation that helps bypass blocked vessels of the heart using a healthy vessel from another part of your body such as your leg. This helps blood flow around the blockage allowing oxygen and nutrients to flow to the heart muscle, reducing pain. |

# 2.3 Hypertension

Hypertension is a very common condition that affects vast swathes of the population. As it is often asymptomatic, most cases are found incidentally when visiting the GP or having their blood pressure checked at the pharmacy. Hypertension is a major risk factor for developing coronary heart disease, kidney disease and strokes. The higher the blood pressure, the more likely the risk of cardiovascular disease. Hence, all newly diagnosed hypertensive patients should be risk stratified using tools such as QRisk2 to assess their 10 year risk of having a cardiovascular event.

---

### Diagnosing Hypertension

According to QoF guidance, 'elevated BP readings of >140/90 on three separate occasions are generally taken to confirm sustained high blood pressure.' The gold standard recommended by NICE is that if the BP is raised greater than 140/90, the patient should be offered ambulatory blood pressure monitoring (ABPM) or home blood pressure monitoring (HBPM) if ABPM is not available or tolerated

| | |
|---|---|
| *ABPM* | Take ≥2 readings every waking hour, and average at least 14 measurements when deciding whether hypertension is present |
| *HBPM* | On each occasion take two consecutive BP measurements (<1 minute apart), with the person seated. Take readings twice daily (morning and evening) over ≥4 days (ideally 7 days) - disregard the first day and then average the rest |
| *<140/90* | Raised normal values i.e. 130-139/85-89 mmHg should be checked annually |

*Ref: Quality and Outcomes Framework guidance for GMS contract 2011/12, April 2011 & Hypertension: management of hypertension in adults in primary care, NICE Clinical Guideline (August 2011)*

### HISTORY

Mild to moderate essential hypertension is usually asymptomatic and hence it is difficult to elicit from the history alone. However, when taking a history, you should include a cardiovascular risk factor assessment. Ensure that you read the notes thoroughly, and note if the patient has had previously raised BP readings.

| | |
|---|---|
| **Open questions** | How can I help you today? |

**Focused questions**

| | |
|---|---|
| *Acceler. HTN* | Have you had any headaches, feeling drowsy, confused, visual disturbances, nausea or vomiting (hypertensive encephalopathy)? |
| *Risk factors* | Elicit relevant risk factors such as diabetes, stroke, raised cholesterol, smoking and a family history of cardiovascular disease |

### RED FLAGS

| | |
|---|---|
| *Malignant HTN* | >180/110mmHg with signs of papilloedema or retinal haemorrhage, or one-off BP with systolic >220mmHg or diastolic >120mmHg |
| *Others* | Microscopic haematuria, very high BP with headache, pregnancy (preeclampsia), signs of end-organ damage, fits, heart failure |

### PAST HISTORY

Although 95% of patients suffer with essential hypertension where there is unknown aetiology, 5% do have an underlying condition i.e. secondary hypertension

| Renal disease | Do you suffer from any kidney problems? |
|---|---|
| Endocrine disease | Do you have any illnesses that affect your endocrine system? |
| CV disease | Have you been diagnosed with any heart problems? |

## Secondary causes of Hypertension (5% of hypertension)

| Renal (80%) | Chronic renal failure, renal artery stenosis, glomerulonephritis, adult polycystic kidney disease, renal tumour |
|---|---|
| Endocrine | Cushing's or Conn's syndrome, acromegaly, hyperthyroidism, phaeochromocytoma |
| Others | Coarctation of the aorta, aortic valve disease, pregnancy |
| Drugs | Steroids, MAOI, OCP |

## DRUG HISTORY

| Medication | Are you taking any medications (COCP, steroids, MAOI)? |
|---|---|

## SOCIAL HISTORY

| Occupation | Are you working at the moment? Any stress at work? |
|---|---|
| Smoker | Do you smoke? How many cigarettes do you smoke per day and for how long? |
| Alcohol | Do you drink alcohol? How much and how often? |
| Stress | How are things at work or at home? Are you experiencing any stress? |

## FAMILY HISTORY

| Hypertension | Has anyone in your family been diagnosed with hypertension? |
|---|---|
| Secondary causes | Has anyone been diagnosed with polycystic kidney disease? |

## IDEA, CONCERNS, EXPECTATIONS

| Idea | What did you think was causing your raised blood pressure today? |
|---|---|
| Concerns | Is there anything worrying you about your raised blood pressure (stroke/heart attacks)? |
| Expectations | How were you hoping I could help you? |

## CSA TIPS

It is unlikely that a patient will attend with hypertension as their presenting complaint in your CSA exam. It is more likely that the patient may harbour underlying concerns about hypertension or have raised blood pressure as a result of a loss of a job or a recent death in the family which should be explored further. You may have a patient presenting with an unrelated complaint but previous notes show two or three consecutively raised blood pressures that may need to be acted upon. A sensible approach in such cases would be to check the patient's understanding and offer a brief explanation of what hypertension is and correct any misconceptions the patient may hold.

## PHYSICAL EXAMINATION

| Blood pressure | 3 separate consecutive readings |
|---|---|

## Stages of Hypertension

| Grade | BP in surgery | ABPM/HBPM |
|---|---|---|
| Grade 1 | ≥140/90 | ≥135/85 |
| Grade 2 | ≥160/100 | ≥150/95 |
| Severe HTN | ≥180/110 | ≥ 180/110 |

| Cardiovascular | Listen for heart sounds, check peripheral pulses (aortic aneurysm) |
| Fundoscopy | Assess the fundi for signs of hypertension |

## Signs of Hypertensive retinopathy

| Grade 1 | Silver wiring, arteriolar narrowing |
| Grade 2 | Arterio-venous (AV) nipping |
| Grade 3 | Flame and blot hemorrhages, Cotton-wool exudates |
| Grade 4 | Papilloedema |

## INVESTIGATIONS

| Bloods | FBC, U&Es including eGFR, fasting lipid profile, glucose |
| Resting ECG | Left ventricular hypertrophy, left atrial enlargement |
| Urine | Haematuria and proteinuria (renal causes), urinary catecholamines (pheochromocytoma) |

## Complications of Hypertension

| Urine | Test for protein in urine i.e. ACR and test for haematuria using a reagent strip |
| Blood | Glucose, U/E, eGFR, serum total cholesterol and HDL cholesterol |
| Eyes | Examine the fundi for the presence of hypertensive retinopathy |
| ECG | Arrange for a 12-lead ECG to be performed (left ventricular hypertrophy) |

## MANAGEMENT

### Conservative

| CV risk | Do QRISK2 score to assess the patient's 10 year risk of having a stroke or heart attack (see hypercholesterol chapter) |
| Aim BP | <140/85, if DM or CVD aim: <130/80 (QOF standard: <150/90) |

## Target Blood pressure (NICE)

| 140/90 | All newly diagnosed patients with hypertension should have a BP of 140/90 |
| 130/80 | Patients with a history of renal, diabetes, cardiovascular disease or end stage organ damage should have a target of less than 130/80 |
| 125/75 | In patients with CKD, if there is proteinuria then target BP of <125/75 |

*Ref: Developed by the joint speciality committee on renal medicine on RCP. Chronic Kidney Disease in Adults: UK Guidelines for Identification, Management and Referral, March 2006*

*Lifestyle*

| Diet | Reduce salt intake (<5-6g/d). Increase fruit & veg (5/d), reduce coffee intake (<5 cups/d) |
| Stress | Encourage relaxation techniques and stress management |
| Exercise | Aim for optimum weight BMI <25, encourage exercise (30min x5/wk) |
| Smoking & Ethol | Smoking cessation advice, reduce alcohol (<21u/wk ♂, <14u/wk ♀) |

| Driving | Should inform the DVLA for group 2 drivers (buses, lorries). Disqualifies if systolic >180mmHg or resting diastolic >100mmHg. May be relicensed if controlled with treatment and no side-effects |

## Medical

### Antihypertensives

| | |
|---|---|
| Step 1 | If patient < 55-years-old: ACE inhibitor or ARB if not tolerated (cough) |
| | If patient > 55-years-old or of African-Caribbean origin: calcium channel blocker |
| Step 2 | If the target blood pressure is not achieved, a combination of an ACE inhibitor with a calcium channel blocker is recommended |
| Step 3 | If target blood pressure still not achieved combine all three medication: ACE inhibitor + calcium channel blocker + diuretic (indapamide 1.5 mg MR od (or 2.5 mg od) or chlortalidone 12.5–25.0mg od |
| Step 4 | If a fourth drug is needed to control blood pressure, add one of the following: alpha-blocker, beta-blocker, another diuretic |

| | |
|---|---|
| Prevention | Aspirin 75mg od if >50 years old & 10 year CVD risk >20% or in DM patients. Statins if >40 years old with raised BP & 10 year CVD risk >20% |
| QoF | Maintain a register of patients with BP. Monitor BP yearly. Ensure patient BP <150/90 |

---

## Side-effects of Antihypertensive Medication

| | |
|---|---|
| ACEI / ARB | Profound BP drop, renal impairment, dry cough (ACEI), angioedema, rash (urticaria), ↑K, ↑Glu. Consider ARB if ACEI not tolerated i.e. dry cough |
| Beta blocker | Bradycardia, bronchospasm, impotence. Avoid in asthma, COPD, HF, heart block, PVD, DM (impaired glucose tolerance). Avoid combining with rate limiting Ca2+ channel blocker (bradycardia / asystole) |
| Ca2+ ch block | Pedal oedema, dizziness, flushing, constipation. Avoid rate limiting agents (diltiazem) in HF or heart block |
| Diuretic | (e.g. thiazide) Avoid in gout (increases uric acid). Impotence, DM/SLE worsens. ↓K , ↑Ca2+, ↑Glu, metabolic acidosis |
| Alpha blocker | (e.g. doxazosin) Urinary incontinence, postural hypotension |

---

## SAFETY NETTING

| | |
|---|---|
| Follow up | Review can be performed by practice nurse if controlled. If initiating treatment review in 1 month, if controlled review 3-6 monthly. Patient will need follow-up U&E's within 1-2 wks if on ACE-I or 4-6wks if on diuretic |
| Refer | Refer if young patient (<30yr requiring treatment) for investigation of secondary HTN |
| Admit | Arrange same-day admission if BP 220/120mmHg or signs of malignant hypertension |

## EXPLANATIONS

| | |
|---|---|
| Hypertension | The heart is a pump that moves blood around your body. The pressure at which your blood flows is known as the blood pressure. It is normally expressed as a fraction, with the upper number representing the systolic pressure (pressure when the heart is pumping) and the lower number, the diastolic pressure (pressure when the heart is at rest). High blood pressure is when your blood pressure is above 140 over 90 (140/90). This can put you at risk of having a heart attack, stroke or other serious conditions. |
| Diuretics | These are a group of medications also known as water-tablets. They work by making the kidneys pass more salt and water into your urine, leading you to go to the toilet much more. Too much salt causes the BP to rise, and so passing it out into your urine will make the BP come down. |

ACEI — Angiotensin converting enzyme inhibitor, or ACEI, blocks a protein (enzyme) that helps make a chemical called angiotensin II. This helps relax the blood vessels and also reduces how much water is reabsorbed in the kidney.

Calcium Channel — Calcium channel blockers help reduce your BP by relaxing the vessels that take blood away from the heart. They also reduce the force and speed of each heartbeat therefore reducing your blood pressure.

Palpitations describe the abnormal awareness of a heartbeat by a patient. It may be caused by a wide range of clinical conditions including anaemia, cardiac disease or even anxiety. In most cases the cause is unknown. However, it is important to be able to distinguish life threatening causes from the more benign. This can sometimes be difficult as the severity of the symptoms rarely correlate with the seriousness of the underlying condition. For example, significant palpitations may be felt despite the patient being in sinus rhythm; conversely, a patient in VT may remain asymptomatic.

## Causes of Palpitations

| | |
|---|---|
| *Cardiac* | Atrial (AF/atrial flutter, WPW, sick sinus syndrome, ectopic beats), Ventricular (VT,VF), sinus tachycardia |
| *Metabolic* | Hyperthyroidism, hypoglycaemia, hypo/hypercalcemia, hypo/hyperkalaemia |
| *Drugs* | Alcohol, amphetamines, anticholinergic, caffeine, nicotine, cocaine, nitrates |
| *Structural abn.* | Left heart failure, aortic aneurysm, cardiomegaly, congenital heart disease (ASD, PDA, VSD), mitral prolapse, pericarditis, PE |
| *High cardiac output* | (Cardiac outputs) Anaemia, fever, pregnancy, thyrotoxicosis |
| *Psychogenic* | Panic attacks, anxiety disorders, depression, phobia |
| *Other* | Emotional distress, hyperventilation, migraine, PMS |

## HISTORY

**Open questions** Can you tell me more about the symptoms you are experiencing? Could you tell me about what has been troubling you?

## Focused questions

| | |
|---|---|
| *Palpitations* | Clarify what they mean by palpitations? When did it start? How long did it last for? What were you doing at the time? |
| Character | Can you describe the palpitations? |
| Rhythms | Ask the patient to tap out the rhythm. Do you feel it as a heavy beat, missed beat or an extra beat? Did you feel your heart was beating fast? Was it beating regularly or irregularly? |
| Frequency | How often have you felt it in the past day/week/month? |
| Exac & relieving | Does anything make the palpitations better or worse? |

## Triggers for Palpitations

| | |
|---|---|
| *Lifestyle* | Caffeine, chocolate, cheese, cigarettes, GORD, heavy meals, alcohol |
| *Drugs* | Beta-agonist (salbutamol), vasodilators (nifedipine) |

## Associated history

| | |
|---|---|
| *SOB* | Have you had any shortness of breath? |
| *Chest pain* | Have you experienced any chest pain? |
| *LOC* | Have you had any dizziness or loss of consciousness? |

## Differentials

| | |
|---|---|
| *Cardiac* | Have you had any chest pain? Does it come on when you are exercising? |

| Anaemia | Do you feel tired all the time? Do you suffer from shortness of breath? |
|---|---|
| Hyperthyroidism | Any weight loss, sweating, diarrhoea or tremor in the hands? |
| Panic attacks | Have you been feeling stressed recently? Have you noticed any tingling in your mouth, lips (perioral) or fingers? Do you experience these symptoms when in a crowded place or in a lift? |

**RED FLAGS**

| Cardiac | Chest pain with PMHx cardiovascular disease, structural heart disease |
|---|---|
| Syncope | Loss of consciousness (VT, SVT, FHx of sudden death - cardiomyopathy, long QT syndrome) |

---

**Loss of Consciousness Guidelines**

Refer all patients with total loss of consciousness for a specialist cardiovascular assessment by the most appropriate local service. Exceptions are:

| Firm Diagnosis | People with a firm diagnosis, after initial assessment of uncomplicated faint, situational syncope, orthostatic hypotension |
|---|---|
| Epilepsy | People whose presentation is strongly suggestive of epileptic seizures |

*Ref: NICE guidelines: Transient loss of consciousness in adults and young people, August 2010*

**PAST HISTORY**

| Previous | Have you ever experienced these symptoms before? |
|---|---|
| Cardiac | Do you suffer from any heart problems such as a heart attack or angina? Have you had cardiomyopathy, heart failure or rheumatic fever? |
| Anxiety | Have you had any panic attacks in the past or suffered from any phobias? |

**DRUG HISTORY**

| Medication | Are you taking any medications? (salbutamol, theophylline, TCA, thyroxine, nitrates, ca channel blocker) |
|---|---|
| OTC | Have you taken any over the counter medications such as cough or cold remedies? (sympathomimetic agents - ephedrine) |

**SOCIAL HISTORY**

| Occupation | Are you currently working at the moment? Any stress there? |
|---|---|
| Diet | Do you drink tea, coffee, cola or energy drinks? Do you eat lots of chocolate? |
| Alcohol | Do you drink alcohol? How much and how often? |
| Smoker | Do you smoke? How many cigarettes do you smoke per day? |
| Elicit drugs | Have you ever used any recreational drugs such as amphetamines or cocaine? |

**FAMILY HISTORY**

| Cardiac | Anyone in the family suffer from heart problems or have a history of unexpected sudden death? |
|---|---|

---

**Risk Stratification for Palpitation**

| Green | Skipped beats, thumping or pounding, normal ECG, no FHx, no structural heart disease, No risk factors for ischaemic heart disease |
|---|---|
| Management | Reassure patients |
| Amber | Hx of recurrent tachyarrhythmia, CP/SOB, abnormal ECG, structural heart disease, HTN, AF |

| Management | Refer patients to cardiology |
| Red | Palpitation during exercise, syncope/near syncope, FHx structural heart disease, high grade AV block, VT |
| Management | Urgent referral to cardiology |

## IDEA, CONCERNS, EXPECTATIONS

| Idea | What did you think was causing your palpitations? |
| Concerns | Was there any thing in particularly that was worrying you about your symptoms? |
| Expectations | How were you hoping I could help you? |

## CSA TIPS

Palpitations are an alarming symptom for patients as they are often presumed to be due to severe heart dysfunction. Subsequently, patients may present with concerns around sudden death or whether they have suffered a heart attack. Be aware that the patient's symptoms of palpitations may only be a cue to discuss more complex and challenging underlying psychological stressors.

## PHYSICAL EXAMINATION

| Vitals | BP, pulse (regular, irregular, tachycardia, bounding), temperature |
| General | Signs of anaemia (pale conjunctiva) |
| Cardiovascular | Listen for heart sounds (murmurs), lung bases (heart failure) |
| Thyroid | Perform a focused thyroid examination – palpate the thyroid gland, check for tremor – hands out stretched), eye signs (stand behind the patient - exophthalmos) |

## INVESTIGATIONS

| Bloods | FBC, ferritin, U&E, TFTs, fasting glucose |
| ECG | 12 lead ECG, 24 hour tape, event recorder (sinus tachy, SVT, VT, AF, atrial flutter, ectopics) |
| CXR | Cardiomegaly, HF |
| Other | Echo (AF, HF, valvular disease, cardiomyopathy) |

## Types of ECG to do in Palpitations

| Resting ECG | Perform resting 12 lead ECG if symptoms have long duration (several hours or frequent) |
| Signs | ST elevation/depression (IHD), long QT, ectopics, heart blocks, AF, sinus tachycardia or bradycardia |
| Treadmill ECG | Consider if history of ischaemic heart disease or if palpitation brought on by exercise |
| 24hr Monitor | If palpitations short-lived but occur frequently (more than 2-3 times/wk) use a 24 hour Holter monitor |
| Event Recorder | If palpitations are short-lived and infrequent (less than once a week) use an event recorder |

## MANAGEMENT    treat underlying cause
### Conservative

| Lifestyle | Advise to cut down alcohol, and caffeine consumption. Avoid cheese and chocolates |
| Diary | Consider keeping a symptom diary to elucidate trigger factors |
| Admission | Consider admitting the patient if acutely unwell or signs of significant disease |

**Admitting Patient with Palpitations to Hospital**
- Arrhythmias associated with haemodynamic compromise
- Life-threatening arrhythmia requiring rapid control (e.g. VT, SVT)
- Significant heart disease (cardiomyopathy, CCF)
- Associated with angina or syncope or severe SOB

| | |
|---|---|
| *Panic Attacks* | Reassure and advise relaxation and re-breathing techniques. Avoid any precipitants or stressors. Consider beta-blocker (propranolol) for symptomatic relief if no contraindications (asthma). Try SSRI or psychotherapy (CBT) |
| *Hyperthyroidism* | B-blocker for symptomatic relief. Carbimazole, radioactive iodine or surgical removal of thyroid gland. These options often initiated by secondary care |
| *SVT* | Try and get an ECG where possible and consider admitting patient. Can try carotid sinus massage (except if IHD, TIA, elderly) or Valsalva manoeuvre. If attack terminates refer to cardiology |
| *AF*<br>*Symptomatic* | Find and treat cause of AF (hyperthyroidism, pneumonia, HF, alcohol etc.)<br>Consider a beta-blocker or antiarrhythmic drug (initiated by specialist care) |

**Rate or Rhythm Control in AF -** *Ref: NICE Guidance: Atrial fibrillation June 2006*

| | |
|---|---|
| *Rate control* | Over 65, CHD, Contra-indications to antiarrhythmic therapy, unsuitable for cardioversion |
| Drugs | Beta-blockers, calcium channel blockers, digoxin (patients with sedentary lifestyles) |
| *Rhythm control* | Symptomatic, younger (<65), First episode of AF, Secondary to treated or corrected precipitant (e.g. infection/alcohol), CCF |
| Drugs | Sotalol, amiodarone, flecainide |

| | |
|---|---|
| *Anticoagulation* | Start aspirin or warfarin to reduce the risk of thromboembolism |

**Anticoagulation in Atrial Fibrillation – CHADS2 score**

| | Condition | Points |
|---|---|---|
| C | Congestive heart failure | 1 |
| H | Hypertension (or treated) | 1 |
| A | Age > 75 years | 1 |
| D | Diabetes | 1 |
| S2 | Stroke or TIA | 2 |

| Score | Anticoagulation |
|---|---|
| 0 | Aspirin (Aspirin 75 to 300 mg/day) |
| 1 | Discuss with patient pros and cons of either aspirin or warfarin |
| 2-6 | Warfarin (if not contraindicated) |

| | |
|---|---|
| *QoF* | Maintain a register of AF patients and maintained yearly. Ensure patients with a CHADS2 score of 1 are on anticoagulation or antiplatelet therapy. Those with a CHADS2 >1 to be on anti-coagulation |

**AF and cardioversion** - *Ref: NICE Guidance: Atrial fibrillation June 2006*

| | |
|---|---|
| *Onset < 48hrs* | If AF <24 hrs, refer to hospital to be heparinised, transthoracic echocardiogram done to exclude a thrombus. Patients can be cardioverted, either electrically (DC cardioversion) or pharmacology using amiodarone (structural heart disease) or flecainide (no structural heart disease) |
| *Onset > 48hrs* | If AF >48 hrs, refer to cardiology clinic. Patients should be anticoagulated for 3 weeks before cardioversion (aim INR 2.5). After cardioversion continue anticoagulation for at least 4 weeks |

| | |
|---|---|
| *Driving* | Advice regarding DVLA depends on cause |
| Arrhythmias | Sinoatrial disease, Significant AV conduction defect. Atrial flutter/AF, Narrow or broad complex tachycardia |
| Group 1 | Driving must cease if the arrhythmia has caused or is likely to cause incapacity. Driving may be permitted when underlying cause has been identified and controlled for at least 4/52. DVLA need not be notified unless there are distracting/disabling symptoms (no structural heart disease) |
| Group 2 | Disqualifies from driving if the arrhythmia has caused or is likely to cause incapacity. Driving may be permitted when: the arrhythmia is controlled for at least 3/12, or the LV ejection fraction is = to or > 0.4. or there is no other disqualifying condition |
| Syncope | A simple faint requires no restriction. An unexplained syncopal attack with low risk of recurrence 4 weeks off driving. Explained and treated cause of syncope needs 4 weeks off. Unexplained syncope should avoid driving for 6 months |

**SAFETY NETTING**

| | |
|---|---|
| *Follow up* | Seek medical advice if any red flags symptoms such as chest pain, loss of consciousness or severe dyspnoea |

**DIFFERENTIAL DIAGNOSIS**

| Conditions | Characteristic exam feature |
|---|---|
| **Ectopic beats** | Worse at rest. Patients feel a missed, skipped or 'extra beat' |
| **AF** | Irregularly irregular pulse, may be paroxysmal. Can start suddenly. May be due to thyrotoxicosis, pneumonia |
| **SVT** | Sudden onset, feels pounding heart with rapid pulse, dyspnoea, chest tightness and dizziness. Confirmed tachycardia |
| **Hyperthyroidism** | Heat intolerance, weight loss, diarrhoea, eye symptoms, tremor. OE: goitre, AF on pulse, eye signs, sweaty palms |
| **Panic attacks** | Sweating with hyperventilation, perioral tingling. Short lived. Associated with stress. Feeling of impending doom. OE: sweaty palms, tachycardia, tachypnoea |

## EXPLANATIONS

*Palpitations*

Palpitations describes the uncomfortable feeling we can get when our heart thumps or beats heavily. It is an extremely common problem and in most cases is not because of any serious heart condition.

*Ectopic beats*

The heart has a pacemaker that controls the heartbeat. An ectopic beat occurs when a few cells in the heart can infrequently discharge their own electrical impulse causing an extra beat. Although this may sound and feel quite serious, they are quite common and are usually harmless.

*AF*

Atrial fibrillation is when the normal heart pacemaker is overridden by electrical impulses that originate from the upper chamber of the heart (atrium). This causes the heart to quiver and beat in an irregular way.

*ECG*

An electrocardiogram is a special device that painlessly monitors your heart through leads that are placed on your chest and limbs. The heart works by sending out electrical signals from the natural pacemaker, and this passes to the remainder of the heart through special cells that act as wires. As the signals moves through the heart, the heart muscles squeeze and contract and this causes the heart to beat. The ECG is able to pick up these electrical signals and tells us if the heart is working well.

# 2.5 Hypercholesterolaemia

Hypercholesterolaemia describes the presence of raised cholesterol levels in the blood. It is an important feature, as it can increase the risk of heart disease in the form of angina, MI or even strokes. The most common cause of raised cholesterol is dietary due to eating high levels of saturated fats. However, it may also occur genetically in the form of familial hypercholesterolaemia.

---

**Targeted Cholesterol levels**

| | |
|---|---|
| *Normal Risk* | Total Cholesterol <5.0 mmol/L, LDL <3mmol/L, HDL >1mmol/L, TGs <1.7mmol/L |
| *High Risk* | Total Cholesterol <4.0 mmol/L, LDL <2mmol/L, Total chol : HDL ratio <4 |

---

**HISTORY**

Focus should be on gathering information so that an accurate cardiovascular risk assessment can be performed. Analyse the patient notes closely for risk factors and blood results. Is the patient obese? Do they smoke or drink? Is there family history of IHD?

| | |
|---|---|
| **Open questions** | Tell me how can I help you today? |

**Focused questions**

| | |
|---|---|
| *Cardiac* | Do you have any chest pain? Does it occur at rest or on exertion? Do you experience pain on walking (PVD)? |
| *Stroke* | Do you have any weakness or numbness in your arms or legs? |
| *ED* | Do you have any problems maintaining an erection? |

**PAST HISTORY**

| | |
|---|---|
| *Hypertension* | Do you suffer from high blood pressure? |
| *Diabetes* | Have you been diagnosed with diabetes? |
| *CVD* | Have you had any heart problems in the past? Heart attacks or angina? |
| *Secondary causes* | Do you have any kidney problems (CKD) or thyroid problems (hypothyroidism)? |

---

**Cardiovascular risk assessment: QRISK2 & Framingham**

| | |
|---|---|
| *Framingham* | NICE no longer recommends the use of the Framingham equations as they can overestimate the risk by 50% in UK populations especially people living in affluent areas and underestimate high risk areas i.e. socially deprived. If used, multiply the score by 1.4 in South Asian ethnicities and by 1.5 if history of 1st degree premature heart disease |
| *QRISK2* | QRisk is a cardiovascular risk calculator that was developed using UK primary care data. It calculates the 10yr CV risk based upon the patient's age, BMI, BP, cholesterol, ethnicity, deprivation score, smoker, presence of RA, CKD or AF and FHx of premature IHD |
| Explanation | A 10 year score of 20% means that you have a 20% chance (i.e. 1 in 5) of developing a cardiovascular disease (heart attack or stroke) within the next 10 years |
| Classify Risk | The score is classified into low (<10%), moderate (10-20%) or high risk (>20%) with low risk patients followed up after 5yrs, moderate risk after 3yrs and high risk yearly. High risk patients should be initiated on a statin |

**DRUG HISTORY**

Medication          Are you taking any medications? (steroids, B-blockers, thiazides, COCP, antipsychotic treatment, amiodarone)

**SOCIAL HISTORY**

Occupation          Are you currently in employment? What type of work do you do (sedentary lifestyle, restaurant worker)? Is it stressful at work?

Smoker          Do you smoke? How many cigarettes do you smoke per day and for how long have you been doing this?

---

**Calculating Pack Years**

A person smoking 20 cigarettes a day (a pack of cigarettes) for one year is a pack year. Hence a patient smoking 10/d for 10 years has a smoking habit of 5 pack years

---

Alcohol          Do you drink alcohol? How much and how often?

Diet          What type of foods do you eat? Do you eat fried or fast food much? Tell me about your diet for a typical day

Exercise          How much exercise do you do?

---

**Assessing the Patient's Level of Exercise**

The GPPAQ (General Practice Physical Activity Questionnaire) is a screening tool to assess an adult's physical activity levels (16-74 years). The questionnaire takes into account the patient's occupation and level of physical intensity that arises from that. It also scores the patient's degree of exercises across 5 domains including physical exercises (football, jogging, swimming), cycling, walking, housework or child care and gardening or DIY. Patients are asked if over the domains they spend 0, <1, 1-3, >3+ hours in the past week doing these activities. The final question enquires about the pace at which the patient regularly walks, i.e. slow, steady, brisk or fast. The answers are aggregated and the patient is classified on the Physical Activity Index (PAI) as active, moderately active, moderately inactive, or inactive.

---

**FAMILY HISTORY**

CVD          Does anyone in your family suffer from heart problems? Patients with family history of premature cardiovascular disease (<55 men, <65 women) or sudden death should be routinely screened for hypercholesterolaemia

Familial          Do anyone in your family have raised cholesterol? How old are they?

---

**Familial Hypercholesterolaemia**

This is an autosomal dominant condition that has an incidence of 1 in 500. It causes early cardiovascular disease with persistently high LDL levels. Patients can be referred to specialist lipid clinics for screening and treatment. Diagnosed using the Simon Broom criteria:

- Adults total cholesterol (TC) > 7.5 mmol/l and LDL-C > 4.9 mmol/l plus
- FHx of tendon xanthoma (1st or 2nd degree relatives)
- Or possible FHx: MI <50 yrs age in 2nd degree relative or <60 in 1st degree or FHx raised cholesterol

---

**IDEA, CONCERNS, EXPECTATIONS**

Idea          Why do think that you have raised cholesterol levels?

Concerns          Is there anything that is worrying you about your cholesterol levels?

Expectations          What were you hoping we could do to lower your raised cholesterol?

**CSA TIPS**

It is unlikely for patients to attend with symptoms of raised cholesterol but rather present enquiring about the results of routine blood tests. In such cases you would be expected to risk stratify the patient whilst offering an appropriate explanation and management of the condition. Patients may present following an unexpected family bereavement or a family member diagnosed with hypercholesterolaemia. In all such cases, negotiating a shared management plan with the patient and ascertaining their willingness to follow lifestyle advice or take medication will be necessary.

**PHYSICAL EXAMINATION**

| | |
|---|---|
| *Vitals* | BP, BMI, waist circumstance |
| *General* | Eyes – Corneal arcus, face - xanthelasma, tendons - xanthomata |
| *Cardiovascular* | Listen to the heart, assess peripheral pulses |
| *Screening* | The DoH commissioned the NHS health check to screen asymptomatic patients aged 40-74 without any pre-existing conditions for cholesterol and glucose check up |

**INVESTIGATIONS**

| | |
|---|---|
| *Bloods* | Fasting lipids, fasting glucose, U&Es, LFTs (fatty liver), TFTs |
| Other | Consider CK if experiences muscle pain whilst on a statin |
| *ECG* | If history of chest pain or erectile dysfunction |

---

**Ratio of Total Cholesterol : HDL**

The total cholesterol is rarely used on its own when advising a patient regarding their cardiovascular risk. A better measure is to calculate the total cholesterol (TC) / HDL ratio to predict risk. The higher the HDL, the lower the ratio and subsequently, the lower the cardiovascular risk. High risk is defined as >= 6

---

| **MANAGEMENT** | *treat underlying cause* |
|---|---|
| **Conservative** | |
| *Diet* | |
| Avoid fatty food | Avoid fried foods & fatty meats (meat pies), full-fat butter, cheese, cream. Grill, bake, poach or steam instead of roasting or frying foods. If frying, use vegetable oils (sunflower/olive) |
| Healthy foods | Introduce starch-based foods i.e. wholegrain brown bread, potatoes, rice, pasta, cereals. If meat-eater, consider lean meat or chicken |
| Fruit | Encourage eating at least 5 portions of fruit and vegetable daily |
| Fish | Eat at least 2 portions of fish with at least 1 oily fish weekly |
| | |
| *Exercise* | Advise 30 minutes of moderate exercise 5x/week – 'until you feel your heart racing or you become slightly short of breath' |
| *Smoking* | Offer smoking cessation advice |
| *Alcohol* | Reduce intake to <21units /week for men, <14units/week for women |

---

**Cardioprotective Diet** - *Ref: NICE guidelines, Lipid modification, 2010*

- People at high risk of or with CVD should be advised to eat a diet in which total fat intake is <=30%, saturated fats <=10% or less of total energy intake. Intake of dietary cholesterol should be <300 mg/day and saturated fats should be replaced by monounsaturated and polyunsaturated fats
- Do not routinely recommend to take plant sterols and stanols for the primary prevention of CVD

---

## Lipid Modification - Statins

Statins inhibit the action of HMG-CoA reductase within the liver, the rate-limiting step in cholesterol synthesis. They should be taken in the evening as most of the cholesterol synthesis occurs overnight. Side effects include myalgia, myositis and rhabdomyolysis and liver impairment.

- Risk factors for myopathy include old age, female, low BMI, DM and medication (erythromycin, Ca ch. blockers, fibrates, amiodarone). Simvastatin and atorvastatin more likely to cause myopathy compared with rosuvastatin, pravastatin. If CK level is 5x upper limit stop statin
- Concurrent grapefruit juice consumption can increase serum concentration of some statins by affecting the P450 enzyme
- NICE guidelines (2008) recommend baseline liver enzymes be checked prior to initiation and repeated 3 months and 12 months after initiation. If AST remain 3x upper limit then discontinue statin
- CI: Pregnancy, breastfeeding, liver disease. Can potentiate the effects of warfarin

*Alternative*              Consider titrating up to 80mg if patient tolerates or initiate alternative statin (atorvastatin), fibrate or ezetimibe if not tolerated. Do not routinely give omega 3 fatty acid supplements for the primary prevention of cholesterol

## Statins Guidelines for patients on amlodipine & simvastatin

According to the latest MHRA recommendations, there is a risk of myopathy or rhabdomyolysis with this combination. Avoid prescribing 40mg of simvastatin with amlodipine. Consider either reducing the dose or changing the statin i.e. to atorvastatin

*Ref: MHRA Drug Safety Update: Updated prescribing advice for simvastatin 2012*

*Prevention*              Consider aspirin if >50 years old, DM, 10 year CVD risk >20%

Primary                  Patients aged 40-75 who have increased risk of CVD i.e. 10-year risk of 20% or greater, should be offered a statin (simvastatin 40mg on). There is no target level for primary prevention

Secondary                Patients with a history of CVD (angina, MI, stroke, TIA, PVD) should be initiated on a statin irrespective of cholesterol levels. Patients should be started on simvastatin 40mg and can increase to 80mg. A total cholesterol <4 mmol/l or LDL <2 mmol/l should be targeted. Other groups who should be considered for a statin include >75 years old, south Asians, diabetics, 1st degree relative with premature heart disease

*Review*                 Review LFTs after 3mths and 1 year after starting statin

*Refer*                  Options include dietician, smoking cessation clinic, health trainers, exercise / weight loss programme (active for life/ /weight watchers)

## Community Health Trainers

The NHS community health trainer scheme is an innovative idea by which local people are trained to offer lifestyle advice and signposting to other service. They support patients over a 6 week period and help encourage and implement personalised goal setting around a healthy lifestyle

**EXPLANATIONS**

Hypercholesterolemia Cholesterol is the name of the fatty substance found in your blood. It is made in the body (liver) after breaking down the saturated fats from your diet. Too much cholesterol in the blood can build up in your arteries, fur them and slowly over time cause a blockage. This can increase the risk of a blockage in the vessels of the head - known as a stroke, or in the vessels of the heart - known as a heart attack.

LDL                LDL means Low Density Lipoprotein, it is sometimes known as the 'bad cholesterol' as it can build up on the walls of your arteries causing a blockage.

HDL                HDL means High Density Lipoprotein, it is sometimes known as the 'good cholesterol' as it carries away the bad cholesterol from the arteries to the liver to be broken down.

Statins            Statins work by reducing your cholesterol by blocking the way cholesterol is made in the liver. As this process normally occurs at night we advise all patients to take the tablet at this time.

QRisk score        A 10 year score of 20% means that you have a 20% chance (i.e. out of 100, 20 people...) of developing a cardiovascular disease (a heart attack or stroke) within the next 10 years.

# 2.6 Intermittent Claudication

Peripheral arterial disease (PAD), also known as peripheral vascular disease, refers to the narrowing or occlusion of the arterial blood supply to the legs. It is primarily caused by atherosclerosis. Although the majority of patients with PAD are asymptomatic, blood flow may become restricted during exercise or activity giving rise to the classical presentation of intermittent claudication. In severe occlusions, patients may also feel pain at rest. Patients diagnosed with PAD have an increased risk of significant mortality, or morbidity from myocardial infarction and / or a CVA.

## HISTORY

| | |
|---|---|
| **Open questions** | Can you describe the pain you are feeling in your leg? |

**Focused questions**

| | |
|---|---|
| *Claudication* | When did you first notice it? How long have you had it for? |
| Location | Where exactly do you feel the pain? Is it felt in your buttocks, thigh or calf? |

---

**Possible Location of Occlusion**

| | |
|---|---|
| *Thigh pain* | Occlusion in femoral or common inguinal artery |
| *Calf pain* | Occlusion in popliteal or tibial artery |
| *Foot pain* | Occlusion in posterior tibial or dorsalis pedis artery |

---

| | |
|---|---|
| Character | How would you describe the pain? Is it a cramping, burning or a numbness feeling? |
| Severity | How severe is the pain on a scale of 1 to 10, ten being the most severe? |
| Aggr. / relieve | Does anything make it better, such as rest or hanging your leg off the edge of the bed? Does anything make it worse, such as walking long periods or after taking medication? (beta blockers) |
| Claud. distance | How far can you walk before the pain comes on? |
| Rest pain | Do you ever experience the pain at rest? |
| Associated | Have you noticed any changes to your leg? Like change in colour, feeling cold or any skin changes? |

**Associated history**

| | |
|---|---|
| *Assoc. sympt* | Have you noticed any shortness of breath, chest pain, palpitations, ankle swelling? |
| *Erectile Dysfunction* | Do you have any problems with having or maintaining an erection? |

**Differentials**

| | |
|---|---|
| *Sciatica* | Do you have any shooting pains that starts from your back moving down to your foot? Do you have any problems passing urine or stools? |
| *Spinal Stenosis* | Do you get numbness and weakness in the legs when walking? Is it more difficult to walk uphill? Do you get pain over the buttocks? Does it affect both sides? |
| *DVT* | Have you noticed your calf has swollen? Have you flown recently or had an operation? |

---

**Classification of PAD (Fontaine classification)**

I    Asymptomatic

II   Intermittent claudication

    a    Pain-free, claudication when walking >200 metres

b  Pain-free, claudication when walking <200 metres
III  Pain while resting / nocturnal pain
IV  Necrosis / gangrene

## RED FLAGS

| | |
|---|---|
| *Critical ischaemia* | Pain at rest, pallor, paraesthesiae in foot, cold legs, gangrene |

## PAST HISTORY

| | |
|---|---|
| *Previous* | Have you ever experienced these symptoms before? |
| *CVD* | Have you ever had a heart attack, high blood pressure, cholesterol or diabetes? |

## DRUG HISTORY

| | |
|---|---|
| *Medication* | Are you taking any medications? (B-blocker) |

## SOCIAL HISTORY

| | |
|---|---|
| *Occupation* | Are you currently in employment? Do you stand for long periods at work? |
| *Smoker* | Do you smoke? How many cigarettes do you smoke per day? |
| *Alcohol* | Do you drink alcohol? How much and how often? |
| *Diet* | What type of foods do you eat? Do you eat fast food much? |
| *Exercise* | How much exercise do you do? |

## FAMILY HISTORY

| | |
|---|---|
| *IHD* | Anyone in the family suffer from heart problems? |
| *PAD* | Has anyone in your family had similar symptoms as you described? |

## Risk factors for Peripheral Arterial Disease

Gender (M>F), age (>50yr), BP, DM, smoking, raised cholesterol, FHx of PAD/IHD, BMI >30, physical inactivity

## IDEA, CONCERNS, EXPECTATIONS

| | |
|---|---|
| *Idea* | What did you think may be causing your leg pain? |
| *Concerns* | How has it affected you? (Stopping normal activities - sports/walking/gardening) |

## CSA TIPS

Patients suffering from claudication may have significant disability affecting their day to day functioning. It may restrict them from performing sports and hobbies that they enjoyed in the past or it may even cause problems when climbing hills or inclines. It is also easy to confuse the presenting complaint with alternative diagnoses if a clear history including PMHx and FHx of cardiac disease is not identified.

## PHYSICAL EXAMINATION

| | |
|---|---|
| *Vitals* | BP, pulse, BMI |
| *Cardiovascular* | Listen for heart sounds |
| *Abdomen* | Palpate the abdomen for an aortic aneurysm |
| *Arterial leg exam* | |
|   Inspection | Inspect the legs for colour change (white, blue, purple, black), trophic changes (shiny skin, hair loss, ulcers) and other signs (gangrenous, amputated toes). Inspect the pressure points (heel, malleoli) for ulcers |
|   Palpation | Check temperature of the legs and capillary refill |
|     Pulses | Palpate the posterior tibial, dorsalis pedis artery, popliteal artery and femoral artery |

| Special test | Consider performing Buerger's test. Have the patient on the couch, establish the angle of elevation of the leg where it becomes pale. Angle >30 degrees suggests severe ischaemia. Sit them up with leg hanging off the edge of the bed. Time how long it takes for the leg to return to normal colour. Redness suggests reactive hyperaemia (chronic lower limb ischaemia, 2-3 min to return colour) |
|---|---|

## INVESTIGATIONS

| Bloods | FBC, U&E (excl renal artery stenosis), fasting lipids, fasting glucose |
|---|---|
| ECG | Look for signs of ischaemia |
| ABPI | Perform an ABPI or refer to vascular clinic to be done |
| Other | Doppler studies to establish site of disease |

### Interpreting Ankle Brachial Pressure Index

In diabetics, the ABPI can be falsely elevated due to vessel wall calcification

| ABPI | > 1.0 | Normal |
|---|---|---|
| ABPI | 0.5 - 0.9 | Claudication |
| ABPI | < 0.4 | Critical Ischaemia |

## MANAGEMENT    *treat underlying cause*
### Conservative

| Smoking | Offer smoking cessation advice |
|---|---|
| Diet | 5 fruit and vegetable a day, less red meat and dairy products. Eat normal healthy diet |
| Weight reduction | If BMI>30 refer to intense weight loss programme |
| Alcohol | Reduce alcohol intake (<21u/wk in men, <14u/wk in women) |
| Exercise | Encourage increase exercise primarily by walking as far as possible within their pain threshold. Attempt to extend their maximum walking distance over time. Evidence shows that supervised exercise therapy has more success |
| Foot hygiene | Avoid tight shoes or socks that may injure or reduce the blood supply to the foot. Avoid any trauma or accidents to the foot |

### Medical

| Treat risk factors | Patients with DM, HTN and hypercholesterolaemia should be optimally controlled |
|---|---|
| Aspirin | Consider offered aspirin (75mg – 150mg) with symptomatic peripheral vascular disease. If contraindicated try clopidogrel or dipyridamole |

### Aspirin in Peripheral Vascular Disease - *Ref: SIGN, Diagnosis and management of PVD, 2006*

Antiplatelet therapy is recommended for patients with symptomatic peripheral arterial disease. In trials comparing different aspirin regimens in patients with cardiovascular disease, doses of 75-150mg were as effective as higher doses: overall aspirin produced a 23% reduction in vascular events. The gastrotoxic side effects from aspirin appear to be greater with increasing dose, so 75-150mg is the dose of choice

| Statin | Offer a statin to the patient i.e. simvastatin 40mg |
|---|---|
| Refer | Consider referral to podiatry for foot hygiene including cutting nails or treating corns or callous. Refer to vascular for diagnosis and further treatment options i.e. Naftidrofuryl, angioplasty or bypass |

## SAFETY NETTING

| Follow-up | To seek medical advice if they notice any pain at rest or features of critical ischaemia |
|---|---|

## Features of Critical Ischaemia

Painful, Pulseless, Pallor (pale), Paralysis, Paraesthesia (numbness), Perishing with cold. Acute limb ischemia is any sudden decrease in limb perfusion that causes a threat to limb viability. It can be caused by thrombosis, emboli or trauma

## DIFFERENTIAL DIAGNOSiS

| Condition | Characteristic exam feature |
|-----------|-----------------------------|
| Intermittent claudication | Calf, buttock or thigh pain worse on exertion and relieved by rest. Claudication distance. Associated with erectile dysfunction |
| OA hip | Hip pain radiating to thigh or buttock. Worse on weight bearing. Can occur at rest (less intensity) or certain positions. OE: antalgic gait, reduced ROM at the hip joint |
| Lumbar radiculopathy | Hx of back pain. Burning sensation back of leg. Worse on bending or carrying. OE: reduced SLR. Altered sensation in lower leg. Reduced ankle reflexes |
| Chronic Compartment sy. | Tight bursting pain in the calf muscle. Common in athletes. Starts after exercise. Relief on elevation of leg. OE: ABPI normal |
| Spinal Stenosis | May present with slowly worsening back pain. Worse on exercise but patient has to sit down for a few minutes to relieve the pain. Numbness and tingling may also be associated. OE: pain reduced on spiral flexion forward. No weakness |

## EXPLANATIONS

*PVD*

This is a condition that affects the blood vessels in your lower legs. Over time fat in the blood can build up and fur the arteries causing a narrowing of the vessels and reduced blood flow to the muscles. If there is decreased blood flow, the muscle is starved of the necessary oxygen and nutrients to work. As a result, you feel pain particularly when you are exercising as your muscles need more blood and oxygen.

*ABPI*

ABPI stands for arterial brachial pressure index. It compares the blood pressure in yours arms against that of your legs using a blood pressure cuff and a Doppler ultrasound probe. This allows the doctor to decide how severe your condition is.

# *2.7 Varicose Veins*

Varicose veins are engorged, tortuous superficial veins found in the leg which are often unpleasant to the eye. They usually present with venous insufficiency due to incompetent valves. Although they are unsightly, they rarely present as medical emergencies. However, they may cause medical symptoms shall as pain, skin ulcers, bleeding and superficial infection.

**HISTORY**

**Open questions**  Can you tell me more about the symptoms you have noticed in your leg?

**Focused questions**

*Varicose veins*  When did you first notice it? How long have you had it for?

   Location  Where exactly have you noticed it? Is it in your thigh or lower leg?

   Pain  Have you felt an aching, heaviness or pressure in your leg? When did the pain start?

   Aggr. / relieve  Does anything make it better (sitting down, elevating leg) or worse (standing for long periods)?

**Associated history**

*Oedema*  Do you have any swelling in the leg or ankles?

*Skin changes*  Have you noticed any skin changes, itch or ulcers over your legs?

**RED FLAGS**

*DVT*  Calf swelling, recent travel or operation

*Abdominal mass*  Abdominal swelling or lump

**PAST HISTORY**

*Pregnancy*  Have you been pregnant previously? How many children do you have?

*Pelvic tumour*  Have you been told you suffer from any cancers?

*Surgery*  Have you had any previous treatments for varicose veins?

**DRUG HISTORY**

*Medication*  Are you taking any medications? (COCP, HRT)

**SOCIAL HISTORY**

*Occupation*  Are you currently in employment? Do stand for long periods at work (teaching, hairdressing)?

*Smoker*  Do you smoke? How many cigarettes do you smoke per day?

*Alcohol*  Do you drink alcohol? How much and how often?

**FAMILY HISTORY**

*DVT*  Anyone in the family suffer from blood clots in the leg?

*Varicose veins*  Has anyone in your family had similar symptoms as you described?

---

**Risk factors for Varicose Veins**

Gender (F>M 6:1), age (young/middle aged), pregnancy and parity, occupation (prolonged standing), DVT, abdominal mass, AV fistula, FHx of varicose veins  or varicose veins, thrombophlebitis, OCP/HRT

---

## IDEA, CONCERNS, EXPECTATIONS

| | |
|---|---|
| *Idea* | What did you think may be causing your leg symptoms? |
| *Concerns* | Do you have any worries about your symptoms? (appearance, wearing clothes, DVT) |
| *Expectations* | How were you hoping I could help you with your varicose veins today? (surgery) |

## CSA TIPS

Varicose veins are unsightly veins that can be found in the lower limbs. Most patients attending with such problems usually want them removed. However, the NHS does not offer surgical intervention for purely cosmetic reasons. You should explain to patients what varicose veins are, and reassure them that in most cases they are non-life threatening. If on examination, the patient has severe skin changes or pain that affects their quality of life, then you should consider onward referral to a local vascular clinic.

## PHYSICAL EXAMINATION

| | |
|---|---|
| *Vitals* | BMI |
| *Abdomen* | Examine for any pelvic or abdominal masses |
| *Venous leg exam* | |
| Inspection | Inspect the gaitor area (above medial malleolus), long (groin to medial malleolus) and short saphenous vein (popliteal to lateral malleolus) for eczema, ulcers or oedema. Check for hemosiderin pigmentation or lipodermatosclerosis |
| Palpation | Palpate along long and short saphenous vein for tenderness (phlebitis) or hardness (thrombosis). Check for peripheral oedema |

## INVESTIGATIONS

| | |
|---|---|
| *Bloods* | Not routinely performed |
| *Doppler studies* | Establish site of disease |
| *ABPI* | ABPI may be performed to exclude peripheral vascular disease prior to offering support stockings |

## MANAGEMENT

### Conservative

| | |
|---|---|
| *Reassure* | If mild varicose veins then reassure |
| *Weight reduction* | If BMI>30 refer to intense weight loss programme |
| *Exercise* | Encourage to increase exercise primarily by walking as far as possible within their pain threshold |
| *Pain* | Place a hot flannel over the vein to reduce pain |
| *Position* | |
| Avoid standing | Avoid prolonged uninterrupted standing. Intersperse periods with walking or sitting |
| Elevate legs | Elevate legs where possible particularly at night or when seated which may also provide temporary symptomatic relief. Put pillows under your foot when lying in bed or use a footstool when seated |

### Medical

| | |
|---|---|
| *Support stockings* | Offer graduated compression stockings to control symptoms and reduce the risk of ulceration. Advise patient to wear them first thing in the morning just before they get out of bed (veins collapsed, easier to put on) and to remove before sleeping at night. Class I stockings are used for mild symptoms. However, in the presence of significant ankle oedema or to prevent recurrent ulceration then Class 2 stockings should be provided |

**Types of Compression Stockings**
3 different grades according to the pressure they exert upon the ankle. They work by reducing venous reflux via increasing venous pressure in the legs: Class 1 stocking can be purchased OTC whilst grade 2 and 3 require a prescription. Avoid in PVD (pressure necrosis). Support stockings come in two sizes: below knee and thigh length. They can also be made to measure as required. Thigh length are useful for varicose veins in the thigh as well as during pregnancy. Knee length are recommended for varicose veins in the lower leg, swollen ankles and ulcers

| | |
|---|---|
| *Class 1 Compression* | Mild varicose veins with aching legs & mild ankle swelling e.g. for long flights |
| *Class 2 Compression* | Moderate to severe varicose veins, moderate ankle swelling, after vein surgery prevent recurrent ulcerations |
| *Class 3 Compression* | Severe varicose veins or ankle swelling, active leg ulcers |

*Complications*

| | |
|---|---|
| Eczema | Varicose eczema can be offered simple moisturising emollients and/or topical mild steroids |
| Thrombophlebitis | Consider antibiotics if infected or NSAIDs. Thrombophlebitis increases the risk of an underlying DVT by 25% particularly if it is along the course of the long saphenous vein |

**Complications of Varicose Veins**
Pain & heaviness, DVTs, haemorrhage from trauma, varicose eczema, venous ulceration, skin pigmentation, thrombophlebitis, lipodermatosclerosis, oedema, atrophic blanche

**Surgery**

| | |
|---|---|
| *Operation* | Refer to low priority panel if relevant depending on your area protocol. Consider in severe varicose veins. Option include stripping, sclerotherapy. Newer techniques include foam therapy and radiofrequency ablation |

**Safety netting**

| | |
|---|---|
| *Follow-up* | Advise patient to seek medical advice if they notice any pain at rest or features of critical ischaemia. If the varicose veins bleed, recommend the patient to lift leg above the heart and apply pressure |

**Referral to a Vascular service -** *Ref: NICE: Varicose veins in the legs: 2013*
Refer people with bleeding varicose veins to a vascular service immediately. Refer people to a vascular service if they have any of the following;
- Symptomatic primary or symptomatic recurrent varicose veins
- Lower-limb skin changes (pigmentation or eczema, thought to be caused by chronic venous insufficiency
- Superficial vein thrombosis (hard, painful veins) and suspected venous incompetence
- A venous leg ulcer (a break in the skin below the knee that has not healed within 2 weeks)
- A healed venous leg ulcer

## DIFFERENTIAL DIAGNOSIS

| Condition | Characteristic exam feature |
|-----------|----------------------------|
| Varicose veins | Unpleasant tortuous veins in leg along saphenous distribution. Aching, heaviness worse at the end of the day, worse on standing, improved with rest and elevation. OE: dilated veins in the long / short saphenous vein distribution. Pedal oedema and skin changes |
| Saphena varix | Enlarged saphenous vein at the sapheno-femoral junction. OE: cough impulse, lump in groin. Bluish tinge, disappears on lying down. May appear with varicose veins |
| Thrombophlebitis | Superficial inflammation of a vein. May cause pain, redness, swelling. OE: tender and hard vein |

## EXPLANATIONS

*Varicose veins*

Varicose veins are twisted enlarged veins that run just under the skin of the legs. Veins usually have one way valves (doors) that help push blood back to the heart. Unfortunately, when the valves become leaky or weak, blood pools in the veins because of gravity. This is why they are worse when you are standing and get better when you raise your legs.

*Thrombophlebitis*

This is when the superficial veins, usually of the legs become inflamed. We do not know why this happens, but often it is because of slight damage or injury. If you have varicose veins then these may also get affected. When the veins becomes inflamed, they may get mildly swollen, red and cause pain.

*Compress. Stockings*

These are special stockings the doctor can give you that help the blood move in the lower legs. They work by putting pressure at the ankle and the legs and squeeze the veins to help the blood return to the heart.

When wearing the stockings, you should put them on first thing in the morning and take them off, before you go to bed. You should try and wear the stockings properly for them to give you the most benefit. Sometimes they may cause your skin to become dry or feel uncomfortable in hot weather.

# *3.1 Cough*

A cough reflex is the body's first line of defence to prevent any foreign bodies from entering the respiratory tract. Coughing is a non-specific symptom that is due to irritation of the airways anywhere from the pharynx to the lungs. It may be caused by a number of unrelated conditions such as infections, gastric reflux, airway obstruction or foreign body aspiration. When taking a history it is often useful to distinguish between acute (<3wks) and chronic (>8wks) causes whilst also attempting to rule out the more sinister causes such as lung cancer and PE.

**HISTORY**
**Open questions**  Can you tell me more about your cough?

**Focused questions**
*Cough*        When did you first notice it? How long have you had it for? Is it dry or wet (chesty)?
  Frequency      Is it there all the time or does it come and go?
  Aggr. / relieve  Does anything makes it better (inhaler) or worse (NSAIDs)?
  Better         Changes with the season, being away from work, after eating or using an inhaler
  Worse          Exercise, stress or pets

**Causes of Cough based upon Duration**
*Sudden onset*  Inhaled foreign body, acute pulmonary embolism
*Acute*        URTI, LRTI, acute bronchitis, croup
*Chronic*      Asthma, COPD, lung cancer, GORD, TB, post nasal drip, ACE inhibitors, bronchiectasis

**Associated history**
*SOB*          Do you feel short of breath? Did it come on suddenly?
*Chest pain*   Have you had any chest pain? Is it worse on breathing in or coughing?
*Weight loss*  Have you had a reduced appetite or weight loss?

**Differentials**
*Pneumonia*    Do you bring up any phlegm or sputum? What colour is it (white, grey, yellow, green)? Any fevers or sweats?
*PE*           Did it come on suddenly? Were you short of breath or coughing up any blood up? Do you have any leg pain? Did you fly recently?
*GORD*         Do you get any heartburn? Is it worse if you lie flat? Do you ever get excessive saliva (water brash) or an acidic taste in your mouth (acid brash)?
*Asthma*       Is it worse in the morning or late at night? Is it associated with a wheeze? Do you suffer from hay fever or eczema?
*TB*           Have you had any night sweats? Have you lived abroad for a prolonged period? Do you cough up any blood?
*Lung cancer*  Have you noticed any hoarseness to your voice? Have you coughed up any blood? How much?

**RED FLAGS**   Confusion, pleuritic chest pain, weight loss, hoarseness of voice haemoptysis

## Admission for Community Acquired Pneumonia

The British Thoracic Society suggests using the CRB-65, 4 point score to gauge the severity of a community-acquired pneumonia helping GPs to decide when to admit patients. Each area has a score of 1 point if present; with a total score of 0 not requiring hospital admission, 1 - 2 – consider hospital referral, 3+ needing urgent hospital admission.

**CRB-65:** **C**onfusion (disorientation to time, place, person), **R**R >30/mins, **B**P <90/60, **65** yrs or older

*Ref: BTS guidelines for the management of community acquired pneumonia in adults (2007)*

## PAST HISTORY

| | |
|---|---|
| *PE* | Have you ever had a blood clot in the chest (PE) or leg (DVT)? |
| *Asthma/COPD* | Do you suffer from asthma or COPD? |
| *Atopy* | Have you suffered from hay fever, eczema or any allergies? |

## DRUG HISTORY

| | |
|---|---|
| *Medication* | Are you taking any medications? Are you on an ACE inhibitor? |
| Asthma | *Triggers* - Aspirin, B-blocker, NSAIDs |
| GORD | *Worsens* - NSAIDs, steroids, bisphosphonates, nitrates, calcium channel antagonists |
| PE | *Associated* - OCP, HRT |

## SOCIAL HISTORY

| | |
|---|---|
| *Occupation* | Are you working at the moment (wood industry, chemicals)? Have you ever worked in the manufacture of concrete? |
| Occ. asthma | Do you find that if you are away from work your symptoms get better? |
| Alveolitis | Have you worked in the following occupations, as a farmer with animals (pigeons), coal miner, in a dockyard or as a builder (asbestosis exposure)? |
| *Smoker* | Do you smoke? How many cigarettes do you smoke per day? |
| *Alcohol* | Do you drink alcohol? How much and how often? |
| *Travel* | Have you been on any long haul flights? |
| Pets | Do you have any pets at home (cat, dog, rabbit, birds)? |

## FAMILY HISTORY

| | |
|---|---|
| *Asthma* | Anyone in the family suffer from asthma? |
| *Cystic Fibrosis* | Has anyone in your close family been diagnosed with CF? |

## IDEA, CONCERNS, EXPECTATIONS

| | |
|---|---|
| *Idea* | What did you think was causing the cough? |
| *Concerns* | What were you worried about your cough? (lung cancer) |
| *Expectations* | How were you hoping I could help you with your cough? (cough meds, inhalers, CXR, referral) |
| *Impact* | How have your symptoms affected your life? |

## CSA TIPS

Taking a cough history may reveal red flags for serious underlying pathology such as lung cancer. It may be necessary to take a very brief cough history and dedicate more time on breaking the news to the patient that one of the possible causes of their cough could be lung cancer. Please see breaking bad news for further guidance on how to do this. A possible cue in a cough history could be the nature of the patient's employment. Symptoms that are related to occupation should be explored as they may reveal more useful information. Patients who have been exposed to asbestos may need advise regarding the financial benefits available to them.

---

## Asbestos Benefits
Merely being exposed to asbestos or the presence of pleural plaques on a CXR does not automatically entitle a patient to benefits. Rather the government offers compensation to those who develop complications from asbestos exposure including mesothelioma, asbestosis, pleural thickening with disability, lung cancer from asbestos. Patients will need to submit an application using FORM BI 100(PN), which is available from their local benefits office

---

## PHYSICAL EXAMINATION

| | |
|---|---|
| *Vitals* | BP, pulse (AF-pneumonia), temperature, respiratory rate (PE), O2 sats (reduced in PE, pneumonia), weight (loss – cancer, TB) |
| *Respiratory* | |
| Hands | Clubbing (lung cancer, bronchiectasis), peripheral cyanosis |
| Percussion | Check for percussion note or vocal fremitus (pneumonia) |
| Auscultation | Listen to chest for crepitations, wheeze, reduced air entry |
| *Lymph nodes* | Examine the head and neck lymph nodes (URTI, TB) |
| *Cardiovascular* | Listen for heart sounds. Palpate legs for oedema (HF) and DVT (PE) |

## INVESTIGATIONS

| | |
|---|---|
| *Bloods* | FBC, U&E, ESR, CRP, LFTs, proBNP (CCF) |
| *Sputum* | MCS, cytology, ZN staining (TB) |
| *ECG* | CCF (LVH), PE (AF, RBBB, S1Q3T3) |
| *CXR* | Exclude chest infection, TB, lung cancer |
| *Peak flow* | Asthma – reversibility with B-agonist |
| *Spirometry* | COPD (lacks reversibility) |
| *Other (specialist)* | ABG, VQ scan or CTPA, bronchoscopy, CT chest, blood cultures |

## MANAGEMENT  *treat underlying cause*
### Asthma

| | |
|---|---|
| *Conservative* | Avoid allergens – pets, pollen, dust. Education re inhalers |
| *Medical* | Salbutamol, inhaled steroids. Follow BTS guidelines. Consider oral steroids in acute exacerbation (see asthma chapter) |

### COPD

| | |
|---|---|
| *Conservative* | Stop smoking (most important), pulmonary rehabilitation |
| *Medical* | Ipratropium bromide, LABAs, LABA + ICS, oral steroids (see COPD chapter) |

| | |
|---|---|
| **PE** | If suspected, start on LMWH. If confirmed, start warfarin (INR 2-3) for 3mth if transient risk factors (surgery, trauma, transient immobility) or 6mth if permanent risk factors |

### Dyspepsia

| | |
|---|---|
| *Conservative* | Avoid chilli and spicy food. Cut down on caffeine and alcohol. Stop smoking. Eat small, regular meals and ensure that the last meal is several hours before bedtime |
| *Medical* | Alginates – Gaviscon, H2 Antagonist - Ranitidine, PPI – Omeprazole |

| Post Nasal drip | Avoid triggers / allergens. Trial of oral antihistamines or nasal steroids |
|---|---|
| **TB** | Refer to specialist, contract tracing, triple therapy, DOT (directly observed treatment) |
| **Drug induced** | Stop ACE inhibitor and change to an ARB. May take a few months to settle down |
| **LRTI** | Initiate antibiotics, consider Amoxicillin, or erythromycin |
| **URTI** | Reassure self-limiting, OTC meds (no evidence), paracetamol or NSAIDs, fluid hydration |

## Immediate Antibiotic Prescribing

Antibiotics are recommended if the patient is felt to be developing complications. Other criteria include:

* Systemically very unwell
* Symptoms of serious illness / complications (e.g. pneumonia, mastoiditis, peritonsillar abscess, peritonsillar cellulitis)
* High risk of complications due to comorbidity (heart, lung, renal, liver, immunosuppression, CF, premature babies)
* >65 years with cough plus >=2 of following or >80 years with cough plus >=1 features - hospitalisation in previous yr, DM type 1 / type 2, CCF, oral glucocorticoids

| *Refer* | Refer to speciality (chest clinic) as appropriate |
|---|---|

## Cancer Referral Guidelines 2005 - *Ref: NICE*

| *Immediate* | Stridor, signs of superior vena caval obstruction |
|---|---|
| *Urgent* | Persistent haemoptysis (smokers/ex-smokers in >40yrs) |
| | CXR suggestive of lung cancer (pleural effusion, persistent consolidation) |
| | Normal CXR but high suspicion of lung cancer |
| | Asbestos exposure with chest pain, SOB or unexplained systemic symptoms + CXR (pleural effusion, pleural mass, suspicious lung lesion) |
| *Urgent CXR* | Haemoptysis, Persistent cough (>3wks): chest or shoulder pain, SOB, weight loss, chest signs, hoarseness, finger clubbing, cervical/supraclavicular lymphadenopathy, cough, metastatic lung cancer (brain, bone, liver, skin mets) |
| | Unexplained change to chronic respiratory problem |

## SAFETY NETTING

| *Follow up* | If cough persist for 3-4weeks review. If any red flag symptoms request to seek medical advice urgently i.e. cancer referral symptoms |
|---|---|
| *Referral* | Refer if unsure of diagnosis. Admit if haemodynamically unstable (tachycardia, tachypnoea, BP <90/60, reduced O2 sats or altered consciousness) |

## DIFFERENTIAL DIAGNOSIS

| Conditions | Characteristic exam feature |
|---|---|
| **URTI** | Acute cough, coryzal symptoms, fever, myalgia, pharyngitis, otorrhoea. OE: red throat, bulging eardrum, pyrexia. Cervical nodes |

| | |
|---|---|
| **Postnasal drip** | Feeling of liquid running down the back of the throat, sneezing, nasal congestion or blockage. OE: inflamed turbinates |
| **GORD** | Burning sensation over epigastrium moving up to the neck. Worsened by lying down or bending over. Acid brash and water brash may be present. Can cause painful swallowing or nocturnal asthma. Relieved by antacids but related to spicy food, alcohol or hot caffeine drinks. OE: epigastric pain |
| **Pulmonary embolism** | Sudden shortness of breath with pleuritic chest pain. May also have haemoptysis and tachycardia. Risk factors: DVT, travel, trauma, OCP, malignancy. OE: tachypnea with calf tenderness |
| **TB** | Night sweats, haemoptysis, lymphadenopathy, weight loss. OE: cachectic appearance, LN bilaterally in the cervical chain |
| **Pneumonia** | Pleuritic chest pain associated with fever, productive cough and dyspnoea. OE: coarse crackles with dull percussion note and fever |
| **Asthma** | Diurnal variation, wheeze, shortness of breath, reversibility with salbutamol / steroids. OE: expiratory wheeze, reduced PF |
| **COPD** | Heavy smoker, productive cough, >35 yr old, lacks reversibility on spirometry. OE: cyanosis, hyperinflation, wheeze |
| **Lung cancer** | Heavy smoker, weight loss, haemoptysis, hoarseness of voice, clubbing. OE: cachectic appearance, LN in the neck, supraclavicular area |

**EXPLANATIONS**

*Lung Cancer*      This is a growth that is found in your lungs. It normally affects older people and the majority of cases are because of smoking. Over time, the chemicals in the smoke cause the normal cells in your lungs to change and they may become cancerous. As they grow uncontrollably, this gives rise to cancer.

*TB*      This is an infection (usually of the lungs) caused by a type of bug called Mycobacterium tuberculosis. You normally catch it from close contact with other people who have the disease as the bacteria spreads through breathing in the bug from others. The bug does not always cause problems straight away and may sit sleeping in the lung for many years.

*URTI*      An URTI refers to an infection that affects the upper airways that include the throat, ear, nose or sinuses. They are usually caused by viruses and occasionally by bugs known as bacteria. When one catches an URTI, we feel tired, suffer with body aches and may have symptoms like a sore ear or throat. However, usually with simple symptomatic treatment the body clears the infection itself.

| | |
|---|---|
| *Pneumonia* | This simply refers to a chest infection. It is very common and affects people of all ages. Usually a bacterial infection enters the lungs and causes the small sacs at the end of the breathing tubes called bronchioles to get inflamed and fill up with fluid. Most pneumonias can be treated quite comfortably with antibiotics. |
| *PE* | A pulmonary embolism refers to a blockage of the vessels that carry blood to the lungs from the heart. This sometimes can happen because of a blood clot that has formed in your legs. There are things that can make this more likely to happen such as not moving after a serious operation, being seated for long periods in a long-haul flight or because of a blood defect. |
| *Asthma* | Asthma is a condition that affects your lungs. Your lungs are made up of lots of small tubes that allow air and in particular oxygen to pass freely. In asthma certain triggers, also known as allergens, may irritate these airways and cause them to narrow. As a result, air may become trapped inside your lungs making you feel short of breath. The narrowed airways also restrict the flow of air through them making your chest feel tight as well as producing a high-pitched sound known as a wheeze. |
| *COPD* | COPD stands for Chronic Obstructive Pulmonary Disease, it is an umbrella term that describes both chronic bronchitis and emphysema. Your airways become narrowed and obstructed due to lung damage caused by smoking. As the damage gets worse, the lungs lose their ability to stretch (elasticity) and air becomes stuck in the lungs which leads to the feeling of shortness of breath. |
| *Post Nasal drip* | This is when fluid and mucus builds up at the back of the nose and throat. It describes a process rather than a medical condition. The fluid may build up because of an infection or irritation (allergen). As it builds up, it trickles down into the throat and may give rise to a sore throat, a stuffy nose or a cough. |

# 3.2 Shortness of breath

Dyspnoea can be quite an anxiety-provoking symptom for the patient. Some may describe a feeling of tightness or pressure in the chest, swelling over the throat or an inability to breathe. Dyspnoea is entirely a subjective experience that may vary widely between patients. The intensity by which it is described may not necessarily correlate to the severity of underlying pathology. It may be as a result of disease in the cardiac or respiratory systems, or may be due to other conditions such as anaemia, obesity or even as a result of a panic disorder.

---

**Causes of Shortness of Breath based upon Duration**

| | |
|---|---|
| *Sudden onset* | Upper airway obstruction (inhaled FB, anaphylaxis), PE, pneumothorax |
| *Acute (hrs)* | Asthma, pneumonia, pulmonary oedema |
| *Chronic* | COPD, lung cancer, heart failure, pleural effusion, pneumoconiosis, anaemia |

---

**HISTORY**

**Open questions**      Can you tell me more about the shortness of breath you are experiencing?

**Focused questions**

| | |
|---|---|
| *Dyspnoea* | When did you first notice it? How long have you had it for? Did it come on suddenly? |
| *Nature* | Does it come and go or is it there all the time? |
| *Trigger* | Does anything make it better or worse? |
| Better | Using inhalers, period away from work, sitting down and resting |
| Worse | Lying down, walking, allergens (cats, pets, grass) |
| *Exercise* | How far can you walk before you get breathless? How are you with stairs? How far could you walk before all of this started? |

---

**New York Heart Association Functional Classification**

The New York Heart Association is a tool recommended by NICE and QOF to grade the severity of heart failure. The degree of exertion required to elicit the symptoms does not necessarily equate with the severity of the underlying heart problem i.e. a patient with mild symptoms can in fact have profound damage to the heart.

| Class | Symptoms |
|---|---|
| *I* | No limitation in ordinary physical activity. Does not cause SOB, fatigue |
| *II* | Slight limitations during ordinary activity symptoms such as walking, climbing stairs |
| *III* | Marked limitation in activity due to symptoms, even during less than ordinary activity e.g. walking short distances (20–100m); comfortable only at rest |
| *IV* | Severe limitations – experiences symptoms even while at rest (mostly bed-bound patients) |

---

**Associated history**

| | |
|---|---|
| *Sleep* | Does it affect your sleep? |
| *Chest pain* | Have you noticed chest pain? Is it worse when you breathe in? |
| *Cough* | Have you been coughing as well? |

## Differentials

| | |
|---|---|
| *Heart failure* | Is it worse when you lie down (orthopnoea)? Does it ever wake you up in the middle of the night (PND)? Do you have any swelling of your legs? How many pillows do you sleep on? Has this changed recently? |
| *Pneumonia* | Do you bring up any phlegm or sputum? What colour is it (white, grey, yellow, green)? Any fevers or sweats? |
| *PE* | Did it come on suddenly? Were you coughing up any blood up? Do have any leg pain? |
| *Asthma* | Is it worse in the morning or late at night? Is it associated with wheeze? Do you suffer from hay fever or eczema? |
| *Panic attack* | Do you experience any palpitations, sweaty palms or pins and needles around your lips? Would you describe yourself as an anxious person? |
| *Cardiac* | Did you experience your heart beating heavier or faster when the breathlessness started? |

## RED FLAGS

| | |
|---|---|
| *Anaphylaxis* | Acute severe, shortness of breath, angioedema, stridor |
| *Asthma* | Inability to complete sentences, silent chest |
| *MI / ACS* | Cardiac chest pain |
| *PE* | Haemoptysis |

## PAST HISTORY

| | |
|---|---|
| *Cardiac* | Do you suffer from high blood pressure, raised cholesterol, angina, or DM? Have you ever had a heart attack? |
| *PE/DVT* | Have you had a blood clot in your lung or leg? |
| *Atopy* | Have you suffered from asthma, hay fever, eczema or any allergies? |

## DRUG HISTORY

| | |
|---|---|
| *Medication* | Are you taking any medications? |
| Asthma | *Triggers* - Aspirin, B-blocker, NSAIDs |
| PE | *Associated* - OCP, HRT |
| *Allergies* | Do you suffer from any drug allergies? |

## SOCIAL HISTORY

| | |
|---|---|
| *Occupation* | Are you working at the moment? |
| Occ asthma | Do you find that if you are away from work your symptoms get better? |
| Alveolitis | Have you worked in the following occupations, as a farmer with animals (pigeons), coal miner, in a dockyard or as a builder (asbestosis exposure)? |
| *Smoker* | Do you smoke? How many cigarettes do you smoke per day? |
| *Alcohol* | Do you drink alcohol? How much and how often? |
| *Travel* | Have you been on any long haul flights (PE)? Did you stay in any hotels (legionnaires)? |

## FAMILY HISTORY

| | |
|---|---|
| Asthma | Does anyone in the family suffer from asthma? |

## IDEA, CONCERNS, EXPECTATIONS

| | |
|---|---|
| *Idea* | What do you think may have caused your shortness of breath? |
| *Concerns* | Were you worried about your shortness of breath (MI, dying, limitation of activity)? |
| *Impact on life* | How has it affected your life or your family? |

## Medical Research Council Dyspnoea Scale

The MRC Dyspnoea Scale is used to assess the degree of disability caused by breathlessness rather than the severity of the underlying pathology.

1   Not troubled by breathlessness except on strenuous exercise
2   Short of breath when hurrying or walking up a slight hill
3   Walks slower than contemporaries on level ground because of breathlessness, or has to stop for breath when walking at own pace
4   Stops for breath after about 100m or after a few minutes on level ground
5   Too breathless to leave the house or breathless when dressing or undressing

## CSA TIPS

It is important to appreciate the impact that the shortness of breath has on the patient particularly in the elderly. These patients may not be initially forthcoming in revealing their difficulties and a more detailed social history may be required to establish if they are having problems coping or whether they have assistance in the form of a carer or relative. Also determine whether they can perform simple activities of daily living such as going to the toilet, walking up and down stairs or whether they can go shopping unaided.

## PHYSICAL EXAMINATION

| | |
|---|---|
| *Vitals* | BP, pulse (irregular), temperature, respiratory rate (PE), O2 sats (reduced in PE, pneumonia), weight (increased in HF) |
| *Respiratory* | |
| Hands | Clubbing (lung cancer, bronchiectasis), peripheral cyanosis |
| Palpate | Tracheal deviation |
| Percussion | Check for percussion note or vocal fremitus (pneumonia, fluid) |
| Auscultation | Listen to chest for crepitations, wheeze, reduced air entry |
| *Lymph nodes* | Examine the head and neck lymph nodes (URTI, TB) |
| *Cardiovascular* | Listen for heart sounds (AS). Palpate legs for oedema (HF) and DVT (PE) |

## INVESTIGATIONS

| | |
|---|---|
| Bloods | FBC (low Hb, raised WCC), U&E, LFTs, ESR, CRP |
| Other | D-dimers (PE), proBNP (CCF), TFTs (AF), Troponin T (MI) |
| *Sputum* | MC&S |
| *ECG* | CCF (LVH), PE (AF, RBBB, S1Q3T3), arrhythmias |
| *CXR* | Exclude chest infection, lung cancer |
| *Peak flow* | Asthma – reversibility with B-agonist |
| *Spirometry* | COPD (lacks reversibility) |
| *Echo* | Heart failure, valvular dysfunction |
| *Other (specialist)* | VQ scan or CTPA, bronchoscopy, CT chest, ABG, Lung function tests |

---

**ProBNP and Heart Failure-** *Management of chronic heart failure, SIGN 2007*

BNP and NT-pro BNP are amino acids that are secreted when the heart muscle is stretched. They are raised in heart failure and have been recommended by NICE & SIGN to rule out heart failure before an echo. They may be raised in MI, valvular disease, PE, DM & CKD (GFR<60). They may be reduced due to ACEI, ARBs & diuretics.

| | | |
|---|---|---|
| *High levels* | BNP > 400 pg/ml | NTpro BNP > 2000 pg/ml |
| *Raised levels* | BNP 100–400 pg/ml | NTpro BNP 400–2000 pg/ml |
| *Normal levels* | BNP < 100 pg/ml | NTpro BNP < 400 pg/ml |

---

*Ref: Management of chronic heart failure in adults in primary and secondary care, NICE August 2010*

| MANAGEMENT | *treat underlying cause* |
|---|---|
| **Heart failure** | |
| Conservative | Mx risk factors and comorbid conditions (BP, IHD). Lose weight, avoid alcohol |
| Immunisation | Offer annual flu jab and one-off pneumococcal injection |
| Medical | Initiate on ACEI and beta-blocker 'start low & go slow'. 2nd line treatment includes aldosterone antagonist, ARB, hydralazine with nitrates (African-Caribbean) |
| QoF | Diagnosis made by specialist and/or ECHO confirmation. Ensure patient is on ACE-I and/or beta-blocker |

| **Asthma** | |
|---|---|
| Conservative | Avoid allergens – pets, pollen, dust. Education re inhalers |
| Medical | Salbutamol, inhaled steroids. Follow BTS guidelines. Consider oral steroids in acute exacerbation (see asthma chapter) |

| **COPD** | |
|---|---|
| Conservative | Stop smoking (most important), pulmonary rehabilitation |
| Medical | Ipratropium bromide, LABAs, LABA + ICS, oral steroids |

| **PE** | If suspected, start on LMWH. If confirmed, start warfarin (INR 2-3) for 3mth if transient risk factors (surgery, trauma, immobility) or 6mth if permanent risk factors |
|---|---|

| **Palpitations** | |
|---|---|
| SVT | Perform ECG and consider admitting patient. Can try carotid sinus massage (except if IHD, TIA, elderly) or Valsalva manoeuvre. If attack terminates refer to cardiology |
| AF | Find cause of AF if relevant (hyperthyroidism, pneumonia, heart failure, alcohol etc.) |

| **LRTI** | Initiate antibiotics, consider Amoxicillin, or erythromycin |
|---|---|

| **URTI** | Reassure, OTC meds (no evidence), paracetamol or NSAIDs, fluid hydration |
|---|---|

| **Refer** | Refer to speciality for management of shortness of breath if poorly controlled |
|---|---|
| Admit | Consider admission if red flags, MI, PE or reduced O2 sats (<92%), tachycardia (>130bpm), tachypnoea (>30/min), PF 33% of normal |

---

**Heart failure Referral Guidelines** - *Ref: Mx of chronic HF in adults in primary & secondary care, NICE 2010*
*Specialist advice*
Refer patients to the specialist multidisciplinary heart failure team in the following situations;

- Initial diagnosis of heart failure
- Management of severe heart failure (NYHA class IV), heart failure that does not respond to treatment, heart failure due to valve disease, or heart failure that can no longer be managed at home
- Advice and care of women who are planning a pregnancy or are pregnant. Care of pregnant women should be shared between the cardiologist and obstetrician

*Patients with previous MI*
Refer patients with suspected heart failure and previous myocardial infarction (MI) urgently to have transthoracic Doppler 2D echocardiography and specialist assessment within 2 weeks

---

*Follow up*  If any red flag symptoms request to seek medical advice i.e. cancer referral symptoms

## DIFFERENTIAL DIAGNOSIS

| Conditions | Characteristic exam feature |
|---|---|
| Pulmonary embolism | Sudden SOB with pleuritic chest pain. May also have haemoptysis and tachycardia. Risk factors: DVT, travel, trauma, OCP, malignancy. OE: tachypnea with calf tenderness |
| Panic attack | Stressors, perioral tingling, palpitations, hyperventilation, short-lived, anxiety, sweating, feeling of doom |
| Pneumonia | Pleuritic chest pain associated with fever, productive cough and dyspnoea. OE: coarse crackles with dull percussion note and fever |
| Asthma | Diurnal variation, wheeze, shortness of breath, reversibility with salbutamol / steroids. OE: reduced PF, expiratory wheeze |
| COPD | Heavy smoker, productive cough, >35 yr old, lacks reversibility on spirometry. OE: cyanosis, hyperinflation, wheeze |
| Arrhythmias | Sudden onset, feels pounding heart with rapid pulse, dyspnoea, chest tightness and dizziness. OE: tachycardia |

## EXPLANATIONS

*Heart Failure*  Heart failure means that your heart is not pumping blood around the body as well as required. This is usually because the heart muscle has been previously damaged perhaps due to a heart attack or very high blood pressure. As a result you may feel breathless when walking, lying flat or when you are sleeping. You may note some extra fluid around your ankles. It does not mean your heart has 'failed' and is going to stop beating at any time.

Echo  An echocardiogram is a special scan that gives us a lot of information about your heart. It uses sound waves to get a picture of the heart muscles, valves and whether the heart is beating healthily or not. It is similar to the ultrasound that is used when monitoring the baby in pregnant women and is a safe and painless procedure.

*Arrhythmia*  This describes a problem with the heartbeat. Occasionally the heart may beat too fast, too slow or erratically. This change in beat pattern is termed an arrhythmia.

# 3.3 Asthma

Asthma is a chronic respiratory disease, that is characterised by inflammation of the airways, hypersensitivity and reversible, reduced outflow (bronchospasm) obstruction. The exact cause of asthma is not known; however a complex interaction between genes, infections and environmental exposure are believed to play a part. The main symptoms of asthma include breathlessness, chest tightness, wheezing and coughing (worse at night or early morning). An obvious allergen such as pets, pollen or foodstuffs may also be elicited and family history is often positive for asthma. Sufferers may have had eczema as a child or allergic rhinitis (hay fever).

## HISTORY

**Open questions**   Please tell me more about your cough / problems with your breathing?

**Focused questions**

| | |
|---|---|
| *Asthma* | When did it first start? How long does it last for? |
| Diurnal variation | Is it worse at night or in the mornings? |
| Triggers | Does anything make it better or worse? |
| Better | Changes with the season, being away from work, using an inhaler |
| Worse | Exercise, stress or pets, cold weather |

**Associated history**

| | |
|---|---|
| *SOB* | Do you feel short of breath or wheezy when you have the cough? |
| *Chest pain* | Have you experienced any chest pain or tightness? |

### RCP Questions to Assess Asthma

*In the last month…*
- Have you had difficulty sleeping because of your asthma symptoms? (including cough)
- Have you had your usual asthma symptoms during the day? (cough, wheeze, chest tightness, SOB)
- Has your asthma interfered with your usual activities? (housework, work/school)

Nocturnal walking and activity limitations are considered abnormal in controlled asthma (mild to moderate). Asthma symptoms can occur up to 3d/wk

*Ref: Measuring Clinical Outcome in Asthma: a patient-focused approach. London: RCP, 1999*

**Differentials**

| | |
|---|---|
| *Pneumonia* | Do you bring up any phlegm or sputum? What colour is it (white, grey, yellow, green)? Any fevers or sweats? Do you have any chest pain when you cough? |
| *PE* | Did it come on suddenly? Is there any chest pain when taking a deep breath in? Were you short of breath or coughing up any blood up? Do have any leg pain? |
| *GORD* | Do you get any heartburn? Is it worse if you lie flat? Do you ever get excessive saliva (water brash) or an acidic taste in your mouth (acid brash)? |

## RED FLAGS

| | |
|---|---|
| *Severe asthma* | Severe SOB, incomplete sentences, exhaustion, confusion |

## PAST HISTORY

| | |
|---|---|
| *Atopy* | Do you suffer from hay fever, eczema or urticaria? |
| *Asthma attacks* | In the last year, have you had any asthma attacks? How many? |

| A+E | Have you ever attended A+E with your asthma? |
| ITU | Have you ever been admitted to ITU with your asthma? |

## DRUG HISTORY

| *Medication* | Are you taking any medications? (Aspirin, B-blocker, NSAIDs) |
| Inhalers | How often do you use them? Do you know how to use them properly? |
| Steroids | Have you used oral steroids in the last year? How many times did you have to use them? |

## SOCIAL HISTORY

| *Smoker* | Do you smoke? How many cigarettes do you smoke per day? |
| *Alcohol* | Do you drink alcohol? How much and how often? |
| *Occupation* | Are you working at the moment? Do you find that if you are away from work your symptoms get better (occupational asthma)? |
| *Hobbies* | Do you participate in any sports? Does your symptoms prevent you from competing? |

---

**Occupational & Exercise Induced Asthma** - *Ref: Adapted from SIGN*

| *Occupational* | >400 industrial materials can induce asthma. Often insidious onset taking months to years. Classically symptoms improve whilst away from work (on holiday). Diagnosis with serial PEFR before, during and after work |
| High risk | Baking, pastry making, spray painting, laboratory animal work, healthcare, dental care, food processing, welding/soldering, metalwork, woodwork, chemical processing, textile, plastics and rubber manufacture |
| *Exercise* | Asthma can be precipitated by exercise. Spirometry should be performed before and after exercise for diagnosis |

---

## FAMILY HISTORY

| *Atopy* | Anyone in the family suffer from asthma, eczema or hay fever? |

---

**Probability of Diagnosis of Asthma**

| *High* | Wheeze, SOB, chest tightness, cough, worse at night; early morning or after exercise. Other triggers include cold, allergens or exposure to aspirin/B-blocker. PMHx/FHx of atopy, wheeze on auscultation, unexplained blood eosinophilia or low PEFR/spirometry |
| *Low* | Prominent dizziness, light-headedness, peripheral tingling, voice disturbance, chronic productive cough with no wheeze/SOB, Repeatedly normal examination, smoker (>20 pack yrs), Normal PEFR/spirometry when symptomatic |

---

## IDEA, CONCERNS, EXPECTATIONS

| *Idea* | What did you think was causing your symptoms? |
| *Concerns* | Were you worried that it was going to affect your work/school/sports activities? |
| *Impact on life* | How has it affected your life or your family? |

## CSA TIPS

Patients who are given a diagnosis of asthma may have misconceptions as to what it means and the impact it may have on their life. They may fear from being unable to perform their daily tasks or enjoy their favourite pastimes. Others who have lived with their conditions for several years may be fearful that their condition may deteriorate and they may require ITU admissions. Spend some time explaining the diagnosis and stress the importance of correct inhaler technique where possible.

**PHYSICAL EXAMINATION**

| | |
|---|---|
| *Vitals* | BP, pulse, temperature, respiratory rate, O2 sats |
| *Respiratory* | |
| Inspection | Resp distress, accessory muscles, barrel chest, tachypnea, incomplete sentences |
| Auscultation | Listen to the chest for prolonged expiratory phase, wheeze, silent chest |

**INVESTIGATIONS**

| | |
|---|---|
| *Bloods* | *Often not indicated:* FBC (eosinophilia) |
| *CXR* | Overinflated chest or unclear diagnosis |
| *Peak flow* | Reversibility with B-agonist or inhaled steroids |
| *Spirometry* | Reversibility seen |

---

**Investigations in Asthma**

| | |
|---|---|
| *Reversibility* | If evidence of airflow obstruction assess FEV1 or PEFR before and after trial of inhaled salbutamol; >400ml improvement in spirometry of FEV1 or 15% in PEFR suggests asthma. If no evidence of obstruction, can trial inhaled (beclomethasone 200mcg bd) or oral steroids (prednisolone 30mg od 2wks) and recheck FEV1/PEFR |
| *Spirometry* | Moderate probability of asthma should have a spirometry to diagnose |
| FEV1/FVC < 0.7 | Offer reversibility testing/trial tx |
| FEV1/FVC > 0.7 | No evidence of airway obstruction. Further investigation required |
| *Serial PEFR* | Diagnosis made with serial PEFR (poor sensitivity) over 2wk period. >20% of variation (diurnal) or >60ml/min improvement over 3d/wk is suggestive |
| Diurnal variation | Diurnal variation % = (Highest – Lowest PEFR) / Highest PEFR x 100 |

---

**MANAGEMENT**

***Conservative***

| | |
|---|---|
| *Allergen avoid* | Although many recommend to avoid, SIGN report no improvement |
| Dust mite | Remove carpets, curtains, soft toys. Cover pillows, mattress, regular hovering (get someone else to hoover and return to the room after 20min) |
| Pets | Avoid pets (cats or dogs) |
| *Breastfeeding* | Protective against asthma |
| *Smoking* | Stop smoking and avoid passive smoking where possible |
| *Exercise* | Reduce weight; can recommend exercise programmes |

***Medical***

| | |
|---|---|
| BTS guidelines | Use BTS and SIGN Asthma Guidelines (2011). If the patient is using salbutamol inhaler >3/wk or have nocturnal symptoms |
| Step 1 | Inhaled short-acting beta agonist as required |
| Step 2 | Add inhaled steroid 200–800 mcg/d (beclomethasone). Start at dose of steroid appropriate to severity of disease |
| Step 3 | Add inhaled long-acting agonist (LABA – salmeterol). Assess control |
| Good | If good response – continue LABA |
| Inadequate | Benefit from LABA but control still inadequate – continue LABA and increase inhaled steroid dose to 800 mcg/d |
| No response | If no response, stop LABA and increase steroid to 800 mcg/d. If control still inadequate, institute trial of other therapies, e.g. leukotriene |

| Step 4 | Increase inhaled steroids up to 2000 mcg/d or add 4th drug, e.g. leukotriene receptor antagonist, SR theophylline, beta agonist tablets |
|---|---|
| Step 5 | Use daily steroid tablets in lowest dose providing adequate control. Maintain high-dose inhaled steroid at 2000 mcg/d. Consider other treatments to minimize use of steroid tablets |

| *Immunisation* | If on inhaled/oral steroids offer annual flu vaccinations |
|---|---|
| *QoF* | Patient needs yearly QoF screening with the RCP questions. Patients aged 14-20 should have their smoking status recorded. |
| *Refer* | Refer to specialist if stage 5 or the BTS guidelines. Refer urgently if signs of severe or life threatening asthma |

---

## Severity of Asthma

| *Moderate* | Normal speech, PEFR > 50%, RR < 25 / min, Pulse < 110 bpm |
|---|---|
| *Severe* | Cannot complete sentences, PEFR 33-50%, RR > 25/min, Pulse > 110 bpm |
| *Life threatening* | Silent chest, PEFR < 33%, O2 sats < 92%, cyanosis or feeble respiratory effort, bradycardia, dysrhythmias, hypotension, exhaustion, confusion or coma |

---

## SAFETY NETTING

| *Follow up* | Follow up every 3mths to consider stepping down or change to the lowest inhaled steroid dose if symptoms are controlled |
|---|---|
| *Admission* | If patients are acutely short of breath, chest tightness, wheezing, unable to complete sentences, exhausted, confused or drowsy they should seek medical advice |

## EXPLANATIONS

| *Asthma* | Asthma is a condition that affects your lungs. Your lungs are made up of lots of small tubes that allow air and in particular oxygen to pass freely. In asthma certain triggers, also known as allergens, may irritate these airways and cause them to become narrow. As a result, air may become trapped inside your lungs making you feel short of breath. The narrowed airways also restrict the flow of air through them making your chest feel tight as well as producing a sound known as a wheeze. |
|---|---|
| Inhalers | The reliever (salbutamol) works by relaxing the muscle in the airways to allow air to flow from the lungs more freely. The preventer (steroids) work by reducing inflammation around the airways. Once they are less inflamed they are less likely to narrow because of specific triggers (allergens). Steroids do not work straight away and may take up to 14 days for their effects to be seen. |
| Technique | Before you take the inhaler, it is important to shake it well so that the medicine is mixed with the gas propellant. Exhale fully before using the inhaler, and remove the cap. Hold the inhaler between your thumb and index finger with your index finger on the canister. Make a seal with your lips around the mouth of the inhaler. As you press down on the inhaler, it is important to simultaneously start taking a slow deep breath in over 5 seconds. Close your mouth and hold your breath for another 5 seconds. |
| Peak flow | Stand up and take a deep breath in and place the mouthpiece in your mouth ensuring that you make a tight seal around it with your lips. Hold the peak flow meter making sure your fingers do not interfere with the pointer. Ensure the pointer is placed to zero. Blow as hard and fast as you can; as if you are trying to blow out candles. |

Chronic Obstructive Pulmonary Disease is an umbrella term used to describe chronic lung diseases including emphysema and chronic bronchitis. The main cause of COPD is believed to be due to cigarette smoking (both active and passive); however inherited disorders such as alpha-1 antitrypsin deficiency and air pollution have also been implicated. The classification of COPD into 'blue-bloaters' and 'pink-puffers' has been discarded in recent times. Symptoms vary depending on the stage of the disease; however breathlessness, coughing and excessive sputum production as well as wheeze and recurrent chest infections are often found.

---

**Diagnosing COPD by History**

A diagnosis of COPD should be considered in patients over the age of 35 who have a risk factor (generally smoking) and who present with one or more of the following symptoms:

- Exertional breathlessness
- Regular sputum production
- Chronic cough
- Frequent winter 'bronchitis'
- Wheeze

*Ref: Mx of chronic obstructive pulmonary disease in adults in primary and secondary care – NICE, June 2010*

**HISTORY**

**Open questions**    Please tell me more about your cough / problems with your breathing?

**Focused questions**

| | |
|---|---|
| *COPD* | When did it first start? How long does it last for? |
| Cough | Do you have a cough all the time or does it come and go? Is it dry or wet (chesty)? |
| Sputum | Do you bring up any phlegm? What colour is it (grey, yellow, green)? |
| SOB | Do you feel breathless at rest or on exertion? Do you have a chesty wheeze? |
| Exercise | How far can you walk before you get breathless? How are you with stairs? How far could you walk before all of this started? |

**Associated history**

| | |
|---|---|
| *Mood* | How has it affected your mood? |
| *Weight loss* | Have you felt fatigued or noticed any weight loss? |
| *Sleep* | Do you awake at night as a result of your breathing? |

---

**Medical Research Council Dyspnoea Scale**

The MRC Dyspnoea Scale is used to assess the degree of disability caused by breathlessness in COPD rather than the severity of the underlying pathology.

1   Not troubled by breathlessness except on strenuous exercise
2   Short of breath when hurrying or walking up a slight hill
3   Walks slower than contemporaries on the level because of breathlessness, or has to stop for breath when walking at own pace
4   Stops for breath after about 100m or after a few minutes on level ground
5   Too breathless to leave the house or breathless when dressing or undressing

*Ref: Adapted from Fletcher CM, Elmes PC, Fairbairn MB et al. (1959) The significance of respiratory symptoms and the diagnosis of chronic bronchitis in a working population. BMJ 2: 257–66*

**Differentials**

| | |
|---|---|
| *Asthma* | Is it worse in the morning or late at night? Is it associated with a wheeze? Do you suffer from hay fever or eczema? |
| *Pneumonia* | Do you bring up any phlegm or sputum? What colour is it (white, grey, yellow, green)? Any fevers or sweats? Do you have any chest pain when you cough? |
| *Heart Failure* | Is it worse when you lie down (orthopnoea)? Does it ever wake you up in the middle of the night (PND)? Have you noticed any swelling of your legs? How many pillows do you sleep on? Has this changed recently? |

**RED FLAGS**

| | |
|---|---|
| *Cor Pulmonale* | Ankle swelling, paroxysmal nocturnal dysnopea (PND) |
| *COPD* | Early onset symptoms, non-smoker with FHx (alpha-1 antitrypsin def.) |
| *Other* | Chest pain, haemoptysis – consider alternative diagnosis |

**PAST HISTORY**

| | |
|---|---|
| *Exacerbations* | Have you ever attended A+E with your breathing problems? How many times in the last year? How often do you get chest infections? |
| *Winter attacks* | Do you regularly suffering from a wheezy chest during the winter period? |
| *ITU* | Have you ever been admitted to ITU? |

**DRUG HISTORY**

| | |
|---|---|
| *Medication* | Are you taking any medications? (Aspirin, B-blocker, NSAIDs) |
|   Inhalers | How often do you use them? Do you know how to use them properly? |
|   Steroids | Have you used oral steroids in the last year? How many times did you have to use them? |

**SOCIAL HISTORY**

| | |
|---|---|
| *Smoker* | Do you smoke? How many cigarettes do you smoke per day? |
| *Alcohol* | Do you drink alcohol? How much and how often? |
| *Occupation* | Are you working at the moment? |
|   COPD | Coal miners, hard rock miners (silica, quarks), tunnel workers |
| *Hobbies* | Do you participate in any sports? Does your symptoms prevent you from competing? |

**FAMILY HISTORY**

| | |
|---|---|
| *COPD* | Anyone in the family suffer from chest problems such as COPD? Does anyone have alpha-1 antitrypsin deficiency? |

---

**Differentiating COPD from Asthma**

Some clinicians struggle to differentiate between asthma and COPD. In principle, asthma is a condition of reversible airway obstruction caused by exposure to precipitants, whilst COPD is irreversible airway obstruction caused by damage to the lung parenchyma. Be aware that COPD & asthma may co-exist and approximately 15% of COPD patients will also suffer from asthma.

| *Clinical Features* | *COPD* | *Asthma* |
|---|---|---|
| Smoker or ex-smoker | Nearly all | Possibly |
| Age < 35 years | Rare | Often |
| Chronic productive cough | Persistent & productive | Variable |
| Breathlessness | Uncommon | Common |
| Night waking with SOB or wheeze | Uncommon | Common |

| | | |
|---|---|---|
| Eczema, hayfever, allergies | Uncommon | Common |
| Diurnal day variation in symptoms | Uncommon | Common |

*Ref: Adapted from clinical features differentiating COPD and asthma – NICE, June 2010*

## IDEA, CONCERNS, EXPECTATIONS

| | |
|---|---|
| *Idea* | Did you have any thoughts as to what may be causing your breathlessness? |
| *Concerns* | Were you worried that it was going to affect your daily activities? |
| Other | Need for home oxygen therapy, premature death |
| *Impact on life* | How has it affected your life? How are you coping at home? |

## CSA TIPS

Patients with COPD are usually aware of their diagnosis and the role that their lifelong smoking has impacted upon their health. Despite this you should continue to offer opportunistic smoking cessation advice if the patient continues to smoke as this is still considered the best intervention at reducing overall morbidity and mortality from COPD. Other patients may present with end-stage COPD on home oxygen and seek advice about travelling abroad or within the UK. Having some knowledge about travel guidelines may prevent unnecessary referrals to the respiratory clinic.

---

### Long Term Oxygen therapy & Air Travel

Patients with COPD on long term oxygen or who have an FEV1 <50% of predicted should consult a doctor and be fully assessed before considering or embarking on any flights abroad. Commercial airplanes fly at altitudes of up to 12,500 metres, and require the cabin to be pressurised. This can reduce the pO2 levels on aircrafts and can drop a healthy person's oxygen saturation from 97% to 93%. As a result there is risk of increasing hypoxia in an already hypoxic patient especially if they have COPD. Patients with a pO2 of less than 9.3 kPa at sea level should consult the airline company and receive supplemental oxygen whilst travelling. Patients with significant hypoxia (<6.7 kPa) or hypercapnia are advised not to fly. Patients with bullous disease should be informed of the potential risk of developing a pneumothorax during the flight.

---

## PHYSICAL EXAMINATION

| | |
|---|---|
| *Vitals* | BP, pulse, temperature, respiratory rate, O2 sats, BMI (cachexia) |
| *Respiratory* | |
| Inspection | Respiratory distress, accessory muscles, barrel chest, tachypnea, cyanosis (central/peripheral), pursing of lips on expiration, raised JVP |
| Palpate | Hyperresonance |
| Auscultation | Listen to the chest for crepitations, decreased breath sounds, wheeze |
| | |
| *Cardiovascular* | Pedal oedema |

## INVESTIGATIONS

| | |
|---|---|
| *Bloods* | *Often not indicated:* FBC (anaemia, polycythaemia) |
| *Sputum* | Sputum culture (MC&S) if productive sputum |
| *CXR* | Overinflated chest or unclear diagnosis |
| *Spirometry* | Used to diagnose as well as monitor COPD |

---

### Diagnosing COPD by Spirometry

COPD is clinically diagnosed by spirometry if evidence of irreversible airway obstruction. QoF require evidence of reversibility testing with an inhaled bronchodilator <400ml in FEV1 after a trial suggests COPD

- FEV1/FVC ratio < 0.7 (70%) and FEV1 <80% predicted

- If the FEV1 is >=80 % predicted, then diagnosis made only if symptomatic (i.e. SOB or cough)
- Clinically significant COPD is not present if FEV1 and FEV1/FVC ratio return to normal with drug therapy

| | |
|---|---|
| *Peak flow* | To exclude asthma (COPD – irreversibility). Can underestimate the degree of airflow obstruction in COPD |
| *ECG/Echo* | If cor-pulmonale is suspected |

### Gradation of severity of airflow obstruction

| FEV1/FVC (post bronch.) | FEV1 (of predicted) | Severity |
|---|---|---|
| < 0.7 | > 80% | Stage 1 - Mild |
| < 0.7 | 50–79% | Stage 2 - Moderate |
| < 0.7 | 30–49% | Stage 3 - Severe |
| < 0.7 | < 30% | Stage 4 - Very severe |

## MANAGEMENT
### *Conservative*

| | |
|---|---|
| *Smoking* | Offer smoking cessation advice or refer to smoking cessation clinic |

### Smoking Cessation in COPD
Stopping smoking is the single most beneficial intervention that can be offered to the patient. Although stopping smoking when COPD is established will not reverse any damage already done, it will prolong survival and reduce morbidity compared to those who continue to smoke.

| | |
|---|---|
| *Exercise* | Reduce weight to BMI<25; can recommend exercise programmes |
| *Employment* | Avoid employment that has health hazards that may worsen your COPD |
| *Questionnaire* | Although not widely utilised, NICE recommend COPD patients be monitored using the Clinical COPD (CCQ questionnaire) |
| *Chest physio* | Offer chest physiotherapy if the patient has excessive sputum secretions |

### Active Cycle of Breathing Techniques (ACBT)
ACBT is a series of breathing techniques that has been recognised by NICE to loosen secretions and help improve severe ventilation. It is often taught by a chest physiotherapist. It involves using deep breathing, huffing, coughing and breathing control over 10 to 20 minutes to help clear excessive sputum that may put the patient in distress.

### *Medical*

| | |
|---|---|
| *Bronchodilator* | Initiate an inhaled short-acting 2 agonist (SABA e.g. salbutamol 2 prn) or short-acting muscarinic antagonists (SAMA e.g. ipratropium bromide 1 qds). If patient remains breathless or has exacerbations check FEV1. Consider a spacer device if the patient has severe OA or has problems using the inhaler |
| *FEV1 > 50%* | Add long-acting beta2-agonist (LABA e.g. salmeterol 2bd) or long-acting muscarinic antagonist (LAMA e.g. tiotropium 1od) |
| *FEV1 < 50%* | Add LABA + inhaled corticosteroid (ICS) in a combination inhaler (e.g. seretide or symbicort), or LAMA |
| *SOB* | For those who are still SOB or have recurrent exacerbations switch to an LABA + ICS if already on a LABA. Otherwise offer a LAMA and a LABA + ICS combination inhaler |

| | |
|---|---|
| Theophylline | Offer oral theophylline after a trial of short and long-acting bronchodilators, or in patients who are unable to use inhaled therapy |
| Mucolytic | Consider in patients with a chronic cough or sputum (Carbocisteine 375mg tds) continue if benefits after 4wks. Caution if has peptic ulcer |
| Exacerbations | Increase bronchodilators inhalers, give oral antibiotics if purulent sputum or infection, give prednisolone 30mg 7-14d |
| Rescue Pack | Consider giving a rescue pack of abx and steroids that they can keep at home |
| Nebulisers | Consider in distressing dyspnoea despite maximum inhaler therapy. Only continue if symptom relief, increase in ADLs, better exercise capacity or improvement in lung function |
| Alternative | No evidence to support antitussive, anti-oxidant nor prophylactic abx therapies |
| | |
| Immunisation | Offer annual influenza and one-off pneumococcal vaccination |
| QoF | A register of COPD patients needs to be updated and maintained yearly. Patients should have a yearly FEV1, and be assessed for dyspnoea using MRC scale. Those with MRC $\geq$ 3 should have O2 sats |
| Pulmonary rehab | Consider pulmonary rehab for MRC $\geq$ 3 |
| Oxygen therapy | Consider in end-stage COPD |

---

**Oxygen Therapy in COPD Patients**

Long-term oxygen (LT) therapy can reduce mortality in COPD. Patients who are being considered for LT oxygen therapy, should first be assessed by a respiratory specialist. They must also stop smoking to reduce the risk of fire hazards (burns, fire). They should use O2 therapy for >15hrs/d to see any medical benefits. It is best delivered with a concentrator, via nasal prongs at 2-4 l/min (depends on the patient's clinical presentation and ABGs).

*Indications for initiating Oxygen Therapy*

Initiated if they have an abnormal ABG (pO2 <7.3kPa when stable or pO2 of 7.3-8.0 kPa when stable with other features including secondary polycythaemia, nocturnal hypoxaemia, peripheral oedema or pulmonary hypertension). It should be considered with an abnormal spirometry test (severe airflow obstruction with FEV1 of < 30% of predicted or moderate airflow obstruction FEV1 30–49% predicted), O2 sat <92% on air, evidence of cyanosis, polycythaemia, raised JVP or peripheral oedema.

---

| | |
|---|---|
| Refer | Refer to speciality if there is worsening of symptoms, severe COPD, onset <40yrs, frequent infections/exacerbations. Refer to OT /social services if the patient has poor social support or is having difficulty in mobilising at home with stairs |

**SAFETY NETTING**

| | |
|---|---|
| Admission | If the patient is acutely short of breath, increased frequency of sputum, exhausted, confused or drowsy they should seek medical advice |

**EXPLANATIONS**

| | |
|---|---|
| COPD | COPD stands for Chronic Obstructive Pulmonary Disease, it is an umbrella term to describe both chronic bronchitis and emphysema. Your airways become narrowed and obstructed due to the lung damage caused by smoking. In addition, the smoke damages the stretchiness of the lungs and as the damage gets worse this leads to shortness of breath. |
| Treatments | Unfortunately there is no cure for COPD however the single best thing you can do to help your condition is to stop smoking. It is never too late to stop as this has been |

shown to prevent the disease from worsening. The inhalers we can give you, will help to open up the airways and make you feel better symptomatically.

Spirometry       Spirometry is a test using a handheld machine that measures the amount of air your lung can hold as well as how fast you can breathe it out. You will be asked to wear a nose clip to prevent air from escaping as you breathe through the machine. Whilst sitting, take a deep breath in until your lungs are full. Make a tight seal with your lips and the mouthpiece and then blow as hard and as fast as possible into the machine until you have no more air left in your lungs.

Lung Function    These are special tests that are carried out in the hospital. They help to see how well you can breathe in and out. You will have to blow through a tube into a machine and you will be advised to wear a nose clip to stop air from leaking out of your nose. Sometimes, the test may take place in a see-through cubicle where you will sit and the door will be closed. This helps the machine work more accurately and gives better results.

# 3.5 Smoking cessation

Tobacco smoking is the single most preventable cause of premature death in the UK. Each year it is thought that over 100,000 smokers in the UK die from smoking related causes. Approximately 10 million adults smoke with the majority being male but the rising prevalence of female smokers is rapidly closing the gap. It is the largest preventable cause of cancer and is known to be a significant risk factor for cardiovascular disease. Whilst the majority of smokers profess to wanting to quit (>70%) only a very small number actually go on to do so (<2%/year). Quitting smoking at any age brings much benefit, both immediate and long term. Hence, all patients who smoke should be offered support and advice regarding smoking cessation opportunistically.

---

**Association of Smoking and Disease**

| | |
|---|---|
| *Cancers* | Lung (90%), oropharyngeal, oesophageal, gastric, lip, colon, bladder |
| *CVD* | CHD, CVA/TIA, PVD |
| *Respiratory* | COPD, exacerbation of asthma, chest infections |
| *Obstetrics* | IUGR, preterm delivery, stillbirth, cot death |
| *Other* | Dyspepsia, peptic ulcers, osteoporosis, thrombosis, infertility |

---

**HISTORY**

**Open questions**      Please tell me more about why you want to stop smoking?

**Focused questions**

| | |
|---|---|
| *Smoking cessation* | How many do you smoke a day? And for how long (calculate pack years)? Do you smoke at work or at home? |
| Type | Do you smoke cigarettes, cigars, roll ups or pipes? |
| Why start | Why did you start smoking? (stress, social, habit)? |

**SOCIAL HISTORY**

| | |
|---|---|
| *Smokers* | Does anyone else smoke at home or at work? |
| *Occupation* | Are you working at the moment? |
| *Stress* | Are you suffering from stress? Is everything alright at home or at work? |
| *Alcohol* | Do you drink alcohol? How much? |

**PAST HISTORY**

| | |
|---|---|
| *Prev. attempts* | Have you tried quitting before? What happened? Have you ever been smoke free? Why did you start smoking again? |
| *Other* | Do you suffer from any medical problems? (DM, CVA, HTN, cholesterol, asthma, ca) |
| *Contraindications* | Do you suffer from depression or any other mental health disorders? Have you been diagnosed with epilepsy before? Are you pregnant? |

**DRUG HISTORY**

| | |
|---|---|
| *Prev. attempts* | Any problems with previous treatments? (NRT, bupropion-Zyban, varenicline-Champix) |

**IDEA, CONCERNS, EXPECTATIONS**

| | |
|---|---|
| *Idea* | What made you want to stop now? Has anything happened that made you want to quit? |

| Concerns | Was there anything worrying you about smoking that made you want to stop? |
|---|---|
| Other | Family bereavement (lung cancer/stroke/MI), newborn child, pregnant |
| Expectations | Was there a particular treatment that you were hoping for? |

## CSA TIPS

Patients who wish to quit smoking often attend their surgery quite excited and hopeful, wishing to 'turn over a new leaf.' It is important to enquire as to what the trigger or motivational factor in their decision to stop today i.e. having a newborn baby or a recent family death. This can be used to reinforce the need to stop and act as a reminder when their motivation may wane. All patients who smoke should be offered brief intervention to help them stop smoking and signpost them to the appropriate services. All patients who smoke should be given opportunistic advice about smoking cessation and if patients are able to, be advised to go cold-turkey.

## INVESTIGATIONS

| CO | Smoking cessation clinic often monitor CO levels per every session |
|---|---|

## MANAGEMENT

### Conservative

| Quit date | Fix an agreed date when they should completely stop smoking |
|---|---|
| Motivational | Offer quit smoking tips tailored to the patient |
| Financial | 1 packet of cigarettes cost approximately £7. Can save £2500 in 1yr |
| List | Make a list of reason why you want to quit smoking |
| Relatives | Inform relatives and friends that you wish to quit |
| Paraphernalia | Discard ashtrays, lighters, pipes and cigarettes boxes |
| Avoid situations | Avoid events which could encourage you to smoke i.e. pubs, clubs, parties |
| Food | Quitting smoking can cause increased appetite. Try avoiding fatty or sugary foods i.e. snacks and eat fruit instead |
| Withdrawal sympts | Can cause nausea, headaches, anxiety, irritability, craving, insomnia. Symptoms caused by lack of nicotine in blood. Worse on first day but reduce after 2-4 weeks |
| Relaxation | Consider practicing relaxation techniques - deep-breathing exercises |
| Reduce cravings | Chewing on sugarless gum or carrots, celery. Drinking water |

---

### Benefits of Quitting Smoking

Stopping smoking at any stage of life provides immediate as well as long term health benefits.

| Financial | Cigarettes are heavily taxed and are expensive. By quitting one will have more disposable income to spend |
|---|---|
| Skin | One month post quitting, physical appearance will improve. Wrinkles may fade and the facial grey colour will be replaced as circulation improves |
| Respiratory | After 3mths, breathing should improve and coughing and wheeze should subside. Lung cancer risk falls by 50% 10yrs post quitting |
| Cardiac | 1 year post cessation reduces risk of MI by 50% |

---

### Medical

| Medication | Enquire and offer medication to help stop smoking if appropriate. Do not combine different agents together. If medication is unsuccessful, do not offer repeat prescription within 6mth |
|---|---|
| NRT | Different forms available (gum, inhalator, lozenge, nasal spray, patch). Types can be combined. Increases chances of quitting by 70%. Start higher doses in dependent patients and taper down 2wks before end date (except gum – can stop instantly) |

| | |
|---|---|
| Side effects | Nausea & vomiting, flushing headaches, flu-like symptoms |
| CI | CVA / TIA or MI in last 6mths, arrhythmias |

## Different NRT preparations

Patients should be started with NRTs. Most patients use combination i.e. patches and nasal spray or patches and gum to try to closely mimic the regularity of their cigarette smoking

| | |
|---|---|
| Gum | Two strengths – 2mg/4mg. Chew gum slowly until flavour is strong. Place between cheek and teeth to increase absorption |
| Lozengers | Placed and sucked under the tongue, not swallowed |
| Inhalators | Shaped as a cigarette. Useful if patient accustomed to holding onto a cigarette. Caution in chronic throat diseases, asthma |
| Patches | Daytime (16hrs) / whole day (24hrs) patches available. Discrete. Does not replicate 'highs' of cigarettes. Avoid in skin disorders. High dose patches for those who smoke >10 day and low dose for those <10 day |
| Nasal spray | Rapidly absorbed mimicking the highs of cigarettes. Useful when wanting to suppress strong urges or cravings |

| | |
|---|---|
| Bupropion (Zyban) | Start 150mg od for 6d then 150mg bd for 7-9wks. Doubles the chance of quitting. Initiate medication 1-2wks prior to quit date. If no response after 8wks stop medication |
| Side effects | Dry mouth, insomnia, GI symptoms, anxiety |
| CI | Pregnancy, breastfeeding, epilepsy/seizures, bipolar disorders, eating disorders, MAOI |
| Varenicline (Champix) | Start one week before quit date. Take 0.5mg od for 3d, 0.5mg bd for 4d, 1mg bd for 11wks. Cessation rates more than double |
| Side effects | N&V, headaches, insomnia, stop medication if develops anxiety, depression, suicidal ideation |
| CI | Pregnancy, breastfeeding, psychiatric disorders (depression/suicide) |

## SAFETY NETTING

| | |
|---|---|
| Review | Should attend weekly for monitoring of CO levels |
| Admission | If the patient feels suicidal, low mood or anxious whilst on champix advised them to stop immediately and seek medical advice |
| Refer | Consider referral to a local NHS Stop smoking service |

## EXPLANATIONS

| | |
|---|---|
| NRT | Nicotine replacement therapy is the pills and medicines we use to help people stop smoking. Nicotine is the addictive part of cigarettes, and if we replace it with gums, tablets or an inhaler, we can prevent the other harms that cigarette smoking causes. Gradually over time, we will wean you off and hopefully this will reduce any unpleasant withdrawal symptoms. |
| Zyban | This is a medicine that was first made to help people who had low mood and depression. It was found to also reduce the cravings that smokers get from nicotine. It works by altering the level of chemicals in the brain (neurotransmitters) which helps reduce any withdrawal symptoms people get when trying to stop. |
| Champix | This is a tablet that helps people stop smoking. It works by partially copying the effects nicotine has in the brain so that when you stop smoking, the withdrawal symptoms are reduced. It also reduces the cravings that smoking causes in people. |

# 4.1 Abdominal pain

Abdominal pain is a common complaint in general practice. Its aetiology may be caused by a number of different organs within the abdominal cavity as well as from surrounding structures that may refer in to it such as from the chest, pelvis or loin. You should always attempt to exclude an acute abdomen that may be a surgical emergency as soon as possible. Also consider the patient's age, gender and lifestyle when drawing up a list of differentials.

## HISTORY

| | |
|---|---|
| **Open questions** | Tell me more about the tummy pain that you have experienced? |

## Focused questions

| | |
|---|---|
| *Abdominal pain* | Where exactly is the pain? Can you point to it? When did you first notice it? How long does it last for? |
| Radiation | Does the pain move anywhere, such as to your shoulder, back or groin? |
| Severity | How severe is the pain on a scale of 1 to 10, ten being the most severe? |
| Character | How would you describe it (sharp, dull, burning sensation, cramp)? Does it come and go (colicky) or is it there all the time? |
| Trigger | Does anything makes it better or worse? |
| Better | Gaviscon, fatty food, leaning forwards, defecation, lying still |
| Worse | Spicy or fatty foods, alcohol, lying flat |

## Associated history

| | |
|---|---|
| *Nausea & vomiting* | Do you feel sick or have you vomited? |
| *Fever* | Did you feel hot and sweaty or run a fever? |
| *Appetite* | How has your appetite been? Are you eating more or less than normal? |
| *Bowels* | How are your bowels? Do you suffer with hard stools or diarrhoea? |

## Differentials

| | |
|---|---|
| *Peptic Ulcer* | Is the pain related to meals? Does drinking milk make it better? Do you find spicy foods make it worse? Have you noticed any black tarry stools? Have you vomited up any blood? |
| *Pancreatitis* | Does the pain move to your back? Is it made worse by drinking alcohol or better if you lean forwards? |
| *Gastroenteritis* | Have you eaten out recently? Any diarrhoea or vomiting? Do you get cramping abdominal pains? Have you been abroad? |
| *Gallstones* | Is the pain in the right upper part of the tummy? Does it go to your shoulder? Is it made worse after fatty foods? |
| *Appendicitis* | Has the pain shifted from the middle of your tummy to the lower right side? Is it worse on walking or moving? Any fevers or diarrhoea? |
| *Diverticulitis* | Do you have any cramping pain on the lower left side of your tummy? Do you feel bloated? Do you have any fevers or blood in your stools? Do you have constipation or diarrhoea? |
| *Intest. obstruction* | Have you opened your bowel recently or passed any wind? |
| *Renal Colic* | Have you experienced a dull ache? Does it go to your groin from your back? How bad is the pain? |
| *Ectopic* | Have you missed your period recently? Any pv bleeding? |

**RED FLAGS**

| | |
|---|---|
| *Ectopic* | Pain with PV bleeding and missed period |
| *Intest. obstruction* | Severe colicky pain with no bowel movements or flatus |
| *Upper GI bleed* | Dizziness, melaena, haematemesis |
| *Ruptured AAA* | Tearing central abdominal pain radiating to the back |
| *Peritonitis* | Sharp, constant pain worsened with movement |

**PAST HISTORY**

| | |
|---|---|
| *Previous* | Have you ever experienced these symptoms before? |
| *Medical* | Do you suffer from any medical illnesses (IBD, gallstones, depression)? |
| *Surgery* | Have you had any recent surgery (adhesions)? |

**DRUG HISTORY**

| | |
|---|---|
| *Medication* | Are you taking any medications? |
| GU/PU | Aspirin, steroids, bisphosphonates, ferrous sulphate, erythromycin, NSAIDs |

**SOCIAL HISTORY**

| | |
|---|---|
| *Smoker* | Do you smoke? How many cigarettes do you smoke per day? |
| *Alcohol* | Do you drink alcohol? How much do you drink and how often? |
| *Occupation* | Are you working at the moment? What do you work as? |
| *Stress* | Have you felt particularly stressed recently? |
| *Travel* | Have you been abroad recently? |

**FAMILY HISTORY**

| | |
|---|---|
| *Medical* | Are there any illnesses that run in your family? (IBD, bowel cancer, HNPCC) |

**IDEA, CONCERNS, EXPECTATIONS**

| | |
|---|---|
| *Idea* | What did you think was causing your abdominal pain? |
| *Concerns* | Do you have any worries about the pain you have been experiencing (bowel cancer)? |
| *Expectations* | What were hoping we could do for you today? Were you hoping for a particular treatment or investigation? |
| *Impact* | How have the symptoms affected your life? |

**CSA TIPS**

Patients presenting with abdominal pain may have very vague and non-specific symptoms. However, it is important that a sound, focussed history is performed to narrow down your list of differentials. This may be aided by examining the patient and not forgetting to request to perform a pelvic examination in all females. It may be that the patient has already had an investigation such as an ultrasound or blood test and you will be required to reconfirm the history before offering an explanation of the results.

**PHYSICAL EXAMINATION**

| | |
|---|---|
| *Vitals* | BP (hypotension), pulse (tachycardia), temperature |
| *General* | Inspect for anaemia and jaundice in the eyes. Look at general appearance, is the patient silent, pale and still? |
| *Abdomen* | |
| Inspection | Inspect for swollen abdomen or peristalsis |
| Palpation | Palpate quadrants for pain. Examine for constipation, organomegaly (liver/spleen), pulsatile mass (AAA). Percuss for ascites if present |
| Auscultation | Listen for bowel sounds (tinkling, reduced, absent) |

| PR | Perform if evidence of PR bleeding or melaena |
|---|---|
| *Pelvic exam* | Consider in females pelvic masses, cervical excitation, adnexal pain |

## INVESTIGATIONS

| | |
|---|---|
| *Bloods* | FBC (anaemia), U&E, LFTs, ESR (IBD), fasting glucose (DKA), CRP |
| Other | Amylase (pancreatitis), CEA (bowel cancer), CA125 (ovarian cancer) |
| *Urine* | Leucocytes, nitrates (UTI), blood (renal stones, infection), pregnancy test |
| *Stool* | FOB, H. pylori (peptic ulcer), C&S |
| *HVS* | PID |
| *AXR* | Renal stones, constipation, intestinal obstruction |
| *US* | Gallstones, renal stones, hepatitis, appendicitis |
| *Other (specialist)* | Barium meal/enema, CT abdo, ERCP, endoscopy (OGD, colon-, sigmoidoscopy) |

## MANAGEMENT   *treat underlying cause*
### Gastric/peptic ulcer

| | |
|---|---|
| *Conservative* | Avoid chilli and spicy food. Cut down on caffeine and alcohol. Stop smoking and avoid NSAIDs. Eat small, regular meals and ensure that the last meal is several hours before bedtime |
| *Medical* | Alginates – Gaviscon, Ranitidine, PPI – Omeprazole |
| H. pylori | Initiate triple therapy i.e. 7d ppi, amoxicillin 1g, clarithromycin 500mg bd |

### Gallstones

| | |
|---|---|
| *Conservative* | Lose weight, exercise and adhere to low fat diet. Stop smoking |
| *Medical* | Asymptomatic gallstones do not need removal |

### Acute Cholecystitis
Admit patient for IV abx. Offer analgesia if painful. Refer routinely for cholecystectomy, lithotripsy or ursodeoxycholic acid

### Gastroenteritis

| | |
|---|---|
| *Conservative* | Oral rehydration salts, fluids. Eat lighter foods but more regularly. Avoid fruit juice or fizzy drinks. Wash hands with soap and water. Dry well |
| *Medical* | Antidiarrhoeals (loperamide) are not usually recommended but may help reduce frequency of bowel motions. Antibiotics if only confirmed bacterial infection |

### Constipation
Increase fluids. Regular exercise, more fibre (cereals), less red meat, 5 fruit & veg. See constipation chapter

### Renal stones
Increase fluids, reduce salt intake, reduce dairy products (calcium), animal protein (amino acid), grape juice, apple juice. See renal stones chapter

### Pancreatitis   Treat cause by removing gallstones

| | |
|---|---|
| *Conservative* | Avoid alcohol, high protein, low fat diet. High calorie diet. Refer dietician |
| Acute | Admission for IV fluids, analgesia and nutrition |
| Chronic | Stop smoking and alcohol. Eat a low-fat diet and offer analgesia if pain |
| Creons | Prescribe to help digestion if steatorrhoea |
| Operations | Refer to specialist to consider pancreatectomy |

### Diverticular disease

| | |
|---|---|
| *Conservative* | High fibre diet and fluid intake |
| *Medical* | Admission for IV fluids, analgesia and antibiotics. Consider paracetamol for pain relief and mesalazine (specialist) |

### Safety netting

| | |
|---|---|
| *Follow up* | Seek medical advice if any red flag symptoms |
| *Admission* | If abdominal pain worsens or patient experiences projectile vomiting, absolute constipation or pain on minimal movement (peritonitis), patient should be admitted into hospital |

## DIFFERENTIAL DIAGNOSIS

| Condition | Characteristic exam feature |
|---|---|
| **Appendicitis** | Diffuse central abdominal colic, shifting to the right iliac fossa. Worsened by movement, touch and coughing. Associated with anorexia, nausea and vomiting and occasionally diarrhoea. OE: Low grade fever, tachycardia, tender RIF (McBurney's point), Rovsing's sign (pain in RIF when LIF palpated) |
| **Pancreatitis** | Commonly caused by alcohol or gallstones. Severe epigastric pain radiating to the back or chest. Constant pain for hours, worsened by drinking alcohol or eating a meal. Bending forward provides temporary relief. Severe pancreatitis can have fever, jaundice, a rapid pulse and feel nauseous and vomit. OE: Jaundice, fever, epigastric pain with rigidity, Cullen's (umbilical bruising) and Grey Turney's (flank bruising) signs |
| **Biliary colic** | Right upper quadrant pain radiating to back and interscapular area. Often worse at night. Associated with nausea especially after eating a meal. The pain may be constant but is classically colicky and often presents with obstructive jaundice (pale stools dark urine). Consider risk factors (female, fat, 40s, fair, fertile) |
| **Renal colic** | Sudden onset of a dull ache that is colicky in nature with the passing of blood in urine and often may be severe enough to cause nausea and vomiting. Pain can originate from flank or loin area and radiate to groin |
| **Acute cholecystitis** | Same as above but with local peritonism, fever and vomiting may indicate biliary tract infection (acute or chronic cholecystitis). Raised inflammatory markers (wcc, crp). OE: fever, jaundice, RUQ pain. Murphy's sign positive (patients stops inspiration when 2 fingers on RUQ as patient breaths in, absent on LUQ) |
| **Diverticulitis** | Inflammation of the diverticula causing abdominal pain, bloating and cramps. The most common symptom is tenderness around the left side of the lower abdomen along with fever, nausea, vomiting and constipation |
| **Intestinal obstruction** | History of adhesions (previous surgery), malignancy. Colicky pain, distension, absolute constipation including wind. Bowels not opened. 'Tinkling' bowel sounds |

**EXPLANATIONS**

*Gallstones*          These are small stones usually made out of fat (cholesterol) that are made in the gallbladder in the right upper part of your tummy. Normally, they do not cause any problems, however, sometimes they may get stuck in a tube inside the gallbladder and give rise to the colicky pain that you have. They usually form because of high fat levels in the blood and may be made worse after eating a fatty meal.

*Pancreatitis*        The pancreas is an organ (gland) in the body that helps make proteins (enzymes) that break down and digest food. Sometimes it can become inflamed because of a gallstone, or because of alcohol and as a result it gives rise to central tummy pain and vomiting.

*Diverticulitis*       In the large intestine, over time, small outpouchings or weaknesses in the wall develop called diverticula. They sometimes happen as we get older, but can be because of hard stools or lack of fibre intake. Occasionally, they get inflamed and swollen giving rise to pain, bloating and a temperature.

*Appendicitis*        This is swelling and inflammation of an outgrowth of the large bowel called the appendix. Everyone has an appendix and sometimes it may become blocked because of faecal matter. When it gets blocked, it initially gives rise to pain in the middle of your tummy that comes and goes. After a while the pain becomes more continuous and moves to the lower right side of your tummy.

*Bowel obstruction*   This is where the bowel (large or small) becomes blocked, preventing fluid or food from passing through. As a result you may suffer from pain, vomiting and swelling of the tummy. It can be caused because of previous surgery leaving scar tissue that affects a section of the bowel.

Dyspepsia, as defined by the Rome III criteria refers to persistent or recurrent pain or discomfort centred in the upper abdomen. It is often associated with abdominal fullness, bloating, nausea, belching, and a feeling of satiety. It is an extremely common symptom with 20% of people suffering from it at some point in their lives. Heartburn is often confused with dyspepsia, however, it is synonymous with acid reflux (GORD). Causes of dyspepsia include GORD, peptic ulcer disease, gastritis, non-functional dyspepsia, stomach cancer and oesophagitis.

**HISTORY**

| | |
|---|---|
| **Open questions** | Please tell me more about the symptoms you have experienced? |

**Focused questions**

| | |
|---|---|
| *Dyspepsia* | Have you had any tummy pain, feeling sick or bloatedness recently? When did you first notice it? How long does it last for? |
| Site | Where abouts do you feel the discomfort? |
| Character | How would you describe it? Is it a bloated, crampy or burning feeling? Does it come and go (colicky) or is it there all the time? |
| Triggers | Does anything make your symptoms better or worse? |
| Better | Gaviscon, food, milk |
| Worse | Spicy or fatty foods, alcohol, coffee, citrus fruits |

**Associated history**

| | |
|---|---|
| *Nausea & vomiting* | Do you feel sick or have you vomited? |
| *Belching* | Do you find that you belch or burp a lot? |
| *Cough* | Do you suffer from a persistent cough? |

**Differentials**

| | |
|---|---|
| *GORD* | Is the pain a burning feeling? Does it go to your throat? Do you ever get an acidic taste (acid brash) or excessive saliva (water brash) in your mouth? Is it worse at night? |
| *Peptic ulcer* | Does the pain go to your back? Is it related to meals? Does drinking milk make it better? Do you find spicy foods make it worse? |
| *Stomach cancer* | Have you lost your appetite or any weight recently? Are you vomiting blood (haematemesis) or noticed black stools (melaena)? Any difficulty swallowing? |
| *Biliary* | Is the pain in the right upper area of the tummy? Does it go to your shoulder? Is it made worse after fatty foods? Have you had a fever? |
| *Cardiac* | Do you feel a pressure on your chest? Does the symptoms go to your left arm? Does it come on rest or exercise? |

| | |
|---|---|
| **RED FLAGS** | Progressive dysphagia, persistent vomiting, unexplained iron deficiency anaemia, unintentional weight loss, upper abdominal mass, aged 55 with persistent unexplained dyspepsia |

**PAST MEDICAL HISTORY**

| | |
|---|---|
| *Previous* | Have you had any medical problems in the past (GORD, IBS)? Have you been told you have had a stomach infection (H.pylori)? |
| *Investigations* | Have you had any investigations such as camera tests (OGD) or stool tests? |

## DRUG HISTORY

| | |
|---|---|
| *Medication* | Are you taking any medications (NSAIDS, aspirin, bisphosphonates, calcium antagonists, nitrates, steroids)? |

## SOCIAL HISTORY

| | |
|---|---|
| *Smoker* | Do you smoke? How many cigarettes do you smoke per day? |
| *Alcohol* | Do you drink alcohol? How much do you drink and how often? |
| *Occupation* | Are you working at the moment? What do you work as? |
| *Stress* | Have you felt particularly stressed recently? |
| *Diet* | Tell me about your diet. What types of foods do you eat? Do you drink coffee, tea, energy or fizzy drinks? |

## FAMILY HISTORY

| | |
|---|---|
| *Medical* | Are there any illnesses that run in your family (peptic ulcer, stomach cancer)? |

## IDEA, CONCERNS, EXPECTATIONS

| | |
|---|---|
| *Idea* | Do you have any ideas as to what was causing your symptoms? |
| *Concerns* | Is there anything that is particularly worrying you about your symptoms? |
| *Expectations* | What were hoping we could do for you today (OGD)? |
| *Impact* | How have the symptoms affected your life? |

## CSA TIPS

Dyspepsia is a fairly common symptom and should be taken more seriously as a patient ages. Often cases will be about managing the patient's anxieties and worries against a particular treatment or investigation according to guidelines such as SIGN and NICE. Patients may be overtly worried about cancer and may attend to discuss their risks and be keen to be referred to the specialist to exclude this diagnosis. After excluding red flags and other serious causes of dyspepsia, an attempt should be made to reassure the patient and check and improve their understand of their condition.

Other cases may simply revolve around the patient's reflux symptoms with poor dietary, social habits and stressors directly contributing to their symptoms. A suitable outcome in such scenarios would be to discuss with the patient alternative treatment options, diet and offer lifestyle advice whilst appropriately safely netting the patient.

## PHYSICAL EXAMINATION

| | |
|---|---|
| *Vitals* | Weight, BMI, pulse |
| *Abdomen* | |
|    Inspection | Inspect the conjunctiva for signs of anaemia |
|    Palpitation | Palpate the 4 quadrants for any pain or masses particularly over the epigastric area. Palpate the left supraclavicular area for Virchow's nodes (stomach cancer) |
|    Auscultation | Listen for bowel sounds |
|    PR | Check for melaena (if evidence of PR bleeding/black stools) |

## INVESTIGATIONS

| | |
|---|---|
| *Bloods* | FBC, ferritin (fe def. anaemia), U&E (protein meal) |
| Other | Anti-tissue transglutaminase antibodies (tTGA – coeliac screen), CA125 (ovarian cancer) |
| *Stool* | H. pylori stool antigen test, (or C13 urea breath test) |

---

### H. Pylori testing

Ensure prior to testing for H.pylori (Stool/breath test) that the patient has stopped taking a PPI for 2wks or antibiotics within 4wks. H.pylori can be confirmed via stool, breath or serology testing; however stool testing is the most preferred in the GP setting. For confirmation of eradication, urea breath test is more sensitive.

---

| | |
|---|---|
| *CXR* | Barium swallow (hiatus hernia) |
| *Other (specialist)* | Barium meal, CT abdo (cancer), OGD |

## MANAGEMENT
### Conservative

| | |
|---|---|
| *Position* | Raise the head of the bed or sleep on more pillows |
| *Diet* | Eat smaller regular meals and make sure that your last meal is several hours before you go to bed. Tailor advice to the patient |
| *Diary* | Keep a food diary about what you eat and when you eat it. See if there is any link between what you eat and your symptoms |

---

### Foods and Drinks to avoid in dyspepsia

| | |
|---|---|
| *Foods* | Fatty or fried foods (chicken, pizza, burgers, chips), spicy or chilli foods, garlic, onions, tomato sauce, acid fruits (lemon, lime, orange), chocolate |
| *Drinks* | Tea, coffee, orange juice, grape juice |

---

| | |
|---|---|
| *Smoking* | Stop smoking and offer smoking cessation advice. Refer to smoking clinic |
| *Alcohol* | Reduce intake to < 21 units /wk for men, < 14 units/wk for women |
| *Exercise* | Reduce weight; can recommend exercise programmes |
| *Stress* | Relaxation or breathing techniques, speak to friends, counsellor, CBT |

### Medical

| | |
|---|---|
| *Antacids* | Offer antacids (gaviscon, magnesium trisilicate) |
| *PPI* | Give 1-2 months of PPI (lansoprazole 15mg od) |
| *Ranitidine* | Give H2 antagonist if no response to PPI (ranitidine 150mg bd) for 1 mth |
| *Prokinetic* | Add prokinetic drug – domperidone 10mg tds |
| *Treat H.pylori inf.* | Treat with either PAC500 or PMC250 regimen if penicillin allergic |

---

### Treating H. Pylori infection

| Regimen | Cost | Regimen (for 1 week) |
|---|---|---|
| PAC500 | £36 | PPI (omeprazole 20mg bd), amoxicillin 1gm bd, clarithromycin 500mg bd |
| PMC250 | £25 | PPI (omeprazole 20mg bd), metronidazole 400mg bd, clarithromycin 250mg bd |

---

| | |
|---|---|
| *Refer* | Refer urgently to speciality if there is evidence of chronic GI bleeding; progressive unintentional weight loss; progressive difficulty swallowing; persistent vomiting; iron def. anaemia; epigastric mass or suspicious barium meal |

**SAFETY NETTING**

*Admission*                    If haematemesis or melaena admit into hospital

**EXPLANATIONS**

*GORD*                         When you eat, food passes down your food pipe and into the stomach. There the stomach produces acid that helps breakdown the food into smaller bits that can easily be absorbed. It is believed that acid reflux is caused when a valve or muscle called the lower oesophageal sphincter does not close properly. As a result, some of the stomach's acid and contents leaks back into your food pipe causing acid reflux. This can give you the burning feeling that starts from your stomach and moves up to your throat.

*Treatment*                    Gaviscon works by creating a foam layer that floats on top of the stomach contents reducing the risk of acid leaking back into the food pipe. Proton pump inhibitors (lansoprazole) as well as ranitidine work by reducing the amount of acid produced by the lining of the stomach in the first place thereby reducing your symptoms.

*H. Pylori*                    Helicobacter Pylori is a bug that can be found in the stomach that has been linked with stomach problems such as gastritis, ulcer and stomach cancers. In a lot of people, treating you with a short course of antibiotics may remove the bug and treat your symptoms.

*Endoscopy*                    The upper endoscopy test is a procedure that allows the doctor to look directly at the lining of the food pipe (oesophagus), the stomach and the first part of the bowel (intestine). The endoscope is a long thin flexible tube with a bright light on its tip. The doctor may take a small sample of tissue (biopsy) and look at it under the microscope.

*Barium Swallow*               Barium is a safe, white liquid that shows up clearly in an X-ray. It is used to show up the lower part of the food pipe, stomach and upper gut that are usually difficult to see on a plain film X-ray.

Obesity is rapidly becoming a worldwide pandemic problem. It is classified when a patient has a Body Mass Index (BMI) of greater than 30. It increases the relative risk of a whole range of different conditions including type 2 DM, IHD, gallbladder disease, BP, OA, sleep apnoea, cancer (breast, endometrial, colon), PCOS and back pain amongst others. Over 50% of people are considered to be overweight or obese in the UK and require remedial advice or exercise interventions to buck this trend.

---

**Classification of Obesity -** *Ref: NICE- Obesity guidelines 2010 & WHO 2011*

| BMI | Classification |
|---|---|
| 18.5–24.9 | Healthy weight |
| 25–29.9 | Overweight |
| 30–34.9 | Obesity I |
| 35–39.9 | Obesity II |
| >40 | Obesity III |

---

**HISTORY**

**Open questions**  Can you tell me why do you want to lose weight? Has anything happened recently that made you want to lose weight now? Why do you think that your weight has gone up?

**Focused questions**

*Diet*  What types of foods do you eat? Talk me through a typical day?

  Types of food  How many times do you eat a day? Do you eat fatty foods (chicken, pizza, burgers) or sugary foods (snacks, fizzy drinks)? Do you eat snacks (crisps, biscuits, nuts) just before bedtime?

*Exercise*  How much exercise do you do in a week? Do you do any intense exercise (football, swimming, cycling, jogging)? How long do you spend doing this?

*Prev. attempts*  Have you tried losing weight before? What happened? Have you tried any diet plans or weight loss programmes (weightwatchers, slimfast)?

**Associated history**

*Other*  Do you have any breathing problems (asthma), joint pains (OA), difficulty breathing at night (sleep apnoea) or chest pain (IHD)?

**Differentials**

*Hypothyroidism*  Do you feel tired and cold all the time? Do you have dry skin or hair loss?

*PCOS*  Any problems with your periods? Do you have acne?

**PAST HISTORY**

*IHD*  Do you suffer from high blood pressure, diabetes, strokes or high cholesterol?

*Others*  Do you suffer from arthritis, asthma or sleep apnoea?

**DRUG HISTORY**

*Medication*  Are you taking any medications (steroids, COCP, antipsychotics, pizotifen, sulphonylurea, insulin, COCP, HRT, TCAs, sodium valproate, gabapentin)?

## Causes of Obesity

Diet (fatty, excessive), sedentary lifestyle, genetic, endocrine (hypothyroidism, Cushing's, PCOS), binge eating, smoking cessation, medication (as above)

## SOCIAL HISTORY

| | |
|---|---|
| *Smoker* | Do you smoke? How many cigarettes do you smoke per day? |
| *Alcohol* | Do you drink alcohol? How much do you drink and how often? |
| *Occupation* | Are you working at the moment? Does it involve any physical work? |

## FAMILY HISTORY

| | |
|---|---|
| *Medical* | Are there any illnesses that run in your family? (obesity, IHD, DM)? |

## IDEA, CONCERNS, EXPECTATIONS

| | |
|---|---|
| *Idea* | How do you feel about your weight? |
| *Concerns* | Are you particularly worried about your weight? (low mood, self esteem, stress, organic cause) |
| *Expectation* | Was there anything specific you wanted me to do today? (refer dietician, initiate medication, surgery) |
| *Impact* | How have the symptoms affected your life? |

## CSA TIPS

It is often tempting to run through a detailed management plan with the patient when they attend requesting to lose weight. However, some people may forget to take a thorough history of the patient's lifestyle habits including diet and exercise as well as their beliefs and attitudes towards obesity. Patients may attend requesting a script for orlistat that can 'magically make them lose weight' because of anecdotal advice from a friend or ask to be referred for surgery or gastric banding. However, both options have strict guidelines to adhere to and require a detailed explanation and counselling before being undertaken. It should be reinforced that these are not instant cures to a problem and are usually considered as adjuncts to long term exercise and lifestyle modifications.

## PHYSICAL EXAMINATION

| | |
|---|---|
| *Vitals* | Height, weight, BMI, weight circumference, BP |

## Waist circumference

A more sensitive marker of health risks caused by being overweight is to measure the patient's waist circumference. Waist circumference is checked halfway between the ASIS and rib cage.

| Waist Circumference | Inc. Risk | High Risk |
|---|---|---|
| Male (non-Asian) | 94-102cm (37"-39") | ≥102cm (40") |
| Men (Asian) | ≥90cm (35") | |
| Women (not Asian) | 80-90cm (32"-34") | ≥88cm (35") |
| Women (Asian) | ≥80cm (32") | |

*Ref: WHO, Waist circumference & waist–hip ratio: report of a WHO expert consultation, 2011*

## INVESTIGATIONS

| | |
|---|---|
| *Bloods* | U&Es, LFT, fasting lipids & glucose |
| Others | FSH & LH (PCOS), TFT, cortisol (Cushing's) |
| *Urine* | Glucose, protein |

## MANAGEMENT
### *Conservative*

| | |
|---|---|
| *Target* | Aim to lose 5-10% of their original weight at a rate of around 0.5-1kg/wk |
| *Diet* | Suggest to eat their food slowly. Chew each morsel of food 20x. Spread the food thinly over the plate and do not stack it up. Have small portions. Grill or steam rather than fry |

---

**Diet advice in Obesity** - *Ref: NICE (2010) Obesity*
- Eat five portions of fruit and vegetables each day, in place of foods higher in fat and calories
- Base meals on starchy foods (potatoes, bread, rice, pasta), choose whole-grain if possible
- Eat fibre-rich foods (oats, beans, peas, lentils, fruit & veg, brown bread, brown rice, pasta)
- Eat a low-fat diet, avoid fried foods
- Avoid drinks and snacks high in fat and sugar, (takeaway and fast foods) consider water
- Eat breakfast, watch the portion size of meals and snacks, and how often you are eating

---

| | |
|---|---|
| *Alcohol* | Minimise the calories you get from drinking alcohol by cutting down |
| *Exercise* | 30min/d of exercise 5d/wk, enough to get slightly breathless or to increase the rate at which the heart pumps. Can be done over 10min bursts. Consider pedometer |
| Advice | If takes car to work, park the car a distance away and jog to work. Run up and down stairs for >15min twice a day. If uses the bus get off 1 stop before and walk briskly for the remaining distance |

---

**Exercise advice in Obesity** - *Ref: NICE, Obesity, 2010*
- Make enjoyable activities part of everyday life (walking, cycling, swimming, gym, gardening)
- Minimise sedentary activities (watching television, computer, video games)
- Build activity into the working day (take the stairs instead of the lift, take a walk at lunchtime)

---

| | |
|---|---|
| *Motivational* | Stress health benefits of losing weight and should be achieved over a period of time |
| *Support* | Suggest support groups such as Weight Watchers. Consider counselling therapies if obesity is affecting mood |

---

**Health Benefits of Weight loss** - *Ref: SIGN 2008, Management of Obesity*
- 10kg weight loss is associated with a reduction in systolic BP of 6 mmHg and diastolic BP of around 4.6 mmHg at 2 years and reduction in LDL of around 0.22mmol/L.
- 5 kg weight loss in DM is associated with a reduction in fasting blood glucose of between 0.17mmol/L to 0.24mmol/L at 12mths
- 5 kg weight loss in obese type 2 DM is linked with drop of HbA1c of 0.28% at 12mths

---

### *Medical*

| | |
|---|---|
| *Orlistat* | Offer orlistat as an adjunct to lifestyle advice. Sibutramine has been banned by NICE due the increased risk of CVA / MI |
| Initiate | Consider if patient has a >BMI of 28.0 kg/m2 with associated risk factors (HTN, DM, chol) or a BMI of >30.0 kg/m2 without risk factors |
| Target wt loss | Aim for 5% weight loss after 3mth before continuing. Tx for >12mth if pros and cons discussed with patient |

| | |
|---|---|
| How to take | Take 120mg tds before or with meals (30min before or up to 1hr after). If misses a meal or the meal lacks fat, omit dose. Can be taken with vitamin tablets (reduces absorption of fat soluble vitamins – K, A, D, E) |
| Side effects | Wind, diarrhoea, faecal urgency, faecal incontinence |
| CI | Malabsorption, breastfeeding, cholecystectomy |

## Surgical

| | |
|---|---|
| Surgery | Consider surgery (banding/gastric bypass) in patients with severe obesity i.e. BMI >40, >35 + risk factors, have attempted non-surgical measure for 6mth and failed. Patients receive intensive follow up with specialist team including dietician and counsellors. Patients must be physically fit for surgery. Often long waiting lists |

## Refer

| | |
|---|---|
| Exercise | Can refer patients to local exercise programme |
| Dietician | Refer to dietician for diet advice and support |

## SAFETY NETTING

| | |
|---|---|
| Follow up | Follow up and monitor weight initially fortnightly and then monthly. Consider referral to a nurse run obesity clinic |

## EXPLANATIONS

| | |
|---|---|
| BMI | BMI or Body Mass Index is a ratio that compares your weight against your height. The figure it gives allows us to compare your score against other people. A BMI of more than 25 is considered to be overweight. We would hope to aim for a BMI between 20 and 25 which is in the healthy range. |
| Obesity | A BMI over 30 is considered obese and is associated with health problems such as increased risk of death, heart attacks, breathing problems, diabetes and even some types of cancer. |
| Orlistat | This is a medicine that helps to reduce weight. It works by blocking the absorption of fat in the bowel and so foods containing fat are not taken into the body. However, if you were to eat fatty food then you may suffer from soft, watery motions that are oily. |
| Losing weight | Losing 10% of your weight reduces your blood pressure, sugar, and cholesterol levels significantly and prolongs life. Losing weight is achievable, but needs to be done over a long period of time rather than short-term to achieve the real benefits and improvements in your health. |

# *4.4 Diarrhoea*

Diarrhoea is the passing of loose stool motions. It is defined by the WHO as the passing of 3 or more loose motions per day or having an increased stool frequency for that person. In the UK, the most common cause is due to viral infections; however, persistent diarrhoea in the elderly should be taken seriously and could signify underlying bowel cancer.

Diarrhoea can be a debilitating and embarrassing condition, with patients often soiling their undergarments. It is important to enquire about the impact the patient's symptom is having on their social or work setting. Acute diarrhoea is the presence of symptoms less than 2 weeks duration and chronic is that lasting more than 4 weeks.

## HISTORY
**Open questions**     What do you mean by diarrhoea? (increased frequency or loose stool)

**Focused questions**

| | |
|---|---|
| *Diarrhoea* | When did it start? How long has it been going on for? |
| Frequency | How often are you opening your bowels? |
| Consistency | How are the bowel motions? Are they loose, watery or any mucus? |
| Pain | Have you experienced any pain? Is it cramping in nature? Where is it located? |
| Blood | Have you noticed any blood in your stool? |

**Associated history**

| | |
|---|---|
| *Nausea & vomiting* | Do you feel sick or have you vomited? |
| *Fever* | DId you feel hot and sweaty or run a fever? |
| *Contact* | Did you meet or were you in contact with anyone who had diarrhoea? |

**Differentials**

| | |
|---|---|
| *Food poison* | Have you eaten out recently? Did you eat any uncooked foods? Anyone else unwell? Have you vomited? |
| *Travel* | Did you travel abroad recently? Did you visit a farm? |
| *IBD* | Any mucus or blood in your stools? Any ulcers in the mouth? Have you had a fever or weight loss? Have you had any eye symptoms? |
| *IBS* | Any stress? Do you feel bloated? Is the pain better with bowel motions? |
| *Coeliac* | Are your stools difficult to flush away (steatorrhoea)? Is it related to certain foods (gluten)? Any weight loss? |
| *Cancer* | Any recent change in bowel habits (>50 yrs old)? Any weight loss? Have you lost appetite? Any blood in the stool? |
| *Pancreatitis* | Do you have problems flushing away your stools? Do you have upper tummy pain? Do you drink alcohol? |
| *Hyperthyroid* | Do you feel tired all the time? Do you always feel hot & sweaty? |
| *Appendicitis* | Was there pain that shifted from the middle of your tummy to the lower right side? Is it worse on walking or moving? |
| *Diverticulitis* | Do you have any cramping pain on the lower left side of your tummy? Do you feel bloated? Do you have any fevers or noted blood in your stools? |
| *Overflow* | Were you becoming more constipated before the diarrhoea started? Do you sometimes have no control over it? Do you soil your underwear? |

## Bacterial causes of Gastroenteritis

Below are features and the incubation periods of common bacterial causes of gastroenteritis. If found on stool MC&S testing, the local Health Protection Agency should be notified.

| Time to Symptoms | Organism & Symptoms |
|---|---|
| 1-6 hours | Staph. aureus presents acutely with severe symptoms and is due to undercooked meat (ham, chicken). Bacillus cereus usually contracted from rice consumption. Gives rise to nausea and vomiting before diarrhoea. |
| 12-48 hours | E. coli from undercooked beef, raw milk, contaminated water or recent travelled. Can present with watery stools and abdominal pains. Can cause Haemolytic Uraemic syndrome (HUS). Salmonella is from undercooked chicken or eggs and gives rise to fever, diarrhoea and abdominal cramps. |
| 48-72 hours | Shigella is found on contaminated vegetables or salads. It causes bloody diarrhoea, abdominal cramps and fever. Campylobacter arises from undercooked chicken or unpasteurised milk. Patients present with a flu-like prodrome and diarrhoea. Can cause Guillain-Barré syndrome. |
| >7 day | Giardiasis is a parasite that is found in water contaminated by sewage. It's most common feature is prolonged non-bloody diarrhoea. |

## PAST HISTORY

| | |
|---|---|
| Previous | Have you had any diarrhoea like this before? |
| Medical | Do you suffer from any medical illnesses? (thyroid, IBD, DM, bowel cancer - HNPCC) Have you had HIV in the past or diabetes? Where you admitted to hospital recently (C. diff)? |
| Surgical | Have you had any operations before? (bowel resection, colostomy bags, cholecystectomy) |

## DRUG HISTORY

| | |
|---|---|
| Medication | Are you taking any medications? |
| Improve | Oral rehydration salts (dioralyte), anti-diarrhoeal (loperamide) |
| Worsen | Antibiotics, laxatives (lactulose, senna), digoxin, antacids, cimetidine & PPI, thiazide diuretics, NSAIDs, chemotherapy, metformin, SSRIs |

## SOCIAL HISTORY

| | |
|---|---|
| Smoker | Do you smoke? How many cigarettes do you smoke per day? |
| Alcohol | Do you drink alcohol? How much do you drink and how often? |
| Travel | Any recent travel abroad? |
| Diet | Have you eaten any of the following foods in the past few days? (meat, seafood, eggs, dairy or had a recent picnic or barbecue) |
| Occupation | Are you working at the moment? Do you handle food or do you work in institutions such as hospitals, schools or care homes? |

## FAMILY HISTORY

| | |
|---|---|
| Medical | Are there any illnesses that run in your family? (thyroid, IBD) |

## IDEA, CONCERNS, EXPECTATIONS

| | |
|---|---|
| Idea | Do you have any ideas as to what was causing your diarrhoea? |
| Concerns | Is there anything that is particularly worrying you about it? |

| Expectation | Was there anything specific you wanted me to do today? |
| Impact | How have the symptoms affected your life? |

## CSA TIPS

Whilst many patients may be aware that a short bout of diarrhoea may be caused by gastroenteritis, the presence of chronic symptoms would alarm most of us. Notwithstanding the fact that patients will have to make numerous trips back and forth to the toilet, diarrhoea can be quite an embarrassing and debilitating condition. Patients may be really worried about symptom control such that they can continue in their jobs without drawing attention to themselves. Others may work in environments whereby there is physical contact with vulnerable children or adults. In such cases, any acute infective episodes of diarrhoea may easily be spread to others and appropriate advice about taking time off work should be given.

## PHYSICAL EXAMINATION

| *Vitals* | BP, weight, pulse, temperature |
| *Abdominal* | |
|     Inspection | Inspect for signs of dehydration, anaemia, jaundice |
|     Palpitation | Palpate the 4 quadrants for any pain (gastroenteritis, IBD, IBS, diverticulitis) or masses (colon cancer) |
|     Auscultation | Listen for bowel sounds |
|     PR | Check for fresh blood (if complaining of PR bleeding), rectal mass, impacted faeces (overflow diarrhoea) |
| | |
| *Thyroid* | Inspect outstretched hands (tremor), pulse (AF), thyroid gland (goitre) |

## INVESTIGATIONS

| *Bloods* | FBC, U&E, LFTs |
|     Others | TFTs, coeliac screen (tTGA antibodies – reintroduce gluten diet), ESR + CRP (IBD), B12, red blood cell folate and ferritin (malabsorption screen) |
| *Stool* | MC&S, ova, cysts, parasites, faecal occult blood (FOB), faecal calprotectin |
| *Specialist* | Colonoscopy, sigmoidoscopy + biopsy, jejunal biopsy (coeliac disease), barium enema, ERCP |

| **MANAGEMENT** | *treat underlying cause* |
| **Gastroenteritis** | |
| *Conservative* | |
|     Prevention | Wash your hands thoroughly with soap after going toilet, handling pets or doing gardening. Avoid sharing towels. Wash hands when handling raw meat or prior to eating. Ensure all meats are cooked to the correct temperature with a thermometer |
|     Reassure | Most will improve within 5 days. Occasionally can last up to 2 weeks |
|     Fluids/food | Drink plenty of fluids or oral rehydration salts (dioralyte). Normal diet but small, light meals. Avoid fizzy drinks and fatty, spicy foods |
|     School | Children should not go to school. Should not return until >48hrs after last episode of D&V. They should not swim for 2wks in swimming pool |
|     Work | Doctor, nurses and those working with food should avoid work for 48hrs |
| | |
| *Medical* | |
|     Anti-pyrexic | Take paracetamol or NSAIDS for temperature, body aches or headaches |
|     Anti-motility | Loperamide (avoid if <12yr) or racecadotril can be considered for up to 5d to reduce inconvenience of increase frequency |

| | |
|---|---|
| Antibiotics | If an organism is grown on culture treat with appropriate antibiotics |
| HPA | Inform the Health Protection Agency if you suspect food poisoning |

**Coeliac disease**

| | |
|---|---|
| *Conservative* | Suggest lifelong gluten free diet. Check labels on foods |
| Avoid | Wheat, bread, pastry. pasta, barley, beer, rye, oats (can be tolerated) |
| Gluten free | Rice, potatoes, corn (maize) |
| *Medical* | 1mth supply of gluten free foods (bread, flour, biscuits, pasta, pizza base) can be prescribed |
| **IBD** | Refer for diagnosis. Treat with mesalazine, steroids (oral, topical), azathioprine (2nd line), methotrexate, metronidazole (perianal disease) |

| | |
|---|---|
| **Hyperthyroidism** | Propranolol for symptomatic treatment. Refer for treatment. Consider carbimazole, radioactive iodine |

**Diverticulitis**

| | |
|---|---|
| *Conservative* | Encourage high fibre diet, fluids |
| *Medical* | Admission for IV fluids, analgesia and antibiotics. Consider paracetamol for pain relief and mesalazine (specialist) |

| | |
|---|---|
| **Overflow diarrhoea** | Manual disimpaction, laxatives (macrogol), suppositories (glycerin) or enema (docusate, arachis oil, sodium phosphate) |

| | |
|---|---|
| **Refer** | Refer to speciality if there are signs of red flag symptoms including, diarrhoea for more than 6 weeks in a 60 year old or in a 40 year old or persistent diarrhoea associated with rectal bleeding |
| *Continence clinic* | Refer the patient to nurse-led continence service if elderly and needs pads to prevent soiling |
| *OT* | Consider OT assessment if problems using the toilet for adaptations or the installation of a commode |

**SAFETY NETTING**

| | |
|---|---|
| *Admit* | If signs of severe dehydration |
| *Follow up* | If patients becomes dehydrated, cannot keep fluids down, has blood in vomit or diarrhoea, severe abdominal pain or high fever, seek medical advice |

**DIFFERENTIAL DIAGNOSIS**

| Condition | Characteristic exam feature |
|---|---|
| **Gastroenteritis** | Acute onset of diarrhoea nausea, vomiting, cramping abdominal pain. Diarrhoea often first symptom and abdominal pain often improves after passing motions |
| **Post-Antibiotics** | Any antibiotic (ciprofloxacin) but more so in broad spectrum antibiotics (co-amoxiclav). C.difficile produces offensive smelling diarrhoea particularly after using broad spectrum antibiotics |
| **Irritable bowel** | Extremely common. The most consistent features are abdominal pain relieved from |

| syndrome | defecation, urgency, incomplete evacuation, bloating and change in bowel habit. Symptoms often worse with eating. Patients may be divided into those with diarrhoea predominant IBS and those with constipation predominant IBS. Features such as lethargy, nausea, backache and bladder symptoms may also be present |
|---|---|
| Coeliac disease | Autoimmune, gluten sensitive enteropathy. Intolerance to gluten foods (wheat, barley rye). Presents with fatty diarrhoea (steatorrhoea), abdominal pain, weight loss, fatigue, unexplained iron-deficiency anaemia |
| Crohn's disease | Transmural chronic inflammatory disease, can affect any part of the GI tract from the mouth to the anus. Crampy abdominal pains and diarrhoea and less commonly blood diarrhoea. Other features include perianal tags, fissures and fistulae and with extra-intestinal symptoms such as arthritis, uveitis and erythema nodosum |
| Ulcerative colitis | Ulcerating disease affecting only the mucous membrane of the large bowel. Symptoms include abdominal pain, diarrhoea, rectal bleeding (> Crohn's), growth failure and weight loss. Also present with pyoderma gangrenosum, erythema nodosum, arthritis and spondylitis |
| Diverticulitis | Small outpouchings of the large bowel that become inflamed or infected. Symptoms include abdominal pain, bloating and cramps mainly in left iliac fossa with fever, nausea, vomiting and constipation. Frank blood mixed in with the stools is a complication |
| Colorectal cancer | Weight loss, PR bleeding (mixed with stools), abdominal or rectal mass (can be in right iliac fossa) or looser stools. Unexplained iron deficiency anaemia |
| Hyperthyroidism | Overactive thyroid gland. Presents with heat intolerance, tremor, sweating, irritability, heavy periods, palpitations |

**EXPLANATIONS**

*Gastroenteritis*  Gastroenteritis is an infection of the gut often called the 'stomach flu'. It is most commonly cause by a viral infection but can be spread from one person to another simply by touch. Sometimes it can be caused by a bacterial infection which usually occurs in cases of food poisoning.

*Coeliac disease*  This is a common condition where a person has a sensitivity to gluten. Gluten is a protein that is in a range of foods including primarily in wheat, barley and rye. When you eat food such as pasta, cereals or bread, the gluten is absorbed in the intestine (gut). The body mistakes the gluten to be an infection and attacks it using the immune system. Overtime this damages the lining of the small gut and affects its ability to absorb nutrients from food.

*IBD*  Inflammatory bowel disease describes two conditions, Crohn's disease and ulcerative colitis. It is a condition that results in swelling or inflammation of the lining of the gut. In Crohn's disease the inflammation can take place anywhere in your GI tract i.e. from your mouth to your anus. Whilst in ulcerative colitis, the swelling is limited to the large bowel / intestine.

*Irritable Bowel*    Irritable bowel syndrome is a common condition (20% of people) that affects your bowels. It affects how the bowel works without causing any lasting damage. We call this a functional disorder which means that the workings of the gut are affected, but not because of any damage or abnormality. It is often caused by an overactive bowel sometimes made worse by stress, certain foods and drinks. It gives rise to symptoms including, bloating, tummy pain and change in your bowel motions.

*Stool test*    Place some cling film loosely over the toilet bowl and hold it in place by the weight of the toilet seat. Once you catch the sample, scoop it into the container with the small spoon located in the lid. Once you are done please return the sample to the surgery.

International travel has become much more accessible to all and subsequently, record numbers of people are travelling to different worldwide destinations in recent years. Visiting foreign countries can put a person at risk for a number of illnesses including traveller's diarrhoea, malaria, TB, HIV, and rarer infections such as Typhoid, Dengue fever and Cholera. All patients planning to go abroad should speak to a health professional about need for immunizations and for advice pertaining to preventative measures that can reduce their risk of falling ill.

**HISTORY**

**Open questions**             Tell me more about your travel plans? What do you plan to do when you are there?

**Focused questions**

*Travel*              Where are you going (high risk of malaria)? Which areas in particular (high/low ground, swamp, jungle, urban/rural)?

   Duration              When are you leaving? How long are going for?

   Previous              Have you gone there before?

   Purpose              What is the purpose of your trip? (holiday, business, volunteer)

   Terrain              Is the place you are going to mountainous, woodland, rural or urban?

   Accomodation              WIll you be staying in a hotel, house, ship, campsite or hostel?

**Associated history**

*Immunisations*              Have you taken any travel vaccinations? If so, which ones and when?

*Contraception*              When you go abroad do you intend to engage in casual sex? Have you thought about using contraception?

**RED FLAGS**              Pregnant, young babies, long haul journey, endemic area for malaria/Dengue fever, HIV

**PAST HISTORY**

*Medical*              Do you suffer from any medical problems (DM, COPD, MI)?

*DVT, PE*              Do you suffer from blood clots in your legs or lungs?

---

**Flying and Medical Conditions -** *Ref: Adapted from UK Civil Aviation Authority's Aviation Health Unit (AHU)*

*CVD disease*              Uncomplicated MI may fly >7d, Complicated MI: >4-6 weeks, CABG >10-14 days. PCI: >5d, CVA after 10d

   CI flying              Unstable angina, uncontrolled HTN or arrhythmia, decompensated HF

*Others*              Pneumonia: can fly if treated with no residual infection. If COPD with pO2 <9.3 kPa at sea level then should consult airline and receive supplemental oxygen whilst travelling

   CI flying              Untreated pneumothorax, Hb <7.5, recent ear surgery, active ear effusion, acute psychosis. Patients with significant hypoxia (<6.7 kPa) or hypercapnia are advised not to fly

---

*Immunisations*              Are you up to date with all immunisations?

*Pregnant*              Are you pregnant? How many weeks?

*Children*              Do you have any infants less than 2wks old (advise not to fly)?

**Flying and Pregnancy** - *Ref: Adapted from UK Civil Aviation Authority's Aviation Health Unit (AHU)*

| | |
|---|---|
| *Normal* | Most airline companies will accept pregnant woman to fly up to 36wks but may require a certificate from their doctor after 28wks |
| *Multiple preg* | Twins or multiple pregnancies will be permitted to fly before 32wks |

## DRUG HISTORY

| | |
|---|---|
| *Medication* | Are you taking any medications? (insulin) |
| *Allergies* | Are you allergic to any medicines? (chloroquine) |

## SOCIAL HISTORY

| | |
|---|---|
| *Smoker* | Do you smoke? How many cigarettes do you smoke per day? |
| *Alcohol* | Do you drink alcohol? How much do you drink and how often? |

## IDEA, CONCERNS, EXPECTATIONS

| | |
|---|---|
| *Idea* | Have you read anything about precautions needed when travelling? |
| *Concerns* | Do you have any worries about your trip? (infectious disease, DVT) |

## CSA TIPS

Given that people travel so frequently, it is often easy to forget the potential dangers travellers can befall when abroad. It is an important skill in your health promotion repertoire, to be able to take a full travel history from a potential traveler. It is also important that you have the relevant knowledge to give up-to-date and appropriate preventative advice.

## PHYSICAL EXAMINATION *if returning from travels*

| | |
|---|---|
| *Vitals* | BP, weight, pulse, temperature |
| *General* | General appearance, skin rashes, enlarged LN |
| *Abdominal* | |
|    Inspection | Inspect for signs of dehydration, anaemia, jaundice |
|    Palpitation | Palpate the 4 quadrants for any pain or organomegaly (liver, spleen) |
|    PR | Check for fresh blood (if complaining of PR bleeding) |
| *Respiratory* | Auscultate chest for crepitations |

## INVESTIGATIONS

| | |
|---|---|
| *Bloods* | FBC, U&Es, LFTs, hepatitis screen, blood film, malaria screen |
|    Other | ESR, blood cultures, HIV |
| *Stool* | MCS and parasite |
| *Sputum* | MCS, ZN stain |
| *Xray* | CXR |
| *Swabs* | Chlamydia & gonorrhoea swabs or urine |

## MANAGEMENT
### Conservative

| | |
|---|---|
| *Water* | Drink bottled water or tap water if boiled or treated with sterilising tablets. Avoid ice added to drinks or unpasteurised milk. Sealed fruit cartons or bottled drinks usually safe. Avoid swimming (contaminated) |
| *Food* | Advise good food hygiene as can prevent hepatitis A, typhoid, cholera and diarrhoea (travellers). Avoid buffets and open table arrangements. Stay clear of uncooked meat, |

| | raw shellfish and food containing raw eggs or unpeeled fruit or veg. Ensure all foods are 'piping hot'. Avoid salads and unpasteurised dairy products |
|---|---|
| Sun | Avoid excessive sun exposure to prevent sun cancer/heat stroke. Use broad spectrum sunscreen (>=SPF 15, >= UVA 3). Avoid midday sun. Wear sun hats, full length clothing, sun glasses |
| Jet Lag | Ensure you get plenty of sleep before you travel. If you are travelling east, then for a few days before you fly, try awakening and sleeping a little earlier. If flying west, go to sleep and awake later. When landed, expose yourself to natural sunlight to help regulate the body clock |
| DVT | Advise risk of DVT. Drink plenty of non-alcoholic drinks, regularly walk around or do ankle exercises, consider compression support stockings whilst on the plane |

**Risk and Management of DVT & flying -** *Ref: Adapted from British Heart Foundation (Sept 2010)*

| | |
|---|---|
| Low risk | No PMHx or risk factors |
| Fluids | Drink plenty of non-alcoholic fluids. Avoid caffeine, sleeping tablets |
| Mobile | Do stretches every 30 min. Press the ball of the foot against the foot rest to increase blood flow to leg. Have breaks and walk up and down the aisle |
| Medium risk | PMHx DVT/PE, recent surgery, clotting disorders, pregnancy, or BMI>30 |
| Stockings | Offer compression stockings (graduated class 2). Consider aspirin |
| High risk | PMHx DVT + risk factors i.e. cancer, recent surgery |
| Advice | Offer LMWH before the flight and on next day |

| | |
|---|---|
| Contraception | Advise the need for contraception (condoms) to protect against HIV/STI |
| Insurance | Advise to take travel insurance in case of accidents or sudden illness |
| EHIC | Complete a European Health Insurance Card form for free or reduced costs health care in EEA & Switzerland |
| Home Office | Check Home Office foreign travel advice to see if the country is safe |
| Repeat medications | Up to 3mth repeat medication can be given under NHS. Longer is private |

**Facts about Venous Thromboembolism & flying**

- Evidence suggests increased risk of DVT with flights >4 hours duration
- Risk includes other long journeys such as coach journey, train or car i.e. immobility
- Patients with hip or knee replacement should not travel on long haul flights for up to 3mths
- Patients with a plaster cast should not fly for up to 1-2 days (depending on length of journey)
- Compression stockings can reduce the risk of DVTs (in moderate risk patients). LMWH should be reserved for high risk patients. No supportive evidence for aspirin
- If painful, swollen legs or SOB post flight they should seek urgent medical attention

***Immunisations***

| | |
|---|---|
| Free on NHS | Offer travel vaccinations if patient is travelling to an at risk area and is not immunised. DTP, Typhoid, Hepatitis A & Cholera are available on the NHS |
| Private | Patients will have to pay for other travel immunisations: Hepatitis B, Japanese encephalitis, BCG, Rabies, Yellow Fever, Meningitis ACWY (Hajj) |
| Certificate | GPs may charge for providing a Certificate of Vaccination or Prophylaxis (ICVP) that some countries require as proof (ACW, yellow fever) |

| **Traveller's diarrhoea** | Take paracetamol or NSAIDS for fever, body aches, headaches. Loperamide (avoid in <12yr) can be considered for up to 5d to reduce inconvenience of increase frequency. Stress fluid hydration |
|---|---|
| *Infection* | If an organism is grown on culture seek advice for treatment with appropriate antibiotics. Ciprofloxacin can be considered for most |

## Malaria

*Conservative*

| Nets & sprays | Impregnated mosquito nets (permethrin) provide effective protection against insects (DEET). Lotions, sprays, roll-on are safe and effective when applied to the skin (>2mths old, pregnant, breast feeding) |
|---|---|
| Clothes | Long sleeves and trousers worn at night also provide protection |
| *Medical* | Initiate prophylactic treatment based upon geographic destination and area of malaria resistance. Stress prophylaxis does not offer 100% protection and must be taken before travel and continued upon returning |

---

**Anti-malaria prophylaxis based upon Risk**

Consult the most up to date medical advice. The BNF usually has the latest advice about malaria drug resistance and the degree of risk pertaining to different geographical areas

| *V Low risk* | Chemoprophylaxis not recommended but avoid mosquito bites and consider malaria if fever presents |
|---|---|
| *Variable risk* | Chloroquine + proguanil hydrochloride or (if chloroquine + proguanil not appropriate), mefloquine or doxycycline or Malarone |
| *Substantial risk* | Mefloquine or doxycycline or Malarone |
| *V.risk + drug resistan.* | Doxycycline or Malarone |

---

| Not 100% | Stress prophylaxis does not offer 100% protection |
|---|---|

---

**Anti-Malaria Prophylaxis for short term travel**

Offer anti-malaria prophylaxis based on patient's choice (frequency), local malaria risk, side effects profile, information regarding date of travel as well as duration of use post return

| Medication | Freq | Start | Finish | Side effects |
|---|---|---|---|---|
| Chloroquine 310mg | wkly | 1wk | 4wks | Headache. CI epilepsy |
| Doxycycline 100mg | od | 1-2d | 4wks | Photosensitivity, oesophagitis |
| Proguanil 200mg | od | 1wk | 4wks | GI upset |
| Malarone | od | 1-2d | 7d | GI upset (Atovaquone + proguanil) |
| Mefloquine (Lariam) | wkly | 2.5wks | 4wks | Dizziness, CI epilepsy, neuropsych symptoms |

---

| *Pregnancy* | Offer medication considering side effects and contraindications |
|---|---|

---

**Anti-Malaria Prophylaxis in Pregnancy -** *Ref: Adapted from BNF 2014*

| *Chloroquine* | Safest in pregnancy – becoming resistant |
|---|---|
| *Proguanil* | Safest in pregnancy – becoming resistant. Start also prophylactic 5mg folic acid |
| *Doxycycline* | Contra-indicated during pregnancy |
| *Mefloquine* | Can be used (avoid in 1st trimester) |
| *Malarone* | Should be avoided but can be given if no suitable alternative is found |

---

---

**Prophylaxis for Long Term Travel -** *Ref: Guidelines for malaria prevention in travellers from the UK 2013*

| | |
|---|---|
| Chloroquine | Safe for long term use but check eyes after 6yrs of use |
| Proguanil | Safe for long term use – no duration |
| Doxycycline | Considered safe up to 2yrs of use |
| Mefloquine | Safe up to 3 years |
| Malarone | Licenced only for 28 days but can be used up to 1yr with caution |

---

### *Insulin Diabetics*

| | |
|---|---|
| General | Take more snacks on plane and regularly check sugar levels. Advise about the signs of hypoglycemia (fatigue, sweating, hunger, blurred vision) |
| Timezones | If travelling more than 5 time zones, east (shortens the day - lower dose needed) or west (lengthens the day - increased dose) may affect dose of insulin. Advise not to change their watches until landed and in accommodation to ensure timings of medications are the same |

### SAFETY NETTING

| | |
|---|---|
| Follow up | Review after returning from travel if any illnesses. Advise to seek medical advice if has bloody diarrhoea or signs of dehydration |
| Refer | Consider referral to the practice nurse for more in depth travel advice and immunisation. Refer to Yellow Fever centre |

### DIFFERENTIAL DIAGNOSIS

| Condition | Characteristic exam feature |
|---|---|
| **Malaria** | Spread by mosquito (falciparum most common). Prodromal symptoms of headache, malaria and myalgia. Presents with swinging fever, rigors, sweats lasting up to half a day at a time. Complications include cerebral malaria, coma, anaemia, pulmonary oedema |
| **Travellers diarrhoea** | Watery diarrhoea and abdominal pain from ingesting contaminated food or water whilst travelling. Common. Can last up to 3-5d but some persist up to 1 month |
| **Giardiasis** | Protozoan infection. Delayed presentations (2wks). Presents with foul smelling explosive diarrhoea (watery loose stools with flatus) with absence of fever. Associated with abdominal cramps |
| **Cholera** | Caused by *Vibrio cholerae* due to consumption of contaminated water. Rapid onset (<5hrs). Profuse watery diarrhoea with fever and vomiting. Dehydration common complication |
| **Typhoid** | Spread via contaminated water, presents within 3wks with fever, flu like symptoms with either diarrhoea or constipation. Also can present with epistaxis or bruising. Other features include relative bradycardia, rose-coloured spots on trunk, |

| | splenomegaly |
|---|---|
| **Dengue fever** | Common in tropics, rapid onset of high fever with retro-orbital headache. Can be associated with aching bone pain and maculopapular rash |
| **Hepatitis A** | Spread by contaminated water or shellfish. Prodromal symptoms include flu like symptoms for 2wks before having a fever, fatigue abdominal pain and jaundice |

**EXPLANATIONS**

*Malaria*

Malaria is an infectious disease that is spread by mosquito bites. The parasite travels through the blood within the red blood cells (the part of the blood that makes your blood red). Occasionally it can make these burst making you feel unwell and giving you a high swinging fever. Sometimes it can hide in the liver and give you symptoms much later on (3mths to a 1 yr).

*Traveller's diarrhoea*

This is diarrhoea that may develop during or just after travelling abroad where you may have drunk water or eaten food that was contaminated with gems. However, it often resolves within a few days after drinking plenty of fluids.

*Giardiasis*

This is an infection of the bowels caused by tiny parasites (Giardia lamblia) that often occurs after drinking contaminated water.

# 4.6 Irritable Bowel Syndrome (IBS)

IBS is a chronic (>6 months) relapsing and remitting bowel disorder that presents with gastrointestinal symptoms. It is a functional disorder with no known organic cause. Symptoms typically include abdominal bloating, pain and discomfort, often associated with bouts of diarrhoea and or constipation.

---

**Diagnosing IBS by History** - *Ref: NICE (2008) Diagnosis & management of IBS in primary care*
Consider IBS if the person reports symptoms for at least 6 months:
Abdominal pain or discomfort          Bloating          Change in bowel habit
A diagnosis of IBS should be considered only if the person has
- Abdominal pain or discomfort that is relieved by defecation or
- Associated with altered bowel frequency or stool form
This should be accompanied by at least two of the following four symptoms:
- Altered stool passage (straining, urgency, incomplete evacuation)
- Abdominal bloating (more common in women than men), distension, tension or hardness
- Symptoms made worse by eating
- Passage of mucus
Other features such as lethargy, nausea, backache and bladder symptoms are common in people with IBS, and may be used to support the diagnosis

---

## HISTORY
**Open questions**          Can you tell me more about the diarrhoea/constipation you have been experiencing?
                            Tell me more about the abdominal discomfort you have had?

**Focused questions**

| | |
|---|---|
| *IBS* | How long have you had it for? When did it first start? |
| Abdo pain | Where exactly is the pain? How long does it last for? Does it come and go in waves? |
| Bloating | Do you feel bloated all the time? |
| Defecation | Does the pain get better after you open your bowels? |
| Bowel habits | Have you noticed a change in bowel habits? Do you suffer with diarrhoea, constipation or a bit of both? How often do you go? Do you strain when you are trying to open your bowels? |
| Tenesmus | When you go, do you feel that you have not completely emptied your bowels? |
| Mucus | Have you passed any mucus in your stools? |
| Consistency | Have you noticed your stool form change? (hard lumps, sausage shape, soft, mushy, liquid) |
| Stress | Have you had any recent worries or stress? |

**Associated history**

| | |
|---|---|
| *Fatigue* | Do you feel tired all the time? |
| *Nausea & vomiting* | Do you feel sick or have you vomited? |

**Differentials**

| | |
|---|---|
| *Coeliac* | Have you noticed that the stools are difficult to flush away (steatorrhoea)? Is it related to certain foods (gluten)? Any weight loss? |

| Diverticulitis | Do you have any cramping pain on the lower left side of your tummy? Do you feel bloated? Do you have any fevers or blood in your stools? |
| --- | --- |
| IBD | Any mucus or blood in your stools? Any ulcers in the mouth? Have you had a fever or weight loss? Have you had any eye symptoms? |
| Ovarian cancer | Do you always feel bloated? Do you have continuous pelvic or tummy pain? Do you feel full all the time or sick when you are eating? |

## RED FLAGS

| Colon cancer | Unintentional and unexplained weight loss, rectal bleeding, change in bowel habit to looser or frequent stools persisting >6wks in >60yr old |
| --- | --- |
| Family history | Family history of bowel or ovarian cancer |

## PAST HISTORY

| Previous | Have you ever experienced these symptoms before? |
| --- | --- |
| Medical | Do you suffer from any bowel problems? (IBD) |
| Psychiatry | Have you been diagnosed with GAD or depression? |
| Surgery | Have you had any recent surgery? |

## DRUG HISTORY

| Medication | Are you taking any medications? |
| --- | --- |
| Constipation | SSRIs, TCA, NSAIDs, aspirin, codeine, steroids, loperamide, ferrous sulphate, calcium, buscopan |
| Diarrhoea | Antibiotics, laxatives (lactulose, senna), digoxin, antacids, PPI, thiazide, NSAIDs, chemotherapy |

## SOCIAL HISTORY

| Smoker | Do you smoke? How many cigarettes do you smoke per day? |
| --- | --- |
| Alcohol | Do you drink alcohol? How much do you drink and how often? |
| Occupation | Are you working at the moment? What do you work as? |
| Diet | What type of foods do you eat (wheat)? |

## FAMILY HISTORY

| Bowel | Anyone in the family suffers from bowel problems (IBD, IBS)? |
| --- | --- |
| Cancer | Is there anyone in your family who suffers from bowel or ovarian cancer? |

## IDEA, CONCERNS, EXPECTATIONS

| Idea | What did you think was causing the bowel problems? |
| --- | --- |
| Concerns | Are you worried about your symptoms? |
| Expectations | What were hoping we could do for you today (colonoscopy)? |
| Impact | How have the symptoms affected your life? |

## CSA TIPS

1 in 5 patients suffer with irritable bowel syndrome at some point in their lives. Although not life threatening, the symptoms can be quite debilitating and may cause patients to miss much time off their studies or from work. Essentially, IBS is a diagnosis of exclusion that can be made on the history alone. Be careful from making a rushed diagnosis without having excluding any more serious organic pathology first, particularly in the middle-aged or elderly. Given that stress is associated with the diagnosis, it would be pertinent to explore this in more detail - was there a recent life changing event that precluded the symptoms? How is the patient coping?

## PHYSICAL EXAMINATION

| | |
|---|---|
| *Vitals* | Weight, BMI, Bristol stool chart (assess stool quality) |
| *Abdominal* | |
| Inspection | Inspect for anaemia in the eyes |
| Palpation | Palpate for pain and masses. Examine for organomegaly (liver/spleen) |
| Auscultation | Listen for bowel sounds |
| PR | Do PR for rectal masses, impacted stools or melaena |
| *Pelvic exam* | Consider in females to exclude ovarian cancer |

## INVESTIGATIONS

| | |
|---|---|
| *Bloods* | FBC (anaemia), ESR/CRP (IBD), coeliac disease screen (tissue transglutaminase antibodies), CEA (bowel cancer), CA125 (ovarian ca) |
| *AXR* | Constipation, intestinal obstruction |
| *Stool* | *If diagnosis in doubt.* MC&S, ova, cysts, parasites, faecal occult blood (FOB), faecal calprotectin |

---

### Investigations Not Routinely Required to make Dx of IBS (NICE)

These tests are not necessary to confirm diagnosis in those who meet the IBS diagnostic criteria:
Ultrasound, sigmoidoscopy, colonoscopy; barium enema, TFT, faecal ova and parasite test, FOB, hydrogen breath test (for lactose intolerance and bacterial overgrowth)

*Ref: NICE (2008) Diagnosis and management of IBS in primary care*

---

## MANAGEMENT

### Conservative

| | |
|---|---|
| *Reassure* | Explain the diagnosis and reassure that it is not life-threatening |
| *Diet* | Offer dietary advice depending on symptoms i.e. constipation / diarrhoea |
| Fluids | Drink fluid (8 cups/d), restrict tea & coffee (3 cups/d), avoid alcohol or fizzy drinks |
| Meals | Eat regularly and slowly, do not miss meals, limit high fibre (bran, brown rice, wholemeal bread). Try probiotics for 4wks, restrict fruit & veg 3/d |
| Bloated | Try eating oats or linseeds (1 tablespoon/d) |
| Diarrhoea | Avoid sorbitol (artificial sweetener in sugar free drinks and chewing gum) |
| *FODMAP* | Encourage to eat a low FODMAP diet which may help reduce symptoms |

---

### The low FODMAP diet

FODMAP (Fermentable Oligo-Di-Monosccharides And Polyols) are carbohydrates that are found in some foods which may not be absorbed in the gut and are left to be fermented by intestinal bacteria causing bloatedness, diarrhoea and cramping pain. Common foods to avoid include;

| | Avoid | Alternatives |
|---|---|---|
| *Fruit* | apricot, cherries, peach, apple, pears | orange, lemon, banana |
| *Vegetable* | beet, sprouts, legumes, peas, onion | pepper, cucumbers, carrots |
| *Grains* | wheats, flour tortillas, rye | wheat / gluten free grains |
| *Dairy* | milk, cream, yoghurt, chocolate | cheddar, lactose free dairy |
| *Other* | honey, corn syrup | spices, butter, chives |

---

| | |
|---|---|
| *Exercise* | Encourage exercise 30 minutes 5x/wk |
| *Relaxation* | Suggest relaxation techniques and ways to reduce stress |

### Medical

| | |
|---|---|
| *Bloating* | Mebeverine, hyoscine, peppermint oils. Rotate through the agents separately if no response. If improves then leave the patient on PRN dose |
| *Constipation* | Ispaghula husk first line. Avoid lactulose, consider movicol or senna. Consider a trial of linaclotide (Constella) |
| *Diarrhoea* | Loperamide is first line. Avoid codeine phosphate |

---

### Advice about Treatment (NICE)

People with IBS should be advised how to adjust their doses of laxative or antimotility agent according to the clinical response. The dose should be titrated according to stool consistency, with the aim of achieving a soft, well-formed stool (Bristol Stool Form Scale type 4).

---

| | |
|---|---|
| *Antidepressants* | Consider low dose amitriptyline (5-30mg on). If no response consider SSRIs. If no response after 1yr of treatment should be referred for CBT |

### Safety netting

| | |
|---|---|
| *Follow up* | Review if symptoms persist for >4-6wks. Assess for presence of depressive symptoms |
| *Refer* | Refer urgently if evidence of unexplained anaemia, raised ESR/CRP or abdominal or rectal mass, or symptoms in an over 60 year old |
| Dietician | Refer to dietician for single food exclusion diets |
| Mood | Refer for hypnosis or psychotherapy for persistent low mood |

### EXPLANATIONS

| | |
|---|---|
| *Irritable Bowel* | Irritable bowel syndrome is a common condition (20% of people) that affects your bowels. It affects how the bowel works without causing any lasting damage. We call this a functional disorder which means that the workings of the gut are affected but not because of any damage or abnormality. It is often caused by an overactive bowel sometimes made worse by stress, certain foods and drinks. It gives rise to symptoms including, bloating, tummy pain and change in your bowel motions. |
| Antispasmotics | These medicines work by helping to relax the muscles of the bowels and reduce the abdominal pain you are getting. |
| Antimotility | Loperamide works by slowing down the contractions of the muscles of the gut therefore slowing how fast food travels through the bowels. This then allows your stools more time to harden and help treat the diarrhoea. |
| Laxatives | These work by making your stool softer and easier to pass through your abdomen. |
| Antidepressants | Amitriptyline is a medication that has been shown to work really well in IBS. It works well at blocking messages (nerve impulses) between the gut and brain thereby relaxing the muscles of the gut. In IBS often there is over sensitivity of the gut to these messages from the brain (brain-gut axis). |
| Low FODMAP diet | There is evidence to suggest that in IBS the bowel struggles to absorb certain sugars compared to others. As a result they are broken down (fermented) by normal bugs in the gut producing lots of gas. If we restrict these sugars from your diet we should see an improvement in your symptoms. |

Dysphagia, also known as difficulty in swallowing, affects a large number of patients particularly those who are elderly. It can be quite a distressing symptom to suffer from especially as a result of the choking sensation felt when trying to swallow. There are a number of different causes that may present with dysphagia particularly oesophageal or pharyngeal disorders, however, you should also consider neurological conditions such as strokes and achalasia. Patients suffering with learning disabilities often have associated dysphagia and this should be enquired about.

**HISTORY**

**Open questions**      Please describe to me the problem you have been having with your swallowing?

**Focused questions**

| | |
|---|---|
| *Dysphagia* | When did you first notice it? How long does it last for? |
| Onset | Did it come on suddenly or gradually? |
| Nature | Does it come and go (intermittent) or is it there all the time (persistent)? |
| Site | Is there a particular level where you feel the food gets stuck at? |
| Character | Do you find difficulty swallowing solids, liquids or a combination of the two? |

**Associated history**

| | |
|---|---|
| *Odynophagia* | Do you experience any pain when swallowing? |
| *Cough* | Do you have a bothersome cough? |
| *Choking* | Do you have a choking feeling when you swallow? |
| *Vomiting* | Have you vomited or felt sick with your symptoms? |
| *Weight loss* | Have you lost any weight? |

**Differentials**

| | |
|---|---|
| *GORD* | Do you have a burning feeling in your chest? Does it go to your throat? Do you get an acidic taste (acid brash) or too much saliva (water brash) in your mouth? Is it worse at night? |
| *Achalasia* | Do you find difficulty swallowing both solids and liquids? Do you bring up food? Do you have coughing fits at night when you are trying to sleep? |
| *Pharyngeal pouch* | Have you noticed a bulge in the side of the neck? Do you find that the first mouth full is easy to eat then it gets progressively more difficult to swallow? Do you bring up food? Have you noticed any bad breath? |
| *Globus Pharyngis* | Do you feel as if there is a lump in your throat? Do you otherwise have no problems swallowing? Do you suffer from stress or anxiety? |
| *Oesophageal cancer* | Was it hard to swallow solids (meals) initially, then now affecting liquids (drinks) as well? Have you lost any weight? Do you get discomfort when you swallow? |
| *Bulbar palsy* | Do you find it harder to swallow at the beginning rather than at the end? |
| *CVA* | Did you have slurred speech? Any weakness of your arms or legs? Any problems with your vision? |
| *CREST* | Have you had any tightening or thickening of skin of the hands or feet? Do you notice your hands change colour from white to blue or red? |

## RED FLAGS

| | |
|---|---|
| *Dyspepsia/GORD* | Progressive dysphagia, persistent vomiting, unexplained fe def anaemia, weight loss, upper abdominal mass, >55yr with unexplained dyspepsia |
| *Others* | Weight loss, haematemesis, persistent vomiting, epigastric mass, stroke |

## PAST HISTORY

| | |
|---|---|
| *Previous* | Have you had swallowing problems before? |
| *Medical* | Do you suffer from any medical conditions (Fe anaemia - Plummer-Vinson, GORD, PU, CREST)? |
| *Investigations* | Have you had any tests such as camera tests (OGD) or barium swallow? |

## DRUG HISTORY

| | |
|---|---|
| *Medication* | Are you taking any medications? |
| GORD | NSAIDs, SSRI |
| Xerostomia | (dry mouth) TCAs, antihistamines, anticholinergic inhibitors (buscopan) |

## SOCIAL HISTORY

| | |
|---|---|
| *Smoker* | Do you smoke? How many cigarettes do you smoke per day? |
| *Alcohol* | Do you drink alcohol? How much do you drink and how often? |
| *Occupation* | Are you working at the moment? What do you work as? |
| *Diet* | What type of foods do you eat? |

## FAMILY HISTORY

| | |
|---|---|
| *Cancer* | Anyone in the family suffer from stomach problems such as ulcers or stomach cancer? Does anyone suffer from throat cancer? |

## IDEA, CONCERNS, EXPECTATIONS

| | |
|---|---|
| *Idea* | Did you have any thoughts as to what was causing your swallowing problems? |
| *Concerns* | Are you worried about your symptoms? |
| *Expectations* | What were hoping we could do for you today? |
| *Impact on life* | How have the symptoms affected your life? |

## CSA TIPS

Dysphagia can be caused by a wide range of conditions including pharyngeal, oesophageal and neurological problems. A clear and concise history will help untangle the possible diagnosis and will guide you to be able to share a management plan. Patients with red flags will need to be referred under the 2ww rule to ensure prompt confirmation and management.

## PHYSICAL EXAMINATION

| | |
|---|---|
| *Vitals* | Weight, BMI, pulse |
| *Hands* | Inspect for calcinosis, telangiectasia, sclerodactyly (CREST) |
| *Abdominal* | |
| Inspection | Inspect the conjunctiva for signs of anaemia. Look in the throat for signs of candidiasis |
| Palpitation | Palpate the upper epigastric area for masses |
| *Neurological* | Perform a cerebellar or focused cranial nerve assessment (bulbar palsy) |

## INVESTIGATIONS

| | |
|---|---|
| *Bloods* | FBC, ferritin (iron deficiency anaemia), U&E |

| | |
|---|---|
| *X-Ray* | Barium swallow (achalasia, oesophageal spasm). CXR (mediastinal tumour) |
| *Endoscopy* | OGD (oesophageal web, cancer) |
| *Other (specialist)* | Video fluoroscopy (achalasia) |

| | |
|---|---|
| **MANAGEMENT** | *treat underlying cause* |
| **Conservative** | |
| *Eating habits* | Eat several small meals regularly instead of large meals. After eating, wait 2 hours before lying down. Avoid any late night snacks |
| *Dysphagia* | Alter the consistency of foods consumed (thickeners). Adhere to SALT and dietician advice |
| *Tablets* | Consider substituting tablet preparations to liquid, orodispersible formula, patches or injectable alternatives |

---

**Possible Foods Recommended and to Avoid in Dysphagia**

Below is a list of general points and lifestyle advice for patients with dysphagia. More tailored advice should be sought from the dietician or SALT team

| | |
|---|---|
| *Recommended* | Plain custard, plain yoghurts, pureed meats, fish or poultry, hummus, soft scrambled eggs, pureed fruits and vegetables, mashed potatoes, thickened broths of soup |
| *Avoid* | Cottage cheese, peanut butter, fried foods, unthickened fruit juice, bread slice, waffles, pasta without sauce, rice |

---

| | |
|---|---|
| **Dry Mouth** | Ensure good fluid intake (>2l daily). Stop smoking and reduce alcohol intake. Sip cold drinks frequently or consider sucking ice cubes. Chewing gum helps increase salivation |
| *Medical* | Stop medications that cause xerostomia. Prescribe artificial saliva or pilocarpine 5mg |
| | |
| **Globus pharyngis** | Reassure. Some response to empirical PPI. Often precipitated by anxiety. Offer talking (CBT) therapies. Refer to ENT if persistent |
| | |
| **GORD** | Avoid chilli and spicy food. Cut down on caffeine and alcohol. Stop smoking. Eat small, regular meals and ensure that the last meal is several hours before bedtime |
| *Medical* | Alginates – Gaviscon, H2 Antagonist - Ranitidine, PPI – Omeprazole |
| | |
| **Achalasia/Spasm** | Usually under specialist care for management |
| *Medical* | Consider nitrates or nifedipine to relax the lower oesophageal sphincter (LOS) for symptomatic relief |
| *Surgical* | May require pneumatic dilatation, botulinum injection or surgical resection (myotomy) of the LOS all under GA |
| | |
| **Pharyngeal pouch** | Refer to ENT for further investigations. Surgical repair for incisional and stapling |
| | |
| **Refer** | Patients with dysphagia who show signs of aspiration or choking of unknown cause should be kept NBM and referred to hospital. Patients with red flags should be referred urgently |
| *Dietician* | Consider referring to dietician for advice regarding tailored nutritional advice to prevent dehydration and malnutrition |
| *SALT* | Refer to SALT for swallowing retraining as well as to grade severity of dysphagia. May need assessment for nasal or PEG feeding |

*Follow up*                    A worsening cough or weight loss or persistent dysphagia should seek medical advice

**DIFFERENTIAL DIAGNOSIS**

| Condition | Characteristic exam feature |
|---|---|
| Oesophagitis | Burning sensation with acidic taste in mouth. Odynophagia. Absence of weight loss |
| Oesophageal spasm | Intermittent dysphagia with chest pain |
| Achalasia | Dysphagia of both liquids and solids from the beginning. Gradual onset over years. Associated with heartburn, regurgitation of food and foul belching. Regurgitation can lead to night cough and risk of aspiration pneumonia |
| Oesophageal cancer | Rapid progressive dysphagia of solids then liquids. Regurgitation of foods, haematemesis. Feeling of food stuck at a certain level. Pain is a late feature. Associated with weight loss and appetite change. Risk factors - Barrett's oesophagus, GORD, smoking, alcohol excess, lack of fruit and vegetables |
| Oesophageal candidiasis | Consider in HIV positive patients or steroid inhaler use in asthmatics |
| Pharyngeal pouch | Seen more often in elderly men. Patients complain that first morsel of food swallowed easily whilst later mouthful's are progressively more difficult. Associated with halitosis and regurgitation of foods and are at risk of aspiration. OE: lump protruding to one side (L>R) that gurgles on palpation |
| Globus pharyngeus | Women more than men. Past history of anxiety/depression. Patients report feeling of lump in throat with no swallowing difficulty. Symptoms are intermittent |

**EXPLANATIONS**

*Achalasia*            This is a condition that affects the food pipes ability to swallow. The food pipe uses a system of muscles that squeeze together in unison to help food move down into the stomach. In achalasia there is damage to the nerves that supply these muscles. As a result the lower end of the food pipe remains tight causing your symptoms.

*Pharyngeal pouch*     This is due to weakness in the muscles at the back of your throat that creates a small pocket or pouch. Whenever you eat, food may collect here causing you to have difficulty swallowing and persisting bad breath.

*Scleroderma*          In this condition the tissues of the body become hard and tightened. The body begins to attack its own tissues and when this happens in the food-pipe, the muscles weaken and makes it hard for food to travel down into your tummy causing your swallowing problems.

*Globus pharyngeus*  This is a condition whereby a patient feels as if there is a lump in their throat, but following examination and investigation no lump is found. The feeling usually comes and goes and does not cause problems when eating or drinking. It is not entirely known what causes it, but people who are worried or anxious suffer with it more.

*Barium swallow*  A barium swallow is used to look for problems in your food pipe. The food pipe does not show up very well on ordinary X-ray pictures. However, if barium liquid is swallowed, the outline and functioning of the food pipe shows up more clearly. Barium is a soft white metal drink that shows up on X-rays and is completely safe to drink.

# *4.8 PR bleeding*

PR bleeding describes blood passed per rectum. It includes bleeding that can occur anywhere along the GI tract. It is often classified as upper or lower GI bleed based upon the appearance of the blood. Usually the higher the site of the bleed, the darker the appearance of the blood. Conversely, the closer the site of the bleed is to the anus, the brighter the colour will be. The most common cause for PR bleeding is due to hemorrhoids, however, more serious conditions such as bowel cancer must always be considered particularly in the older persons.

### HISTORY

| | |
|---|---|
| **Open questions** | I can see that you seem a little embarrassed to talk about your problem. Bowel problems are conditions that we see and treat everyday. Please tell me more about the bleeding through your back passage? |

### Focused questions

| | |
|---|---|
| *PR bleeding* | When did you first notice it? How long has it been going on for? |
| Type | |
| Fresh | Does it drip from the back passage? Do you see it on the tissue paper? Has it ever turned the toilet bowl pink or red? |
| Mixed | Is it mixed with your stools? Or separate? |
| Severity | How much blood did you pass? (measured in cup fulls) |
| Colour | Can you describe its colour? Is it bright red or black and tarry? |

### Different Colours of Stools

| | |
|---|---|
| *Dark tarry* (melaena) | Upper GI bleed (peptic, oesophagus), iron, bismuth treatment |
| *Blood red* | Diverticulitis (large volume), colorectal ca (mixed with stool), UC & inf. colitis (blood & mucus mixed in stool), haemorrhoids (painless, fresh blood on stool & pan), anal fissure (painful, fresh blood on paper & stool) |
| *Pale bulky* | (Steatorrhoea) fat malabsorption (coeliac) or pancreatic disease |

### Associated history

| | |
|---|---|
| *Abdominal pain* | Do you experience any abdominal pain? |
| *Bowel* | Have you had any diarrhoea or constipation? |
| *Fever* | Have you had a temperature or fever? |
| *Bloated* | Have you been feeling bloated or full of gas? |
| *Weight loss* | Have you lost any weight? |

### Differentials

| | |
|---|---|
| *Peptic Ulcer* | Do have a burning pain? Does drinking milk make it better? Have you noticed any black tarry stools? Have you vomited up any blood? |
| *Dysentery* | Have you eaten out recently? Any diarrhoea or vomiting? Do you get cramping abdominal pains? Have you recently travelled abroad? |
| *Colon Cancer* | Have you noticed a change in your bowel habits? Any weight loss? Is the blood mixed with the stools? Do you find that when you open your bowels do you feel that you have not completely emptied them? |
| *Anal fissure* | Any soreness in the back passage particularly when you wipe yourself? |

| Piles | Do you strain when you open your bowels? Is there blood bright red on the tissue paper? Is the back passage particularly itchy? Have you been constipated? |
|---|---|
| IBD | Do you ever pass any mucus with the stools? Do you get any abdominal pain or fevers with it? Any ulcers in the mouth or anus? |
| Diverticulitis | Do you have any cramping pain on the lower left side of your tummy? Do you feel bloated? Do you have any fevers? |

## RED FLAGS

| Colon Cancer | >40yrs, weight loss, change in appetite, change in bowel habits for >6wks |
|---|---|
| Upper GI bleed | Melaena, haematemesis, persistent vomiting |
| Fe deficiency | Dizziness, fatigability |
| IBD | More than 4-6 episodes of bloody diarrhoea with fever |

## Assessing Severity of Ulcerative Colitis

| Mild | <4 loose stools/d. No systemic disturbance, no or minimal rectal bleeding |
|---|---|
| Moderate | 4-6 loose stools/d. Moderate rectal bleeding, minimal signs of systemic disturbances, mild ulcerative colitis resistant to treatment |
| Severe | >6 loose stool/d with blood. Systemic disturbance (fever, tachycardia, ↑WCC, ESR, low ↓hb, malnutrition (↓alb), weight loss <10kg |

## PAST HISTORY

| Previous | Have you ever had rectal bleeding in the past or any bowel problems? |
|---|---|
| Medical | Do you suffer from any medical problems? (bowel cancer, diverticulosis, bleeding disorders, constipation) |

## DRUG HISTORY

| Medication | Are you taking any medications? (NSAIDS, aspirin, warfarin) |
|---|---|

## SOCIAL HISTORY

| Smoker | Do you smoke? How many cigarettes do you smoke per day? |
|---|---|
| Alcohol | Do you drink alcohol? How much do you drink and how often? |
| Occupation | Are you working at the moment? What do you work as? |
| Diet | What type of foods do you eat? |

## FAMILY HISTORY

| Medical | Does anyone in the family suffer from illnesses? (bowel ca- HNPCC/FAP, IBD) |
|---|---|

## IDEA, CONCERNS, EXPECTATIONS

| Idea | What did you think was causing the bleeding from your back passage? |
|---|---|
| Concerns | Is there anything that is particularly worrying you about your symptoms? |
| Expectations | What were hoping we could do for you today? |
| Impact | How have the symptoms affected your life? |

## CSA TIPS

Passing blood following defecation may be a worrying symptom that patients suffer from. However, due to the sensitivity of the problem, many patients may present late with quite severe problems due to embarrassment or shyness. You should make your patients feel at rest such that they are willing to discuss their personal matters with you and ensure that your offer a chaperone when examining the rectal area.

## PHYSICAL EXAMINATION

| | |
|---|---|
| *Vitals* | BP (hypotension), pulse (tachycardia), temperature, weight |
| *Chaperone* | Request a chaperone |
| *Abdominal* | |
| Inspection | Inspect the conjunctiva for signs of anaemia |
| Palpitation | Palpate for masses (cancer) or tenderness (ulcer, diverticulitis) |
| *Rectal exam* | |
| Inspection | Look for skin tags, ulcers, fissures, polyps, piles or external haemorrhoids |
| Palpation | Palpate for any masses. Ask patient to strain downwards. Check for blood or mucus |

## INVESTIGATIONS

| | |
|---|---|
| *Bloods* | FBC (anaemia), ferritin (Fe def), U&E (acute bleed), LFTs (oesophageal varices) |
| Other | ESR, CRP (IBD), CEA (bowel cancer), coeliac screen, clotting screen |
| *Stool* | FOB, Helicobacter pylori, MC&S (dysentery) |
| *AXR* | Faecal loading |
| *Specialist* | Barium enema (diverticulum), CT abdo, endoscopy (OGD, colonoscopy, sigmoidoscopy) |

## MANAGEMENT     *treat underlying cause*
### IBD

| | |
|---|---|
| *Conservative* | Offer elemental diet in Crohn's disease particularly in flare ups (settles within 4 wks). Advise to quit smoking. Probiotics in ulcerative colitis |

---

**Elemental Diet in Crohn's disease**

Patients are initially restricted from all foods and the elemental diet is introduced over 3 days to reduce GI symptoms. The diet is a nutritional drink that is strongly weighted with carbohydrates (90%), vitamins, electrolytes and protein.

---

| | |
|---|---|
| *Medical* | Refer to specialist for colonoscopy and diagnosis |
| Crohn's | Consider Mesalazine, steroids (oral, topical) or azathioprine (2nd line). Methotrexate (if cannot tolerate azathioprine or perianal disease). Consider surgery |
| UC | Rectal aminosalicylates (mesalazine) or steroids for distal colitis. Oral aminosalicylates or steroids if severe. Can be offered azathioprine |

### Diverticulitis

| | |
|---|---|
| *Conservative* | Encourage high fibre diet, fluids |
| *Medical* | If severe, refer for admission and IV antibiotics. Can give augmentin or metronidazole with ciprofloxacin (severe). Avoid NSAIDS (risk of perforations). Chronic diverticular disease consider laxatives (ispaghula husk, lactulose) and antispasmodic agents |

### Piles/fissures

| | |
|---|---|
| *Conservative* | Treat constipation by dietary advice. 5 fruit and veg a day, encourage fluid intake and more fibre, lose weight, decrease alcohol and red meat intake. Try not to strain when passing a motion and do not delay passing stools when you feel you have to go |
| *Medical* | Prescribe a stool softener (ispaghula or lactulose). Oral analgesics such as paracetamol. Avoid codeine (worsens constipation) or NSAIDs if pr bleed. Consider Anusol HC, proctosedyl suppositories or topical LA for symptomatic relief. Low dose topical steroids if anal inflammation or eczema present |
| *Invasive* | Refer to surgeons for banding, sclerotherapy (injecting) or haemorrhoidectomy |

| Fissures | Consider topical GTN or diltiazem ointment. Warn about side effects e.g. headaches. May be referred for trial of Botulinum toxin injections if not keen on surgery |

**Refer**

| UC | Refer patients to hospital if >6 stools/d, blood in stools, systemic illness (fever, tachycardia, abdominal pain, distension, reduced bowel sounds) |
| Colon cancer | Refer patients as according to NICE guidelines using 2 week wait |

---

### Colon Cancer referrals guidance NICE

- >40yr with PR bleeding and change of bowel habit (looser stools) or increased stool frequency for >6wks
- >60yr with rectal bleeding >6wks without a change in bowel habit, without anal symptoms
- >60yr with a change in bowel habit (looser) or more frequent stools for >6 wks without rectal bleeding
- Right lower abdominal mass with involvement of the large bowel or palpable rectal mass
- Unexplained fe def. anaemia in men (Hb < 11g/dl ) or non-menstruating women (<10 g/dl)

---

### SAFETY NETTING

| Admission | Refer patients for hospital admission if there are signs of shock |
| Follow up | Review patient if symptoms persist for more than 3-4wks or worsen |

### DIFFERENTIAL DIAGNOSIS

| Condition | Characteristic exam feature |
|---|---|
| Anal fissures | Tear to anal mucosa often posterior to anal canal. Pain on defecation with blood on toilet paper. Associated with constipation. OE: fissure visible. PR exam very tender |
| Haemorrhoids | Background of constipation with fresh blood on tissue paper, surface of stools or dripping into pan. Tenesmus and pruritus ani. OE: Haemorrhoids often visible on PR (except grade 1) |
| Crohn's disease | Transmural chronic inflammatory disease, can affect any part of the GI tract from the mouth to the anus. Crampy abdominal pains and diarrhoea and less commonly blood diarrhoea. OE: Mouth ulcers (lesions from mouth to anus) and mass in RIF. Other features include perianal tags, fissures and fistulas and extra intestinal symptoms such as arthritis, uveitis, erythema nodosum |
| Ulcerative colitis | Ulcerating disease affecting only the mucous membrane of the large bowel. Symptoms include abdominal pain (LIF), diarrhoea, rectal bleeding (> Crohn's), growth failure, tenesmus and weight loss. Also present with pyoderma gangrenosum, erythema nodosum, arthritis and spondylitis |
| Diverticulitis | Small outpouchings of the large bowel that become inflamed or infected. Symptoms include abdominal pain, bloating and cramps mainly in left iliac fossa with fever, nausea, vomiting and constipation. Frank blood mixed in with the stools is a complication |

| | |
|---|---|
| **Polyp** | Common (1/4 of >50yr old) benign growth of lining of colon/rectum. Causes pr bleeding. Can turn cancerous |
| **Colorectal cancer** | Weight loss, change in bowel habit. PR bleeding and abdominal mass (can be in right iliac fossa). Unexplained iron deficiency anaemia |
| **Angiodysplasia** | Cased by small vascular malformation of the colon. Produces painless rectal bleeding and iron deficiency anaemia |

**EXPLANATIONS**

*Diverticulitis*    Diverticulum are out pouches that stick out from the gut wall and is cause by increased pressure in the gut because of a low fibre diet. In diverticulitis, these outpouchings become inflamed or infected as stool gets trapped within them.

*IBD*    Inflammatory bowel disease describes two conditions, Crohn's disease and Ulcerative colitis. It is a condition that results in swelling or inflammation of the lining of the gut. In Crohn's disease the inflammation can take place anywhere in your GI tract i.e. from your mouth to your anus. Whilst in Ulcerative colitis, the swelling is limited to the large bowel and back passage (proctitis).

*Piles*    Piles or haemorrhoids is a common condition that causes bleeding when passing stools. They are swellings of blood vessels that collect in and around the bottom and may be felt as a lump in the anus. They normally start when we exert too much pressure and strain when passing a motion. This may be due to lack of fibre in our diet, or because of constipation.

*Fissure*    This describes a tear in and around the bottom area. They are caused by the passage of hard stools that damage the lining of the anus as they pass out. As a result, they may cause bleeding on the toilet paper and a sharp pain and burning sensation after passing a motion.

*Colonoscopy*    This is a test which allows the doctor to look at your colon more closely. It uses a thin, flexible tube with a camera and bright light on one end that is passed through the back passage and into your lower gut. Using small tweezers a small sample can be taken from the lining of the gut and later looked under the microscope more closely.

*Barium enema*    This is a soft white metal liquid which is placed in the lower bowel though an enema. It outlines the gut (intestines) and allows it to be shown up more clearly on an X-ray.

Pruritus ani describes a sensation of an intense need to itch the anal and perianal areas. It is an uncomfortable feeling and may leave patients feeling acutely embarrassed. If left untreated it may encourage bad hygiene habits and promote infections via the ano-faecal route. The vast majority of causes are believed to be functional, due to faecal material causing itchiness and localised erythema. Other causes include skin infections, eczema, overflow diarrhoea and piles.

## HISTORY
**Open questions** | I just want to reassure that whilst you may feel embarrassed to talk about your problem, it is something that we see and treat everyday. Please can you tell me a little bit about your symptoms?

## Focused questions
| | |
|---|---|
| *Pruritus ani* | When did it start? How long has it been going on for? Does it come and go or is it there all the time? |
| Triggers | Does anything make it better or worse? |
| Worse | Items of clothing, stress, spicy foods, after defecation |
| Better | Topical emollients, anaesthetic creams |
| Severity | Has it affected your sleep or social life? |
| General hygiene | Do you think that you may wash yourself excessively? Do you use any soaps or perfumes? |

## Associated history
| | |
|---|---|
| *PR bleeding* | Any bleeding from your back passage? (toilet paper, dripping) |
| *Pain* | Do you have any pain in the anus? |
| *Strain* | Do you strain when you open your bowel? |
| *Constipation* | Do you suffer with hard stools? |
| *Diarrhoea* | Have you had any diarrhoea? |

## Differentials
| | |
|---|---|
| *Anal fissure* | Does it sting when you wipe yourself with tissue paper? Any blood on it? |
| *Piles* | Have you felt or seen any lumps that come out when you are opening your bowels? Do you strain when passing stools? Any constipation? |
| *Threadworms* | Is the itching worse at night? Have you felt anything move in the back passage? Have you seen any worms or white eggs in your stools? Have you lost any weight? |
| *Crohn's* | Have you noticed any mucus from the back passage? Any fevers or abdominal pain? |
| *Skin* | Have you seen a rash? Are any other family members affected (scabies)? |
| *STI* | Are you in a relationship at the moment? Do you practice anal sex? |

## RED FLAGS
| | |
|---|---|
| *Anorectal cancer* | Change in bowel habits, tenesmus, weight loss, pr bleeding |

## PAST HISTORY
| | |
|---|---|
| *Skin lesions* | Do you suffer from psoriasis, eczema or urticaria? |
| *Other* | Do you suffer from diabetes (predisposes to candidiasis), jaundice (itch)? |

## DRUG HISTORY

| | |
|---|---|
| *Medication* | Are you taking any medications? |
| Worsen | Colchicine, tetracycline, erythromycin, metronidazole |

## SOCIAL HISTORY

| | |
|---|---|
| *Smoker* | Do you smoke? How many cigarettes do you smoke per day? |
| *Alcohol* | Do you drink alcohol? How much do you drink and how often? |
| *Occupation* | Are you working at the moment? What do you work as? Do you sweat a lot at work? |
| *Travel* | Any recent travel abroad (threadworm)? |
| *Diet* | What types of foods do you eat? Do you like spicy food or chilli? |

## FAMILY HISTORY

| | |
|---|---|
| *Medical* | Does anyone in the family suffer from any illness? (IBD) |
| *Ringworm* | Has anyone in the family recently been treated for threadworm? |

## IDEA, CONCERNS, EXPECTATIONS

| | |
|---|---|
| *Idea* | What was going through you mind when you had this problem? (washing up powder, threadworms, antiseptic soaps) |
| *Concerns* | Is there anything that is particularly worrying you about it? |
| *Expectations* | What were you hoping we could do for you today? |
| *Impact* | How have the symptoms affected your life? (sleep, embarrassment) |

## CSA TIPS

An itchy anus is an embarrassing and uncomfortable problem. Although most causes are quite innocuous and rarely due to poor hygiene, patients may blame themselves for the symptoms. You should try and establish the effect it is having on the sufferer's life such as causing social isolation or bullying if at school or college.

## PHYSICAL EXAMINATION

| | |
|---|---|
| *Vitals* | Weight, temperature |
| *Rectal exam* | |
|    Inspection | Look for skin tags, ulcers, fissures, polyps, piles or external haemorrhoids. Look for skin conditions such as psoriasis, candida inf., contact dermatitis, seborrhoeic dermatitis |
|    Palpation | Palpate for any masses if malignancy suspected. Ask patient to strain downwards. Check for blood or mucus |

---

### Grading of internal haemorrhoids

| | |
|---|---|
| *Grade I* | Do not prolapse out of the anal canal |
| *Grade II* | Prolapse on defecation but reduce spontaneously |
| *Grade III* | Can be manually reduced |
| *Grade IV* | Cannot be reduced |

---

## INVESTIGATIONS

| | |
|---|---|
| *Sellotape test* | Perform sellotape test if threadworms are suspected (but not visualised) |

---

### Performing the Sellotape Test

Apply a clear adhesive tape to the anus and leave it in situ overnight. Remove tape in the morning to place on a provided slide. Send off sample for confirmation of threadworms.

---

| | |
|---|---|
| *Bloods* | FBC (eosinophilia – rare in threadworms), ESR (Crohn's) |
| *Stool* | MC&S (ova) |
| *Specialist* | Proctoscopy |

**MANAGEMENT**  *treat underlying cause*

**Pruritus ani**

*Conservative*

| | |
|---|---|
| Hygiene | Wash the anus after each bowel movement and before sleeping. Clean using moist wipes/wet toilet paper. Avoid rubbing vigorously. Avoid soaps or bubble bath scented products. Dry perianal area after bowel motions by gentle patting |
| Underwear | Use cotton underwear. Avoid any tight or synthetic clothing |
| Nails | Try and avoid scratching where possible. Keep nails short and perhaps wear gloves (cotton) at night |
| Hands | Wash hands after every motion |
| Diet | Avoid any foods that exacerbate the problem i.e. spicy, chilli, tomatoes, lemon/orange juice. Cut down caffeine (tea, coffee, cola) and chocolate and reduce fizzy drinks and alcohol |
| Constipation | Drink plenty of fluids, eat 5 fruit & veg/d, reduce weight, have plenty of fibre (cereals) |

| | |
|---|---|
| **Treadworms** | Treat with mebendazole stat and repeat in 2wk if necessary (not licensed for <2yr but can be given). Whole family can be treated. Piperazine is an alternative medicine |

---

**BNF Advice about Threadworms** - *Ref: BNF 2013*

Anthelmintics are effective in threadworm infections, but their use needs to be combined with hygienic measures to break the cycle of auto-infection. All members of the family require treatment. Adult threadworms do not live for longer than 6 weeks and for development of fresh worms, ova must be swallowed and exposed to the action of digestive juices in the upper intestinal tract. Direct multiplication of worms does not take place in the large bowel. Adult female worms lay ova on the perianal skin which causes pruritus; scratching the area then leads to ova being transmitted on fingers to the mouth, often via food eaten with unwashed hands. Washing hands and scrubbing nails before each meal and after each visit to the toilet is essential. A bath taken immediately after rinsing will remove ova laid during the night.

---

| | |
|---|---|
| **Skin conditions** | Apply barrier creams or soothing ointment (bismuth subgallate or zinc oxide). Can trial mild steroid (hydrocortisone) as well as antihistamine (chlorpheniramine 4mg) at night (reduces itch and helps sleep) |
| **Piles** | Treat any constipation if present. Topical local anaesthetic agents include anusol, proctosedyl used for short periods. Suppositories also available |

**Fissures**

| | |
|---|---|
| *Conservative* | 5 fruit and veg a day, encourage fluid intake and more fibre, lose weight |
| *Medical* | Treat constipation (1st line bulk forming – ispaghula husk), barrier cream – petroleum jelly, topical anaesthetics (anusol), sitz baths (remain seated in hot water for several minutes before applying cold water for 1 minute). Chronic fissures try GTN cream |

| | |
|---|---|
| **Refer** | If unresponsive skin condition refer to dermatologist or GPSI. Can refer to a colorectal surgeon if not improving >1mth despite treatment. In piles consider band ligation or sclerotherapy injection if persistent. Fissures can be treated with botulinum injections |

*Follow up*                  Review patient if symptoms persist for more than 3-4wks or worsening

**DIFFERENTIAL DIAGNOSIS**

| Condition | Characteristic exam feature |
|---|---|
| **Anal fissures** | Tear to anal mucosa often posterior to anal canal. Pain on defecation with blood on toilet paper. Associated with constipation. OE: fissure visible. PR exam very tender |
| **Haemorrhoids** | Background of constipation with painless fresh blood on tissue paper, surface of stools or dripping into pan. Tenesmus and pruritus ani. Soling may occur in severe haemorrhoids. OE: Haemorrhoids often visible on examination (except grade 1) |
| **Crohn's disease** | Transmural chronic inflammatory disease, can affect any part of the GI tract from the mouth to the anus. Presents with crampy abdominal pains and diarrhoea which is occasionally bloody. OE: Mouth ulcers can present (lesions from mouth to anus) and mass in RIF. Other features include perianal tags, fissures and fistulas and with extra intestinal symptoms such as arthritis, uveitis and erythema nodosum |
| **Threadworms** | Spread by faecal oral route. Pruritus at night. Other family members may have similar symptoms. Occasionally worms or white ova visualized in stool |
| **Skin conditions** | Contact dermatitis, psoriasis, lichen sclerosis |

**EXPLANATIONS**

*Pruritus ani*          This is the medical term for itchy anus. It is an uncomfortable sensation that has a variety of causes but is rarely due to poor hygiene. Sometimes if we clean the anus very harshly after a motion, or use perfumed scents or tissues, these may irritate the area and cause itchiness. Other common causes include dry skin, worms and piles.

*Piles*                    Haemorrhoids are small swellings found in the back passage. They are usually caused when the normal veins in the back passage become swollen and engorged with blood. As they swell, they may pop out when you strain on the toilet and bleed.

*Threadworms*        Threadworms are small white parasites that can infect the gut. They can lay eggs around the back passage at night giving you an itch. As you scratch your bottom, the eggs may get caught under your fingernails and may cause reinfection.

# 4.10 Constipation

The term constipation may be understood differently between patients and doctors. It is always useful to clarify with the patient what they mean by the word constipation. Constipation is synonymous with the passage of hard stools. However, a health professional may define it as the infrequent passing of bowel motions or incomplete defecation. Stools are usually hard and dry and can fluctuate from being extremely large (blocking the pan) or small (pellet like).

Constipation may be caused by a variety of problems including poor dietary intake, reduced fluids, as a side-effect of medications or due to poor mobility. In the elderly, any prolonged change in bowel habit should trigger the possibility of bowel cancer as a diagnosis.

## HISTORY

**Open questions**   Can you tell more about the problems you are having with your bowel motions? What did you mean when you said you were constipated?

## Focused questions

| | |
|---|---|
| *Constipation* | When did it start? How long has it been going on for? Is it getting worse or better? |
| Frequency | How often are you opening your bowels? |
| Straining | Do you feel as if you are straining when you open your bowels? |
| Pain | Do you experience any pain? Is it cramping in nature? |
| Appearance | Do the stools look like rabbit droppings? Are they often so large that they block the toilet? *Use the Bristol Stool chart to identify the stool type* |
| Blood | Have you noticed any blood in your stool? |

## Associated history

| | |
|---|---|
| *Overflow diarrhoea* | Have you ever soiled your undergarments? |
| *Nausea & vomiting* | Did you feel sick or vomited? |
| *Loading* | Do you sometimes have to use a finger to remove the stool? |
| *Toileting* | Do you have easy access to a toilet? Do you go regularly or hold when you cannot go? |

## Differentials

| | |
|---|---|
| *Diet/functional* | Have you eaten out recently? Anyone else unwell? Have you vomited? |
| *Intestinal obstruction* | Have you opened your bowels, passed any wind or vomited recently? |
| *IBS* | Any stress? Do you feel bloated? Is the pain made worse by eating and better by opening your bowels? |
| *Hypothyroid* | Have you felt tired or cold all the time? Have you noticed any hair loss or dry skin? Have you put on any weight recently? |
| *Cancer* | Are your stools looser than normal? Any recent change in bowel habits to looser stools (in >50 yrs old)? Any weight loss? Any blood mixed with your stools? |
| *Depression* | How is your mood? Do you feel tired all the time or not enjoying the things you used to? |
| *Fissure* | Is there blood on the toilet paper when you've finished? Is it painful when you go? |

## RED FLAGS

| | |
|---|---|
| *Bowel cancer* | Weight loss, PR bleeding, change in bowel habits |
| *Intestinal obstruction* | Abdominal distension, absolute constipation, vomiting |

## PAST HISTORY

| | |
|---|---|
| *Previous* | Have you had any bowel problems? (fissures, diverticular disease, IBS, IBD)? |
| *Medical* | Do you suffer from medical problems? (thyroid, depression, bowel ca)? |

## DRUG HISTORY

| | |
|---|---|
| *Medication* | Are you taking any medications? |
| Worsen | Opioids, ferrous sulphate, SSRIs, calcium ch. antagonists, antacids, anticholinergics (oxybutynin), calcium supplements |
| Improve | Laxatives |

## SOCIAL HISTORY

| | |
|---|---|
| *Smoker* | Do you smoke? How many cigarettes do you smoke per day? |
| *Alcohol* | Do you drink alcohol? How much do you drink and how often? |
| *Diet* | What type of foods do you eat? How is your fluid intake? |
| *Exercise* | Do you exercise? What do you do? |
| *Occupation* | Are you working at the moment? What do you work as? |

## FAMILY HISTORY

| | |
|---|---|
| *Medical* | Anyone in the family suffers from any inherited illnesses? |

## IDEA, CONCERNS, EXPECTATIONS

| | |
|---|---|
| *Idea* | Do you have any ideas as to what was causing your constipation? |
| *Concerns* | Is there anything that is particularly worrying you about it? |
| *Impact on life* | How has it affected you? Do you feel embarrassed by it (overflow)? |

## CSA TIPS

Constipation is a common symptom that patients of all ages can suffer from sometime in their life. Most causes are functional i.e. due to either poor dietary habits or lack of exercise and such patients may only require conservative management to improve their symptoms. Constipation may also be as a result of endocrine or gastrointestinal problems and these should be screened when taking your history.

## PHYSICAL EXAMINATION

| | |
|---|---|
| *Vitals* | BP, weight, temperature |
| *Abdominal* | |
| Inspection | Inspect for signs of peristalsis, distension |
| Palpitation | Palpate the 4 quadrants for any pain, faecal loading and masses (colon cancer) |
| Auscultation | Listen for bowel sounds (tinkling, absence) |
| PR | Inspect for anal fissures and piles. Consider PR if impacted stools |

## INVESTIGATIONS

| | |
|---|---|
| *Bloods* | FBC, ferritin (fe def. – bowel ca), TFTs, PTH, calcium (hypercalcaemia), U&Es (dehydration) |
| *specialist* | Colonoscopy, sigmoidoscopy |

## MANAGEMENT

### Conservative

| | |
|---|---|
| *Water* | Increase oral fluid intake to >2L/d (8 cups). Avoid alcohol and fizzy drinks |

Diet
| | |
|---|---|
| Fruit | Increase fruit and vegetable (x5/d) – e.g. apple, pear, prune, apricot. Dry fruits have higher concentrations of sorbitol. Can be also obtained from fresh fruit juice |
| Fibre | Increase fibre consumption by eating coarse bran, wholegrain bread, flour, brown rice and wholemeal spaghetti. Effects are often rapid but can take as long as 4wks |
| Exercise | Losing weight by exercising can help constipation. Patients who are immobile are more likely to be constipated |

**Medical**

| | |
|---|---|
| Laxatives | Start with bulk forming laxatives. If patient is passing hard stools, consider adding or transferring to an osmotic agent. If the patient still struggles or complains of tenesmus add a stimulant laxative. Be aware of overuse (hypokalemia) and titrating downwards depending on symptoms (diarrhoea) |
| Bulk forming | Increases faecal mass thereby stimulating peristalsis. Takes several days to take effect – e.g. Ispaghula husk, methylcellulose |
| Osmotic | Increases the amount of water in the large bowel – e.g. lactulose, macrogols (movicol), magnesium hydroxide |
| Stimulant | Increases intestinal motility (avoid in obstruction) – e.g. Senna, bisacodyl, sodium docusate |
| Suppositories | Phosphate or glycerol (4g) |
| Impaction | Consider high dose of macrogols in impaction. Add stimulant (senna) if persists. Try suppositories (soft stools – bisacodyl, hard – glycerol/bisacodyl) or mild enema (docusate or sodium citrate). If still poor response, try sodium phosphate enema. Enemas may need to be given several times to release hard impacted stools. Leave on regular laxatives once cleared |

**Refer**

| | |
|---|---|
| Gastroenterologist | Refer for red flags for bowel cancer. Surgical input may be required for anal fissures resistant to treatment. Refer if there is a possible underlying aetiology (e.g. Crohn's) is suspected or no response to treatment |
| Psychiatrist | Psychiatry input may be required if constipation is caused by depression |
| Dietician | Dietician can offer useful advice regarding the patient's diet |

**SAFETY NETTING**

| | |
|---|---|
| Follow up | If symptoms for more than 4-6 weeks re-attend for review. If the patient begins to vomit or suffers and abdominal distension they should seek medical advice |

**DIFFERENTIAL DIAGNOSIS**

| Condition | Characteristic exam feature |
|---|---|
| Anal fissures | Tear to anal mucosa often posterior to anal canal. Pain on defecation with blood on toilet paper. Associated with constipation. OE: fissure visible. PR exam very tender |
| Irritable bowel syndrome | Extremely common. The most consistent features are abdominal pain, bloating and change in bowel habit. Patients may be divided into those with diarrhoea |

| | |
|---|---|
| | predominant IBS and those with constipation predominant IBS. Features such as lethargy, nausea, backache and bladder symptoms may also be present |
| **Colorectal cancer** | Weight loss, PR bleeding and abdominal mass (can be in right iliac fossa). Unexplained iron deficiency anaemia |
| **Intestinal obstruction** | History of adhesions (previous surgery), malignancy. Colicky abdominal pain, distension, absolute constipation including wind. Bowels not opened. 'Tinkling' bowel sounds |
| **Hypothyroidism** | Underactive thyroid gland. Presents with cold intolerance, hair loss, dry skin, fatigability, heavy periods, increased weight, low mood |

## EXPLANATIONS

*Constipation*

Constipation simply means that you are passing stools less often than you normally do. It may also mean you pass painful and hard stools. Sometimes it can cause crampy tummy pain and make you feel bloated or even sick.

Laxatives

Laxatives are medications that help relieve constipation. Some of them work by making the stools bulky and therefore encouraging you to go (bulk forming). Others work by increasing the amount of water in your bowels therefore making the stools pass more smoothly (osmotic). The last type works by encouraging the muscles in the bowel to increase the movement of the stools through your bowels.

Suppositories

Medications can be taken a number of different ways other than by mouth. Special drug preparations that take the form of a pellet can be inserted into the back passage. This is known as a suppository. The best time to insert it is at night before you sleep. Position yourself on your side with one leg straight and the other bent at the knee. Gently insert the capsule about 2–3 cm into your back passage using a finger, making sure it does not slip out immediately. The suppository will then dissolve and be absorbed through the walls of your bowels.

Impaction

Occasionally you can have a very hard stool that gets stuck in the back passage. This can cause very alarming symptoms such as abdominal pain and swelling of your tummy. Sometimes the faeces may leak making you feel that you are having diarrhoea that you have no control over.

# 4.11 Liver disease

The liver is a vital organ what has a wide range of functions including metabolism, detoxification, production of enzymes for digestion and protein synthesis. Given its multiple functions, the liver is prone to disease and damage. It may become infected from hepatitis (A,B,C) damaged, due to alcohol or high fat intake and diseased from overdose of medications (paracetamol). Common symptoms of liver disease include pain, jaundice and malaise.

**HISTORY**

**Open questions**     Can you tell me more about the symptoms you have been feeling? Could you tell me about what has been troubling you?

**Focused questions**

*Jaundice*     Where have you noticed the yellow ting (eyes, skin, mouth)? When did you first notice it? How long have you had it for?

   Onset     Did it come on suddenly (viral) or slowly (cancer)?
   Pruritus     Is your skin itchy?
   Urine & Stools     Have you noticed a change to the colour of your urine (dark) or stools (pale)?

*Lethargy/malaise*     How long have you been feeling tired?
*Bleeding*     Have you noticed any dark blood in your stools? Have you vomited up any blood (varices)?

**Associated history**

*Pain*     Have you experienced any pain anywhere? Can you point to it? Did it come on suddenly (gallstones)?
*Nausea & vomiting*     Do you feel sick or have you vomited? (acute hepatitis)
*Weight loss*     Have you lost any weight recently? (carcinoma)
*Pregnant*     Are you pregnant? (obstetric cholestasis)
*Fever*     Did you feel hot and sweaty or run a fever?

**Risk factors for Hepatitis**

*Blood transfusions*     Have you had any blood transfusions in the past? (<1992)
*Needles*     Have you ever shared needles, had a tattoo or body piercing?
*Travel*     Have you traveled abroad recently (Hep A)? What did you eat (shellfish)?
*Sexual History*     Are you sexually active? Do you have casual sex? Did you use contraception? Do you practice anal sex?

**Differentials**

*Gallstones*     Do you have pain on the right side of your tummy? Does it move to the shoulder tip? Did you notice your urine is darker or your stools are lighter in colour? Did you have an itch?
*Pancreatitis*     Do you have problems flushing away your stools? Do you have upper tummy pain?
*Haemolysis*     Have you been suffering from weakness, dizziness or shortness of breath with your jaundice? Did the problems get worse after taking a medicine or after an infection?
*Primary Biliary Cirrh.*     Do you have itchy skin? Do you have dry mouth and eyes and feel tired all the time?

**RED FLAGS**     Painless jaundice, weight loss

## PAST HISTORY

*Medical*   Have you ever suffered from any medical conditions (raised cholesterol, liver disease, sickle-cell)? Have you had any investigations like an ERCP?

*Surgical*   Did you have any operations for gallstones? Did you have problems after a GA (halothane)?

## FAMILY HISTORY

*Liver*   Are there any illnesses that run in your family (Wilson's disease, haemochromatosis, gallstones, G6PD def.)? Was any of your close family members diagnosed with hepatitis?

## DRUG HISTORY

*Medication*   Are you taking any medications? (aspirin, paracetamol, co-amoxiclav, statins, isoniazid, methotrexate, terbinafine, griseofulvin, quinine, allopurinol, methyldopa, COCP)

## SOCIAL HISTORY

*Alcohol*   Do you drink alcohol? How much do you drink and how often?

*Recreational drugs*   Have you ever used any recreational drugs? Did you ever inject them? Do you share needles?

*Travel*   Did you go abroad? Did you take any immunisations (DTP, Hep A)? Did you have unprotected sexual intercourse when abroad?

*Occupation*   Are you currently working (sewerage worker, health worker, sex worker)?

*Smoker*   Do you smoke? How many cigarettes do you smoke per day?

## IDEA, CONCERNS, EXPECTATIONS

*Ideas*   Have you had any thoughts about what may be causing your symptoms?

*Concerns*   Do you have any worries about the pain you have been experiencing?

*Expectations*   How did you think I could help you today?

*Impact*   How have the symptoms affected your life?

## CSA TIPS

The most common causes of liver dysfunction is due to fatty changes and alcoholic disease. In all patients it is important to try and enquire about diet and alcohol to advise on healthy eating and drinking as part of health promotion. Patients may attend with abnormal liver function tests and you will have to explain the possible causes following a detailed medical history.

## PHYSICAL EXAMINATION

*Vitals*   Temp (fever), BP, pulse, BMI

*Inspection*   Inspect the skin for jaundice (skin, sclera). Look for a scleral Kayser-Fleischer ring (Wilson). Look for signs of liver disease (tremor, clubbing, spider naevi, Dupuytren's, palmar erythema, gynaecomastia, peripheral oedema, ascites)

*Abdominal exam*

Liver   Feel for tenderness and liver edge (smoothy enlarged - hepatitis/cirrhosis, irregular - carcinoma)

Spleen   Feel for an enlarged spleen (malaria, decompensated liver failure)

Gallbladder   Check for palpable gallbladder (gallstones, pancreatic carcinoma)

## INVESTIGATIONS

| | |
|---|---|
| *Bloods* | FBC (low plts), ferritin (haemochromatosis), CRP, Hepatitis serology, LFTs (GGT, ALT, AST, Bili - conjugated and unconjugated, ALP - skeletal and liver isoenzymes), glucose (low), lipids |
| Other | Hb electrophoresis (sickle cell), reticulocytes (haemolysis), viral load, ESR & ANA (PBC), clotting screen (PT/INR), paracetamol levels (overdose), serum copper, malaria screen, alpha-1-antitrypsin levels, AFP, amylase (pancreatitis) |
| *Urine* | Bilirubin and urobilinogen |
| *US* | Liver US |
| *Specialist* | Liver biopsy, Liver MRI/CT, OGD (varices), ERCP, MRCP |

---

### Interpreting Liver function blood tests

| | |
|---|---|
| AST > ALT | Fatty liver, alcoholic hepatitis, cirrhosis, liver cancer, haemolytic jaundice |
| ALT > AST | Acute hepatitis (viral, drug, autoimmune), obstructive jaundice |
| High ALT >500 IU/l | Viral hepatitis, drug induced (paracetamol OD), autoimmune hepatitis |
| >GGT & >MCV | Alcohol abuse. If raised ALT consider alcohol hepatitis |
| >GGT & >ALP | Cholestasis |

### Interpreting Hepatitis B Serology Results

| State | HBsAg | Anti-HBc | Anti-HBs | IgM anti-HBc |
|---|---|---|---|---|
| Susceptible | -ve | -ve | -ve | |
| Immune by infection | -ve | +ve | +ve | |
| Immune by hep B vac | -ve | -ve | +ve | |
| Acute infection | +ve | +ve | -ve | +ve |
| Chronic infection | +ve | +ve | -ve | -ve |
| Resolving infection | -ve | +ve | -ve | |

---

| MANAGEMENT | *treat underlying cause* |
|---|---|
| **Fatty Liver** | Eat a healthy balanced diet. Cut down on fried and fatty foods. Exercise daily. Cut down on alcohol intake (M: 3u/d F:2u/d) or aim to stop |
| **Alcoholic hepatitis** | Aim to stop alcohol intake. See Alcoholism chapter |
| **Hepatitis** | Hepatitis A: Reassure as self-limiting (most <2mth). Avoid alcohol as resolves. Hepatitis B & C: refer to specialist (hepatologist) |
| *Prevention* | |
| Hygiene | Wash hands with soap & water after going toilet or before handling food |
| Needles | Do not share needles. Attend needle sharing program |
| Condoms | Use condoms when having sexual intercourse |
| Tattoos | Go to tattoo parlours that sterilize or use disposable equipment |
| Travel | Ensure you take Hep A, DPT travel vaccines and malaria prophylaxis. Avoid eating raw seafood when traveling |
| *Pain* | Treat pain with paracetamol/NSAIDs or codeine. Reduce dose of paracetamol (1gm bd) and avoid codeine if severe liver dysfunction |
| *Nausea* | Offer metoclopramide for short duration |
| *Pruritus* | Wear loose clothing, avoid hot showers. Give piriton but avoid in severe impairment. Cholestyramine or ursodeoxycholic acid if unresponsive (specialist) |
| *Refer* | Consider referring to GUM, drugs support team for IV users for cause |

| *Haemochromatosis* | Avoid food rich in iron. Regular (weekly) phlebotomy until serum iron in normal range. Then 3 monthly. Consider chelation therapy (specialist) if phlebotomy CI |
|---|---|

| *Cirrhosis* | Refer to a specialist to monitor. Urgent medical team admission if signs of encephalopathy |
|---|---|
| *Immunisation* | Should get yearly influenza and one-off pneumococcus |
| *Specialist led* | 6-12 mth bloods for LFTs, AFP (carcinoma). On waiting list for liver transplant |
| Diet | High protein and high calorie diet. Consider thiamine replacement |
| Ascites | Treat with salt and fluid (<1.5L/day) restriction. Give spironolactone and furosemide Prophylactic abx if Hx of spontaneous bacterial peritonitis |
| Varices | Beta blocker for medium sized varices and consider OGD for ligation |

| *Pancreatitis* | Treat cause by removing gallstones |
|---|---|
| *Conservative* | Avoid alcohol, high protein, low fat diet. High calorie diet. Refer dietician |
| Acute | Admission for IV fluids, analgesia and nutrition |
| Chronic | Stop smoking and alcohol. Eat a low-fat diet and offer analgesia if pain |
| Creons | Prescribe to help digestion if steatorrhoea present |

| *Gallstones* | |
|---|---|
| *Conservative* | Lose weight, exercise and adhere to low fat diet. Stop smoking |
| *Medical* | Do not remove asymptomatic gallstones. If signs of acute cholecystitis admit patient for IV abx. Offer analgesia if painful. Refer routinely for cholecystectomy, lithotripsy or ursodeoxycholic acid |

## DIFFERENTIAL DIAGNOSIS

| Condition | Characteristic exam feature |
|---|---|
| **Hepatitis B, C** | Hx of blood transfusion, IV drugs or tattoo. Hep C may be acquired from travel to Africa, Middle East & Asia. May be engaged in high-risk intercourse (anal). Usually asymptomatic but patients may present with a prodrome of weakness, malaise, fever and tiredness. Later disease causes jaundice, weight loss. OE: jaundice, signs of liver disease |
| **Hepatitis A** | Hx of travel to Africa & Asia. May get a prodrome of weakness, malaise, fever and joint pain. Later may cause jaundice, pale stools and dark urine. OE: fever, jaundice |
| **Gallstones** | Calculi formed in gallbladder or duct. Affects female, >40yr, obese more. Can have FHx. May be asymptomatic. If impacted may cause RUQ pain radiating to shoulder tip, jaundice, N&V and fever. OE: fever, jaundice, RUQ pain. +ve Murphy's sign seen in cholecystitis (2 fingers over RUQ. Ask pt to breathe in, pt stops due to pain. Repeat over LUQ) |
| **Pancreatitis** | Often caused by gallstones or alcohol excess. Patients present with severe epigastric pain radiating to the back along with nausea and vomiting. In chronic pancreatitis, patients may complain of difficulty in flushing away their stools that are paler and offensive. OE: jaundice, fever, epigastric pain with rigidity, Cullen's (umbilical bruising) |

| | |
|---|---|
| | and Grey Turney's (flank bruising) signs |
| **Gilbert's Syndrome** | Inherited condition and may be +ve FHx. Usually asymptomatic but may develop jaundice from time to time especially after an infection or excess exercise. OE: nil to find |
| **Hemochromatosis** | Inherited condition of iron overload. Usually begins in >40yrs. Causes symptoms of fatigue, erectile dysfunction (men), amenorrhea (women), joint pain. Leads to diabetes, liver and heart failure. OE: bronzed skin, hepatomegaly |

**EXPLANATIONS**

*Abnormal LFTs*   We have got your blood tests back and one of them shows that your liver is working a little harder than expected. This may be entirely normal following an infection or taking certain medications (statin); however, in some cases there may be an underlying illness.

*Fatty liver*   This is a condition where there is too much fat in your liver. This can be caused by eating too much fatty food or drinking too much alcohol which the liver has converted into fat. The liver plays an important role in controlling the levels of fat in your the body, however in your case it is working too hard.

*Alcoholic hepatitis*   This is a condition where there is liver damage related to excessive alcohol consumption over a period of time. The liver plays an important role in cleaning poisons and toxins from the body. However in your case it is working too hard. Mild alcoholic hepatitis is often reversible so if we stop drinking your liver can return back to normal function. Severe alcoholic hepatitis can be permanent and cause cirrhosis, which is irreversible damage.

*Cirrhosis*   This is often the last stage of liver disease where the liver tissue has been replaced with scar tissue. Unfortunately, it is not reversible but if you stop drinking immediately this may help to prevent further damage.

*Viral Hepatitis*   This is where your liver is inflamed because of a viral infection. It can cause symptoms such as muscle aches, temperature, feeling sick and give you a yellow tinge to your skin.

Hepatitis A   Hepatitis A is one of the most common causes and is often contracted when traveling abroad and eating something that is contaminated with faeces from someone else with the virus. Symptoms often get better within 3 months.

Hepatitis B   This virus is found within blood and bodily fluids. It can be contracted if someone has unprotected sex, shares needles to inject drugs, or passed from pregnant mother to baby through delivery or breast feeding.

Hepatitis C   This virus is found within the blood and bodily fluids including saliva. It is often spread through blood to blood contact such as sharing injected needles or less often through sex.

| | |
|---|---|
| *Gilberts* | This is not really an illness but a fairly common and harmless condition. It is usually inherited and we find it on routine blood tests. One of the markers of liver function called bilirubin is mildly raised. People with Gilbert's break down bilirubin at a slower rate than others and it may build up in the blood instead of passing out in your 'wee'. Usually you will have no symptoms but occasionally, you may notice a yellow tinge to your eyes or skin (jaundice) after fasting, exercising or suffering an infection. |
| *Haemochromatosis* | This is a disease that is usually inherited as a faulty gene from your parents. It relates to the levels of iron in your body and the faulty gene causes your body to absorb more iron than others. Over time, the iron builds up in the body and is laid down in the skin, joints and sometimes in the heart or liver. People suffering with haemochromatosis may feel tired, or notice that they have a 'tanned appearance' to their skin. Over time, the iron may make the liver and heart work harder, eventually leading to permanent damage and eventually, failure. |

# 5.1 Erectile dysfunction

Erectile dysfunction or impotence is defined as the inability to attain or maintain an erection for satisfactory sexual performance. It is an acutely embarrassing problem for patients, that affects almost 40% of 40-70 year olds. The vast majority of patients are too embarrassed to seek medical advice regarding their problem. It can be due to psychological problems, but a large percentage of patients have some sort of underlying condition. When presenting, it is useful to screen for cardiovascular disease i.e. HTN, hypercholesterolemia, PVD as well as DM as they may be a causal factor in erectile dysfunction.

**HISTORY**

| | |
|---|---|
| **Reassure** | I just want to reassure that whilst you may feel embarrassed to talk about your problem it is something that we see and treat patients with everyday. |
| **Open questions** | Please can you tell me a little bit more about your problems maintaining an erection? |
| *Understanding* | What do you mean by being impotent/erectile dysfunction? Can I just clarify that when you say 'down below' that you mean you have problems with your penis? |

**Focused questions**

| | |
|---|---|
| *Erectile dysfunction* | When did it start? How long has it been going on for? |
| Consistency | Do you have problems initiating or maintaining an erection? Did it come on gradually or slowly? |
| Morning | Do you wake up with erections in the morning? |
| Masturbation | Do you masturbate? Have you had any difficulty getting erections when you do so? |

**Associated history** *if relevant*

| | |
|---|---|
| *Sexual history* | When was the last time you had sex? |
| Partner | Was it with your regular sexual partner? Are they male or female (if they use the term 'partner' without qualifying it)? Did you also have erectile problems with them? |
| STI | Any sexually transmitted infections (STIs) in the past or penile discharge? |

**Differentials**

| | |
|---|---|
| Stress | How has your mood been recently? Do you have any stress at work or in the relationship (performance anxiety, fear of intimacy)? |
| *IHD* | Do you have any chest pain? Do you have raised cholesterol levels? |
| *Back Pain* | Do you have back pain? Does the pain move to the buttocks or legs? |
| *Hypogonadism* | Have you lost your sexual drive? Are your losing body hair? Have you noticed any swellings around your nipples or breast growth? |

**RED FLAGS**   Chest pain, disc prolapse

**PAST HISTORY**

| | |
|---|---|
| *Medical* | Do you suffer from any medical problems? (depression, CKD, DM, prostate cancer, spinal cord injury, polio, Parkinson's disease) |
| *Penile problems* | Do you have any problems with your penis? (small, hypospadias, Peyronie's) |
| *Surgery* | Have you had any recent surgery? (pelvic, prostatectomy - TURP) |

**DRUG HISTORY**

| | |
|---|---|
| *Medication* | Are you taking any medications? |

| Worsen | Antihypertensives (thiazides), antidepressants (TCA, SSRI's), finasteride, cimetidine, beta-blockers, methotrexate, carbamazepine |
|---|---|

## SOCIAL HISTORY

| | |
|---|---|
| *Relationship* | Are you currently in a relationship? How are things? Any arguments or rows? How does your partner feel about your problem? |
| *Occupation* | Are you working at the moment? What do you work as? |
| *Cycling* | Do you cycle more than 3hrs a week? |
| *Smoker* | Do you smoke? How many cigarettes do you smoke per day? |
| *Alcohol* | Do you drink alcohol? How much do you drink and how often? |
| *Illicit Drugs* | Have you experimented with any drugs? (cannabis) |

## FAMILY HISTORY

| | |
|---|---|
| *Cardiac* | Anyone in the family suffer from heart problems? (IHD, DM, PVD) |

## IDEA, CONCERNS, EXPECTATIONS

| | |
|---|---|
| *Idea* | Do you have any ideas as to what was causing your erectile problems? |
| *Concern* | Do you have any specific worries about your problem? Are you worried that you cannot perform as well as you had hoped? |
| *Impact of life* | How has this problem affected you? Has it affected your relationship? |

## CSA TIPS

Erectile dysfunction is a common problem, particularly in the older male. Most patients attending will drop cues or hints that there is some problem with their relationship or performance, hoping that you are able to pick these up and explore further. Try and make the patient feel at ease and provide a reassuring statement that there is no need to feel embarrassed. Although a large percentage of ED is due to psychological disease, ensure that you risk stratify for IHD that is commonly associated especially in the middle-aged.

## PHYSICAL EXAMINATION

| | |
|---|---|
| *Vitals* | BP, Weight, BMI |
| *Genitalia* | Do not perform routinely. Only if structural problems are considered. Hypogonadism, 2ndary sexual characteristics (gynaecomastia, hair distribution), structural abnormalities (Peyronie disease, hypospadia) |
| PR | If prostate problems are considered |
| *Back Exam* | Check for lumbar spine tenderness, reduced SLR, sensation & reflexes |
| *Cardiovascular* | Consider peripheral vascular as well as cardiovascular exam if patient has risk factors |

## INVESTIGATIONS

| | |
|---|---|
| *Bloods* | U&E, fasting lipid profile and glucose. |
| Other | PSA, testosterone (morning), SHBG, FSH, LH, prolactin, LFT |
| *Urine* | Dipstick urine (diabetes) |
| *ECG* | Consider performing a routine ECG (IHD, LVH) |
| *CVD* | 10 year QRisk score |

## MANAGEMENT
### Conservative

| | |
|---|---|
| *Smoking* | Recommend to stop smoking. Refer to smoking cessation clinic |
| *Alcohol* | Reduce intake to < 21 units /wk for men, < 14 units/wk for females |
| *Exercise* | If overweight advise to lose weight and increase exercise |

| Cycling | If cycles >3hrs/wk then advise cessation to see if symptom improves. Advise to use comfortable padded bike seat placed at the correct height |
|---|---|
| Psychogenic | Offer counselling such as psychosexual counselling, couple counselling ('Relate'). Offer self help books: 'Treat yourself to sex' |

**Medical**

| Medication Review | Substitute medications that can cause impotence with alternatives |
|---|---|
| PDE-5 inhibitor | Consider sildenafil (private prescription unless fulfils exemption criteria) or 2nd line vardenafil or tadalafil. Try daily tadalafil if poor response |
| Viagra | Sildenafil (phosphodiesterase type V inhibitor) taken <1hr of planned sexual intercourse with partner engaged in foreplay. Onset is delayed if taken with food. Does not initiate erection, but requires sexual stimulation to facilitate. Diabetics may need to take maximum dose |
| CI | Avoided if unstable angina, strokes, recent MI, ↓BP or if on nitrates |
| Side-effects | Flushing, headaches, gastrointestinal (acid reflux), headache |
| Complications | To seek medical advice if erection >4hrs or sudden loss of vision |
| NHS prescriptions | Available on NHS if being treated for prostate cancer, CKD, spinal cord injury, DM, MS, polio, Parkinson's disease, radical pelvic surgery, prostatectomy (not TURP) or already received medication for impotence <14.9.98. Also prescribe if initiated from specialist services for men suffering severe distress due to erectile dysfunction |

**Comparing PDE5 Inhibitors -** *Ref: Adapted from BHF Factfile: Drugs for Erectile Dysfunction 2005*

| Drug | Peak action | Duration of action | Dose |
|---|---|---|---|
| Sildenafil | 1hr | 4-6hr | 25, 50, 100mg |
| Tadalafil | 2hr | 36-48hr | 10, 20mg |
| Vardenafil | 1hr | 4-6hr | 5, 10, 20mg |

| **Refer** | Offer to refer to erectile dysfunction clinic or endocrinologist if hormone abnormalities. Consider referring to cardiologist if severe IHD |
|---|---|

**SAFETY NETTING**

| Follow up | Review patient if symptoms persist for more than 4-6wks |
|---|---|
| Admission | If prolonged erection or chest pain after using the medication seek medical advice |

**EXPLANATIONS**

| Erectile dysfunction | This is when a person is unable to maintain an erection. Although there are a number of causes including drugs, stress and low mood, the most common cause is due to narrowing of the blood vessels supplying the penis caused by fat build up. |
|---|---|
| PDE-5 inhibitor | This is a tablet that we use to help improve erectile problems in men. When you are sexually excited, the blood supply to the penis increases and this helps make it stand erect. The tablet helps to relax the blood vessels that supply the penis and make the erection stronger. However, they only work if you are sexually excited. They do not make an erection happen on their own. |

# 5.2 Prostate Specific Antigen (PSA)

Prostate Specific Antigen is a glycoprotein that is specifically produced from both healthy as well as malignant prostate cells. It is often used as a screening tool to diagnose prostate cancer even before symptoms have begun. A single PSA result is usually insufficient to make a diagnosis, and a repeat blood test is needed when considering cancer. Whilst it may be a sensitive test, it lacks specificity for prostate carcinomas and can be raised in prostatitis, BPH, following urinary catheterisation and after a PR exam.

---

**Features of Prostate Cancer**

| | |
|---|---|
| *Risk factors* | Age (>65 yrs), FHx: 1st degree relatives or breast ca, African-Caribbean, diet (low fruit intake, high fat and meat) |
| *History* | Often symptomless. Hesitancy, post void dribbling, urinary retention, haematuria |
| *Examination* | Hard asymmetrical irregular non-tender prostate with central sulcus loss |
| *Metastatic* | Weight loss, back pain, fractures, spinal cord compression |

---

**HISTORY**

| | |
|---|---|
| **Open questions** | Can you tell me more about why you would like to have a PSA test? |
| *Understanding* | Can you tell me what you already know about it? |
| *Concerns* | Is there anything in particular that worried you for you to want the test today? |
| *Introduction* | Before I begin explaining what the PSA test is about, can I ask you a few questions about your health? |

**Focused questions**

| | |
|---|---|
| *Urinary* | Do you have any problems passing urine? |
| Frequency | Are you going more often than normal? |
| Stream | Is your urine stream not as strong as it used to be? (hesitancy) |
| Dribbling | After you finish passing urine does some still trickle or dribble out? |
| Nocturia | Do you awake at night to pass urine? |
| Erectile Dysfunc. | Do you have any problems initiating or maintaining an erection? |

**Differentials**

| | |
|---|---|
| *DM* | Do you pass a lot of urine at night? Are you thirsty all the time? Have you lost any weight? |
| *UTI* | Any pain or burning feeling when passing urine? Do you get tummy pain or any fevers? |
| *Prostate cancer* | Have you lost any weight? Do you have any back pain (metastasis)? Any blood in your urine? |

**RED FLAGS**

| | |
|---|---|
| *Metastasis* | Back pain, weight loss, haematuria |

**PAST HISTORY**

| | |
|---|---|
| *Medical* | Do you suffer from any medical problems? (DM, BPH, prostate ca) |

**SOCIAL HISTORY**

| | |
|---|---|
| *Smoker* | Do you smoke? How many cigarettes do you smoke per day? |
| *Alcohol* | Do you drink alcohol? How much do you drink and how often? |

## FAMILY HISTORY

*Cancer*                      Does anyone in your close family suffer from prostate or breast cancer?

## CSA TIPS

The PSA test is not a diagnostic test per se. However, many patients have been conditioned that it is an absolute test for prostate cancer. Men, who are notoriously bad at attending their GPs, may attend demanding this test as part of a general health check-up. It is important to discuss the pros and cons of the test and to explain the role the PSA test has in a way that is neither condescending nor paternalistic. You should communicate the fact that a –ve test does not negate the presence of prostatic cancer, and that 2/3 of patients with a raised PSA, post biopsy has no evidence of cancer.

## PHYSICAL EXAMINATION

*Vitals*          BP, Weight, BMI
*General*         Observe the patient to check if they are cachectic or pale
*PR*              Consider performing after blood test or if has haematuria, back pain, weight loss, erectile dysfunction to exclude prostate cancer

## INVESTIGATIONS

*Urine*           Dipstick urine or MSU to exclude infection
*Bloods*          U&E, and PSA, fasting glucose
*MRI*             Spine for bony mets
*Questionnaire*   Severity of symptoms of prostatism can be assessed by using the International Prostate Symptom Score (IPSS)

---

**Interpreting PSA blood tests**

| Age | PSA level (ng/ml) |
| --- | --- |
| 50-60 years | 3.0 |
| 60-70 years | 4.0 |
| > 70 years | 5.0 |

---

## EXPLANATIONS

*Prostate*        The prostate is a gland that is found under the bladder in men. Its job is to produce fluid that sperm bathes in. Passing through the prostate is your water pipe known as the urethra. Sometimes problems with the prostate may narrow this tube and cause problems such as passing too much urine, dribbling and difficulty when trying to pee with a weak stream.

*PSA Screening test*   The PSA test is a simple blood test that looks at the health of the prostate gland. It is a screening test and not a diagnostic one. It can be raised in a number of conditions including prostate cancer, urinary or prostate infection, or an enlarged prostate.

---

**Pros and Cons of the PSA test**

*Advantage*       Reassurance if blood test is normal, raises awareness of cancer before symptoms occur, finds cancer early permitting treatment to be started earlier
*Disadvantage*    Can occasionally falsely reassure and miss cancer, unnecessary worry and invasive testing if falsely +ve, cannot distinguish between fast and slow growing cancers

---

| Blood tests | When doing the blood test it is important to bear in mind that certain things such as exercise, sex or a urinary infection may affect the results |
|---|---|
| Normal | If the blood test is normal it is unlikely that you have prostate cancer. However, the test is not 100% accurate, and 20% of men with a normal PSA may still have prostate cancer |
| Raised | Having a raised PSA does not necessary mean you have prostate cancer. In fact 2/3 of men with a raised PSA level will not have prostate cancer. However, we can offer you further tests to rule it out |

**Factors that affect the PSA tests**

| Conditions | Delay PSA test until: | Conditions | Delay PSA test until: |
|---|---|---|---|
| Vigorous exercise | 48 hours | Proven UTI | 4 weeks |
| Sex/ejaculation | 48 hours | Prostate biopsy | 6 weeks |
| PR exam | 1 week | | |

| Invasive test | If your PSA level is raised, we can refer you to a specialist to have a prostate biopsy to make sure you do not have cancer. This means taking samples of the prostate through the back passage and then looking at them in detail under a microscope for the presence of cancer cells. |
|---|---|

# 5.3 Haematuria

Haematuria signifies the presence of blood in the urine. It can be an incidental finding on a dipstick (microscopic) or with frank haematuria (macroscopic), an alarming and frightening experience for the patient. It is often difficult to quantify the severity of haematuria as the amount of blood passed may not correlate with the significance of the underlying disorder. However, its presence should warrant thorough investigation. Haematuria could be due to dysfunction at any point of the urinary tract, from the molecular level at the kidneys, down to trauma or damage to the urethra. Non-renal causes should also be consider and include bleeding disorder, trauma, infarction and anticoagulants.

## HISTORY

| | |
|---|---|
| **Open questions** | Tell me more about your problem? |
| *Understanding* | What do you mean when you say 'blood in your urine'? |

**Focused questions**

| | |
|---|---|
| *Haematuria* | When did it start? How long has it been going on for? |
| Colour | What colour is your urine? Is it bright red, pink or brown colour? |
| Duration | When in your stream do you notice the blood? Is it at the beginning of the stream (urethral), the middle (renal/ureter), towards the end (neck of bladder) or throughout? |
| Severity | Have you passed any clots? |

---

**Causes of Haematuria**

| | |
|---|---|
| *Transient microscopic* | UTI, periods, intensive exercise, intercourse |
| *Persistent microscopic* | Cancer (bladder, kidney, prostate), renal stones, BPH, prostatitis, urethritis (Chlamydia), renal (IgA nephropathy) |

---

**Associated history**

| | |
|---|---|
| *Frequency* | Are you passing urine more often than you normally do? |
| *Fever* | Have you had any fever, sweats or shakes (rigors) recently? |
| *Pain* | Do you have any tummy pain? Can you point to it (bladder, loin)? Is it burning, cramping or does it come and go? |

**Differentials**

| | |
|---|---|
| *UTI* | Have you had any abdominal pain? Are you passing urine more often or any discomfort like burning when you are urinating? |
| *Renal stone* | Do you have any pain in your back that moves towards your groin? Is it a dull aching pain? Does it come and go? |
| *Bladder cancer* | Any weight loss? Are you passing clots? |
| *Prostatic* | Is your stream weaker than normal? When you finish do you dribble afterwards? Do you have any back or bone pain (metastasis)? |
| *Pyelonephritis* | Do you have swinging fevers? Do you have pain over your loin area? Have you been feeling sick or vomited? |
| *Glomerulonephritis* | Did you have a sore throat before the urine problems started? Was your urine frothy? Do you have any leg or face swelling? |
| *Vasculitis* | Do you have any joint or muscle pains? Do you feel tired, weak and hot all the time? |

| STI | Have you had unprotected casual sex recently? Any urethral discharge? Any pain or burning when passing urine (chlamydia)? |
|---|---|

## RED FLAGS

| Urinary | Frank haematuria, painless haematuria (>50yr), microscopic haematuria (>40yr) |
|---|---|
| Other | Weight loss, night sweats |

## PAST HISTORY

| Medical | Do you suffer from any medical problems (Sickle cell disease, blood disorders, recurrent UTIs, renal stones, recent illness or sore throats)? |
|---|---|
| Surgery | Have you had any recent surgery (TURP, cystoscopy, prostatectomy)? Did you have a urinary catheter recently? |

## DRUG HISTORY

| Medication | Are you taking any medications? |
|---|---|
| Worsens | Aspirin, warfarin, NSAIDs, rifampicin (orange urine), nitrofurantoin (brown urine) |

## FAMILY HISTORY

| Renal | Does anyone in the family have kidney problems (polycystic, hereditary nephritis)? |
|---|---|

## SOCIAL HISTORY

| Occupation | Are you working at the moment (dye or rubber industry- bladder ca)? |
|---|---|
| Travel | Have you ever been abroad to the tropics or subtropics? Did you swim in any rivers, canals or lakes when there (schistosomiasis)? |
| Smoker | Do you smoke? How many cigarettes do you smoke per day? |
| Alcohol | Do you drink alcohol? How much do you drink and how often? |
| Diet | How is your diet (beetroot, rhubarb - red urine, fava beans - orange urine)? |
| Renal stones | Do you drink lots of water? Do you eat lots of meat or spinach? |

## IDEA, CONCERNS, EXPECTATIONS

| Idea | Do you have any ideas as to what was causing your blood in your urine? |
|---|---|
| Concern | Do you have any specific worries about your problem? |

## CSA TIPS

Haematuria is a frightening symptom for patients and would induce much confusion and anxiety. Attending the surgery, the patient may be quite worried and would be seeking reassurance from the GP. The most common cause of haematuria is due to UTIs and it would be pertinent to take a concise history to confirm or negate this. You should try and educate the patient as to the possible causes and ensure that you safety net clearly so that the patient knows when to seek medical advice if symptoms persist.

## PHYSICAL EXAMINATION

| Vitals | BP (raised), pulse |
|---|---|
| Abdominal exam | Palpate the abdomen for any pain (loin, flank, suprapubic area) |
| PR | If prostate problems are considered |

## INVESTIGATIONS

| Bloods | FBC, haematinics, U&E, eGFR |
|---|---|
| Other | ESR, CRP, complement levels (nephropathy), PSA (prostate), CK (rhabdomyolysis), clotting screening |

| | |
|---|---|
| Urine | Dipstick urine to confirm blood, nitrates (UTI) and protein (glomerulonephritis). MC&S, cytology, ACR |
| Scans | KUB - Renal stones, US - Renal pathology (polycystic kidney), prostate |
| Specialist | CT scan, cystoscopy, blood cultures, renal biopsy |

**MANAGEMENT**    *treat underlying cause*
**UTI**

| | |
|---|---|
| Conservative | Encourage fluids & cranberry juice, urinate often when you feel the urge, wipe from front to back, wear cotton and loose fitting undergarments. Avoid nylon, tight jeans and bubble baths |
| Medical | Initiate antibiotics depending on sensitivity. Consider trimethoprim 1st line (200mg bd for 3/7: F and 7/7: M) nitrofurantoin or cephalexin |
| Pregnant | 1st line, nitrofurantoin (50mg qds) |
| Recurrent | Offer a stand-by course of antibiotics if they suffer with recurrent UTIs. If more than 3x UTI's a year, consider prescribing prophylaxis |
| Sex | If UTIs occur post sexual intercourse advise patient to wash genitals before and after sex. Post sex, advise to empty bladder. Consider stat abx <2hrs prior to intercourse. Stop using spermicide and use condoms |
| Pain | Simple analgesia (paracetamol, codeine) or NSAIDs. Ensure no CI for NSAIDS (PU, asthma) |

| | |
|---|---|
| **Pyelonephritis** | Consider admission if signs of dehydration or sepsis. Treat with antibiotics (co-amoxiclav or ciprofloxacin 500mg bd for 10/7)) |

**Renal stones**

| | |
|---|---|
| Conservative | Increase fluid intake (3L/d). Depending on type offer dietary advice (avoid spinach, red meat). See renal stones chapter |
| Medical | Offer NSAIDS (diclofenac) for pain and antiemetics (cyclizine) |

**Bladder Cancer**

| | |
|---|---|
| Conservative | Stop smoking. Avoid exposure to occupations manufacturing dyes and rubber |
| Medical | Refer urgently within 2 weeks |

| | |
|---|---|
| **Prostatitis** | Treat with antibiotics for up to 4wks (trimethoprim, ciprofloxacin) |
| **Refer** | Refer if red flag symptoms of painless macroscopic haematuria, >40yr with recurrent or persistent UTI associated with haematuria, >50yr with unexplained microscopic haematuria |

**SAFETY NETTING**

| | |
|---|---|
| Follow up | Review patient if symptoms persist for >4-6wks or sooner if red flags symptoms |

**DIFFERENTIAL DIAGNOSIS**

| Condition | Characteristic exam feature |
|---|---|
| **Bladder cancer** | Primarily papillary transitional cell carcinoma. 50% association with smoking or occupation in dye, textile or rubber industry. Presents with painless macroscopic |

| | |
|---|---|
| | haematuria in the absence of fevers |
| **UTIs** | Affects females >males. E. coli most common organism. Lower urinary tract symptoms include abdominal pain, frequency, dysuria and haematuria. Suprabladder infections (i.e. renal) may cause in addition fever, vomiting and general malaise. Confirmed with +ve dipsticks for leucocytes and nitrates |
| **Renal stone** | Most common type is calcium stones. More common in males and associated with medication (e.g. loop or thiazide diuretics) and diet. Presents with sudden onset of loin or flank pain radiating to groin. Often with very severe colicky pain |
| **Prostate cancer** | Usually adenocarcinoma. 2nd most common cancer in men. Symptoms include urgency, frequency, hesitancy and nocturia. Metastatic spread is often characterised by weight loss and bony pain |
| **Pyelonephritis** | More common in females. Patient may have underlying structural abnormalities. Present with uni or bilateral loin pain, fevers, rigors and nausea and vomiting. Lower UTI symptoms of frequency, dysuria and haematuria may also be present. OE: appears pale and unwell. Fever and back pain may be present |

## EXPLANATIONS

*MSU* — Because of the symptoms you have described I wish to carry out a urine test. What this involves is you providing me a fresh specimen of urine in this sterile container. So that we do not get any misleading results it is important that you follow what I say as closely as you can. Before providing the sample of urine, it is important that you clean and wash the area down below well. Do not allow your skin or body to touch the bottle when passing urine. When you begin to pass urine, do not collect the initial part, but when you are mid-stream fill the container from then onwards. Once you are done please return the bottle to me.

*UTI* — A urinary tract infection is an infection that affects the urinary tract; usually the bladder (called cystitis) or the urethra - the tube that carries the urine out of the body. The infection is normally from a bacteria but we don't always know why it happens. Sometimes bugs that sit on the skin, or those from the back passage passes into the urinary tract, or after having sex. Once inside, they give symptoms of going to the toilet frequently, pain or burning and you may even have a fever.

*Pyelonephritis* — This is the medical term that describes a kidney infection. It happens when an infection travels up from the lower urinary tract (urethra, bladder) and infects the kidney. It usually presents with similar symptoms to a UTI but is usually more severe. Patients may feel very hot and may even get pain over the outer tummy areas.

# 5.4 Renal stones

Urinary tract stones or kidneys stones are common; with one person in twenty suffering from a stone at some point in their life. Although stones are commonly associated with dehydration or dietary intake, they can also be caused by a number of medical conditions including gout, hyperparathyroidism, renal tubular acidosis and by inherited metabolic conditions including cystinuria and hyperoxaluria. Renal stones usually present with sudden onset, colicky abdominal pain with the passing of blood in urine and may be severe enough to cause nausea and vomiting.

## Features of Renal Stones

| | |
|---|---|
| *Risk factors* | FHx, dehydration, chronic UTI, gout, hypercalcaemia, cystinuria, hyperoxaluria, abnormal kidneys (horseshoe) |
| *History* | Acute colicky abdominal pain but can be constant, often described as a dull ache. Has been described as the worst pain experienced (worse than childbirth). Loin pain (kidney), suprapubic (bladder), pain radiates to groin (ureteric) |
| *Examination* | Tender flank or loin area. Can be writhing in pain. Haematuria on dipstick |

## HISTORY

**Open questions**       Tell me more about the tummy pain you have been experiencing?

**Focused questions**

| | |
|---|---|
| *Renal stones* | When did it start? How long has it been going on for? |
| Site | Where exactly is the pain (loin, flank)? |
| Radiation | Does the pain move anywhere, such as to your groin? |
| Severity | How severe is the pain on a scale of 1 to 10, ten being the most severe? |
| Character | How would you describe it? Does it come and go (colicky) or is it there all the time? |
| Triggers | Does anything make it better or worse? |

**Associated history**

| | |
|---|---|
| *Haematuria* | Have you noticed any blood in your urine? |

**Differentials**

| | |
|---|---|
| *UTI* | Have you had any abdominal pain, passing urine more often or discomfort when you are urinating? |
| *Pyelonephritis* | Any fever, sweats or shakes? Have you felt sick or vomited? |

## RED FLAGS

| | |
|---|---|
| *Obstruction* | Urinary hesitancy, poor stream or oliguria |
| *Other* | Haematuria, intolerable severe abdominal pain (aortic aneurysm), pain not responding after 1hr of medication, pregnant, CKD |

## PAST HISTORY

| | |
|---|---|
| *Previous* | Have you ever had any similar symptoms or renal stones in the past? |
| *Medical* | Do you suffer from any medical problems? Abnormal kidney (horseshoe kidney or medullary sponge kidney), metabolic problems (gout, hypercalcaemia, hyperparathyroidism, cystinuria)? |

## DRUG HISTORY

| | |
|---|---|
| *Medication* | Are you taking any medications? |
| Worsen | Adcal - calcium + Vit D, steroids, NSAIDs, diuretics (loop, thiazide) |

## SOCIAL HISTORY

| | |
|---|---|
| *Occupation* | Are you working at the moment? (dye or rubber industry- bladder ca) |
| *Smoker* | Do you smoke? How many cigarettes do you smoke per day? |
| *Alcohol* | Do you drink alcohol? How much do you drink and how often? |
| *Diet* | How is your diet (too much meat, in particular liver, spinach, rhubarb, chocolates)? |
| Fluids | Do you drink a sufficient amount of water (2L+)? |

## IDEA, CONCERNS, EXPECTATIONS

| | |
|---|---|
| *Idea* | Do you have any ideas as to what may be causing your abdominal pain? |
| *Concerns* | Do you have any specific worries about your problem? |

## CSA TIPS

Renal stones usually present out of the blue and with excruciating pain. Patients presenting acutely should be initially rehydrated and offered IM pain relief, before taking a history once they settle. Recurrent or chronic stones may require secondary care referral for operative treatments. However, in all cases, take a thorough fluid and diet history and offer conservative advice to reduce the risk of recurrence.

## PHYSICAL EXAMINATION

| | |
|---|---|
| *Vitals* | BP, pulse, temperature |
| *Abdominal exam* | Palpate the abdomen for any pain (loin, flank, suprapubic area). Exclude aortic aneurysm |

## INVESTIGATIONS

| | |
|---|---|
| *Bloods* | FBC, U&E, calcium & phosphate, CRP, uric acid, LFTs (albumin, ALP) |
| *Urine* | Dipstick (pH-urate stones, haematuria, proteinuria, nitrates). MSU |
| *KUB* | Renal stones (90% radio-opaque) |
| *US* | Underlying renal pathology |
| *Sieve* | Sieve the urine to capture stones (difficult to do) |
| *Specialist* | IVU, spiral CT scan, cystoscopy |

## MANAGEMENT

### Conservative

| | |
|---|---|
| *Reassure* | Most stones <5mm pass spontaneously |
| *Fluid intake* | Increase fluid intake to >3L/d and reduce salt intake (<3g/d). Avoid tea (calcium oxalate) or alcohol (particularly binge) |
| *Diet* | Recommend balanced diet with lots of fruit and vegetables. Avoid grapefruit juice. Offer specific dietary advice depending on type of stone |

---

### Dietary Advice depending on Type of Stone

| | |
|---|---|
| *Calcium oxalate* | Avoid tea, rhubarb, chocolates, nuts, spinach, strawberries, beetroot |
| *Calcium phosphate* | Avoid calcium and Vitamin D supplements. Dietary calcium should not be restricted due to inverse proportional relationship with stone formation |
| *Urate* | Avoid liver, sardines, anchovies, herring with skin |
| *Cystinuria* | Avoid animal meat |

---

### Medical

| | |
|---|---|
| *Analgesia* | Offer diclofenac 75mg im. Consider opioid (diamorphine 5mg) if severe |
| *Antiemetics* | Metoclopramide or cyclizine im. Some recommend antispasmodic |
| *Expulsive therapy* | Can offer tamsulosin or nifedipine to facilitate stone passage |
| *UTI* | Initiate antibiotics depending on sensitivity. Common antibiotics include trimethoprim, nitrofurantoin, cephalexin |
| *Preventative* | Consider thiazide diuretics (for calcium) or allopurinol (uric acid stones) |

### Surgery

On occasions stones persist. These need to be reduced and broken to prevent complications. Procedures such as extracorporeal shock wave lithotripsy, percutaneous nephrolithotomy may be employed by secondary care

### Refer

| | |
|---|---|
| Urology | Refer as per red flag symptoms or for chronic renal stones that need surgical input or lithotripsy |
| Dietician | Can refer to dietician for tailored advice to the patient |

### Safety netting

| | |
|---|---|
| *Follow up* | If symptoms recur, patient may need to be referred for more investigations (recurrence is high) |

## DIFFERENTIAL DIAGNOSIS

| Condition | Characteristic exam feature |
|---|---|
| **Renal stone** | Most common type is calcium stones. More common in males and associated with medications (e.g. loop or thiazide diuretics) and diet. Presents with sudden onset of loin or flank pain radiating to groin. Often with very severe, colicky pain |
| **UTIs** | Affects females >males. E. coli most common organism. Lower urinary tract symptoms include abdominal pain, frequency, dysuria and haematuria. Suprabladder infections (i.e. renal) may cause fever, vomiting and general malaise. Confirmed with +ve dipsticks for leucocytes and nitrates |
| **Pyelonephritis** | More common in females. Patient may have underlying structural abnormalities. Present with uni- or bilateral loin pain, fevers, rigors and nausea and vomiting. Lower UTI symptoms of frequency, dysuria and haematuria may also be present. OE: appears pale and unwell. Fever and back pain may be present. |

## EXPLANATIONS

*Renal stones*    The kidneys act as filters to purify the blood from impurities. Sometimes if there is too much of a particular mineral in the blood, these can go on to build up to form crystals that collect within the urinary tubes very much like limescale does in the sink. If these become big enough, they can develop to form stones which can cause pain and discomfort. Renal stones usually come about due to either passing too much concentrated urine (dehydration, hot weather) or eating certain foods that have too much minerals.

# 5.5 Urinary incontinence (female)

Urinary incontinence is defined as being the involuntary passage of urine. It can be an acutely embarrassing and distressing problem that can significantly impact on the patient's quality of life. Broadly speaking, there are 3 different types of urinary incontinence including stress, urge (with or without overactive bladder) or a mixed picture.

---

**Types & Definitions of Urinary Incontinence** - *Ref: NICE (2013) Urinary incontinence*

| | |
|---|---|
| *Stress UI* | Involuntary urine leakage on effort or exertion, or on sneezing or coughing |
| *Urge UI* | Involuntary urine leakage accompanied or immediately preceded by urgency (a sudden compelling desire to urinate that is difficult to defer) |
| *Mixed UI* | Involuntary urine leakage associated with both urgency and exertion, effort, sneezing or coughing |
| *Overactive bladder* | Urgency that occurs with or without urge UI and usually with frequency and nocturia. OAB that occurs with urge UI is known as 'OAB wet'. OAB without urgency is known as 'OAB dry'. These combinations of symptoms are suggestive of the urodynamic finding of detrusor overactivity, but can be the result of other forms of urethrovesical dysfunction. |

---

## HISTORY
**Open questions**

| | |
|---|---|
| **Open questions** | |
| | Tell me more about the problems you've had passing urine? |
| *Understanding* | What do you mean when you say the 'urine leaks'? |

**Focused questions**

| | |
|---|---|
| *Incontinence* | When did it start? How long has it been going on for? |
| Frequency | How often does it happen? |
| Volume | How much urine do you pass? |
| Severity | Do you wear incontinence pads? How often do you change them? Have you had to change your garments because of any leakage? |

**Associated history**

| | |
|---|---|
| *Stress* | Does it occur when you are sneezing, coughing, bearing down or exercising? |
| *Urge* | Do you sometimes get a sudden urge to go to the toilet and pass urine? How often does this happen? Have you had any accidents? Do you go at night (nocturia)? |
| *Overflow* | Do you struggle to pass urine when you try (hesitancy)? Or strain when you go? When you do pass urine do you have a poor stream? Any dribbling at the end? |
| *Bowels* | Do you have a similar problem when you pass bowels? Does it leak as well? |
| *Toileting* | Do you have easy access to the toilet? Do you go regularly or hold when you cant go? |

**Differentials**

| | |
|---|---|
| *UTI* | Have you had any abdominal pain? Are you passing urine more often or do you have discomfort when you are urinating? |
| *DM* | Do you feel thirsty all the time? Have you lost any weight or have reduced appetite? Do you pass urine often? |
| *Fistula/overflow* | Do you find that you pass urine without even realising it? |
| *Constipation* | How are your bowels? How often do you open your bowels? |

## RED FLAGS

| | |
|---|---|
| *Urinary* | Visible or microscopic haematuria (>50yrs), recurrent UTI |
| *Other* | Weight loss, pelvic mass |

## PAST HISTORY

| | |
|---|---|
| *Medical* | Do you suffer from any medical problems? (strokes, MS, DM, spinal cord lesions, Parkinson's, dementia, bladder cancer) |
| *Surgery* | Have you had any operations? (pelvic, hysterectomy) |
| *Obstetric* | Have you given birth recently? How many children do you have? How were they delivered (C-sections, forceps)? |

## DRUG HISTORY

| | |
|---|---|
| *Medication* | Are you taking any medications? |
| Worsen | Diuretics, alpha blockers, TCAs, hypnotics/sedatives, antihistamines |

## SOCIAL HISTORY

| | |
|---|---|
| *Occupation* | Are you working at the moment? What type of work do you do? |
| *Smoker* | Do you smoke? How many cigarettes do you smoke per day? |
| *Alcohol* | Do you drink alcohol? How much do you drink and how often? |
| *Diet* | How is your diet? Do you drink lots of water? Do you drink tea, coffee or cola? |

## IDEA, CONCERNS, EXPECTATIONS

| | |
|---|---|
| *Idea* | Do you have any idea as to what was causing your urine problems? |
| *Concerns* | Do you have any specific worries about your problem? |
| *Impact on life* | How has your symptoms affected you? |
| Other | Do you find that you have plan your journeys or keep a record of all the local toilets (toilet mapping)? Do you feel embarrassed about it? Has it affected your social life or your relationships? |

## CSA TIPS

Urinary incontinence is a common condition that many people suffer in silence with. It can be quite debilitating leading sufferers to reduce the frequency of going out, and if they do, having to map out the location of toilets incase they have the urge to go. The impact of this condition should not be underestimated and it is important to empathise with the patient when they present. Ensure that your take a thorough history to exclude other causes such as DM, UTIs or constipation, before considering treatment options.

## PHYSICAL EXAMINATION

| | |
|---|---|
| *Vitals* | BP, pulse, temperature |
| *Abdominal exam* | Palpate the abdomen for any pain (suprapubic area), masses or constipation |
| *Pelvic exam* | |
| Inspection | Vulva atrophic vaginitis, fistula, prolapse, leakage of urine when coughing |
| Palpation | Palpate the vaginal wall, cervix and both adnexae for pelvic masses. Before withdrawing your digits, ask them to squeeze down feeling for tone of the pelvic muscles |

---

### Types of Pelvic Organ Prolapses

| | |
|---|---|
| *Cystocele* | Bulging of the bladder into the upper two thirds of the anterior vaginal wall |
| *Urethrocele* | Bulging of the urethra into the lower one third of the anterior vaginal wall. Often occurs together with a prolapse of the bladder (cystourethrocele) |

| | |
|---|---|
| Enterocele | Herniation of the pouch of Douglas into the upper posterior vaginal wall. Often occurs with a rectocele or uterine prolapse |
| Rectocele | Prolapse of the rectum into the lower posterior vaginal wall. Unlike a rectal prolapse (rectal prolapse out of the anus) |
| Uterine | Uterus drops down into the vagina. Graded according to level of descent |
| Primary | Uterus drops slightly. Cervix remains within the vagina |
| Secondary | Uterus drops further. Cervix protrudes through the introitus |
| Tertiary | Uterus lies entirely outside the introitus (procidentia) |
| Vaginal Vault | The top of the vagina (vault) sags or bulges down into the vaginal canal. Often secondary to a hysterectomy |

## INVESTIGATIONS

| | |
|---|---|
| Bloods | U&E, eGFR, fasting glucose |
| Urine | Dipstick urine (DM, UTI), MSU |
| Diary | Urinary diary for 1 week (passage of urine and fluid consumption) |
| US | Bladder residual volume (outflow obstruction) |
| Specialist | Cystoscopy, urodynamic studies |

## MANAGEMENT
### Conservative

| | |
|---|---|
| Weight loss | Lose weight, BMI<30 and encourage exercise |
| Fluid restriction | Reduce caffeine, alcohol and high fluid intake |
| Constipation | Encourage 5x/d fruit & veg, water intake, increase fibre, reduce red meat |
| Pads | Offer absorbent pads or bed covers. Inco pads not available on FP10 only supplied by local NHS trusts – DN/continence nurse |
| Bladder retraining | (Urge) Over 6wks gradually increase interval between voiding |
| Pelvic floor exercises | (Stress) Recommend pelvic floor exercises (8 contractions 3x day) or use vaginal cones |

### Medical

| | |
|---|---|
| Stress | If pelvic floor exercises fail consider referral to surgery. If patient declines surgery consider using duloxetine 40mg bd (can titrate up from 20mg bd) |

---

**Duloxetine in Stress incontinence** - *Ref: NICE: Urinary incontinence, 2013*

Duloxetine is not recommended as a first-line treatment for women with predominant stress UI. Duloxetine should not routinely be used as a second-line treatment for women with stress UI, although it may be offered as second-line therapy if women prefer pharmacological to surgical treatment or are not suitable for surgical treatment. If duloxetine is prescribed, women should be counselled about its adverse effects

| | |
|---|---|
| Side effects | GI symptoms, dry mouth, constipation, palpitations/anxiety, hot flush, drowsiness |
| Contraindications | Elderly, uncontrolled HTN, mania, seizures, glaucoma |

---

| | |
|---|---|
| Urge +/- OAB | Offer oxybutynin 5mg tds (titrate upwards) immediate release as first line. If not helping consider antimuscarinic drugs (darifenacin, solifenacin, tolterodine) or Oxybutynin MR. Advise that must try for at least 4wks before seeing any relief |

**Adverse Effects of Antimuscarinics Agents** - *Ref: SIGN: Mx of Urinary incontinence in primary care, 2004*
The most common side effects of antimuscarinic drugs are dry mouth, blurred vision, abdominal discomfort, drowsiness, nausea and dizziness. Urinary retention is a potentially serious but less common side effect.

| | |
|---|---|
| *Prolapse* | Consider ring pessary or surgery |
| *UTI* | Treat depending on organism use empirical therapy (trimethoprim, nitrofurantoin, cefalexin) |
| *Catheter* | Severe incontinence refer for catheterisation |

**Refer**

| | |
|---|---|
| *Physiotherapy* | Refer to physio for bladder retraining programme or pelvic floor exercise, incontinence |
| *Incontinence nurse* | Refer for incontinence nurse for further evaluation of patients or those needing specialised incontinence pads |
| *Surgery* | Refer urogynaecology for consideration of botulinum toxin, operations (urogenital fistula), severe pelvic prolapse (prolapse visible below the introitus), pelvic masses, overflow incontinence, large postvoid residual volume |

**SAFETY NETING**

| | |
|---|---|
| *Follow up* | If not improving within 4 weeks request to review by GP |

**DIFFERENTIAL DIAGNOSIS**

| Condition | Characteristic exam feature |
|---|---|
| **Stress incontinence** | Passage of small amounts of urine related to coughing, sneezing, lifting, exercises. RF: childbirth, menopause, obesity. Rare in men (usually after prostatectomy) |
| **Urge incontinence** | Urgency, frequency with overwhelming sensation to void. Passage of large volume, and nocturia. RF: Stress, neurological (spinal injury, PD, stroke, MS), bladder (stones, cancer) |
| **Overflow incontinence** | Intermittent leaking or dribbling of urine throughout the day. Can be due to constipation. Can also occur in men (BPH, prostate ca, stricture). Anticholinergic medication (Oxybutynin) can worsen symptoms |
| **UTI** | Abdominal pain, dysuria, frequency, urgency with cloudy urine and positive dipstick |
| **Prolapse** | Symptoms depend on type. Can include incontinence, frequency, urgency and incomplete bladder emptying (cystocele, cystourethrocele), constipation (rectocele, enterocele), heaviness or dragging sensation in pelvis, i.e. 'my insides are falling out' (uterine prolapse). OE: bulge in the posterior (enterocele, rectocele) or anterior (cystocele, urethrocele) vaginal wall |

## EXPLANATIONS

*Stress incontinence*    Stress incontinence is when you can leak a bit of urine when you cough, sneeze or do some exercise. It is often caused by weakness of the (pelvic) muscles around the bladder. The muscles are usually made weak following childbirth.

*Urge incontinence*    Urge incontinence is when you have a sudden desire to pass urine or urge and leak a bit of urine before you get to the toilet. It is often caused by an overactive bladder.

*OAB*    An overactive bladder (otherwise known as irritable bladder) is when the bladder squeezes suddenly without your control. It can even occur when the bladder is not completely full. It may occur with or without leaking even before you can get to the toilet.

*Pelvic floor exercise*    Pelvic floor exercises help to strengthen the muscles around the bladder. It is recommended that you clench your pelvic muscles below your bladder. This can be done by imagining that you are passing urine and that you have to squeeze to prevent this. Hold this position for 5 seconds and release. Repeat the exercise everyday to improve the muscle strength. You should do at least 8 contractions, 3 times a day for 6 weeks to gradually improve your symptoms.

*Bladder retraining*    This is designed to slowly stretch the bladder so that it can hold more urine. You should try and cut down the number of trips you take to the toilet to pass urine. At the beginning simply try and hold your urine in for 5 more minutes and slowly increase this up to 10 and more until you are going every 3-4 hours. Alternatively schedule visits to the toilet even if you do not have the urge to go.

# 5.6 Chronic Kidney Disease (CKD)

Chronic kidney disease is a condition that is often symptomless and is usually picked up on routine blood tests or from a urine dipstick. It is diagnosed using the estimated glomerular filtration rate (eGFR) as a guide to the degree of renal dysfunction or damage. There are 5 stages, ranging from mild (stage 1) to severe (stage 5). Patients who cross an eGFR of less than 60 are classified as stage 3 and require medical input with closer monitoring to prevent further deterioration possibly leading to dialysis or in severe cases transplantation.

## HISTORY

CKD is usually asymptomatic and hence it is difficult to elicit from the history alone. However, when taking a history you should include a cardiovascular risk factor assessment as there is an association with IHD. Ensure that you read the notes thoroughly, and note if the patient has had previously low eGFR readings, anaemia or evidence of proteinuria.

| | |
|---|---|
| **Open questions** | Tell me more about your problem? Do you why you had your blood tests? |

**Focused questions**

| | |
|---|---|
| *CKD* | When did it start? How long has it been going on for? |
| Fatigue | Have you been feeling more tired than usual? |
| Urinary | Do you find that you are going to the toilet more often than normal? Do you go a lot at night? How often? |
| N&V | Do you feel sick or have you actually vomited? |
| Fluid retention | Have you noticed any swelling of your legs or ankles? Any shortness of breath? Do you get any puffiness around your face or eyes? |

**Associated History**

| | |
|---|---|
| *Pruritis* | Do you feel itchy all over your body? |
| *Anorexic* | Have you lost any weight? Are you off your food or have a reduced appetite? |
| *Sexual dysfunction* | Are you having problems obtaining an erection? Are you no longer interested in sex? |

**RED FLAGS**

| | |
|---|---|
| *Urinary* | Haematuria, proteinuria, rapid deterioration in eGFR, eGFR <30, anaemia, nephritic syndrome (panda face) |
| *Other* | Weight loss, malignant HTN, hyperkalaemia, pulmonary oedema |

**PAST HISTORY**

| | |
|---|---|
| *Medical* | Do you suffer from any medical problems? (HTN, CVA, DM, recurrent UTIs, connective tissue disease, renal disease-polycystic, glomerulonephritis) |

**DRUG HISTORY**

| | |
|---|---|
| *Medication* | Are you taking any medications? |
| Worsen | NSAIDs, ACEI (renal stenosis), Ca2+ ch blockers, diuretics, lithium, metformin |

**SOCIAL HISTORY**

| | |
|---|---|
| *Occupation* | Are you working at the moment? What type of work do you do? |
| *Smoker* | Do you smoke? How many cigarettes do you smoke per day? |
| *Alcohol* | Do you drink alcohol? How much do you drink and how often? |

## FAMILY HISTORY

| | |
|---|---|
| *Renal* | Does anyone in your family have kidney problems? (CKD, polycystic kidneys) |

## IDEA, CONCERNS, EXPECTATIONS

| | |
|---|---|
| *Idea* | Do you have any idea as to what may be causing your kidney problem? |
| *Concern* | Do you have any specific worries about it? |
| *Understanding* | What do you know about chronic kidney disease? (CKD) |

## CSA TIPS

Patients presenting at a consultation with newly diagnosed CKD are likely to be asymptomatic. Most cases would be found after the patient had attended for a blood test either through A&E or the GP surgery and they are attending for the results. Once diagnosed, patients should be screened for any underlying renal abnormality or associated risk factors for IHD. When speaking to the patient, they would naturally be quite distraught to find their kidneys were not working as expected and you should be empathetic and sensitive when breaking the news and explaining the diagnosis.

## PHYSICAL EXAMINATION

| | |
|---|---|
| *Vitals* | BP (raised), weight (fluid retention), temperature |
| *Abdominal exam* | |
| Inspection | Inspect for yellow 'lemon' tinge (uraemia) |
| Palpation | Palpate the abdomen for ascites or palpable bladder, enlarged kidneys |
| *Respiratory exam* | Auscultate the lung bases for pleural effusions or signs of peripheral oedema |

## INVESTIGATIONS

| | |
|---|---|
| *Bloods* | U&E (creatinine, Na, K), eGFR |
| Other | FBC, ESR, glucose, cholesterol. Measure calcium, phosphate and PTH concentrations in people with stage 4 or 5 |

---

**Advice about the eGFR -** *Ref: NICE (2008) Chronic Kidney Disease*
- Patients should not eat any meat in the 12 hours before eGFR blood test
- Patients with extremes of muscle mass (bodybuilders, amputees or people with muscle wasting disorders) interpret the eGFR with caution. Reduced muscle mass will lead to overestimation and increased muscle mass to underestimation of the GFR
- Multiply correction factor of 1.21 for African-Caribbean ethnicity

---

| | |
|---|---|
| *Urine* | Dipstick urine to exclude UTI, ACR or PCR (morning sample) |
| *US* | Renal pathology (consider if CKD 4/5) |

---

**Screening for CKD -** *Ref: NICE (2008) Chronic Kidney Disease*
*Offer people testing for CKD if they have any of the following risk factors:*
- DM, HTN, CVD (IHD, HF, PVD, CVA), structural renal tract disease, renal calculi or prostatic hypertrophy, multisystem diseases with potential kidney involvement – SLE, FHx stage 5 CKD or hereditary kidney disease, opportunistically in haematuria or proteinuria
- If no risk factors, do not use age, gender or ethnicity as markers to test for CKD. If no metabolic syndrome, DM, HTN, do not use obesity alone as a risk marker to test for CKD

---

## MANAGEMENT

### Conservative

| | |
|---|---|
| Smoking | Encourage to stop smoking. Refer to smoking cessation clinic |
| Alcohol | Reduce alcohol intake <21u/wk for men, <14u/wk for women |
| Exercise/wt loss | Encourage exercise so that they can lose weight |
| Diet | Consider protein restriction, initiated by dietician, if CKD 4 or above. Recommend salt restriction |
| QoF | Maintain a register of patients with CKD stages 3-5. Monitor BP (<140/85) yearly and perform urine ACR. Ensure patients with concurrent BP and proteinuria are on ACE-I |

### Medical

| | |
|---|---|
| Avoid drugs | Avoid nephrotoxic drugs (e.g. NSAIDS). Caution with drugs utilising renal clearance (i.e. stop metformin if GFR<30) |
| ACEI | Initiate ACEI or ARB as per NICE guidelines |

---

**When to initiate ACEI** - *Ref: Adapted from NICE (2008) Chronic Kidney Disease*

| | |
|---|---|
| Diabetic | ACR >2.5 mg/mmol in men, or >3.5 mg/mmol in women |
| Non-diabetic | ACR >70 mg/mmol |
| | HTN with > ACR 30 mg/mmol |
| | HTN with < ACR 30 mg/mmol treat BP according to NICE BP guidance. No need ACEI if not indicated |

---

| | |
|---|---|
| Monitor | Monitor eGFR after 2wks and urine (urine dipstick & ACR). If evidence of proteinuria exclude UTI. If K+ >6mmol stop ACEI |
| CVD disease | Treat HTN (target 130/80), cholesterol and DM |
| Anaemia | Monitor for anaemia. If low, consider referral for erythropoietin injections |

### Refer

| | |
|---|---|
| Dietician | Refer if mildly raised potassium levels |
| Nephrologist | Refer in stage 4/5 CKD, Proteinuria (PCR >100, ACR >70), sudden deterioration of GFR (>10ml/min/1.73m2 drop in 5yrs) with UTI excluded, anaemia (<11g/dL), persistent haematuria in <50yr, refractory HTN) |

## SAFETY NETTING

| | |
|---|---|
| Follow up | Monitor U&Es regularly. Urgent referral for red flags |

---

**Measurement of eGFR: how often** - *Ref: Adapted from NICE (2008) Chronic Kidney Disease*

Annually in all at risk groups as well as during intercurrent illness or preoperatively in all patients with CKD. The frequency of testing may be reduced where eGFR levels remain stable but will need to be increased if there is rapid deterioration

| Stage | eGFR range | Testing frequency |
|---|---|---|
| 1 | ≥ 90 + evidence of kidney damage | 12 monthly |
| 2 | ≥ 60 + evidence of kidney damage | 12 monthly |
| 3A & 3B | 30–59 +/- evidence | 6 monthly |
| 4 | 15–29 +/- evidence | 3 monthly |
| 5 | <15 (renal failure) | 6 weekly |

---

# EXPLANATIONS

*CKD*

The kidney plays an important role in cleaning the blood of any dangerous chemicals/impurities. It also helps to clear excess amounts of fluid in the body. In chronic kidney disease, the kidneys are not working as well as they are supposed to. Most patients with CKD may not even know they suffer from it, as it is often symptomless and only picked up on a blood test. We do not always know what the cause is, but commonly as we age, the kidneys no longer work as well as they did when we were younger.

*ACEI*

Angiotensin converting enzyme inhibitor, or ACEI, works by blocking a protein (enzyme) that helps make a chemical called angiotensin II. This helps relax the blood vessels and reduces how much water is reabsorbed in the kidney. By taking this tablet, it can protect your kidney from further damage and keep your body healthy.

*Dialysis*

Dialysis is a type of treatment that is used in severe forms of chronic kidney disease. It is machine that is attached to a tube connected to your arm that helps takes over the kidney's role in cleaning the blood and removing the harmful impurities that build up.

# 5.7 Vasectomy

Vasectomies are a near permanent form of contraception for men that results in sterilisation. It is usually performed as a day case procedure under local anaesthetic whereby the two ends of the vas deferens are severed and tied so that no sperm can pass. Whilst the initial sterilisation procedure is freely available on the NHS, if the patient has a change of heart then any subsequent reversal procedures must be privately funded. Whilst it is good practice for both partners to be actively involved in the decision making process, informed consent should only be sought from the male partner and there is no legal requirement for the female partner's opinion to be considered.

## HISTORY

| | |
|---|---|
| **Reassure** | I just want to reassure that whilst you may feel embarrassed to talk about your problem it is something that we see and treat everyday |
| **Open questions** | Can you tell me more about why you would like to have a vasectomy? |
| *Understanding* | What do you already know about the vasectomy? Can I just clarify what you mean when you say 'snip'? |

## Focused questions

*Vasectomy*

| | |
|---|---|
| Relationship | Are you currently in a relationship? |
| Family | Do you have any children with your current or previous partner? How many? |
| Contraception | Are you using any forms of contraception? Any problems with it? |
| Counselling | Have you discussed your decision with your partner? How would they feel? If you have not, is there any particular reason why you have not told your partner (relationship problems)? |
| Life events | Have you had any big changes in your life recently? (new baby, mortgage, miscarriage) |

| | |
|---|---|
| *Concerns* | Is there anything worrying you about having the operation? (impotence, reversibility) |

| | |
|---|---|
| **YELLOW FLAGS** | Young (<20yr), not previously fathered children, unhappy relationship, partner pressurisation |

## PAST HISTORY

| | |
|---|---|
| *Medical* | Do you suffer from any medical problems? |
| *Surgery* | Have you had any previous surgery? |

## SOCIAL HISTORY

| | |
|---|---|
| *Occupation* | Are you currently working at the moment? What do you work as? |
| *Home* | Does anyone live with you at home? |
| *Financial* | Do you have any financial worries? (loss of job, mortgages, debt, CSA costs) |
| *Smoker* | Do you smoke? How many cigarettes do you smoke per day? |
| *Alcohol* | Do you drink alcohol? How much do you drink and how often? |

## CSA TIPS

Attending for the 'snip' may be quite a nerve-racking experience for the male patient. They may not have really thought through the implications about what it means for them, their partner or for future relationships having simply heard about the procedure from a pub-friend or being pressured into it by a tired partner. It is important for such patients, to explain what the possible implications are, and ensure that they have material to read and digest at home, before returning with a concrete decision. It is advisable, but not essential, for them to include their partner in the decision making process, especially since reversibility may be expensive and is not always successful.

## PHYSICAL EXAMINATION

| | |
|---|---|
| *Vitals* | BP, BMI |
| *Genital* | *Not usually performed.* Inspect for any abnormalities |

## EXPLANATIONS

| | |
|---|---|
| *Vasectomy* | Vasectomy is a small operation that cuts the tubes (vas deferens) that join the testes, where the sperm is made, to the penis. This prevents the male sperms from passing into the semen when you ejaculate during sex. As there is no longer any sperm in the ejaculate, the chances of making a baby when it meets the female's egg are almost nil. |
| *Reliability* | It is a safe and quick procedure (might take up to 30 minutes) that is usually done as a day case. It is a very reliable operation with only 1 person in a 1000 not being successful. |
| *Risks* | After the operation, you may feel some pain / ache around the area as well as some bruising. This often settles with time. Having a vasectomy should not affect your sex drive as the operation does not interfere with your testes/sex hormones. |

## Risks of Vasectomies

| | |
|---|---|
| *Pain* | Temporary pain or ache in groin postoperative |
| *PVPS* | Post-vasectomy pain syndrome occurs in 1 in 20 cases post op. Patients may experience a chronic dull ache in the groin or pain when ejaculating |
| *Inflammation* | Inflammation, infection, abscess in the skin, testicles. Tx with antibiotics |
| *Hematoma* | Bruises or blood clots. Often settle with time |
| *Adhesion* | Risk of fistula between skin and vas. May require surgery |
| *Hydrocele* | Fluid collection in scrotum. Often resolves. May need draining |
| *Spermatic granuloma* | Swelling caused by seeping of sperm from the vas deferens forming a lump. May cause pain. Often resolves spontaneously. May need drainage |
| *Recanalisation* | Reconnection of two ends of vas deferens. Very rare. Fertility may return |
| *Reduced libido* | Reduced sex drive or impotence (4/1000). Usually psychological |

| | |
|---|---|
| *Sex* | You can have sex soon after the operation. However, we normally advise to wait a few days to let the pain and swelling subside before doing so. If you do decide to have sex, we advise to use condoms as there still may be some sperm left in the tubes. We advise to keep using condoms until you are given the all-clear by your doctor. |
| *All clear* | Once the vasectomy is done, you still have a small chance of being fertile up to 4 months after the procedure. For this reason we would like to check your sperm count 3 and 6 weeks after the operation to confirm that there are no sperms getting through. In the mean time I would recommend using condoms until we have done this. |

| | |
|---|---|
| *Reversibility* | Some people may change their minds after the procedure and want to start a family again. Although this is possible, it is not done on the NHS. Chances of reversal are only 50% in the first 10 years dropping down to 25% thereafter. |
| *STI risk* | It is important to remember that whilst vasectomies offer excellent contraception they do not protect against catching STIs. You should consider using barrier contraception if you are at risk. |
| *Concerns* | I appreciate that you are worried where the sperm go after the operation. Everyday we make millions of sperm and when we are not having sex or ejaculating these build up. However, they never seem to cause any problems as they are broken down and reabsorbed by the body. The same thing will happen after you have had your operation. However, in some rare cases, the sperm may build up and form hard lumps in your testes. If this happens, it is important to return and see your Dr to discuss what can be done to help. |

# 5.8 Testicular problems

Testicular problems often create the greatest anxiety and angst in male patients probably more than any other symptom. Males are particularly sensitive to testicular problems as there is a social perception that masculinity and virility are linked to the health of their testicles. Unfortunately as a result, men often present late to their GP and can find it an acutely embarrassing to discuss.

A scrotal lump does not automatically equate to cancer of the testes; nor does it have to necessarily originate from the scrotum. When examining, it is important to decide initially where the lump arises from and whether it is solely confined to the testes; doing so will help you distinguish between a mass and a hernia.

## HISTORY

| | |
|---|---|
| **Reassure** | I just want to reassure that whilst you may feel embarrassed to talk about your problem, it is something that we see and treat everyday |
| **Open questions** | Can you tell me more about the pain/swelling you have noticed? |

**Focused questions**

| | |
|---|---|
| *Testicular pain* | When did you first notice the pain? How long does it last for? |
| Onset | Did it come on suddenly? |
| Radiation | Does the pain move anywhere? Does it come from your tummy going into your groin or does it move from the groin upwards? |
| Character | How would you describe it? Is it a severe, sharp pain or a dull ache? |
| | |
| *Swelling* | When did you first notice it? How did you notice it? |
| Site | Is it affecting one side or both? |
| Onset | Did it come on suddenly or gradually build up? |
| Position | Does the swelling go when you lie down? (inguinal hernia) |
| Inflammation | Is it red, hot or painful? |

**Associated history**

| | |
|---|---|
| *Nausea & vomiting* | Have you felt sick or vomited? |
| *Trauma* | Have you had any injury to the scrotum? |

## SEXUAL HISTORY *if relevant*

| | |
|---|---|
| *Partner* | When was the last time you had sex? Was it with your regular partner? Are they male or female (if they say 'partner' without qualifying)? |
| Type | Do you engage in anal sex? |
| STI | Have you had any sexually transmitted infections in the past? |
| Penile discharge | Have you noticed any unusual discharge from the penis? |

**Differentials**

| | |
|---|---|
| *Testicular torsion* | Did the pain come on suddenly? How severe is it? Do you feel sick at all? |
| *Prostatitis* | Do you have any pain passing urine? Do you go often? How is your stream? Do you have any pain whilst having sex? |
| *Epididymo-orchitis* | Do you have pain in only one of your testicles? Any blood in your semen (haematospermia) or any discharge? Did you have your MMR vaccine when you were younger (mumps)? Any temperatures? |

| | |
|---|---|
| *Strangulated hernia* | Do you have pain in your tummy? Any problems opening bowels or passing wind? |
| *Varicocele* | Do you have a dragging or aching feeling in your scrotum? |
| *Testicular cancer* | Have you had any weight loss? Is there no pain with it? Is it getting bigger? Do you have tummy or back pain? Have you noticed your chest (breast) getting bigger? |

**RED FLAGS**            Haematuria, acute pain (torsion), weight loss, vomiting, lethargy

**PAST HISTORY**

| | |
|---|---|
| *Medical* | Do you suffer from any medical or testicular problems (TB, hernia, undescended testis, mumps)? Any previous STIs (Chlamydia, gonorrhoea, HIV)? |
| *Surgical* | Have you had any operations on your testes? (orchidopexy, vasectomy) |

**SOCIAL HISTORY**

| | |
|---|---|
| *Occupation* | Are you working at the moment? What type of work do you do? |
| *Hobbies* | Do you do any hobbies? (trauma - football, rugby, martial arts) |
| *Smoker* | Do you smoke? How many cigarettes do you smoke per day? |
| *Alcohol* | Do you drink alcohol? How much do you drink and how often? |

**FAMILY HISTORY**

| | |
|---|---|
| *Cancer* | Anyone in the family have testicular problems (testicular cancer)? |

**IDEA, CONCERNS, EXPECTATIONS**

| | |
|---|---|
| *Idea* | Do you have any ideas as to what was causing your pain/swelling? Have you had any thoughts about what may be causing it? |
| *Concern* | Do you have any worries about it? (cancer) |

**CSA TIPS**

Lumps or masses in the testicular area may cause much stress and anxiety in the male patient. Despite increased awareness through social and mainstream media about the seriousness of testicular lumps, men are still quite embarrassed to attend their doctor for assessment and evaluation. Hence, when they do attend, it is vital that your put them at ease and deal with them in an empathetic way before examining them.

**PHYSICAL EXAMINATION**

| | |
|---|---|
| *Vitals* | BP, pulse |
| *Abdominal exam* | Palpate for generalised tenderness (obstruction) as well as for pain or swellings in the inguinal region (inguinal hernia) |
| Cough impulse | Check for cough impulse if hernia suspected |
| | |
| *Testicular exam* | *seek chaperone* |
| Inspection | Observe position of testicles (held transverse – torsion) or swelling |
| Palpation | Palpate testes (testicular cancer), epididymis (cysts, pain – epididymitis), spermatic cord (varicocele, spermatocele) |
| LN | Palpate the inguinal and para-aortic lymph nodes if cancer is suspected |
| Transluminate | Shine a light (pen torch) through the scrotum and observe from the other end using a tube. Check for illumination seen in hydrocele |

**INVESTIGATIONS**

| | |
|---|---|
| *Urine* | Dipstick urine or MSU to check for UTI, urine STI screen |
| *Swabs* | Urethral swabs to exclude STIs (chlamydia, gonorrhoea - epididymitis) |

| US | Consider scrotal US if lesion suspected |
| Bloods | AFP (Alpha fetoprotein), bHCG, LDH for testicular cancer |

**MANAGEMENT**  *treat underlying cause*

***Conservative***

| Self examination | Recommend self examination or partner to examine to monitor for testicular cancer |
| Support | Wear supportive undergarments when engaged in contact sports |
| Trauma | If you get trauma you should take pain relief and apply ice packs to the area |
| Contraception | Use condoms to prevent STI risk |
| MMR | Recommend that all children have their MMR vaccine to prevent mumps |

***Medical***

| Epididymo-orchitis | Treat with antibiotics ceftriaxone plus doxycycline if gonococcal or chlamydia is suspected. Quinolones (ofloxacin) can be initiated if caused by E. coli |
| Torsion | Refer immediately for surgical review (especially within 6 hours) |
| Hydrocele | Infantile hydrocele should be repaired if not resolved by age 1-2. Monitoring in adults unless severe where can be drained |
| Varicocele | Conservative manage. Consider surgery if painful |
| Prostatitis | Treat with antibiotics for up to 4wks (trimethoprim, ciprofloxacin) |
| Testicular cancer | If suspecting cancer then refer to specialist as 2WW. For further investigations and possible surgery +/- radio or chemotherapy |
| Inguinal Hernia | See inguinal hernia chapter |

**SAFETY NETTING**

| Follow up | If not improving within 2-4 weeks request to review by GP |

**DIFFERENTIAL DIAGNOSIS**

| Condition | Characteristic exam feature |
| --- | --- |
| **Testicular cancer** | Commonest cancer in young. Two types; seminoma (30–50yrs) and teratomas (20–30yrs). Presents as painless swelling of the testis. OE: lump limited to the scrotum, irregular, nodular and hard with no evidence of translumination. Enlarged LNs (para-aortic) seen in secondary spread |
| **Hydrocele** | Collection of fluid within the tunica vaginalis. Primary (idiopathic) or secondary (trauma, cancer, infection). OE: there is a unilateral, non-tender scrotal swelling. Testicle may be impalpable (must exclude testicular cancer). There may be a fluid thrill and it is transilluminable. Can get above swelling |
| **Epididymal cyst** | Fluid filled swellings in the epididymis. OE: often a smooth bilateral, multilocular cyst located above and behind the testis clearly distinct and separate to it associated with polycystic kidney disease or CF |
| **Epididymo-orchitis** | Infection (E.coli, STIs - Chlamydia, Gonococcus) of the epididymis. Presents with unilateral pain and swelling to the testes. May also have pain on ejaculation. OE: Prehn's sign– pain relief on elevating the affected testicle |

| | |
|---|---|
| **Varicocele** | Collection of dilated veins in the pampiniform plexus due to problems in the valves. OE: they appear tortuous and distended on standing and are often described as a 'bag of worms.' Classically, on lying down they disappear and become impalpable. Can be linked to subfertility |
| **Testicular torsion** | Usually occurs in the young adult (15-30 yr old). Sudden onset of pain, swelling and vomiting. OE: the affected testis is held transversely and at a higher position compared with the other testicle. Testicle is hard, tender and enlarged |
| **Inguinal hernia** | Herniation of the contents of the abdomen through the inguinal region. OE: a lump in the groin that may pass into scrotum. Presents with pain & swelling in the groin. If obstructed can present with acute pain, vomiting and absolute constipation |

## EXPLANATIONS

*Testicular torsion*     This is when the testicle twists on itself blocking the blood supply to it similar to a hose pipe tube that is twisted blocking the flow of water. It is an emergency that requires urgent surgical attention to ensure no permanent damage is caused.

*Hydrocele*     This describes a collection of fluid within a sac that surrounds your testes. It is usually due to a blockage in the spermatic cord perhaps due to infection or swelling, that is found above the testicles. They normally go away themselves and are harmless. If they keep increasing in size and cause discomfort, then we may need to remove them.

*Varicocele*     This is a condition that causes a collection of enlarged veins found above the testicles in the scrotum. It is thought that they are caused by leaky valves, similar to those that give rise to varicose veins in the legs. Because the valves are leaky, the blood does not go back quickly upwards and builds up in the scrotum causing a swelling. They are harmless and usually do not cause any problems.

*Epididymal cyst*     It is a collection of fluid in a small sac/cyst found within the collecting tubes behind the testicles. It is very common and harmless. It usually does not cause any problems and does not require any treatment.

*Epididymo-orchitis*     This is inflammation or swelling of the testicles as well as the tubes behind it caused by an infection (STI, E. coli). It may cause pain when passing urine or give you a discharge.

*Self-Examining*     It is important to be able to check yourself to pick up any signs of lumps in your testes. To do this, it is best performed after having a bath or shower to get relaxed. Stand in front of a mirror and look at the skin over your balls. Ensure that there are no obvious swellings or redness. Next check each testis in turn using your index and middle finger. Gently roll the testis and feel for any lumps. Move behind the testis and feel for a soft, tube like structure (epididymis). There should be no pain when doing this.

If you do feel a lump it is best to speak to a doctor. However, any lump that is not linked to your testis or is free-floating in the sac is unlikely to be cancer. It is normal to find that one of your testis is bigger than the other, and may be located higher up in the scrotal sac than the other.

# *5.9 Inguinal hernia*

A hernia is a protrusion of an organ through its cavity into another space. They may be present at birth but may develop later in life due to weaknesses of the abdominal wall. Inguinal hernias are hernias of abdominal contents that pass through the inguinal canal and are more common in men. They are classified as direct and indirect. The majority of hernias are indirect arising from the internal ring and exiting through the superficial ring. Direct hernias pass through a defect in the posterior wall of the inguinal canal and out into the abdominal cavity.

## HISTORY
Enquire about why the patient has presented by asking several open questions before moving on to ask closed questions:

| | |
|---|---|
| **Open questions** | Tell me more about why you attended today? Tell me more about the problems you are having with the lump in your groin |

## Focused questions
| | |
|---|---|
| *Lump* | When did you first notice the lump? What were you doing at the time (lifting, coughing)? |
| Site | Where is the lump (groin, scrotum)? Is it on both sides or just one? |
| Size | Has the lump changed in size since then? |
| Change | Is it there all the time or does it come and go? |
| Trigger | What makes it come out (coughing, bending, standing)? What makes it go away (lying down, pushing it back)? |

## Associated history
| | |
|---|---|
| *Pain* | Is there any pain or tenderness over the lump? Does anything make the pain better or worse? Did it ever become red? |
| *Vomiting* | Have you been vomiting with the lump? |
| *Bowels* | How are your bowels? Do you have constipation? Have you had problems passing flatus? |

## RED FLAGS
| | |
|---|---|
| | Obstruction (Severe pain, vomiting, distention), absolute constipation (inability to pass flatus/faeces), inability to reduce |

## PAST HISTORY
| | |
|---|---|
| *Medical* | Have you had any problems with a chronic cough? (COPD, asthma) |
| *Operation* | Have you had any previous operations for hernias? |

## DRUG HISTORY
| | |
|---|---|
| *Medication* | Are you taking any medications? (codeine, iron, calcium) |

## FAMILY HISTORY
| | |
|---|---|
| *Inguinal Hernia* | Has anyone in your family suffered from similar problems? Have they been diagnosed with inguinal hernia? |

## SOCIAL HISTORY

| | |
|---|---|
| *Occupation* | Are you currently in employment? (builder, bricklayer, delivery) |
| *Hobbies* | Do you do any hobbies? (football, golf, weightlifting) |
| *Smoker* | Do you smoke? How many cigarettes do you smoke per day? |
| *Alcohol* | Do you drink alcohol? How much do you drink and how often? |

## IDEA, CONCERNS, EXPECTATIONS

| | |
|---|---|
| *Ideas* | What do you think may be causing your symptoms? |
| *Concerns* | Do you have any worries about the problems you have been experiencing? |
| *Impact* | How have the symptoms affected and impacted upon your life? |

## CSA TIPS

Inguinal hernias are almost 10x more common in men than women. Patients may present with symptoms and request information around an inguinal hernia repair. In such cases it is important to assess the patient and warn them about red flags symptoms that may mean they need emergency care. In patients who wish to proceed for an operation, you should discuss with them the complications and give them advice when they can return to basic duties following the procedure.

## PHYSICAL EXAMINATION

| | |
|---|---|
| *Vitals* | BP, BMI |
| *Chaperone* | Request a chaperone |
| *Inspect* | Have the patient standing. Look for obvious lumps. Observe for a cough impulse and its location (above inguinal ligament - inguinal hernia, below - femoral) |
| *Palpate* | Feel from the side with one hand on the patient's back. Feel the lump and note its location, size, shape and whether it is hard or soft. Check its temperature. Ask the patient to cough away from you and feel for an impulse |
| *Reduce* | Request the patient to reduce the hernia and place 2 fingers over the deep ring (1.5cm above midpoint of ASIS to pubic tubercle). Ask them to cough. If you see the hernia appear then likely a direct hernia. If it does not appear then likely an indirect hernia |
| *Auscultate* | Listen over the hernia with a stethoscope for bowel sounds |
| *Scrotum* | Feel the scrotum for any lumps or swellings |

## INVESTIGATIONS    *often performed by secondary care*

| | |
|---|---|
| *US / MRI scan* | May be performed to confirm the presence of a hernia |
| *Herniography* | Injection of X-ray contrast may be used for diagnostic uncertainty |

## MANAGEMENT

### Conservative

| | |
|---|---|
| *Reassurance* | Reassure patient if the hernia is small and not strangulated |
| *Lifestyle* | Recommend exercise and eating healthy to lose weight. Take plenty of fibre through fruit and vegetable and drink fluids to reduce constipation |
| *Smoking* | Advise to cut down or stop smoking |
| *Lifting* | Be careful when carrying heavy objects or bending down to lift. Try lifting with your knees rather than your back and do not carry objects which need >1person |
| *Truss* | Refer to surgeons to provide. No evidence that it prevents the hernia from increasing in size but helpful if the patient is having problems managing with the hernia |

### Medical

| | |
|---|---|
| *Constipation* | Use bulk-forming (ispaghula), osmotic (lactulose) or osmotic laxatives (senna) |

| | |
|---|---|
| Pain | Simple analgesia or NSAIDs. Ensure no CI for NSAIDS (ulcers, gastritis or asthma) |
| Cough | Rationalise treatments for asthma or COPD |

**Surgical**

| | |
|---|---|
| Hernia Repair | Often a day-case with laparoscopic guidance. May be under LA or GA. Surgeons locate the hernia and place a mesh to allow tissue to grow and strengthen the weakness |
| Risks | Local pain, infection and haematoma. 1 in 200 have recurrence and 1 in 20 suffer with post herniorrhaphy pain syndrome |
| Post op | Remain active and take OTC pain relief. Shower for 10 days then bath. Return to work within 2wks unless involves heavy lifting - then return at 6wks. Drive after 1-2wks or when you perform an emergency stop |

**SAFETY NETTING**

| | |
|---|---|
| Follow up | Review in 4wks for response to treatment |
| Red flags | If any signs of strangulation (severe pain, vomiting, irreducible mass) or obstruction (absence of flatus or faeces, vomiting, pain, distention) seek emergency advice |
| Referral | Refer to specialist if poor response or according to guidelines below |

**DIFFERENTIAL DIAGNOSIS**

| Conditions | Characteristic exam feature |
|---|---|
| **Inguinal Hernia** | Men 10x compared to women. RIsk factors included chronic cough and prolonged heavy lifting, obesity, constipation. OE: Inguinal swelling that lies above the inguinal ligament that may pass into the scrotum, often has cough impulse and reducible. If red, hot, tender and absolute constipation may be strangulated |
| **Femoral Hernia** | More common in elderly females. Located below the inguinal ligament. Does not disappear when the patient lies flat |
| **Saphena Varix** | Dilatation of the saphenous vein. OE: Cough impulse over the saphenofemoral junction demonstrates valve incompetence. Disappears when lies down |
| **Scrotal Mass** | Hydrocele, spermatocele and lumps in testes. If you can get above them then scrotal mass. If you cannot then probable hernia |

**EXPLANATIONS**

| | |
|---|---|
| Inguinal Hernia | This is a lump that may appear in your groin area. It is usually due to a weakness of the lower tummy muscles that allow the intestine / gut from behind to push through. It may be because of a weakness you were born with or more commonly develop later in life due to straining or heavy exercise. |
| Strangulated | Sometimes when the lump passes through the weakness it may get stuck in that position. Over time, the hernia may get squeezed and the blood supply to it may be reduced. This may cause the tissue inside to begin to die and give you severe pain, constipation and make you feel sick. You should seek medical help immediately if this ever happens. |

# 6.1 Diabetes

Diabetes is characterized by a syndrome of disordered metabolism resulting in hyperglycaemia. Glucose levels are tightly controlled in the body through a complex interaction of chemicals and hormones. Persistently raised blood glucose levels can cause a person to suffer acutely with symptoms of thirst, tiredness, polyuria and weight loss. However, more worryingly, diabetes can cause quite serious long-term complications including raising cardiovascular disease, chronic kidney failure, retinopathy, neuropathy, erectile dysfunction and poor wound healing.

The long-term complications of diabetes can be reduced with tight blood glucose control which can be objectively measured through the HbA1c blood test. The tighter the HbA1c control the less likely the patient will develop complications.

## HISTORY

**Open questions**       Can you tell me more about the symptoms you have been having?

**Focused questions**

*Diabetes*                When did it start? How long has it been going on for?
  Polydipsia             Have you been feeling more thirsty than normal?
  Polyuria               Have you been going to the toilet and passing urine more often?
  Nocturia               Do you awake at night to pass urine? How many times?
  Tiredness              Do you feel tired all the time?
  Weight loss            Have you lost any weight?

**Complications**

*Recurrent Inf.*          Have you had any kind of infection (i.e. UTI, bacterial or fungal – i.e. recurrent thrush) that has been difficult to treat?
*Vision*                  Have you noticed any change in your vision?
*Neurological*            Have you felt any pins and needles in your hands or feet?
*Erectile dysfunction*    Have you had any problems maintaining an erection?
*Acanthosis nigricans*    Do you have any dark skin patches in the arm, neck or groin?

## RED FLAGS

*DKA/HONK*                Abdominal pain, nausea & vomiting, shortness of breath
*Cardiac*                 Chest pain

## PAST HISTORY

*Medical*                 Do you suffer from any medical problems? (IHD, CVA, PVD, CKD, Cholesterol, PCOS)
*Pregnancy*               Did you ever suffer from gestational DM during any of your pregnancies?

## DRUG HISTORY

*Medication*              Are you taking any medications?
  Worsen                 Steroids, thiazides, beta blockers, olanzapine
*Compliance*              Do you take your medications regularly?
*BM monitoring*           How do you monitor your sugar levels?

## SOCIAL HISTORY

| | |
|---|---|
| *Occupation* | Are you working at the moment? What type of work do you do? |
| *Smoker* | Do you smoke? How many cigarettes do you smoke per day? |
| *Alcohol* | Do you drink alcohol? How much do you drink and how often? |
| *Diet* | How is your diet? (excess- sweets, cakes, fizzy drinks) |
| *Exercise* | Do you do much physical activity? |
| *Mood* | How has your mood been recently? |

---

## Depression Screening in Diabetes (QoF)

Patients with DM or heart disease should be screened on one occasion during the previous year using 2 screening questions for depression. A positive to both questions is suggestive of depression and a PHQ9 should be undertaken.

*During the past month:*
- Have you often been bothered by feeling down depressed or hopeless?
- Have you often been bothered by little interest or pleasure in doing things?

---

## FAMILY HISTORY

| | |
|---|---|
| *Diabetes* | Does anyone in the family suffer from diabetes? |

## IDEA, CONCERNS, EXPECTATIONS

| | |
|---|---|
| *Idea* | What did you think was going on when you had your symptoms? |
| *Concerns* | Do you have any specific concerns about being diagnosed with diabetes? (driving, insulin, lifestyle changes) |
| *Impact on life* | How has your symptoms affected you? |

## CSA TIPS

Diabetes is a chronic disease than can have disabling consequences if it is not controlled such as blindness, MI, CVA or even amputation. It is unlikely in the CSA that you will be faced with having to convert a person from oral hypoglycemic agents to injectable insulin. It is more likely that patients will present with poor control of diabetes due to a lack of understanding, poor medication compliance, or poor social support to encourage and help their control. HGV2 drivers may also present with hypoglycemia or poorly controlled DM that may threaten their ability to continue in their jobs.

## PHYSICAL EXAMINATION

| | |
|---|---|
| *Vitals* | BP, pulse, BMI |
| *Eye* | Assess visual acuity, fundoscopy |
| *Foot* | Examine the feet for ulcers, charcot foot |
| Skin | Ulceration or infections |
| Neurological | Check for peripheral neuropathy assessing sensation (vibration, touch) and reflexes |
| Pulse | Check peripheral pulses |

## INVESTIGATIONS

| | |
|---|---|
| *Bloods* | FBC, U&E, fasting glucose, HbA1c, lipid profile |

---

## Diagnosing Diabetes

| | |
|---|---|
| *Screening* | Diagnosis should not be made from a reading from a BM test or urine dipstick. These should only be used for screening for diabetes |

| Diagnosis | Diagnosis requires 1 abnormal glucose blood test if symptomatic (polyuria, polydipsia, weight loss) or 2 abnormal tests on separate dates if asymptomatic |
|---|---|
| Random | ≥ 11.1 mmol/l |
| Fasting | ≥ 7.0 mmol/l |
| OGTT | Consider in impaired fasting glycaemia (6.1 – 7 mmol/l). Ask patient to fast from night before and have blood test in morning 2hr after given sugar load (75g of glucose or 350ml Lucozade) |
| Diabetic | ≥ 11.1 mmol/l 2hrs after sugar load |
| IGT | ≥ 7.8 and <11.1 mmol/l (Impaired glucose tolerance) |
| Non-diabetic | < 7.8 mmol/l |
| HbA1c | ≥ 48 mmol/mol is cut-off point for diagnosing diabetes. Requires 1 abnormal in symptomatic and 2 abnormal if asymptomatic |
| Alters | Fe or B12 deficiency, CKD, alcoholism, splenectomy, hyperbilirubinemia, chronic liver disease, haemoglobinopathies |

| Urine | Glucose, ketones, microalbuminuria, albumin:creatinine ratio (ACR) |
|---|---|
| Other | Oral Glucose tolerance test (OGTT) |

## Impaired fasting glycaemia (IFG) and Impaired glucose tolerance (IGT)

- Impaired fasting glycaemia is a 'borderline' fasting glucose     ≥ 6.1 and <7 mmol/l
- Impaired glucose tolerance is an equivocal OGTT     ≥ 7.8 and <11.1 mmol/l
- IFG and IGT are risk factors for developing DM and CVD. Advise lifestyle modification (i.e. diet, increased exercise, weight loss). Annual fasting glucose tests are recommended

## MANAGEMENT
### Conservative

| Diet | Recommend high fibre, low fat and low glycaemic index foods (brown rice & bread, boiled potatoes). 5 fruits and veg/d and oily fish |
|---|---|
| Avoid | Processed foods, ready meals, alcohol, refined sugars (sweets, cakes) |
| Weight loss | Aim to lose 5-10% in obese patient, can help reduce blood glucose levels |
| Exercise | Recommend 30mins/5x wk. Encourage brisk walking, hobbies i.e. cycling, swimming |
| Smoking cessation | Offer smoking cessation advice |
| DVLA | Diet controlled diabetics need not inform the DVLA. Patient should notify if requires insulin, develop complications (polyneuropathy, vision), >1 episode of hypoglycaemia in a year or has impaired awareness of it |

## Diabetics and the DVLA

| Insulin | G1 Must be able to recognise warning symptoms of hypoglycaemia |
|---|---|
| | G2 Independent medical assessment every year and submit 3mth of continuous readings. No hypos in past year and be able to recognise warning symptoms of hypoglycaemia. Cannot drive emergency vehicles |
| Oral tablets | G1 No restrictions (including exenatide or gliptin) |
| | G2 Licence unless complications |
| Hypoglycaemia | If has frequent ↓BP episodes or has Impaired hypoglycaemia awareness |
| | G1 Stop driving until has control. If have 2x hypos in past year which required assistance then to notify DVLA and stop driving |

Check your levels at least twice per day at times relevant to driving. The results should be recorded on the BM meter memory. If has 1x hypo in past year which required assistance then to notify DVLA and stop driving

*QoF*            Maintain a register of patients with DM. Monitor BP (<140/80) yearly and perform urine ACR. Ensure patient with microalbuminuria are on ACE-I. Maintain HbA1c% (<59, 64 or 75). Yearly foot examination and risk classification (pulses, neuropathy). All new DM should be referred to structured educational programme within 9mth

**Medical**

*Prescription*            Diabetics are offered free prescriptions for their medications

*Type 2 diabetes*            Consider lifestyle advice and oral medications

  Metformin            First line treatment. Initiate if HbA1c% > 6.5 (48) despite lifestyle modifications. Monitor U&E and LFTs. Gradually increase to minimise side effects

    SE            Diarrhoea, nausea and vomiting (GI symptoms) consider Metformin MR

    CI            CKD 4 (GFR<30), liver disease, alcohol excess, recent MI

  Sulphonylurea            2nd line or 1st line if not overweight or metformin is contraindicated

    SE            Hypoglycaemia, weight gain, mild GI symptoms, impaired liver function

    CI            Avoid in severe renal failure, liver impairment, breast feeding, pregnancy

  Pioglitazones            Helps increase sensitivity and secretion of insulin. Monitor LFTs. Continue if HbA1c is reduced by 0.5% within 6 months

    SE            Weight gain, fluid retention, impaired LFTs, hypoglycaemia, fracture risk

    CI            Heart failure, pregnancy

  Acarbose            Delays absorption of starch often combined with metformin or gliclazide

    SE            Flatulence, diarrhoea, abdominal distension, impaired LFTs

    CI            IBD, CKD 4, liver failure, breast feeding & pregnancy

  Sitagliptin            Works by increasing 2 chemical messengers in the body GLP-1 & GIP. Helps to control sugar levels. Licensed to be used as monotherapy or triple therapy with metformin and sulfonylurea or pioglitazone

    SE            Pancreatitis, weight gain, nausea and vomiting, tachycardia

  Combination            The patient can be offered a combination of the above medication

  Other            Exenatide (BMI >35), gliptins

*Type 1 diabetes*            Start insulin typically if HbA1c > 7.5 (58). Begin with intermediate acting insulin (isophane) taken at night or twice daily according to need. Refer to diabetic clinic or diabetic nurse. Aim for pre-prandial glucose level of 4-7 mmol/l and postprandial levels of <9 mmol/l

*1° prevention*            Consider initiating medication to prevent modifiable risk factors

  Aspirin            Initiate in all diabetics >50 years old or <50yrs with risk factors

  BP            Aim < 140/80 or < 130/80 if end organ damage (i.e. eye, kidney, CVA)

      ACE inhibitors are first-line then Ca2+ channel blockers (amlodipine)

| Cholesterol | Simvastatin 40mg if >40yrs and CVD risk >20% over 10 yrs or risk factors |
| | Aim for total cholesterol <4 mmol/l & LDL <2 mmol/l. If not reached consider |
| | increasing to 80mg or trialling another statin (Atorvastatin) or ezetimibe |
| Triglyceride | If triglyceride levels > 4.5 mmol/l consider fenofibrate |

| *Neuropathy* | Consider treatment with amitriptyline, duloxetine, gabapentin or pregabalin. If patient |
| | is unable to tolerate oral, consider capsaicin 0.075% cream |
| Amitriptyline | Off label. Start with 10mg (on) and titrate up to a max of 75mg over 6-8wks. When |
| | discontinuing, step down over 4wks to prevent SE |
| SE | Dry mouth, drowsiness, altered taste, hypotension, bradycardia |

| Duloxetine | NICE recommend this as first line treatment for all neuropathic pain except for |
| | trigeminal neuralgia. Start with 60mg daily increasing to 60mg bd if necessary. Trial for |
| | 8 weeks before assessing if effective. When discontinuing, step down over 2wks to |
| | prevent SE |
| SE | Dry mouth, sleepiness, headache, nausea, dizziness |

| Gabapentin | Fast titration involves 300md on day 1, then bd day 2 then tds day 3. Can be increased |
| | every 3 days to a maximum of 1200mg tds. Slow titration (elderly) start with 100mg |
| | daily, increased 100mg daily up to 1200mg tds. Trial for 8 weeks before assessing if |
| | effective. When discontinuing, step down over 2wks to prevent SE |
| SE | Dizziness, fever, sleepiness, movement disorder, gait problems |

| *Immunisations* | Offer flu vaccine each autumn and also single pneumococcal vaccine |
| *Support groups* | Offer patient contact details of support groups or education programmes (DESMOND) |
| *Safety netting* | Seek medical advice if any red flags symptoms |

**Refer**

| *DM eye screening* | All diabetics should be referred to a local diabetic eye screening programme |
| *Chiropody* | Consider referring patients with increased and high risk feet for assessment by a foot |
| | specialist |

**SAFETY NETTING**

| *Monitor* | Monitor HbA1c% initially every 2-6mths (aim for <48mmol/mol) and every 6mth if |
| | stable. Offer annual eye, feet and kidney check up (more frequently if indicated) |

**EXPLANATIONS**

| *Diabetes type 2* | Diabetes is a condition that affects the body's ability to control sugar levels. Your |
| | sugars levels are controlled by a hormone or chemical messenger called Insulin. |
| | Unfortunately, your body is not responding to the insulin as well as it used to. As a |
| | result the sugar levels in your blood are consistently high consequently causing your |
| | symptoms of tiredness, weight loss and passing urine more often. |

| Metformin | This is a type of medicine called a biguanide. It works well in diabetes by blocking and |
| | reducing how sugar is made in the liver and also increases the body's sensitivity to |
| | insulin. |

| Sulphonylurea | This a medicine that helps reduce the sugar levels in diabetics. It works by helping the |
| | release of insulin from the pancreas that lowers blood sugar. |

| | |
|---|---|
| Pioglitazones | This helps lower blood sugar levels in diabetics by making your cells more sensitive to the insulin so more sugar can be moved into cells for the same amount of insulin. |
| *Diabetes type 1* | Type 1 diabetes, in most cases, is an autoimmune condition. This is where your immune system, that normally protects the body from bacteria and viruses, instead makes antibodies that attack parts of the body. This includes cells within the organ (pancreas) that make insulin which helps bring your sugar levels down. |
| *Complications* | Unfortunately poorly controlled sugar levels over a long period of time can damage the blood vessels in your body. It can damage the vessels in back of the eye and affect your vision as well as give you feet problems from poor circulation. It can also fur the arteries putting you at risk of having angina, heart attacks or a stroke. Other effects include kidney damage, nerve damage and impotence. |
| *Pre-diabetes* | Your blood tests suggest that you could have pre-diabetes. This is when your sugar levels in your body are raised but not sufficiently enough to be diabetic. However, this can put you at risk of developing diabetes and heart problems in the near future. |

# *6.2 Hypothyroidism*

Hypothyroidism is a condition caused by underactivity of the thyroid gland producing less of the thyroid hormones, T4 and T3. It is more common in elderly women and affects 2% of people over the age of 60 years. The commonest form is Hashimoto thyroiditis which is an autoimmune disease affecting late middle aged women. Other causes including damage to the thyroid gland due to treatment for an overactive gland using radioactive iodine or following surgery. Internationally, a lack of dietary iodine is a common cause of hypothyroidism.

## HISTORY

**Open questions**    Tell me a little bit more as to why you had your blood tests? Can you tell me more about your symptoms?

## Focused questions

| | |
|---|---|
| *Hypothyroidism* | When did it start? How long has it been going on for? |
| Cold intolerance | Do you feel cold when others are feeling hot? |
| Tiredness | Do you feel tired or exhausted all the time? |
| Weight | Have you recently put on any weight unintentionally? |
| Constipation | How are your bowel motions? Do you open your bowels less frequently? |

## Associated history

| | |
|---|---|
| *Low mood* | How has your mood been like? How is your concentration? |
| *Dry skin* | Have you seen any changes to your skin or hair? (hair loss, dry skin) |
| *Myalgia* | Do you have any muscle aches? |
| *Hoarse voice* | Have you noticed a huskier or hoarseness to your voice? |
| *Menorrhagia* | Have you noticed any changes to your periods? (menstrual irregularity) |
| *Pregnancy* | Are you currently pregnant? |
| *Carpal Tunnel* | Do you have any pins and needles or tingling in your hands? Is it worse at night? |

## RED FLAGS

| | |
|---|---|
| *Myxoedema* | Deterioration in mental state, late presentation, exaggerated features (hypothermia, psychosis, ataxia, coma) |

## PAST HISTORY

| | |
|---|---|
| *Medical* | Do you suffer from any medical problems? (DM type 1, Addison's, pernicious anaemia, Down's syndrome, vitiligo) |
| *Surgery* | Have you ever had surgery or radiation therapy for your thyroid? (thyroidectomy, radioiodine) |

## DRUG HISTORY

| | |
|---|---|
| *Medication* | Are you taking any medications? (amiodarone, lithium, tamoxifen) |
| *Compliance* | Do you take your thyroid medications regularly? |

## SOCIAL HISTORY

| | |
|---|---|
| *Occupation* | Are you working at the moment? What do you work as? |
| *Smoker* | Do you smoke? How many cigarettes do you smoke per day? |
| *Alcohol* | Do you drink alcohol? How much do you drink and how often? |

## FAMILY HISTORY

*Hypothyroidism*        Does anyone in the family suffer from thyroid problems?

## IDEA, CONCERNS, EXPECTATIONS

| | |
|---|---|
| *Idea* | What did you think was going on when you had your symptoms? |
| *Concerns* | Do you have any specific concerns about them? (putting on weight, long term medication) |
| *Impact on life* | How has your symptoms affected you? |

## CSA TIPS

The symptoms of thyroid disease are quite nonspecific and may present in a wide range of different conditions. Females have a 2% prevalence for overt hypothyroidism and around 8% have subclinical signs. In the CSA exam patients may simply present with one overt symptom such as bowel changes, wt increase or menstrual disorders, and you will have to tease out the associated symptoms and make the diagnosis. Failure to take a comprehensive history, may lead you to make an incorrect diagnosis and subsequent shared management plan.

## PHYSICAL EXAMINATION

| | |
|---|---|
| *Vitals* | Pulse (bradycardia), BP (hypotension) BMI (obesity), temp (hypothermia) |
| *Thyroid exam* | |
|    Inspection | Inspect for dry skin, thinning of temporal hair, eyebrows and neck for goitre |
|    Palpation | Stand behind the patient. Offer glass of water to see if goitre moves up and down with swallowing. Feel for a goitre (tenderness – thyroiditis) as well as its size and nodularity |
|    Percussion | Can percuss down for retrosternal extension if SOB or dysphagia |
|    Reflexes | Slowly relaxing reflexes |
| *Neurology* | Check for slow relaxing reflexes |

## INVESTIGATIONS

*Bloods*      TFT (TSH, T3, T4), FBC & CRP (thyroiditis), cholesterol, thyroid antibodies (antithyroid peroxidase antibodies – Hashimoto's)

---

### Interpreting TFTs

| TSH | T4 | Interpretation |
|---|---|---|
| ↑ | ↓ | Hypothyroidism – initiate on medication |
| ↑ | ↔ | Subclinical hypothyroidism. Recheck after 3-6mth and annually if asymptomatic. If has symptoms initiate levothyroxine. If on medication likely poor compliance |
| ↓ | ↓ | Hypothyroidism caused by pituitary failure |
| ↑ | N | If patient is on treatment check medication compliance. If pt omits T4 for a few days/weeks TSH gradually rises. If patient then remembers and takes T4 on date of test, the serum t4 will be normal with a raised TSH |

---

*US*      Ultrasound scan of thyroid gland if mass or goitre palpable

---

### TFT Screening

- Asymptomatic patients should not be routinely tested for hypothyroidism
- Measuring TSH is indicated in patients with goitre, DM, AF, hypercholesterolaemia, radioactive iodine or surgery, congenital hypothyroidism, Down's/Turner's syndrome, drugs (amiodarone, lithium), postpartum depression, dementia

## MANAGEMENT
### Conservative
Prescription     Hypothyroid patients are offered free prescriptions

### Medical
Levothyroxine    Initiate on levothyroxine 50-100mcg od (preferably before breakfast). Recheck TFTs after 3mths and titrate dose accordingly. Aim to get TSH within normal range. Once stable monitor annually. Advise patient the need to take medication for life

 Elderly      Start with low dose 25mcg and titrate upwards mthly depending on TFTs. Consider B-blocker in elderly as levothyroxine can precipitate angina

Subclinical     Repeat TFT after 3-6mths. Levothyroxine can be considered if presence of goitre, elevating TSH. Consider trial if also symptomatic

### Refer
Endocrinologist   Refer if <16 yrs, subacute thyroiditis, pituitary disease, pregnant, persistent TSH despite increasing medication

## SAFETY NETTING
Follow-up     If symptoms not improved after 4-6wks with medication then review

## EXPLANATIONS
Hypothyroidism   Hypothyroidism is a condition where your thyroid gland found at the base of your neck is underactive and not making enough of a hormone (chemical messenger) called thyroxine. This hormone helps control the body's metabolism and energy levels. When there is too little thyroid hormone, your body's metabolism slows down and as a result you may get some of the symptoms you have described.

# 6.3 Hyperthyroidism

Thyrotoxicosis is a condition that is caused by overactivity of the thyroid gland due to an overproduction of the thyroid hormones, T4 and T3. It affects 1% of women and 0.1% of men. Symptoms include sympathetic overactivity (tremor, tachycardia, sweating), onycholysis (separation of nail from nail bed), palmar erythema, proximal myopathy and lid retraction.

The most common form of thyrotoxicosis is Grave's disease. It is a condition that commonly affects young people and presents with an enlarged smooth goitre, eye changes (exophthalmos, ophthalmoplegia), acropachy and pretibial myxoedema. It is also associated with myasthenia gravis and pernicious anaemia.

**HISTORY**

| | |
|---|---|
| **Open questions** | Tell me a little bit more as to why you had your blood tests? Can you tell me more about your symptoms? |

**Focused questions**

| | |
|---|---|
| *Hyperthyroidism* | When did it start? How long has it been going on for? |
| Heal intolerance | Do you feel hot when others feel cold? |
| Weight loss | Have you recently lost some weight despite having an increased appetite? |
| Palpitations | Do you feel that your heart beats faster than normal? |
| Diarrhoea | How are your bowel motions? Are they more frequent? |

**Associated history**

| | |
|---|---|
| *Tiredness* | Do you feel tired or exhausted all the time? |
| *Sweaty* | Do you feel sweaty more than normal? |
| *Tremor* | Do you feel your hands more shaky than usual? |
| *Irritability* | How is your mood? Do you feel more anxious or irritable than normal? |
| *Menorrhagia* | Have you noticed any changes to your periods? (infrequent) |

**RED FLAGS**

| | |
|---|---|
| *Thyrotoxic crisis* | Fever, agitation, confusion, diarrhoea & vomiting, acute abdomen, coma, tachycardia |
| *Graves disease* | Thyroid eye disease (double vision, lid lag, eye discomfort, eye protrusion) |

**PAST HISTORY**

| | |
|---|---|
| *Medical* | Do you suffer from any medical problems? (myasthenia gravis) |

**DRUG HISTORY**

| | |
|---|---|
| *Medication* | Are you taking any medications? (amiodarone, levothyroxine excess) |

**SOCIAL HISTORY**

| | |
|---|---|
| *Occupation* | Are you working at the moment? What do you work as? |
| *Smoker* | Do you smoke? How many cigarettes do you smoke per day? |
| *Alcohol* | Do you drink alcohol? How much do you drink and how often? |

**FAMILY HISTORY**

| | |
|---|---|
| *Hyperthyroidism* | Does anyone in the family suffer from thyroid problems? |

## IDEA, CONCERNS, EXPECTATIONS

| | |
|---|---|
| *Idea* | What did you think was going on when you had your symptoms? |
| *Concerns* | Do you have any specific concerns about them (losing weight, surgery)? |
| *Impact on life* | How has your symptoms affected you? |

## CSA TIPS

The signs and symptoms of hyperthyroidism may be subtle. A patient may simply attend feeling tired, irritable or with change in bowel habits but have tachycardia and a tremor on examination. In most cases, the diagnosis may not be obvious without further investigations; however, it is important that you signpost to the patient and subsequently the examiner, your thoughts about what the possible diagnoses may be.

## PHYSICAL EXAMINATION

| | |
|---|---|
| Vitals | Pulse (tachycardia, AF), BP (hypertension), BMI (low) |
| *Thyroid exam* | |
|    Inspection | |
|       Hands | Have hands outstretched (tremor), clubbing (Graves), acropachy, onycholysis, palmar erythema |
|       Eye | Look for exophthalmos, loss of hair outer 1/3 of eyebrow, lid lag/retraction, ophthalmoplegia |
|       Neck | Inspect the neck for presence of goitre |
|    Palpation | Stand behind the patient. Can offer glass of water to see if goitre moves up and down with swallowing. Feel for goitre (tenderness - thyroiditis) as well as its size and nodularity |
|    Percussion | Can percuss down for retrosternal extension if SOB or dysphagia |
|    Auscultate | Listen for a thyroid bruit |
| *Legs* | Palpate the legs for evidence of pitting oedema |

## INVESTIGATIONS

| | |
|---|---|
| *Bloods* | TFT (TSH, T3, T4), FBC (anaemia – Graves' disease), thyroid antibodies (anti-TSH-receptor antibodies - Graves' disease), ESR (Graves' disease, subacute thyroiditis) |

---

### Interpreting TFTs

| TSH | T4 | Interpretation |
|---|---|---|
| ↓ | ↑ | Hyperthyroidism – initiate on medication |
| ↓ | ↔ | Subclinical hyperthyroidism. Observe and monitor every 3-6 months. Treatment if converts into frank hyperthyroidism |
| ↑ | ↑ | Suspect pituitary microadenoma, erratic levothyroxine compliance |

---

| | |
|---|---|
| *US* | Ultrasound scan of thyroid gland if mass or goitre palpable |
| *Scintigraphy* | Specialist initiated, often pre-operation |

## MANAGEMENT

### Medical

| | |
|---|---|
| *B Blocker* | Can start on a beta blocker (propranolol, metoprolol) to control symptoms (palpitations, anxiety, tremor) until antithyroid medication is initiated. If contraindicated can consider diltiazem (specialist advice) |

| | |
|---|---|
| *Carbimazole* | Antithyroid drug that inhibits synthesis of thyroid hormones. Refer to specialist for carbimazole (often started at 40mg) or propylthiouracil to be initiated. Often given for 12-18mths but high risk of relapse (50%) |
| Side effects | Alopecia, cholestatic jaundice, pruritus, rash |
| Complications | Agranulocytosis. Advise to observe for fever, sore throat, mouth ulcers or feeling generally unwell. If noted contact doctor straight away. May be necessary to stop medication |
| | |
| *Other* | Radioiodine and surgery options offered by specialist to the patient |
| Radioiodine | Most become hypothyroid and require thyroxine for years |
| CI | Pregnant or breast-feeding and avoid up falling pregnant up to 6mths following treatment and 4mths in men trying to father children. Avoid in thyroid eye disease as can worsen the condition |
| Surgery | Can be partial or total thyroidectomy especially if large goitre. Risk of hypothyroidism with lifelong thyroxine if too much excised |
| SE | Recurrent laryngeal nerve palsy and damage to the parathyroids post surgery |
| | |
| *Subclinical* | Repeat TFT after 3-6 months and refer once it becomes hyperthyroidism or if subclinical position persists after several blood tests. Refer for specialist management if a goitre is present as well |
| | |
| *Eye symptoms* | Consider lacrilube or artificial tears to lubricate dry eyes. If periorbital oedema, elevating the head of the bed often helps reduce symptoms |
| ***Refer*** | |
| *Ophthalmology* | Refer to ophthalmology if evidence of thyroid eye disease |
| *Endocrinologist* | Refer to specialist if wanting to initiate medication i.e. carbimazole |

**SAFETY NETTING**

| | |
|---|---|
| *Follow-up* | If symptoms not improved after 4-6wks with medication then review |

**EXPLANATIONS**

| | |
|---|---|
| *Hyperthyroidism* | Hyperthyroidism is a condition where the thyroid gland found at the base of your neck is overactive and making too much of a hormone (chemical messenger) called thyroxine. This hormone helps control the body's metabolism and energy levels. If you have too much hormone, then you may get some of the symptoms you have described. |
| | |
| *Carbimazole* | This medication blocks the way the thyroid messengers or hormone is made by your thyroid gland. It may take up to 1-2 months to work and is must be taken for up to 1.5 years. |
| | |
| *Iodine therapy* | It involves taking a capsule or drink that contains a small amount of iodine that is radioactive. Iodine is taken up by the thyroid gland and is normally used to make the thyroid hormone (thyroxine). As the radioactive iodine collects within the gland it destroys some of the tissue meaning that your body will produces less thyroid hormone in the future and reduces your symptoms of hyperthyroidism. |

# 6.4 Galactorrhoea

Galactorrhoea refers to the inappropriate secretion or discharge of milk from the female breasts that is not associated with breastfeeding or pregnancy. The most common cause is raised prolactin levels that can originate from a prolactin secreting pituitary tumour. However, a number of drugs have also been implicated. Whilst galactorrhoea may be physiological in women it is more likely to be pathological in men. It can also be seen in the neonates, along with breast enlargement, who have been affected by the temporary effects of the maternal oestrogen.

## HISTORY

**Open questions**         Can you tell me more about your symptoms?

**Focused questions**

| | |
|---|---|
| *Galactorrhoea* | When did it start? How long has it been going on for? |
| Region | Does it affect both breasts or just one side? |
| Discharge | Is it only a milky discharge or have you notice any blood or pus? |
| Volume | How much milk has been produced? |
| Breast pain | Are your breasts painful? |
| Trigger | Does anything increase the flow such as stimulating or sucking the breast? Or taking tablets? |

**Associated history** *in men*

| | |
|---|---|
| *Impotence* | Have you noticed any problems getting an erection? |
| *Libido loss* | Have you lost interest in having sex? |
| *Gynaecomastia* | Have you notice any abnormal breast tissue? |

**Gynaecology history** *in women*

| | |
|---|---|
| *Menstrual disturb.* | When was your last period? Are they regular? |
| *Infertility* | Have you had any problems getting pregnant? |
| *Contraception* | Are you using any forms of contraception? Have you recently started using the pill? |

**Differentials**

| | |
|---|---|
| *Pregnancy* | Do you think you are pregnant? Have you had any terminations? |
| *Breast feeding* | How many children do you have? Are you currently breast feeding? |
| *Hypothyroidism* | Do you feel tired all the time? Have you put on any weight? Do you feel cold when others feel hot? |
| *Pituitary adenoma* | Do you get blurring of the peripheries of vision or any other visual disturbances? Do you get headaches? |

## RED FLAGS

| | |
|---|---|
| *Pituitary adenoma* | Visual disturbances, severe headaches |
| *Breast cancer* | Unilateral, bloody discharge, lump |

## PAST HISTORY

| | |
|---|---|
| *Medical* | Do you suffer from any medical problems (hypothyroidism, acromegaly, CKD, liver cirrhosis)? |

## DRUG HISTORY

| | |
|---|---|
| *Medication* | Are you taking any medications? |
| *OTC / Herbs* | Are you taking any OTC medication / herb supplements? (fennel, thistle, nettle, marshmallow) |

## Drugs that can Cause Galactorrhoea

- Metoclopramide, domperidone, TCAs, haloperidol, risperidone, methyldopa, oral contraceptive pill, SSRIs, bendroflumethiazide, ranitidine, spironolactone, cimetidine, beta blockers
- Drug induced galactorrhoea do not cause a rise in prolactin levels >2500 mU/L. Such levels warrant a full examination and further investigation to exclude pituitary pathology

## SOCIAL HISTORY

| | |
|---|---|
| *Occupation* | Are you working at the moment? What do you work as? |
| *Stress* | Are you feeling more stressed than normal? Do you have any financial worries (mortgage, debt) or relationship problems? (breakup, divorce) |
| *Smoker* | Do you smoke? How many cigarettes do you smoke per day? |
| *Alcohol* | Do you drink alcohol? How much do you drink and how often? |
| *Illicit Drugs* | Have you ever used any recreational drugs? (cannabis, amphetamines) |

## FAMILY HISTORY

| | |
|---|---|
| *Endocrine* | Does anyone in the family suffer from thyroid problems? Does anyone suffer from Multiple Endocrine Neoplasia? |

## IDEA, CONCERNS, EXPECTATIONS

| | |
|---|---|
| *Idea* | What did you think was going on when you had your symptoms? |
| *Concerns* | Have you had any particular worries about it? (pregnancy, breast cancer) |
| *Impact on life* | How has it affected you day to day? How are you coping with it? How have you been managing it (pads, regular change in clothing)? |

## CSA TIPS

Patients who have never been pregnant and suffering with a milky breast discharge may be quite distraught and confused about what is causing their symptoms. Patients may have to go to the toilet discretely quite often during working hours, to replace pads or change their clothes causing disruption of and interruption to their daily routine. It is important to take a clear history and empathise with the patient about their problem. Always enquire about headaches and visual loss to exclude any possible prolactinoma and about a unilateral lump and bloody discharge for breast cancer. Do not forget that physiological galactorrhoea can persist up to 2 years following the cessation of breast feeding.

## PHYSICAL EXAMINATION

| | |
|---|---|
| *Vitals* | BP (hypothyroidism), weight (hypothyroidism, acromegaly, pregnancy) |
| *General* | Examine the skin for signs of hirsutism, hair loss or acne |
| *Breast* | Observe for any skin changes (peau d' orange) & palpate to exclude any breast lumps |
| Express | Request the patient to express any milk from their nipples |

| | |
|---|---|
| *Neurology* | |
| Visual fields | Assess visual fields by confrontation if pituitary lesion is suspected. Map the visual fields and observe for bitemporal hemianopia (pituitary adenoma, craniopharyngioma) |

## INVESTIGATIONS

| | |
|---|---|
| *Bloods* | Prolactin levels (hyperprolactinoma >500 requires investigation, >4000 is pathological), TFTs |
| *MC&S + cytology* | Breast discharge |
| *Urine* | Pregnancy test |
| *Other* | MRI/CT head (pituitary adenoma/ craniopharyngioma) |

## MANAGEMENT *treat the underlying cause*

| | |
|---|---|
| ***Medication*** | Identify precipitating drug and stop or change to an alternative |

### Hyperprolactinemia

| | |
|---|---|
| *Microadenoma* | Monitor pituitary adenomas with MRI scans and prolactin blood tests |
| *Bromocriptine* | Refer to specialist for initiation of bromocriptine. Stimulates dopamine receptors in the brain and inhibits release of prolactin in the pituitary |
| Dosage | 2.5 mg on day 1 (prevention) or daily for 2–3 days (suppression); then 2.5 mg bd for 14 days. Always be taken with food |
| SE | Sleepiness, postural ↓BP, dizziness, nasal congestion, lung fibrosis |
| CI | Pre-eclampsia, HTN in postpartum women/puerperium, CHD, serious mental disorder. Discontinue immediately if HTN, unremitting headache, or signs of CNS toxicity develop |
| ***Idiopathic*** | Treat symptomatic galactorrhoea with bromocriptine |
| ***Hypothyroidism*** | Start levothyroxine depending on TFTs (refer to hypothyroidism chapter) |

### Refer

| | |
|---|---|
| *Endocrinologist* | Refer to specialist if suspicion of a brain lesion causing the galactorrhoea |

## SAFETY NETTING

| | |
|---|---|
| *Side effects* | if symptoms are not improving or visual disturbances, headaches, dizziness whilst taking bromocriptine then stop driving or using power tools or machines |

## DIFFERENTIAL DIAGNOSIS

| Condition | Characteristic exam feature |
|---|---|
| **Physiological** | Breast feeding, pregnancy, stress |
| **Prolactinoma** | Can be caused by pituitary adenoma or craniopharyngioma. Presents with headache, visual disturbances (bitemporal hemianopia), irregular periods (amenorrhoea), infertility and reduced libido. OE: reduced peripheral vision, papilloedema |
| **Hypothyroidism** | Patients complain of tiredness, weight gain, cold intolerance, constipation and menstrual irregularities. OE: dry skin, thinning hair and reduced reflexes. A goitre may be present |
| **Acromegaly** | Rare condition due to increased growth hormone. Causes large hand and feet, prominent jaw and facial features, enlarged tongue. Patients may have oily coarse skin |

| | and complain of low libido, impotence (men) or menstrual disturbances |
| --- | --- |
| **PCOS** | Hirsutism, obesity, acne. Irregular periods and fertility problems |

**EXPLANATIONS**

*Prolactinoma*    Prolactinoma is a non-cancerous lump or swelling found in the part of the brain that controls your hormone levels (pituitary gland). It releases too much of a hormone or chemical messenger called prolactin. As a result you may experience headaches, changes in your vision and milk secretion as it is the hormone responsible for priming the breasts for breastfeeding.

# 6.5 Gynaecomastia

Gynaecomastia describes the abnormal enlargement and development of breasts in males. Although it may be present physiologically in the newborn, adolescence and elderly, it usually causes much distress and angst in the male sufferer.

## HISTORY

**Open questions**          Can you tell me more about your symptoms?

## Focused questions

| | |
|---|---|
| *Gynaecomastia* | When did it start? How long has it been going on for? |
| Region | Does it affect both sides of your chest or just one side? |
| Discharge | Have you noticed any discharge from it? |
| Breast pain | Are they painful? |
| Sexual function | Have you lost interest in having sex? Do you struggle to get erections? |

## Differentials

| | |
|---|---|
| *Testicular cancer* | Have you noticed any lumps in your testicles? Have you lost any weight? |
| *Hyperthyroidism* | Do you feel tired all the time? Have you lost any weight recently? Do you feel hot when others feel cold? Any problems with your periods? |

## RED FLAGS

| | |
|---|---|
| *Breast cancer* | FHx of breast ca, rapidly growing lesion, >5cm, irregular firm mass, unilateral |
| *Other* | Testicular cancer (testicular mass), liver disease (jaundice, weight loss) |

## PAST HISTORY

| | |
|---|---|
| *Medical* | Do you suffer from any medical problems? (hyperthyroidism, adrenal cancer, liver disease - cirrhosis, renal failure, Hypogonadism - Klinefelter syndrome) |

## DRUG HISTORY

| | |
|---|---|
| *Medication* | Are you taking any medications? |
| Worsens | Spironolactone, cimetidine, digoxin, antipsychotics (phenothiazine, risperidone), furosemide, finasteride, anabolic steroids, COCP |

## SOCIAL HISTORY

| | |
|---|---|
| *Smoker* | Do you smoke? How many cigarettes do you smoke per day? |
| *Alcohol* | Do you drink alcohol? How much do you drink and how often? |
| *Illicit drugs* | Have you ever taken any drugs (heroin, cannabis)? |
| *Mood* | How would you describe your mood? |

## FAMILY HISTORY

| | |
|---|---|
| *Breast cancer* | Does anyone in the family suffer from breast problems? |

## IDEA, CONCERNS, EXPECTATIONS

| | |
|---|---|
| Idea | What did you think was going on when you had your symptoms? |
| *Concerns* | Have you had any particular worries about it (breast cancer)? |

| Impact on life | How has it affected you? How do you feel in yourself? Has anyone commented about it? How did they make you feel? |
|---|---|

## CSA TIPS

The development of breast tissue can be an embarrassing time for any male. Particularly, those who are obese or passing through adolescence, it may make their already turbulent time even more problematic. The teenage times are notoriously difficult for children who may appear different or abnormal compared to their peers. Young males with excess breast development may be teased or bullied at school, causing them to avoid sporting activities such as swimming for fear of being insulted. It is important to ask about the patient's psychological state and mood as relevant.

## PHYSICAL EXAMINATION

| *Vitals* | BMI (Obesity) |
|---|---|
| *Breast* | |
| Inspection | Inspect for enlargement of the breasts. Check for unilateral or bilateral presentation. Any skin changes (peau d' orange, nipple retraction) |
| Palpation | Palpate four quadrants for masses. Ascertain the size and shape. Feel for axillary lymphadenopathy |
| | |
| *Abdomen* | |
| Inspection | Inspect for liver disease signs (spider naevi, jaundice, palmar erythema) |
| Palpation | Palpate the liver for signs of hepatomegaly or irregular edge (cirrhosis) |
| | |
| *Testicular exam* | |
| Inspection | Inspect for hypogonadism, Klinefelter synd. ($2^0$ sexual characteristics) |
| Palpation | Palpate the testicles for any masses |
| | |
| *Thyroid exam* | Palpate the thyroid for signs of a goitre |

## INVESTIGATIONS

| Bloods | U&Es, LFTs, TFTs, Karyotype (Klinefelter's) |
|---|---|
| Hormone | LH & FSH, testosterone, oestradiol, prolactin, ALF, bHCG (testicular ca) |

---

### Interpreting LH & Testosterone levels in Gynaecomastia

| LH | Test. | Interpretation |
|---|---|---|
| N | N | Idiopathic gynaecomastia |
| N | ↓ | Pituitary or hypothalamic disease |
| ↑ | ↓ | Testicular failure (hypogonadism), Klinefelter's |
| ↑ | ↑ | Androgen resistance or neoplasm secreting gonadotrophins |
| ↓ | ↓ | Increased oestrogen (testicular/adrenal cancer, liver failure, hyperthyroidism, obesity) |

---

| *US* | Testes or breast tissue |
|---|---|
| *CXR* | Lung cancer |
| *Specialist (other)* | FNA or biopsy, CT scan adrenal lesions |

## MANAGEMENT *treat the underlying cause*

| *Medication* | Identify precipitating drug and stop |
|---|---|
| *Physiological* | Most common form, seen in elderly, neonates, teenagers, obesity. Reassure |

| | |
|---|---|
| *Obesity* | Encourage weight loss. Refer to exercise programme to get BMI <25 |
| *Adolescent* | Majority resolves within 3 years |

**Treatment**

| | |
|---|---|
| *Medication* | Specialist may initiate anti-oestrogens (tamoxifen and clomiphene; di-hydrotestosterone). Consider testosterone replacements in hypogonadal men |
| *Surgery* | Surgical reduction via mammoplasty if the gynaecomastia does not get better or patient cannot tolerate appearance |

**Refer**

| | |
|---|---|
| *Counselling* | Consider referring to counsellor or psychotherapy for support |
| *Urologist* | Refer urgently if suspect testicular cancer |
| *Endocrinologist* | Refer to specialist if suspicion of a brain lesion causing the galactorrhoea |
| *Breast surgeons* | Refer urgently as per cancer guidelines |

---

**Referral Guidance Gynaecomastia 2ww**

Unilateral enlargement. hard or irregular breast tissue, rapidly enlarging, recent onset, fixed mass, nipple or skin abnormalities, painful, >5 cm, axillary lymphadenopathy

---

**EXPLANATIONS**

| | |
|---|---|
| *Gynaecomastia* | All men naturally have a small amount of breast tissue. In gynaecomastia, this breast tissue has increased in size and is more pronounced. It is commonly seen in newborn babies, teenagers as well as in the elderly. |
| *Physiological* | Newborn babies can have enlarged breasts after birth as mum's hormones (maternal oestrogens) may still be circulating in the baby's blood. This can cause a small amount of harmless discharge of milk known by some people as witch's milk. It often disappears after a few weeks. |
| Teenagers | Because of the hormonal changes during puberty, sometimes boys (14yr old+) may get gynecomastia affecting one or both sides. This normally disappears later in puberty and is usually nothing to worry about. |

# 6.6 Tiredness all the time

Tiredness and fatigue are extremely common symptoms that a wide range of patients present with. In the UK, it is believed that up to 20% of people suffer with tiredness lasting longer than a month. Tiredness and fatigue may be caused by psychological problems such as stress, insomnia or depression, physical problems such as hard manual labour or due to a number of physiological conditions such as obesity, thyroid dysfunction, DM etc. However, fatigue that persists may suggest that something more sinister such as cancer or inflammation is at play. It is important to take an extensive history of the patient's complaint, before examining and tailoring investigations to locate the route cause.

## HISTORY
**Open questions**  How can I help you today? Tell me more about the problems you are having. What do you mean by tiredness (physical, mental)?

**Focused questions**
*Fatigue*
Onset  When did your tiredness start?
Frequency  How often do you get tired? Is it all the time or does it come and go?
Triggers (ideas)  Have you noticed anything that makes you feel tired (stress, new tablet)? Did you have a recent illness?
*Function*  Has it affected your ability to do things? (walking, cooking, climbing stairs, dressing)

**Associated history**
*Sleep*  How is your sleep? What time do you wake up and go to sleep? Do you nap during the day? Do you feel refreshed after you wake up?
*Cognitive*  Are you able to concentrate? Do you get distracted easily?
*Dizziness*  Do you feel dizzy or faint? Do you feel sick as well? Have you vomited?
*Flu-like*  Do you suffer with a sore throat, fevers or flu-like symptoms? (post viral)
*Weight*  Have you noticed any change in weight?

**Differentials**
*Organic*
*Anaemia*  Have you noticed any hair loss or headaches? Do you feel lightheaded?
  Menstrual  When was your last period (LMP)? Are they regular or irregular? Heavy?
*Thyroid*  Have you put on weight recently? Do you feel cold when others feel hot?
*Diabetes*  Do you feel thirsty? Do you pass more urine than normal?
*Sleep Apnoea*  Do you snore at night? Do you choke or stop breathing when you sleep?
*Malabsorption*  Have you had any diarrhoea? Is it related to any specific types of food (coeliac)? Have you noticed any mucus or blood in stools (IBD)?
*Myositis*  Do you suffer with pain or weakness of muscles? (shoulder or pelvis)
*PMR*  Is there any pain or tenderness in both of your shoulders? Are your muscles painful to touch? Have you had any stiffness of the joints? Is it worse in the morning?

*Cancer*  Have you passed any blood when coughing (lung ca, TB, sarcoid)? Vomiting (stomach ca)? Passing stools (bowel ca)? When passing urine (renal tumour, infection)?
*Blood*  Have you had any weight loss? Or noticed any lumps in the body? Do you sweat a lot at night time?

## Infections

| | |
|---|---|
| *Glandular Fever* | Did you have a high temp (>38)? Did you have swollen neck glands? |
| *Hep B* | Are you sexually active? Do you use protection? Do you use injectable recreational drugs? Do you share needles? |
| *TB/Sarcoid* | Have you lost weight? Do you have drenching night sweats? Do you have a dry cough or blood in the phlegm? |

## Psychological

| | |
|---|---|
| *Depression* | Have you been feeling low recently? Do you feel disinterested in life or worthless? |
| *CFS* | Do you suffer from tiredness or fatigue after carrying out any activity? |

## RED FLAGS

Weight loss, night sweats, persistent fevers, haemoptysis, PR bleeding, postmenopausal PV bleeding, dysphagia, swollen LN

## PAST HISTORY

| | |
|---|---|
| *Medical* | Have you ever suffered from any medical conditions (cancer, TB)? |

## DRUG HISTORY

| | |
|---|---|
| *Medication* | Are you taking any medications (B-blockers, SSRIs, TCA, BDZs, antihistamines)? |

## FAMILY HISTORY

| | |
|---|---|
| *Medical* | Does anyone in your family suffer from similar symptoms? |

## SOCIAL HISTORY

| | |
|---|---|
| *Travel* | Have you recently travelled anywhere (malaria, Hep A,B,C, tics- lyme disease)? |
| *Relationships* | Are you currently in a relationship? How are things? |
| *Support network* | Who lives with you at home? Do you have any close friends or family? |
| *Occupation* | Are you working or studying at the moment? Have you had to miss these activities due to your symptoms? How is work? How many hours do you work? Do you work nights or shift patterns? |
| *Diet* | Tell me about your diet? Do you eat a balanced diet with fruits, meat and veg? Are you vegetarian or vegan? |
| *Smoker* | Do you smoke? How many cigarettes do you smoke per day? |
| *Alcohol* | Do you drink alcohol? How much do you drink and how often? |
| *Recreational drugs* | Have you ever used any recreational drugs (cannabis, cocaine)? |

## IDEA, CONCERNS, EXPECTATIONS

| | |
|---|---|
| *Ideas* | Have you had any thoughts what may be causing your tiredness? Was there anything significant that happened before your symptoms started? |
| *Concerns* | Do you have any worries about the tiredness you have been feeling? |
| *Expectations* | How did you think I could help you today? |
| *Impact* | How have the symptoms affected your life? |

## CSA TIPS

A feeling of general tiredness is an extremely common presenting complaint in general practice. 20% of people feel tired at any given time and 10% will suffer with prolonged, chronic tiredness. The list of differentials for tiredness is very long, and it may be due to organic illness in any system, but also importantly can be due to psychological stress. It may even be physiological due to overweight or lifestyle considerations such as over and under-eating, poor sleeping habits and being overworked.

## PHYSICAL EXAMINATION

| | |
|---|---|
| *Vitals* | Temp, BP, weight, pulse |
| *General* | Does the pt appear sad, irritable or anxious? |
| *Examination* | Do a complete physical examination focussing on systems where symptoms may be present |
| Inspect | Look for general health, signs of anaemia (pale conjunctiva, atrophic glossitis, tachycardia) |
| Palpate | Perform focused thyroid examination. Feel for lymphadenopathy |
| *Questionnaires* | Offer PHQ-9 if symptoms of depression |
| | Complete the (ESS Epworth Sleepiness Scale) if suspecting OSA |

## INVESTIGATIONS

| | |
|---|---|
| *Bloods* | FBC (anaemia), ESR, CRP, TFT, fasting glucose |
| Other | *If clinically indicated:* ferritin, U&E's, LFTs, Vit D, calcium, tTGA antibodies |
| Myeloma screen | Consider urine Bence Jones protein and protein electrophoresis |
| Viral screen | HIV, Hep B and C, monospot test |
| *Sputum* | 3x early morning samples for ZN stain, MC&S |
| *Urine* | Dipstick for protein, blood, glucose. MC&S for infection |
| *Stools* | MC&S If recent travel and chronic diarrhoea |
| *X-ray* | Chest to exclude infection, TB, sarcoid, lung cancer |

## MANAGEMENT

### Conservative

*Lifestyle*

| | |
|---|---|
| Exercise | Take regular exercise i.e. walk, stretching, aerobic |
| Diet | Cut down alcohol. Eat a balanced diet including red meat, red kidney beans |
| Sleep hygiene | Relax in a dark room with minimal distraction. Go to sleep at the same time every night and have a light snack. No sleeping during the day |
| Rest | Ensure any rest periods are not more than 30 minutes |
| Relaxation | Use breathing techniques or guided visualisation to help relax during rest period |
| Weight | Advise patients to reduce weight to BMI <25m² to help reduce tiredness symptoms |

| | |
|---|---|
| *Sick Certificate* | Offer short fit-note if severe symptoms. Consider amended duties or altered hours if finding it difficult to carry out certain tasks or to attend work. Advise to go to the Jobcentre for advice around benefits, income support and disability |
| *Occup. Adviser* | Advise the patient to attend a work based occupational adviser or physician if the patient is having problems due to work |

*Talking therapies*

| | |
|---|---|
| CBT | Consider cognitive behavioural therapy for mild / moderate depression |
| GET | Consider referring for graded exercise therapies or activity management programs |

| | |
|---|---|
| **Medical** | *Treat the underlying cause* |
| *Anaemia* | Consider ferrous supplements if evidence of low iron |
| *Dysmenorrhoea* | See dysmenorrhoea chapter |
| *Diabetes* | See diabetes chapter |
| *Thyroidism* | See hypothyroidism chapter |

| | |
|---|---|
| *Myositis* | Refer to rheumatology to consider treatment with steroids or immunosuppressive agents (azathioprine) |
| *TB* | Refer to respiratory team for triple therapy abx (isoniazid, rifampicin, pyrazinamide) for 6mths |
| *Depression* | Try SSRI (fluoxetine, sertraline) to treat stress/depression. See depression chapter |

**Referral**

| | |
|---|---|
| *OT* | Speak to OT about adaptations that can be made or regarding adaptations at work to maintain ability to stay in employment |
| *Pain Clinic* | Consider referring to pain clinic to maximise treatment |
| *Rheumatologist* | Refer to a rheumatologist or specialist CFS service if available locally |
| *2WW* | Refer patients according to the 2WW pathways if any red flags of cancer suspected |

**SAFETY NETTING**

| | |
|---|---|
| *Follow up* | Review in 4-6wks for response to treatment or to check the diagnosis |

**EXPLANATIONS**

| | |
|---|---|
| *Fe Def Anaemia* | Iron deficiency anaemia is when the body has low iron levels that lead to low numbers of red blood cells. Red blood cells are needed to help carry oxygen to the tissues and cells of the body. When these cells become fewer, less oxygen is carried and may lead to symptoms such as tiredness, dizziness, shortness of breath and headache. |

# 7.1 Headache

Headaches are an extremely common symptom that patients present with. The vast majority of headaches are due to migraine and tension. However, a small minority are due to more sinister and serious causes such as an intracranial bleed, or a space occupying lesion. The key to a good consultation is to take a comprehensive history about the headache and identify any associated features.

**Differentials of headaches**

| | |
|---|---|
| *Sudden* | Subarachnoid haemorrhage, minor viral headache, postcoital migraine, migraine, meningitis |
| *Periodic* | Migraine, cluster headaches, sinusitis, glaucoma, hypertension, cervical spondylosis |
| *Continuous* | Temporal arteritis, brain tumour, depression |

**HISTORY**

**Open questions**   Can you tell me more about your headache?

**Focused questions**

| | |
|---|---|
| *Headache* | When did your headache first start? How long has it been going on for? How long does the pain last for? |
| Onset | Did the headache come on suddenly (subarachnoid) or gradually? |
| Frequency | Is it always there (continuous) or does it come and go (episodic)? |
| Site | Where exactly is the pain? (unilateral/bilateral/always same side) |
| Severity | How severe is the pain? (pain score) |
| Character | How would you describe the headache? (sharp, dull, throbbing, band) |
| Timing | Are they worse at a particular time of day ?(evening - tension) |
| Relieving | Does anything make the pain better? (standing, lying, posture) |
| Aggravating | Does anything make the pain worse? (stress, head movements, coughing, periods) |

**Associated history**

| | |
|---|---|
| *Fever* | Have you had a fever, sweats or shakes? (rigors) |
| *Nausea & vomiting* | Do you feel sick or have you vomited with the headaches? |
| *Visual disturbances* | Have you had any visual symptoms such as zigzag lines, blurring or loss of vision? Do you have problems when looking at the light (photophobia)? |
| *Eyes* | Do you wear glasses? Have you had your eyes tested? |

**Differentials**

| | |
|---|---|
| *Migraine* | Do you get throbbing headache? Any visual symptoms (flickering lights, spots, zig-zag lines, fortification spectra)? Do you feel sick or vomited? |
| *Cluster* | Do you get an intense pain around your eye? Is it always the same side? Does your eye water or you get a runny nose shortly after? |
| *Tension* | Have you been under a lot of stress recently? |
| *Sinusitis* | Are the headaches worse when you lean forward? |
| *Postcoital* | Do they come on after having sex? |
| *Glaucoma* | Do you see halos around bright lights? Is it really painful especially when you move your eyes? Do you feel sick? Do you have problems with the light? |

| Meningitis | Have you had any fever, rash, neck stiffness? |
| Malignant BP | Do you have any blurred vision or nausea? Have you noted any swelling in the legs or feet? |
| Subdural | Have you had any recent head injuries? |
| Brain tumour | Have you noticed a change in your personality? Have you had any fitting? |
| Raised ICP | Do your headaches wake you up in the morning? Are they worse on sneezing, coughing or standing up? Do you feel sick or nauseous? |
| Temporal Arteritis | Are your headaches worse on chewing food or combing your hair? |

**RED FLAGS**    Sudden onset of severe pain (thunderclap), blurring of vision, focal neurology, head injury, change in personality, signs of meningitis, drowsiness, scalp tenderness, seizure, wakes up from sleep

**PAST HISTORY**

| Medical | Do you suffer from any medical conditions? (migraines) |
| CVD | Do you suffer from high blood pressure or have you had a stroke before? |

**FAMILY HISTORY**

| Headaches | Does anyone in your family suffer from headaches? (migraines, brain tumours) |

**DRUG HISTORY**

| Medication | Are you taking any medications (nitrates, Ca channel blockers, codeine, COCP)? Do you take any painkillers? How often are you taking them (overuse)? |

**SOCIAL HISTORY**

| Occupation | Are you working at the moment? Do you have any stress at work? Do you have any financial worries (loss of job, mortgages, debt)? |
| Relationships | Are you currently in a relationship? How are things? |
| Smoker | Do you smoke? How many cigarettes do you smoke per day? |
| Alcohol | Do you drink alcohol? How much do you drink and how often? |
| Diet | How is your diet? (cheese, chocolate, caffeine) |

**IDEA, CONCERNS, EXPECTATIONS**

| Idea | Do you have any idea what may be causing your headache? |
| Concerns | Do you have any worries about it? (cancer)? |
| Expectations | How were you hoping I could help you? (MRI, referral) |
| Impact | How have your symptoms affected your life? |

**CSA TIPS**

Headache is a common problem that many patients complain of in primary care. Although most cases are benign and may be simply due to poor eyesight, or tension, other more serious causes always should be excluded. The headache may be quite debilitating and impacting on the patient's work or life and it is important that you should enquire about this.

**PHYSICAL EXAMINATION**

| Vitals | BP (hypertension), pulse, temp |
| Eyes | Inspect the pupils & examine the fundi (papilledema), if indicated press on the eyeballs (IOP- glaucoma) |
| Rheumatology | Palpate the temporal arteries for tenderness if headache in >50yr |

| MSK | Examine the neck for muscle tenderness and stiffness (tension) |
|---|---|
| Neurological | Perform a focused CN examination (e.g. CN 2,3,4,6) and neurological assessment (dependent of symptoms: Kernig's & Brudzinski's (meningitis), pupillary reflexes, gait) |

## INVESTIGATIONS

| Bloods | FBC, Fe (anaemia), ESR, CRP (temporal arteritis) |
|---|---|
| X-Ray | Facial sinuses (sinusitis) |
| CT/MRI | Brain scan if suggestive of pathology |
| Specialist | LP (subarachnoid) |

## MANAGEMENT

### Conservative

| Diary | Offer a headache diary to monitor symptoms |
|---|---|

### Treat cause

| Migraine | See migraine chapter |
|---|---|
| Sinusitis | See facial pain chapter |
| Tension | |
| Conservative | Manage stress – reassure, offer CBT, relaxation techniques and recommend exercise. Avoid missing or delaying meals and poor sleep patterns. Recommend fluid hydration and avoid caffeine |
| Medical | Offer paracetamol, aspirin or NSAIDS, avoid opioids or triptans. If frequent consider amitriptyline (75mg up to 150mg) or nortriptyline if CI, acupuncture |
| Cluster | |
| Conservative | Avoid triggers such as alcohol or fumes (solvents, oil products) |
| Medical | For acute attacks offer 100% oxygen (ambulatory), sumatriptan (sc/intranasal). Avoid alcohol during headaches. Prophylaxis give verapamil 240-960 mg daily |
| Medication overuse | Attempt to stop medication completely for at least 1mth (opioids/BDZ gradually). Advise headaches may worsen before improving (2-10d). May experience withdrawal symptoms for 7-21d (nausea, vomiting, restlessness, anxiety, sleep problems). Consider antiemetics or topiramate |
| Postcoital headache | If first presentation consider excluding subarachnoid haemorrhage. Recommend NSAIDs (indomethacin) or propranolol as prophylaxis. Some evidence support triptan use |
| Temporal Arteritis | Refer urgently to hospital. Consider prednisolone (40-60mg without visual symptoms, 60-80mg with visual symptoms) with low dose aspirin and PPI. May warrant bone bisphosphonates if on long term steroids |
| Acute Glaucoma | See red eye chapter |

### Referral

| Cluster | For first episode consider neuroimaging. If not responding to verapamil or requiring treatment during pregnancy, refer for specialist advice |
|---|---|
| Temporal arteritis | Refer urgently to ophthalmologist for temporal biopsy |
| Tension | Refer if poor response to treatment |

---

**Urgent referral pathway -** *Ref: NICE (2005). Referral Guidelines for Suspected Cancer*
*Urgent referral to neurologist under 2-week rule*

| Brain tumour | Progressive neurological deficit, new onset seizures, CN palsy, unilateral sensorineural deafness |
|---|---|

| ICP | Headaches with vomiting, drowsiness, pulse-synchronous tinnitus, headache related to posture, focal neurology, change in personality or memory |

**SAFETY NETTING**

*Follow up*      Review 2-4 weeks if symptoms not improving

| Condition | Characteristic exam feature |
|-----------|------------------------------|
| Migraine | Unilateral throbbing frontal or temporal headaches more common in women than men. May present with or without an aura (flashing lights, loss of vision) but invariably patients suffer with nausea, vomiting and photophobia. Classically patient's sleep it off. Rarely presents with hemiplegia. Occasionally triggered by certains foods (caffeine, chocolate), drugs (OCP), stress and periods |
| Tension headaches | Stress induced headaches. Often bilateral, moderate intensity that is felt as a band (frontal/occipital) across head that worsens through the day. Can last from 30min to 7d, not worsened with activity, nor associated with N&V. Absence of neurological signs |
| Cluster headaches | Common in 30-40yr olds males. Recurrent attacks of unilateral pain (temporal/eye) lasting 45-90 min often described as most severe pain ever felt. Can awaken from sleep but usually occurs same time every day (night). Can be triggered by alcohol. Associated with rhinorrhoea, lacrimation, flushing, pupil constriction, drooping eyelid. Attacks occur in clusters lasting several weeks with periods of remission (>1mth) |
| Medication overuse | More common in women. Often affects people with migraines or tension headache who suffer from chronic headache present >14d per month that worsens with analgesia. Likely if taking analgesia for >3mths. At risk if taking triptans or opioids for >= 10d/mth or paracetamol, aspirin or NSAIDs for >= 15d/mth |
| Temporal arteritis | Inflammation of the walls of medium/large arteries. Often in elderly (>50yr) presents with temporal headache, malaise, fever, scalp tenderness (combing hair), jaw claudication (chewing). OE: temporal tenderness and decreased temporal pulse, CN palsy (III, IV, VI). Can cause sudden blindness. Associated with raised ESR (>50) and polymyalgia rheumatica. Confirmed with biopsy |

**EXPLANATIONS**

*Migraine*      This is a type of headache that causes pain on the front or the side of the head. It is usually one sided and may be associated with other symptoms such as feeling sick or vomiting. Sometimes the headache presents with a warning sign called an aura which may include flashing lights. We do not know what the cause is, but it is thought that it is due to the blood vessels tightening and then relaxing in the head.

*Tension*      A tension headache is the most common cause of headache. Most people suffer from it at some point in their lives. It is thought that they may be triggered due to stress, poor sleep or not eating well. However, they are not life threatening.

| | |
|---|---|
| *Cluster* | These are one sided headaches that recur in clusters (bouts) over a few weeks and can be extremely painful. It is thought that they occur when the brain releases chemicals that trigger the pain receptors in the head causing the pain. They may be triggered by alcohol or strong-smelling scents. |
| *Temporal arteritis* | This is a condition where there is swelling or inflammation of a blood vessel that supplies the scalp of the head known as the temporal artery. This leads to tenderness over the area and headache. If it is left untreated for a long time it may cause damage to your vision and eventually can lead to blindness. |

# 7.2 Migraine

Migraine is a condition that causes episodic headaches that at times can be debilitating. They are the commonest cause of headaches and often affect teenage women more than men. Most experience moderate to severe pain that can affect their ability to work or function. They often present with headaches that last between 4-72hrs which are throbbing, unilateral and aggravated by performing daily physical activities. They can also cause nausea or vomiting with sensitivity to light (photophobia) or sound (phonophobia). They can also occur with auras (visual, sensory, speech disturbance) that can last up to 1hr.

## HISTORY

**Open questions**   Can you tell me more about your headache? Could you tell me more about what has been troubling you?

## Focused questions

*Migraine*   When did your headache first start? How long has it been going on for? How long does it last?

Site   Where exactly is the pain? (unilateral)
Onset   Did the headache come on suddenly or gradually?
Frequency   How often do you get the headaches? Every day or weekly?
Character   How would you describe the headache? (throbbing)
Aggravating   Does anything make the pain worse? (food, lack of sleep, emotion)
Relieving   Does anything make the pain better? (medication)
Severity   How severe is the pain? (pain score)

## Associated history

*Nausea & vomiting*   Do you feel sick or have you vomited with the headaches?
*Neurological*   Do you get any numbness or weakness in your arms or legs? Any speech problems (dysphasic)? Do you get dizzy spells with the headaches (vertigo)?
Visual   Have you had any visual symptoms? (flickering lights, spots, zig-zag lines, fortification spectra, blurring, loss of vision)
Photophobia   Do you have problems when looking at light?
Phonophobia   Do you have an increased sensitivity to sounds during the headaches?
*Prodromal*   Do you get a warning before they start? (change in mood, appetite or temperature, sensitivity to light, sound, smell)

## Triggers

*Diet*   What foods do you enjoy eating (cheese, chocolate, caffeine)? Do you ever miss meals?
*Alcohol*   Do you drink alcohol? How much do you drink and how often?
*Menstrual*   Are the headaches related to your periods?
*Sleep*   Have you changed your sleep pattern recently?
*Stress*   Any stress at work or home?
*Exercise*   Have you been doing more exercise than normal recently?
*Others*   Do certain smells or bright lights bring it on?

## RED FLAGS

Migraine with aura whilst on COCP, atypical features (weakness, diplopia, unilateral visual symptoms, ataxia, reduced level of consciousness), worsening migraine

## PAST HISTORY

| | |
|---|---|
| *Migraines* | Have you suffered from migraines in the past? |

## FAMILY HISTORY

| | |
|---|---|
| *Migraines* | Does anyone in your family suffer from migraines? |

## DRUG HISTORY

| | |
|---|---|
| *Medication* | Are you taking any medications? (COCP, HRT) |

## SOCIAL HISTORY

| | |
|---|---|
| *Occupation* | Are you currently working at the moment? (flicking lights) |
| Time off | Have you taken time off work, university or school because of your headaches? |
| *Relationships* | Are you currently in a relationship? How are things? |
| *Smoker* | Do you smoke? How many cigarettes do you smoke per day? |

## IDEA, CONCERNS, EXPECTATIONS

| | |
|---|---|
| *Idea* | Do you have any idea about what may be causing your headaches? |
| *Concerns* | Do you have any worries about it? |
| *Expectations* | How were you hoping I could help you? |
| *Impact* | How have your symptoms affected your life? |

## CSA TIPS

Migraines can be quite severe and lead a sufferer to miss much time off work or their studies. Patients may present with a headache, and on further questioning your should be able to establish whether it is a migraine or not. Once established, you should discuss potential triggers and advise on the treatment options. Establish the impact the headaches are having on the patient's life.

## PHYSICAL EXAMINATION *Should have no signs during attacks*

| | |
|---|---|
| *Vitals* | BP |
| *Eyes* | Inspect the pupils & examine the fundi |
| *Neurological* | *If clinically indicated:* Perform a focused CN examination (e.g. visual fields, CN 2,3,4,6) and neurological assessment (pupillary reflexes, gait- ataxia, sensory, power of limbs) |

## INVESTIGATIONS

| | |
|---|---|
| *None* | Investigations usually not indicated |

## MANAGEMENT

### Conservative

| | |
|---|---|
| *Diary* | Offer a headache diary to monitor symptoms for 8 weeks |
| *Occupation* | Avoid jobs that can affect your sleep pattern (shift-work) or expose you to triggers (DJ) |
| *Avoid triggers* | |
| Diet | Advise to eat regular meals and avoid dieting too quickly. Avoid cheese, chocolate, citrus fruits, alcohol (red wine) |
| Environment | Avoid flickering lights (night clubs) or TVs, loud sounds or strong smells. Stop smoking and avoid smoky rooms |
| Stress | Consider relaxation techniques to improve stress, anger or anxiety |

*Medical*

| | |
|---|---|
| *Avoid* | Stop COCP or HRT |
| *Acute* | Monotherapy (preferred) or combined therapy (triptan + NSAIDs) |
|    Simple | Consider offering aspirin (900mg 4-6hrly), paracetamol or NSAIDs with antiemetic (e.g. Paramax, Migraleve). If vomiting affects oral consumption consider buccal (buccastem) |
|    Triptans | Offer sumatriptan (50/100mg) taken during attacks. If vomiting, consider nasal or SC. Others include zolmitriptan, naratriptan |
|     SE | Sensations of tingling, heat, heaviness, pressure on any part of body - due to vasoconstriction. Flushing, dizziness, fatigue, N&V |
|     CI | CVA, TIA, PVD, severe HTN, CVD |
| | |
| *Preventative* | Offer propranolol or topiramate as first line. Consider if >1 attack/mth that causes disability lasting >=3d or at risk of developing medication overuse headaches (analgesia used more than 2d per week) |
|    Propranolol | Start 40mg bd titrating up to 240mg in divided doses depending on symptom control. Consider if suffers from anxiety or HTN |
|     CI | Asthma, COPD, PVD, uncontrolled HF |
|    Topiramate | Start 25mg on for 1wk then increase in 25mg steps at wkly intervals to 50-100mg in 2 divided doses |
|     Advice | Increased risk of fetal malformations and reduce COCP effectiveness |
| | |
|    Other | Consider Gabapentin (1.2gm/d) or acupuncture. If on amitriptyline can continue with dose. Riboflavin (400mg od) can reduce intensity and frequency |
| | |
| *Pregnancy* | Recommend paracetamol. NSAIDs to be avoided 3rd trimester. Triptans avoided but sumatriptan if used. Aspirin avoid when conceiving, in early and late (3rd trimester) pregnancy |
| | |
| *Menstrual migraine* | Offer NSAIDs (mefenamic acid) during period (if menorrhagia or dysmenorrhea) or triptan (frovatriptan 2.5mg bd) starting 2d before and until end of menstrual migraine. Consider COCP for migraines without aura or progesterone (cerazette) |
| | |
| *Referral* | |
| *Migraine* | Refer if atypical features (weakness, diplopia, unilateral visual symptoms, ataxia, reduced level of consciousness) or become chronic, on maximal treatment |
|    Urgent | Refer urgently if patient has severe, uncontrolled status migrainosus (>72hr) |

**SAFETY NETTING**

| | |
|---|---|
| *Follow up* | Review after completing first pack of triptans (6 doses) or if change in symptoms (frequency, severity), poor tolerance to medication |

**DIFFERENTIAL DIAGNOSIS**

| Condition | Characteristic exam feature |
|---|---|
| **Migraine** | Unilateral throbbing frontal or temporal headaches more common in women than men. May present with or without an aura (flashing lights, loss of vision) but invariably patients suffer with nausea, vomiting and photophobia. Classically patients sleep it off. |

| | Rarely presents with hemiplegia. Occasionally triggered by certains foods (caffeine, chocolate), drugs (OCP), stress and periods |
|---|---|
| **Menstrual related migraines** | Headaches that occur 2d before or 3d after beginning of period. Occurs in 2 out of 3 consecutive cycles |

**EXPLANATIONS**

*Migraine*        This is a type of headache that causes pain on the front or the side of the head. It is usually one sided and may be associated with other symptoms such as feeling sick or vomiting. Sometimes the headache presents with a warning sign called an aura which may include flashing lights. We do not know what the cause is, but it is thought that it is due to the blood vessels tightening and then relaxing in the head.

# 7.3 Temporal Arteritis

Temporal arteritis is an immune mediated vasculitis that is characterized by granulomatous inflammation in the walls of medium-size and large arteries i.e. aorta, extracranial branches. It is more common in the elderly (>50yr) and in women of northern European descent. There is a clear association with polymyalgia rheumatica. If can present with recent onset of temporally located pain, scalp tenderness, jaw claudication and potentially transient visual symptoms. There may be tenderness to the temporal artery and a reduced temporal artery pulse. Often the ESR is raised with diagnosis confirmed with a temporal artery biopsy.

## HISTORY

**Open questions** — Can you tell me more about your headache? Could you tell me more about what has been troubling you?

## Focused questions

| | |
|---|---|
| *Temporal arteritis* | When did your headache first start? How long has it been going on for? How long does the pain last for? |
| Onset | Did the headache come on suddenly? |
| Site | Where exactly is the pain? (temporal) |
| Severe | How severe would you describe the headache? (pain score) |
| Triggers | Does anything make the pain better or worse? |
| Scalp tend. | Does it hurt when you comb or wash your hair? |
| Jaw claudi. | Is it painful when you chew food or brush your teeth? |
| Vision | Have you ever had any visual disturbances? (partial/total loss, diplopia) |
| | |
| *PMR* | Is there any pain or tenderness in both of your shoulders? |
| Stiffness | Have you had any stiffness of the joints? Is it worse in the morning? Do you struggle to turn over in bed? |
| Frequency | Does anything make it better (>45min being active) or worse (rest)? |

## Associated history

| | |
|---|---|
| *Fatigue* | Do you feel extremely tired all the time? |
| *Fever* | Have you noticed any fever or night sweats? |
| *Weight loss* | Has it affected your appetite or caused any weight loss? |
| *Oedema* | Have you had any swelling of your hands or legs? |

## Differentials

| | |
|---|---|
| *Migraine* | Do you get a throbbing headache? Any visual symptoms (flickering lights, spots, zig-zag lines, fortification spectra)? Do you feel sick or have you vomited? |
| *Tension* | Have you been under a lot of stress recently? |
| *Trigeminal Neuralgia* | Do you get stabbing pains over your face? Do you have trigger points? Is it worse when shaving or brushing your teeth? |

## RED FLAGS

Visual - diplopia or loss, CVA, neuropathy

## PAST HISTORY

| | |
|---|---|
| *Medical* | Have you ever suffered from any medical conditions? (PMR) |

## FAMILY HISTORY

| | |
|---|---|
| PMR | Does anyone else in your family have similar symptoms? (temporal arteritis, PMR) |

## DRUG HISTORY

| | |
|---|---|
| Medication | Are you taking any medications? (steroids) |

## SOCIAL HISTORY

| | |
|---|---|
| Home | Who lives with you at home? |
| Occupation | Are you currently working? Has it affected you at work? |
| Smoker | Do you smoke? How many cigarettes do you smoke per day? |
| Alcohol | Do you drink alcohol? How much do you drink and how often? |

## IDEA, CONCERNS, EXPECTATIONS

| | |
|---|---|
| Ideas | Have you had any thoughts what may be causing your symptoms? |
| Concerns | Do you have any worries about the pain you have been experiencing? |
| Expectations | How did you think I could help you today? |
| Impact | How have the symptoms affected your life? |

## CSA TIPS

Temporal arteritis is a vital diagnosis to be made in middle-aged patients presenting with headaches and muscle pains. If it is suspected, admission for biopsy and subsequent steroid treatment will save any potential visual loss and blindness.

## PHYSICAL EXAMINATION

| | |
|---|---|
| Vitals | Temp (fever), BP (unequal upper limb BP - large vessel involvement), pulse |
| Inspection | Inspect for ulcerations of scalp skin |
| Palpation | Check for tenderness, prominence, thickening or pulseless of artery |
| Auscultation | Listen for bruits over carotids |
| Fundoscopy | Ischaemic changes: optic disc pallor/oedema, small hemorrhages, cotton-wool sports |

*If clinically indicated:*

| | |
|---|---|
| MSK | Examine the shoulder for muscle tenderness or stiffness |
| Neurological | Perform CN examination (III, IV, VI). Check for power (hemiplegia) and sensation (mono/polyneuropathy) |

---

**Diagnosis Criteria of Temporal Arteritis -** *Ref: American College of Rheumatology*

| | |
|---|---|
| >50yr | Symptoms start when pt >50yr |
| New headache | New onset or localised head pain |
| Temporal artery | Tenderness, reduced pulse of temporal arteritis |
| ESR | >50mm/hr |
| Biopsy | Vasculitis (granulomatous inflammation, multinucleated giant cell) |

---

## INVESTIGATIONS

| | |
|---|---|
| Bloods | ESR (>50 mm/hr) and CRP. Hb (anaemia, thrombocytosis), LFT (AP) |
| Specialist | Duplex US, CT/MRI, Temporal artery biopsy confirms diagnosis |

## MANAGEMENT
### Medical
*Steroids*

| | |
|---|---|
| Jaw claudication | Start 60mg prednisolone and seek specialist advice |
| Visual sympt. | Start 60mg prednisolone, for urgent same day review by ophthalmologist |
| No visual sympt. | Start 40-60mg prednisolone od. Initiate aspirin 75mg (with PPI) |

| | |
|---|---|
| *Ongoing Mx* | Continue high dose steroids until symptoms and ESR/CRP normalise, then reduce dose 2wkly by 5-10mg until 20mg od is reach. Reduce dose in smaller quantities by 2.5mg every 2-4wk until 10mg od then reduce by 2mg every 1-2mths. Continue aspirin and PPI |
| Blood test | Monitor inflammatory markers regularly |
| Bone protection | Offer bisphosphonate if >65yr or fragility fracture or DEXA scan (-1.5) |

### Referral
| | |
|---|---|
| *Specialist* | Refer urgently (within 2wks of starting steroids) to specialist (local pathway - ophthalmologist, medics, rhem, geriatrics) if diagnosis suspected. Requires temporal artery biopsy |
| *Ophthalmology* | Immediate referral to ophthalmologist if sudden loss of vision |

## SAFETY NETTING
| | |
|---|---|
| *Follow up* | Advise if develops visual symptoms seek immediate advice. Review 2d after initiating prednisolone as response often rapid. If poor response, review diagnosis and refer to specialist |

## EXPLANATIONS
| | |
|---|---|
| *Temporal arteritis* | This is a condition where there is swelling or inflammation of the wall of the large arteries particularly those affecting the head and neck. One of these branches is known as the temporal artery on the side of your head. This can lead to tenderness over the area and cause headaches. If it is left untreated for a while it may cause damage to your vision and can lead to blindness. |
| Steroids | Often we treat it with steroid medication that reduces the swelling or inflammation. This is a different steroid to that which bodybuilders use. After taking it you should feel much better quite quickly (2-3d). We hope to reduce the medication over a few months once your symptoms get under control. |

# 7.4 Trigeminal Neuralgia

Trigeminal neuralgia is a rare but chronic debilitating condition that gives rise to intense excruciating painful episodic facial pain. It is due to a neuropathy or disorder of one or more branches of the trigeminal nerve causing unilateral discomfort. Episodes may occur infrequently to over one hundred times a day, lasting anything from a few seconds to many minutes. Classically there are trigger points and certain actions that bring on the attacks such as shaving, eating or brushing the teeth.

---

**Types of Trigeminal Neuralgia**

| | |
|---|---|
| *Classic (Type 1)* | Usually idiopathic with relapsing and remitting symptoms of piercing stabbing pain |
| *Atypical (Type 2)* | Constant throbbing pain with burning sensation or associated sensory loss |
| *Symptomatic* | Symptoms are due to an underlying condition such as MS |

---

**HISTORY**

| | |
|---|---|
| **Open questions** | Can you tell me more about the pain you are experiencing on your face? Could you tell me about what has been troubling you? |

**Focused questions**

| | |
|---|---|
| *Trigeminal Neuralgia* | When did your face pain first start? How long has it been going on for? |
| Onset | Did it come on suddenly? |
| Site | Where exactly is the pain? (cheek, forehead, chin) |
| Character | What does the pain feel like? (stabbing, burning, electric shock) |
| Timing | How long do the episodes last? Do they come and go? How long did you have no symptoms for? When did they begin again? |
| Severe | How severe would you describe the pain? (pain score) |
| Triggers | Does anything make the pain better or worse? Does anything bring it on (chewing, eating, talking, washing, shaving, brushing teeth)? |

**Associated history**

| | |
|---|---|
| *Paresthesia* | Do you get any tingling or burning in your face before the pain starts? |

**Differentials**

| | |
|---|---|
| *Migraine* | Do you get a throbbing headache? Any visual symptoms (flickering lights, spots, zig-zag lines)? Do you feel sick or have you vomited? |
| *TMJ dysfunction* | Do you have pain just in front of the ear? Do you have problems eating? Does your jaw ever lock whereby you cannot open it fully? |
| *Temporal arteritis* | Are your headaches worse on chewing food or combing your hair? |
| *Postherpetic neural.* | Did you have a skin rash come up in the same area you have the pain? |
| *MS* | Have you had any eye problems? Have you had different symptoms over a period of time? Any urine or bowel problems? |

| | |
|---|---|
| **RED FLAGS** | Optic symptoms (MS), herpetic lesions, <40 |

**PAST HISTORY**

| | |
|---|---|
| *Medical* | Have you ever suffered from any medical conditions (MS, BP, brain tumour)? Did you have shingles in the past? |

## FAMILY HISTORY

*Medical*                Are there any inherited disorders that run in your family?

## DRUG HISTORY

*Medication*             Are you taking any medications (analgesics)? Have they helped?

## SOCIAL HISTORY

*Home*                   Who lives with you at home?
*Occupation*             Are you currently working? Has it affected you at work?
*Smoker*                 Do you smoke? How many cigarettes do you smoke per day?
*Alcohol*                Do you drink alcohol? How much do you drink and how often?

---

### Diagnostic Criteria for Trigeminal Neuralgia

A.  Paroxysmal attacks of pain lasting from a fraction of a second to two minutes, affecting one or more divisions of the trigeminal nerve, and fulfilling criteria B and C

B.  Pain has at least one of the following characteristics:
1. Intense, sharp, superficial, or stabbing
2. Precipitated from trigger zones or by trigger factors

C.  Attacks are stereotyped in the individual patient

D.  There is no clinically evident neurologic deficit

E.  Not attributed to another disorder

---

*Ref: International Headache Society Diagnostic Criteria for Classical Trigeminal Neuralgia*

### IDEA, CONCERNS, EXPECTATIONS

*Ideas*              Have you had any thoughts what may be causing your symptoms?
*Concerns*           Do you have any worries about the pain you have been experiencing?
*Expectations*       How did you think I could help you today?
*Impact*             How have the symptoms affected your life?

### CSA TIPS

Patients with trigeminal neuralgia may suffer with severe debilitating symptoms. Attacks, although short lived, may persist for many months before subsiding and then returning in force. Many patients are misdiagnosed as having migraines and it is important to take a full history including triggers to make the correct diagnosis. In the young, ensure that you take a fuller neurological history to exclude MS or a brain tumour.

### PHYSICAL EXAMINATION

*Vitals*            Temp (fever), BP (unequal upper limb BP - large vessel involvement), pulse
*Inspection*        Inspect for vesicles of scalp skin
*Palpation*         Check for tenderness, prominence, thickening or pulseless of artery. Feel over the TMJ joint for crepitus. Request patient to open, close and move side to side the jaw and look for restricted movements

*If clinically indicated:*

*MSK*               Examine the shoulder for muscle tenderness
*Neurological*      Perform CN examination (brain tumour). Check for power (hemiplegia) and sensation (mono/polyneuropathy)

| | |
|---|---|
| **INVESTIGATIONS** | *to exclude other causes* |
| *Bloods* | ESR (exclude TA) and CRP |
| *Specialist* | TMJ / Dental X-ray, MRI (brain tumour, MS) |

## MANAGEMENT
### Conservative

| | |
|---|---|
| *Lifestyle* | Complete a pain diary and record triggers |
| *Reassure* | Reassure not a life-threatening condition but can be debilitating |
| *Support group* | Suggest to join Trigeminal Neuralgia Association UK (TNA) for support |

### Medical

| | |
|---|---|
| *Carbamazepine* | Start at 100mg bd and titrate according to response |
| Maximum | Max daily dose is 1200mg |
| Maintenance | Usual dose is 200mg tds |
| Remission | When pain is in remission, titrate down to lowest possible dose |
| Night | Consider MR preparation for night pain |
| Blood test | Monitor FBC, LFTs, U&E's before commencement and 6 monthly |
| Side effects | Advise SE of nausea, vomiting, dizziness, skin reactions or mood changes. Warn of signs of agranulocytosis (fever, sore throat, rash, bruising, bleeding) |
| *Alternative* | Alternatives initiated by specialist. Oxcarbazepine can be considered in treatment failure. Others include baclofen, lamotrigine, phenytoin, topiramate, clonazepam or TCA |

### Referral

| | |
|---|---|
| *Atypical* | Refer to neurologist if atypical symptoms (burning sensation between paroxysms, numbness, neuro signs), <40yr old, or unsure of diagnosis i.e optic neuritis, FHx MS, ophthalmic involvement only |
| *Uncontrolled sympt.* | If severe symptoms, uncontrolled with carbamazepine refer to specialist. Can consider surgery using gamma knife, rhizotomy or decompression of trigeminal nerve |

## SAFETY NETTING

| | |
|---|---|
| *Follow up* | Review 6-8wks for response to treatment. If poor response review diagnosis and refer to specialist |

## DIFFERENTIAL DIAGNOSIS

| Condition | Characteristic exam feature |
|---|---|
| **Trigeminal Neuralgia** | Affects women 2x c.f. men. Usually found in patients above 50 years. Common symptoms include unilateral face pain that comes and goes and is lanciating in nature. May be associated with other conditions such as MS |
| **Post Herpetic Neuralgia** | Occurs following shingles eruption. Burning stabbing and gnawing pain that persists for 3 months once the rash has faded |
| **TMJ Dysfunction** | Causes pain and limited movement around the joint. May note crepitus. Multifactorial aetiology due to muscle overactivity, dental problems and underlying OA |

| Temporal Arteritis | Inflammation of the walls of medium/large arteries. Often in elderly (>50yr) presents with temporal headache, malaise, fever, scalp tenderness (combing hair), jaw claudication (chewing). OE: temporal tenderness and decreased temporal pulse, CN palsy (III, IV, VI). Can cause sudden blindness. Associated with raised ESR (>50) and polymyalgia rheumatica. Confirmed with biopsy |
|---|---|

**EXPLANATIONS**

*Trigeminal neuralgia*    Trigeminal neuralgia is a condition that affects one of the nerves of the face. Pressure on the nerve leads it to be overactive and gives rise to the sharp pain that you are experiencing.

*Carbamazepine*    As the pain is due to a nerve, normal painkillers do not always work very well. However, there is a medicine that is more commonly used to treat epilepsy that works very well called, carbamazepine. The dose of carbamazepine used for your condition is much lower than that required to treat epilepsy and by taking it, it does not mean that you suffer from epilepsy. Carbamazepine works by dulling or slowing down the excess nerve signals being sent out and hence stops the pain.

# 7.5 Transient Ischaemic Attack (TIA)/Stroke (CVA)

Transient ischaemic attacks (TIA) are focal neurological events that are caused by vascular ischaemia from a microemboli or occlusion. By definition, symptoms last less than 24 hours with complete resolution. Strokes present with symptoms that persist for more than 24 hours and can be ischaemic (85%) or haemorrhagic (15%). They often present with unilateral weakness, numbness, slurred speech, dysphagia and visual symptoms (hemianopia). Headaches are not typical features of a TIA. It is important to treat TIA's as there is a 20% risk of a stroke in the first month with the highest risk in the first 3d.

## HISTORY

**Open questions**         Can you tell me more about the symptoms you are experiencing? Tell me more about what has been troubling you?

**Focused questions**

*TIA/CVA*                  When did your symptoms first start? How long has it been going on for? Are they slowly improving?

  Weak/numbness   Have you noticed any numbness or weakness affecting your arms, face or legs? Which side does it affect?

  Dysphasia       Have you had any slurring of your speech? Have you recently struggled to find the right name for common things (expressive)?

  Dysphagia       Have you had any problems eating or swallowing food or water?

  Vision          Have you had any visual symptoms? (loss of vision, curtain falling down - amaurosis fugax, diplopia)

  Coordination    Have you felt unbalanced or lacked co-ordination in our actions?

---

**FAST screen to diagnose Stroke or TIA** - *Ref: NICE (2008) Stroke*

Use a validated tool to screen for a stroke or TIA

*Face*      Has your face fallen on one side? Can you smile?
*Arms*      Can you raise your arms and keep them there?
*Speech*    Is your speech slurred?
*Time*      Call 999 if any of these symptoms

---

## Associated history

*Previous episodes*   Has it happened before? When exactly?
*Head injury*         Have you had a head injury or fall recently (subdural, haemorrhagic)?
*Mood*                How is your mood now? How do you feel in yourself?

## Differentials

*Hypoglycemia*    Do you suffer from diabetes? Are you on any medications (gliclazide)? Do you feel drowsy? Have you had any palpitations? Did you feel sweaty or hungry?

*Migraines*       Have you had any headaches? Do you get a warning before the symptoms come on? Do you feel sick or vomit when it starts?

*Labyrinthitis*   Do you feel as if the room is spinning around? Have you had a recent URTI?

*Epilepsy*        Did you have a fit? Did you bite your tongue or wet yourself?

## RED FLAGS         Prolonged symptoms >1wk

## PAST HISTORY

| | |
|---|---|
| *Ischaemic* | Do you suffer from any medical conditions? (TIA/CVA, AF, DM, HTN, CVD, cholesterol) |
| *Haemorrhagic* | Do you suffer from any blood disorders? |

## FAMILY HISTORY

| | |
|---|---|
| *Ischaemic* | Does anyone in your family suffer from any illness? (CVA, DM, HTN, CVD, cholesterol) |

## DRUG HISTORY

| | |
|---|---|
| *Haemorrhagic* | Are you taking any medications? (NSAIDs, Aspirin, warfarin) |

## SOCIAL HISTORY

| | |
|---|---|
| *Occupation* | Are you working at the moment? |
| *Home* | How are things at home? Do you have any carers? |
| *Relationships* | Are you currently in a relationship? How are things? |
| *Smoker* | Do you smoke? How many cigarettes do you smoke per day? |
| *Alcohol* | Do you drink alcohol? How much do you drink and how often? |
| *Drive* | Are you driving at the moment? |
| *ADLs* | Are you having problems with looking after yourself? Are you able to cook? Can you feed yourself? Are you washing yourself regularly? Are you able to control your passing of urine? Are you able to to walk unaided? |

## IDEA, CONCERNS, EXPECTATIONS

| | |
|---|---|
| *Idea* | Do you have any idea about what may be causing your symptoms? |
| *Concerns* | Do you have any worries about it? |
| *Expectations* | How were you hoping I could help you? |
| *Impact* | How have your symptoms affected your life? |

## CSA TIPS

Suffering from a TIA or a CVA may be a frightening experience for the patient and carer alike. Not being able to swallow food, see clearly or move your limbs, even for a short period of time, may cause a person to become dependent on others, having previously been fiercely independent. Patients often become withdrawn and depressed due to disability and it is important that you enquire about low mood in such patients.

## PHYSICAL EXAMINATION

| | |
|---|---|
| *Vitals* | BP (hypertension), pulse (irregularly irregular - AF), BMI |

| | |
|---|---|
| *Neurological* | *Perform a focused examination based on clinical findings:* |
| Inspect | Look for signs of VII nerve palsy/drooping face |
| Tone | Check for hypertonia |
| Power | Check power of limbs compared to normal side |
| Reflexes | Consider biceps, tricep, supinator, knee or ankle |
| Cranial nerves | CN examination (e.g. visual fields, V, VII) |
| Sensation | Check light touch compared to normal side |
| Cerebellar | Check for inattention, dysdiadokinesis, past pointing |
| Gait | Hemiplegic gait, broad based gait (cerebellar) |

| | |
|---|---|
| *Cardiovascular* | Listen for heart murmurs, carotid bruits. Check peripheral pulses |

## INVESTIGATIONS

| | |
|---|---|
| *Bloods* | Hb (anaemia), fasting glucose (DM), lipids |
| Others | Coagulation screen, thrombophilia if haemorrhagic, ESR, U&Es |
| *ECG* | AF |
| *Echo* | Heart murmurs |
| *Specialist* | CT/MRI (urgent), carotid doppler (endarterectomy) |

## MANAGEMENT

### Suspected TIA

| | |
|---|---|
| *Risk Assessment* | Assess the risk of stroke after a TIA. If high risk, refer immediately for specialist review and CT scan within 24hrs. If low risk refer for review by specialist and CT scan within 1 week |
| High risk | ABCD2 score >=4, AF, >1 TIA in a week, TIA while on anticoagulant |
| Low risk | ABCD2 score <=3, attend >1wk after symptoms, not in AF |
| ABCD2 | |
| **A**ge | More than or equal to 60yr (1 point) |
| **B**P | Blood pressure more or equal to 140/90 (1 point) |
| **C**linical | Unilateral weakness (2 point), speech disturbance without weakness (1 point) |
| **D**uration | Duration of symptoms: 10-60min (1 point), >=60min (2 point) |
| **D**M | History of diabetes (1 point) |
| Other risks | AF, more than 1 TIA in 1wk |

*Medical*

| | |
|---|---|
| Statin | Initiate on simvastatin 40mg unless contraindicated |
| Antiplatelet | Offer stat aspirin 300mg. Give PPI if risk of GI bleed |

| | |
|---|---|
| *Driving* | Advise not to drive and inform DVLA |
| *Refer* | Refer for same day review if high risk or within 1wk if low risk |
| *Safety netting* | If low risk and awaiting appt in the week, advise to seek urgent medical attention if further episode during that time or focal neurology persists |
| *Follow up* | Follow up 1 month after the event |

| | |
|---|---|
| **Suspected CVA** | If suspected CVA refer urgently (<1hr) to specialist stroke unit. If diagnosed on phone advise them to contact 999. Do not start antiplatelet treatment until had brain scan to exclude hemorrhagic stroke. Patients should be nil by mouth (NBM) until review by speech and language |

### Secondary prevention for TIA

*Lifestyle advice*

| | |
|---|---|
| *Smoking* | Offer smoking cessation advice |
| *Alcohol* | Suggest to cut down to safe limits (F: 2u/d, M: 3u/d) |
| *Diet* | Recommend cardioprotective diet (low fat, 5x fruit & veg, 2 fish portions, low salt) |
| *Exercise* | 30min of aerobic exercise 5x a day. Aim for BMI<25 |
| *Driving* | If driving car (group 1) must not drive for 4wks. If multiple TIAs over short period must be 3mths free of further attacks |

*Medical*

| | |
|---|---|
| Antiplatelet | Offer aspirin with MR dipyridamole (asasantin retard) or MR dipyridamole if aspirin is not tolerated. If dyspepsia give PPI |

| | |
|---|---|
| Statin | Ensure statin has been prescribed. Recheck lipids 1-3mths after initiating medication and aim for total cholesterol <4 mmol/l & LDL <2 mmol/l |
| Immunisation | Offer annual influenza immunisation |
| Conditions | Ensure optimal control of: |
| AF | Offer anticoagulation (warfarin) for AF unless CI. Consider aspirin next |
| DM | Control DM |
| HTN | Aim to reduce to <=140/90. Ideally 130/80 |

## CVA management

| | |
|---|---|
| *Health care needs* | Assess the patient's neurological symptoms, pain, cognitive, speech and visual impairments. Assess for bladder and bowel problems, swallowing issues or sexual dysfunction. Assess ability to do activities of daily living |
| Depression | Perform depression screen |
| *Lifestyle advice* | As per TIA |
| *Driving* | For group 1 no driving for 4wks. Notify DVLA if residual deficit >1mth after (visual, cognitive, limb function) |
| *Medical* | Ensure aspirin 300mg given once haemorrhagic stroke excluded for 2weeks. Give low dose clopidogrel or aspirin & dipyridamole only if CI. If dyspepsia give PPI. Ensure already on a statin |
| Conditions | As per TIA, control risk factors (lipids, BP) |
| Immunisation | Offer annual influenza immunisation |
| *QoF* | Maintain a register of patients with TIA/CVA. Refer new pts within 3mths of presenting. Monitor BP (<150/90) yearly and offer flu jab. Ensure those without haemorrhagic stroke are on antiplatelet treatment |

## Referral

| | |
|---|---|
| *Physiotherapy* | To assess mobility and treat weakness or poor balance |
| *OT* | Assess and offer equipment (ZF, walking aids), adaptations if reduced ADLs |
| *Speech & language* | SALT can assess and treat communication or swallowing difficulties |
| *Dietician* | Can offer advice about healthy diet |
| *Continence adviser* | Can assess and manage urinary or faecal incontinence |

## DIFFERENTIAL DIAGNOSIS

| Condition | Characteristic exam feature |
|---|---|
| **TIA/Stroke** | TIA <24hr, strokes >24hr neurological symptoms of contralateral motor or sensory disturbance, ipsilateral visual signs, amaurosis fugax (curtain coming down). Other symptoms (vertebrobasilar) vertigo diplopia, dysarthria, weakness, numbness affecting limbs. OE: hemiplegia, homonymous hemianopia, dysphagia, hemisensory loss, neglect, carotid bruit |
| **Hypoglycemia** | Rare in non-diabetics (addisons, severe liver disease, alcohol excess), often seen in diabetics on new medication (gliclazide, insulin) or concurrent illness. Presents with sweating, tremor, anxiety, confusion, slurred speech, personality change or hunger |

| Migraine | Unilateral throbbing headaches. May present with or without an aura (flashing lights, loss of vision) but invariably patients suffer with nausea, vomiting and photophobia. Classically patient's sleep it off. Can presents with slowing evolving hemiplegia lasting several days in contrast to acute TIA symptoms |
|---|---|
| Labyrinthitis | Inflammation of the vestibular nerve or labyrinth. Caused by recent onset of URTI. Often affects 20-30yr olds. Presents with severe acute onset of vertigo and nausea and vomiting that recurs for several days. Head movements can precipitate symptoms. Hearing loss may be present. Nystagmus fast direction to healthy side. Patients sway to ipsilateral side during Romberg's or on gait assessment |
| Subdural haemorrhage | Brain injury after trauma. More common in elderly or alcoholics. Presents with fluctuating conscious levels with lucid periods along with headaches, personality change and confusion. Can present with ipsilateral hemiparesis (false localising sign). Can have latent phase of wks to mths |
| Bell's palsy | Facial paralysis caused by latent viral infection. Presents with acute unilateral facial paralysis often after a bout of post auricular pain. OE: inability to frown or close eye with loss of wrinkles of the brow. The corner of mouth may drop and drool |

## EXPLANATIONS

*TIA / CVA*  A transient ischaemic attack, otherwise known as TIA or mini-stroke, is a condition that causes a temporary lack of blood flow to parts of the brain. This can cause symptoms similar to a stroke that are short lived and last for no more than 24 hours with full recovery. However, it is often a warning sign that you are at risk of a possible stroke.

*Antiplatelet meds*  Aspirin or clopidogrel help reduce the stickiness of the blood (platelets) and prevent blood clots from forming inside the blood vessels.

*Carotid endarterect.*  This is where the doctor performs surgery to open up the artery to take out the fatty lumps (atheroma) that develop inside the lining of the arteries causing a narrowing in the vessel.

*Carotid A. Angioplasty*  This is where the doctor will make a small cut in the vessel in the groin (femoral artery) and pass a wire up to the neck. They will then inflate a small balloon and clean out the blocked artery, almost like a pipe cleaner. They will then leave a small stent or mesh-like tube to keep the vessel open and unblocked.

# 7.6 Loss of Consciousness

Transient LoC or a blackout episode may be due to a number of different conditions. Most commonly it is due to low cerebral oxygenation as a result of impairment of cerebral perfusion because of postural hypotension, cardiac causes or hypoglycaemia. In such cases the symptoms are acute, short lived and the patients will eventually return to full consciousness without any loss of function. Other causes of loss of consciousness include epilepsy or less commonly, a TIA/mini-stroke and these may recur if the patient is not diagnosed or managed correctly.

## HISTORY
Begin by making your first few questions designed to put the patient at ease.

| | |
|---|---|
| **Open questions** | Can you tell me more about the symptoms you are experiencing? Could you tell me more about what has been troubling you? |

## Focused questions

| | |
|---|---|
| *Loss of Consciousness* | Clarify what they mean by LoC or blackout. When did it happen? |
| Pre-LoC | Did you know you were going to blackout (warning)? Did you have an odd taste in your mouth? |
| Posture | Had you been lying down and then suddenly stood up? Were you standing for a long period of time before it occurred? |
| Circumstances | What were you doing before you felt faint (passing urine, coughing, exercising)? Were you stressed or in pain? Was there any flashing lights around you? |
| Prodromal | Did you have any chest pain or palpitations (arrhythmia)? Did you feel sweaty and hot (panic, hypoglycaemia)? Did your slur your speech (TIA)? |
| | |
| During LoC | If the patient is unsure then try and obtain witness statements |
| Duration | How long where you unconsciousness for? |
| Onset | Did it start slowly or come on suddenly? (cardiac) |
| Fit | Did your whole body shake? or just a single part? |
| Symptoms | Did you bite your tongue or pass urine? Did your face go pale? Did you notice weakness of your limbs? |
| | |
| Post LoC | Find out how the patient felt after recovering |
| Recovery | When you came round, how did you feel (confused, headache)? Did you get better quickly (syncope)? |
| Amnesia | Are you able to remember everything that happened? |

## Associated history

| | |
|---|---|
| *Previous episodes* | Has it happened before? When exactly? |
| *Head injury* | Did you have a head injury or fall recently? (subdural, haemorrhagic) |

## Differentials

| | |
|---|---|
| *Syncope* | Did it happen when you stood from sitting or lying down? |
| *Situational* | Where you shaving at the time (carotid sinus)? Where you passing urine? |
| *Panic Attack* | Have you had any stress? Any pins & needles around your lips? Did your body feel hot and your heart begin to race? Were you breathing quickly? |

| Hypoglycemia | Do you suffer from diabetes? Are you on any medications (gliclazide, insulin)? Do you feel drowsy? Have you had any palpitations, feel sweaty or hungry? |
| Epilepsy | Do you get warning signs beforehand (prodromal - taste, smell)? Did your body go stiff and then shake? Did you bite your tongue or wet yourself? |
| Cardiac | Did you have any palpitations or chest pain (arrhythmia)? Were you exercising (AS)? Did you fall and bang your head when it happened? |
| TIA | Did you have slurred speech? Any weakness of your arms or legs? |

**RED FLAGS**    Sudden onset, recent head injury, exercise induced LoC, focal neurology

## PAST HISTORY
| Ischaemic | Do you suffer from any medical conditions? (AF, DM, HTN, CVD, epilepsy) |
| Panic | Have you ever had panic attacks in the past? |

## DRUG HISTORY
| Medication | Are you taking any medications? (antihypertensives, diuretics, nitrates - postural hypotension, hypoglycaemics, antiarrhythmics) |

## FAMILY HISTORY
| Epilepsy | Does anyone in your family suffer from epilepsy? |
| Early Death | Did anyone in your family have a premature sudden death <40yrs? (berry aneurysm, congenital aortic stenosis, HOCM, long QT syndrome) |

## SOCIAL HISTORY
| Occupation | Are you currently working? |
| Home | How are things at home? |
| Smoker | Do you smoke? How many cigarettes do you smoke per day? |
| Alcohol | Do you drink alcohol? How much and how often (hypoglycaemia)? |
| Drive | Are you driving at the moment? |
| Diet | How is your appetite? Are you eating well and drinking fluids regularly? |

## IDEA, CONCERNS, EXPECTATIONS
| Idea | Do you have any idea what may be causing your symptoms? |
| Concerns | Do you have any worries about it? |
| Expectations | How were you hoping I could help you? |
| Impact | How have your symptoms affected your life? |

## CSA TIPS
Loss of consciousness (LoC) can be a frightful experience for the patient. However, there are a wide range of causes and it is paramount you take a systematic history to distinguish the more serious from a simple faint or blackout.

## PHYSICAL EXAMINATION
| Vitals | Lying and standing BP (hypotension), pulse (AF, bradycardic), BMI |
| Inspect | Look at general appearance (anxious, pale) |

| Neurological | *Perform focused examination based on clinical findings:* |
| Tone | Check for hypertonia |
| Power | Check power of limbs compared to normal side |

| Reflexes | Consider biceps, triceps, supinator, knee or ankle |
|---|---|
| Cranial nerves | CN examination (e.g. visual fields, V, VII) |
| | |
| *Cardiovascular* | Listen for heart murmurs (AS), enlarged heart (HOCM), carotid bruits |

## INVESTIGATIONS

| | |
|---|---|
| *Bloods* | Hb (anaemia), glucose (DM), U&Es (dehydration), LFTs (liver damage) |
| *CXR* | Enlarged heart |
| *Cardiac* | ECG - Arrhythmia, WPW, Long QT, bradycardia, 24 ECG - If ECG normal and cardiac sounding, Echo - Heart murmurs, HOCM |
| *Specialist* | CT/MRI (subdural, subarachnoid), carotid doppler (TIA), tilt-table, carotid sinus massage, EEG - epilepsy |

## MANAGEMENT — *treat underlying cause*

*Driving*

| | |
|---|---|
| Vasovagal | No restrictions and no need to inform DVLA |
| Cardiac cause | Licence revoked for 6mths if no cause or 1mth if identifiable cause |
| Seizure markers | Strong suspicion of epilepsy (not diagnosed) - 6mths off driving, 12mths if PMHx epilepsy or solitary seizure |
| No markers | If LOC but investigated and no abnormality detected - 6mths revoked |

### Postural Hypotension

*Lifestyle*

| | |
|---|---|
| Fluids | Drink plenty of fluids (>2l) and reduce alcohol intake |
| Diet | Do not miss meals. Add salt to meals (low BP). |
| *Prevent* | Sit up for a short period first before standing |
| Standing | Avoid standing for long periods. Do not go out if it is very hot |
| Bending | Squat down with your knees (not bending at your waist) to pick things up |
| Stockings | Wear leg compression stockings to stop pooling of blood in the legs |
| | |
| *Polypharmacy* | Rationalise medications if on multiple medications for BP |
| *Medication* | Fludrocortisone to increase salt and water retention - specialist initiated |
| *Referral* | Refer to an endocrinologist if you suspect autonomic neuropathy |

### Cardiac

| | |
|---|---|
| *Bradycardia* | Consider changing medications if on beta blockers |
| *AF* | Find cause if relevant (hyperthyroidism, pneumonia, HF, alcohol). Consider a beta-blocker or antiarrhythmic drug (specialist initiated) |
| *Referral* | Cardiology referral for LOC with abnormal ECG, HF, LOC with exertion, FHx sudden death <40yrs, unexplained SOB, heart murmur or LOC >65yr without prodromal symptoms |

### Epilepsy

| | |
|---|---|
| *Referral* | Urgent neurologist referral if first seizure with LOC (bitten tongue, prolonged limb jerking, confusion after event, deja vu/jamais vu) |

### Panic Attacks — See panic attack chapter
### TIA — See TIA / CVA chapter

**DIFFERENTIAL DIAGNOSIS**

| Condition | Characteristic exam feature |
|---|---|
| Vasovagal syncope | Simple faint. Precipitated by prolonged standing, stress, pain, strenuous exercise, micturition, coughing, dehydration. Often experiences prodromal symptoms i.e. sweating, feeling hot prior. During episode can appear pale and clammy |
| Cardiac syncope | History of cardiac condition (murmur, HOCM). Can have FHx of sudden death. Chest pain or palpitations may precede syncope |
| Generalised seizures | Require >1 seizure for diagnosis of epilepsy. Episodes can last for seconds to minutes. May present with clonic, myoclonic, tonic, tonic clonic seizures or absences. Can get warning auras (smell, tastes, deja vu, jamais vu) |
| Postural hypotension | Dizziness or blackouts due to impaired cerebral perfusion, precipitated by postural change, prolonged standing (hot places) and improved lying flat. Often caused by medication (antihypertensives, diuretics), big meal, dehydration, anaemia or autonomic affecting conditions (PD). OE: drop of BP >20/10mmHg within 3mins of standing |
| TIA/Stroke | Neurological symptoms of contralateral motor or sensory disturbance, ipsilateral visual signs, amaurosis fugax (curtain coming down), vertigo, diplopia, dysarthria |
| Hypoglycemia | Rare in non-diabetics (Addisons, severe liver disease, alcohol excess), often seen in diabetics on new medication (gliclazide, insulin) or concurrent illness. Presents with sweating, tremor, anxiety, confusion, slurred speech, personality change or hunger |
| Panic attack | Unpredictable, recurrent, panic attacks with severe anxiety, palpitations, tremor, SOB, chest pain or paraesthesia. Often lasts 5-10 minutes but can last for few hours |

**EXPLANATIONS**

*Postural Hypotension*  This is a condition that results in reduced blood flow to the brain causing dizzy spells often when someone stands too quickly. It can also be caused by medications that reduce the blood pressure or by taking a water tablet that makes you pee more.

*Syncope*  This is a sudden brief loss of consciousness that a patient may experience due to reduced blood supply to the head / brain. It may be triggered by pain, emotion or a specific circumstance like passing urine, coughing or shaving but is usually not serious.

*Epilepsy*  This is a condition that affects the brain and leads to fitting. In most cases we do not know what the cause is, but abnormal brain impulses or signals are sent in an uncontrolled manner and gives rise to the symptoms. Some people may only fall into a short trance-like state, whereas more commonly, these signals cause the person to go stiff and fit.

Epilepsy is a chronic brain disorder that causes seizures. Almost 500,000 people have been diagnosed with epilepsy making it the second most common neurological condition in the UK. Although in most cases (66%) we do not know the cause, some people suffer from epilepsy due to a head injury, brain cancer, stroke or as a result of alcohol or drug abuse. It is diagnosed when a person has had at least 2 seizures and other causes are excluded. Seizures may be generalised or partial with generalised giving rise to tonic-clonic, absence or myoclonic seizures.

### HISTORY

**Open questions**  Can you tell me more about the symptoms you are experiencing? Could you tell me about what has been troubling you?

**Focused questions**

*Seizure*  What exactly happened? When did it occur? How did it start?

  Before  What were you doing before you felt faint? Were you stressed or exposed to flashing lights?

    Aura  Did you get any warning symptoms before the fit? Did you have an odd taste in your mouth or smell? Did you get a feeling that an event had occurred in the past even if it hadn't (deja vu)? Have you had a feeling of unfamiliarity with usually familiar places or people (jamais vu)?

  During

    Witness  Did anyone see you fit? What did they say happened? How long did it last?

    Fit  Did your whole body shake (clonic) or go firm (tonic)? Did it spread gradually over the body (Jacksonian march)?

    Symptoms  Did you bite your tongue or pass urine? Did you have any weakness of your limbs?

    Absence  Did you have a brief period where you lost awareness or went into a blank stare?

    Partial  Did you have any jerks or odd sensations in your arm or leg?

  Recovery  Did you feel drowsy or have a headache afterwards? How long did it take to go back to normal (post-ictal)? Do you remember what happened (amnesia)? Did your muscles ache afterwards?

**Associated history**

*Previous episodes*  Has it happened before? When exactly?

*LOC*  Did you lose consciousness when it happened?

*Head injury*  Did you have a head injury or fall recently? (subdural, haemorrhagic)

**Differentials**

*Brain tumour*  Do you get a headache when you cough or sneeze? Has anyone said that your behaviour or personality has recently changed?

*Meningitis*  Have you had a fever or rash recently? Any neck stiffness?

**RED FLAGS**  Sudden onset, recent head injury, focal neurology, prolonged fit (>30min)

**PAST HISTORY**

*Epilepsy*  Do you suffer from any medical conditions? (CVA, brain tumour, epilepsy)

## DRUG HISTORY

| | |
|---|---|
| *Medication* | Are you taking any medications (TCA, clozapine)? |

## FAMILY HISTORY

| | |
|---|---|
| *Epilepsy* | Does anyone in your family suffer from epilepsy? |

## SOCIAL HISTORY

| | |
|---|---|
| *Occupation* | Are you working at the moment? (bus, train driver, DJ) |
| *Home* | How are things at home? Do you live with anyone? |
| *Smoker* | Do you smoke? How many cigarettes do you smoke per day? |
| *Alcohol* | Do you drink alcohol? How much and how often? |
| *Recreational drugs* | Have you ever used any recreational drugs? Have you used heroin or cannabis? |
| *Drive* | Are you driving at the moment? |

## IDEA, CONCERNS, EXPECTATIONS

| | |
|---|---|
| *Idea* | Do you have any idea about what may be causing your symptoms? |
| *Concerns* | Do you have any worries about it? (unable to drive, swim) |
| *Expectations* | How were you hoping I could help you? |
| *Impact* | How have your symptoms affected your life? |

## CSA TIPS

Having a fit is extremely distressing for the patient, relatives and passer-bys alike. Patients may attend having fitted in the street wanting to find out if they are suffering from a brain injury or tumour. It is important to take a detailed history from such patients to tease out what actually happened. If a diagnosis of possible epilepsy is made, then the patient should be given clear guidelines about performing everyday activities such as swimming, driving and advice around undertaking certain jobs such as working in the army, operating machinery and working at heights.

## PHYSICAL EXAMINATION

| | |
|---|---|
| *Vitals* | BP, pulse, GCS, temperature |
| *Inspect* | Look at general appearance (anxious, pale) |
| *Neurological* | *Perform a focused examination based on clinical findings.* Patient should be asymptomatic after the fit. Exclude features of a brain tumour |
| Tone | Check for hypertonia |
| Power | Check power of limbs |
| Reflexes | Consider biceps, tricep, supinator, knee or ankle |
| Cranial nerves | CN examination (e.g. nystagmus, visual fields, III, IV, VII) |
| Cerebellar | Intentional tremor, dysdiadokinesis, past pointing |
| Fundoscopy | Exclude raised intracranial pressure |

## INVESTIGATIONS

| | |
|---|---|
| *Bloods* | Hb, ESR, glucose, U&Es, LFTs, Calcium. Do drug levels if poor compliance |
| *Cardiac* | ECG - Arrhythmia, WPW, Long QT, bradycardia, 24 ECG - If ECG normal and cardiac sounding, Echo - Heart murmurs, HOCM |
| *Specialist* | CT/MRI (brain tumour), EEG |

## MANAGEMENT
### *Conservative*

| | |
|---|---|
| Emergency | Prevent injury by cushioning the head. Remove any harmful or sharp objects from their surroundings. When they recover protect the airway and place in recovery position. Call 999 if the fit >5 minutes |
| Drugs | Buccal midazolam / PR diazepam |

*Safety*

| | |
|---|---|
| Occupation | Avoid working at heights or heavy machinery |
| Driving | Stop driving, inform insurance company and DVLA. No driving for 1yr or 3yrs if fits during sleep. If withdrawing medication no driving during period and 6mths after. Avoid cycling |
| Others | Avoid bathing a baby alone. Better to have a shower, however if using a bath keep door open. Avoid swimming alone |

*Lifestyle*

| | |
|---|---|
| Alcohol & drugs | Advise to cut alcohol to safe limits. Stop using recreational drugs |
| Triggers | Reduce stress and ensure good sleep. Avoid flashing light/flickering TVs |
| Other | Do not miss meals. Eat regularly. Suggest to wear a MedicAlert bracelet |

### *Medical*
Specialist initiated after 2nd seizure. Entitled to free prescriptions

| | |
|---|---|
| *Medication* | Do FBC if mouth ulcer, bruising or infection (sore throat). Check LFTs, U&E |
| Sodium valproate | SE: Pancreatitis, liver toxicity, blood dyscrasias, tremor, weight gain |
| Carbamazepine | SE: Blood dyscrasias, liver toxicity, rash, drowsiness, fluid retention |
| Phenytoin | SE: Blood dyscrasias, drowsiness, rash, gum hyperplasia, cerebellar symptoms |
| Withdrawal | If fit free for 2-3yrs consider withdrawing medication |

| | |
|---|---|
| *COCP* | Can affect the efficacy of the COCP (except Na valproate). Barrier methods be considered. Consider 50mcg (up to 100mcg if breakthrough bleeding) of oestrogen or tricycling (3 packs with no breaks) |
| *Preconception* | Drugs are teratogenic. Carbamazepine has the least risk. Try and rationalise patient to single agent if on polypharmacy. Take extra folic acid (5mg) until 12wks of pregnancy |
| *Pregnancy* | Refer early for shared care (obstetrician & neurologist). Increased risk of miscarriage if fitting and teratogenicity risk is increased with or without treatment. Give Vitamin K 20mg tablets after 36wks gestation |
| *Breastfeeding* | Safe to breastfeed on medications |

| | |
|---|---|
| *Referral* | Urgent neurologist referral if first seizure to exclude any underlying pathology (tumour) and to get advice |

## EXPLANATIONS

| | |
|---|---|
| *Epilepsy* | This is a condition that affects the brain and leads to fitting. In most cases we do not know what the cause is, but abnormal brain impulses or signals are sent in an uncontrolled manner and gives rise to the symptoms. Some people may only fall into a short trance-like state, whereas more commonly, these signals cause the person to go stiff and fit or make them look at if they are staring into space. |
| *EEG* | This is a special test that records the electrical signals of the brain. It can check for abnormal wave patterns that could suggest that you suffer from epilepsy. The brain |

specialist will place some electrodes on your head and ask you to take slow deep breaths. They may show you some flashing lights and check how your brain responds using an EEG machine.

*MRI*

An MRI scan uses strong magnetic fields and radiowaves to create detailed pictures of your brain. The radiographer will ask you to lie still on a bed that moves inside a tube or scanner. As it scans the head it will however make a loud noise. You should be given headphones or earplugs to wear.

# 7.8 Multiple Sclerosis (MS)

MS is an inflammatory disease affecting the insulating covers of the central nervous system (brain and spinal cord). It's cause is not clear but the body's immune system is directed against itself, attacking the white matter and continued destruction leads to disruption of the conduction pathways of the nerves causing signs and symptoms in the areas it affects. It is usually suspected when a person suffers distinct neurological symptoms that are disseminated in space and time. It largely affects young people between the ages of 20 and 40 and presents in 4 distinct patterns.

## Types of Multiple Sclerosis

| | |
|---|---|
| *Relapsing / Remitting* | Symptoms come and go with periods of remission interspersed with relapse. This is the most common |
| *Primary progressive* | Symptoms begin and gradually worsen over time |
| *Secondary progressive* | Initially relapsing / remitting go on to have less remissive periods and more longer relapses |
| *Benign* | Symptoms present less frequently and cause no permanent damage |

## HISTORY

**Open questions**   Can you tell me more about the symptoms you are experiencing? Tell me what has been troubling you?

**Focused questions**

| | |
|---|---|
| *Eye Symptoms* | Tell me more about the eye symptoms you have been suffering? Is it affecting one eye or both eyes? |
| Optic Neuritis | Did you feel pain in your eye? Was the pain worse when you move them? |
| Visual Loss | Did you have problems with your vision (red colour loss)? Did you have blurry vision? Did you lose sight in a small part of the vision (scotoma)? |
| Diplopia | Do you notice any double vision when looking to one side or the other? |
| | |
| *Sensory* | Do you have an odd sensation in your body? |
| Numbness | Do you have any areas of reduced feeling? |
| Pain | What does it feel like, burning or shooting? (trigeminal neuralgia) |
| Lhermitte's sign | Do you feel shooting pain down your spine when you bend your neck forwards? |
| | |
| *Motor* | Have you had any symptoms affecting your muscles? |
| Tremor | Did you experience any tremors? (hands, arms, face, legs) |
| Spasm | Do your muscles feel stiff? Do they ever go into spasm or an unintentional contraction? |
| Ataxia | How have your movements been (clumsy)? Are you able to walk? |
| | |
| *Other* | |
| Bowel / Bladder | Do you have any problems going toilet? Do you pass urine more often? Does it leak? Do you suffer from constipation or bad diarrhoea? |
| Speech | Have you ever had slurred speech? |
| Erectile Dysfunc. | Do you have problems performing during sex? |

*Timing*

| | |
|---|---|
| Onset | When did all this start? Does it come and go or is it there all the time? |
| Remission | How long did you have no symptoms for? |
| Relapse | When did they begin again? |

**Associated history**

| | |
|---|---|
| *Cognition* | How is your memory? Are you able to concentrate? |
| *Depression* | Have you been feeling low recently? |
| *Function* | Do you have problems with looking after yourself? (cook, feed, wash, dress, mobilise) |

**Differentials**

| | |
|---|---|
| *Transverse myelitis* | Did your problems come on quickly and affect the lower half of your body? Do you also have problems with your urine and bowels? |
| *Migraine* | Do you get throbbing headaches? Any visual symptoms (flickering lights, spots, zig-zag lines)? Do you feel sick or have you vomited? |
| *TIA* | Did you have slurred speech? Any weakness of your arms or legs? |
| *Labyrinthitis* | Do you feel as if the room is spinning around? Did you feel sick? Have you had a cold recently? |

**RED FLAGS**

Transverse myelitis, persistent neurological dysfunction (spine, brain tumour, infarction)

**PAST HISTORY**

| | |
|---|---|
| *Autoimmune* | Do you suffer from any medical conditions? (thyroid, type 1 DM, IBD) |
| *Vitamin D* | Have you ever had low vitamin D levels? |

**DRUG HISTORY**

| | |
|---|---|
| *Medication* | Are you taking any medications (TCA's, anticholinergics - similar symptoms)? Have you ever taken infliximab for RA? |

**FAMILY HISTORY**

| | |
|---|---|
| *MS* | Does anyone in your family suffer from MS? |

**SOCIAL HISTORY**

| | |
|---|---|
| *Diet* | How is your diet? Do you eat vegetables (B12)? |
| *Occupation* | Are you working at the moment? |
| *Home* | How are things at home? Do you have any carers? |
| *Smoker* | Do you smoke? How many cigarettes do you smoke per day? |
| *Alcohol* | Do you drink alcohol? How much and how often? |
| *Drive* | Do you drive? |

**IDEA, CONCERNS, EXPECTATIONS**

| | |
|---|---|
| *Idea* | Do you have any idea about what may be causing your symptoms? |
| *Concerns* | Do you have any worries about it? |
| *Expectations* | How were you hoping I could help you? |
| *Impact* | How have the symptoms affected your life? |

**CSA TIPS**

MS can present with a number of different symptoms that may appear unrelated. In such cases you should read the patient notes clearly to see if the patient attended previously with neurological symptoms at the surgery or in A&E. It is unlikely that you will have to inform a patient that they have multiple sclerosis as NICE recommends that the patient is explained the diagnosis by a neurologist (SPR level or above). However, you should be confident in being able to explain what it is as part of a possible diagnosis.

## PHYSICAL EXAMINATION

| | |
|---|---|
| *Vitals* | BP, pulse, BMI |
| *Inspect* | Look at general appearance, tremor |
| *Eyes* | Inspect the pupils, nystagmus, diplopia, check for scotoma, colour plates (red colour) |
| Fundoscopy | Examine the fundi (pale discs) |
| | |
| *Neurological* | *Perform focused examination based on clinical findings:* |
| Tone | Check for hypertonia |
| Power | Check power of limbs compared to normal side |
| Reflexes | Consider increased biceps, tricep, supinator, knee or ankle reflexes |
| Sensory | Check for reduced sensation (pain, light touch, vibration) in affected areas |
| Cranial nerves | CN examination (e.g. III, IV, VI) |

## INVESTIGATIONS

| | |
|---|---|
| *Bloods* | Hb (anaemia), ESR (sarcoid), B12, glucose (DM), U&Es (dehydration) |
| *Specialist* | MRI (sclerotic lesions in brain or spine), CT (exclude other causes), Evoked potentials, CSF (oligoclonal bands) |

## MANAGEMENT

### Conservative

| | |
|---|---|
| *Driving* | Must inform DVLA but usually no restrictions. Consider driving adaptations (hand controls - no pedals, wheelchair access) |
| *Support group* | Suggest to join Multiple Sclerosis Society for support |
| | |
| *Lifestyle* | |
| Exercise | Regular exercise such as jogging, swimming, cycling helps reduce stress and release tension. Also helps build muscle strength, tone and balance |
| Reduce stress | Recommend relaxation techniques and try and reduce stress |
| Keep cool | MS symptoms are worse when feeling hot. Use A/C, swimming and cold water to cool down |
| Rest | Ensure you have plenty of rest when feeling fatigued |
| Diet | Eat a healthy balanced diet. Take foods which have high Vit D content (sunlight, dairy, fish, mushroom) and Linoleic acid (sunflower, corn, soya) |

### Medical

| | |
|---|---|
| *Refer* | Refer to neurologist to confirm diagnosis. Specialist would consider IV/oral methylprednisolone in relapse and Interferon beta as disease modifying therapy (reduce frequency of relapses) |
| Other | Consider referring to physiotherapy, continence nurse, OT, SALT, CBT, neurorehabilitation |
| | |
| *Spasticity* | Consider baclofen (SE: drowsy, weakness). Refer to physiotherapy |

| | |
|---|---|
| *Incontinence* | Offer oxybutynin or TCAs (amitriptyline). If nocturia, consider desmopressin. Consider urinary catheter |
| *Bowel* | Suggest fibre diet, laxative (docusate). Offer incontinence pads if serious |
| *Erectile Dysfunc.* | Initiate with sildenafil 25-100mg prn |
| *Pain* | Simple analgesia (paracetamol, codeine) or NSAIDs can be prescribed as topical creams or oral. Ensure no CI for NSAIDS (ulcers, gastritis or asthma). Add PPI in the elderly |
| *Neuropathic* | Treat with gabapentin, carbamazepine or amitriptyline, TENS |
| *Vitamin D* | Some studies advise to give vit D supplements to reduce relapse rates |
| *Immunisation* | They should get an annual influenza vaccine |

**Acute Symptoms**

| | |
|---|---|
| *Optic Neuritis* | Refer to ophthalmologist as an emergency for corticosteroids |
| *Transverse Myelitis* | Refer as emergency to neurologist to consider corticosteroids |

## DIFFERENTIAL DIAGNOSIS

| Condition | Characteristic exam feature |
|---|---|
| **Multiple Sclerosis** | Affects women 3x c.f. with men. Usually in young 20-40 years. Neurological symptoms in different time and space. Common symptoms include visual (optic neuritis, hemianopia, diplopia, nystagmus), muscle spasticity, neuropathic pain, paresthesia, bladder (incontinence) and bowel dysfunction (faecal incontinence - rare) |
| **Transverse Myelitis** | Rare disorder that comes on acutely affecting the lower spine. Patients present with sharp shooting pain, with numbness and tingling over the legs or abdomen. May also be associated with limb weakness and urinary dysfunction |

## EXPLANATIONS

| | |
|---|---|
| *Multiple Sclerosis* | MS is a condition that affects the nerves fibres of the brain and spinal cord in patches. Nerves fibres are like copper wires; they send electrical impulses along them. In order to do this well they need insulation (myelin) to protect and help send messages quickly. In MS this insulation is damaged disrupting electrical signals from being sent to and from the brain. It can affect your vision (diplopia, optic neuritis), cause stiffness to your muscles (spasticity) and difficulties with your balance (ataxia). |
| *Optic neuritis* | This is often the first symptom seen with MS. It is where the nerve to the eye is inflamed causing pain with eye movements, double or blurry vision or occasionally some loss of vision. |
| *Transverse Myelitis* | This is a condition that comes on quickly and affects the back. It can cause problems like tingling and numbness in the legs and issues with passing urine. You need to see a specialist quickly to see what the cause is and give treatment if needed. |

# 8.1 Ear pain

Ear pain or otalgia is a fairly common presentation in primary care. It is usually caused by local aural disease processes or can be referred from external sites radiating into the ear. Whilst it is a common symptom, it is often transient in nature particularly affecting children when presenting with URTIs or ear infections.

## HISTORY

| | |
|---|---|
| **Open questions** | Can you tell me more about the pain in your ear? How did it start? |

**Focused questions**

| | |
|---|---|
| *Otalgia* | When did it start? How long has it been going on for? |
| Side | Which side is affected? Does it affect both ears? |
| Character | What does the pain feel like? (sharp, lancinating, fullness or boring) |
| Severity | How bad is the pain? |
| Radiation | Does the pain go anywhere? |
| Referred pain | Do you have pain anywhere else in your head/neck? (tooth, throat, jaws) |
| Worsens | Does anything make the pain worse? (moving neck, swallowing, chewing) |
| Trauma | Did you suffer any injury to your ear? (cotton bud, slap, loud noise) |

**Associated history**

| | |
|---|---|
| *Dizziness* | Have you had any dizziness, fever or recent coughs or colds? |
| *Tinnitus* | Any ringing in your ears? |
| *Hearing* | Did you notice any change in your hearing? (muffled or loss) |
| *Discharge* | Any liquidy discharge from the ear? (blood, purulent, waxy) |

## Differentials

| | |
|---|---|
| *Otitis externa* | Any smelly discharge from the ear? Do you often go swimming or visit humid countries? Is the ear itchy? |
| *Otitis media* | Have you noticed any high fever or sweats with it? Any coughs or colds? |
| *Dental* | Is there any pain when you eat? Or when you drink cold fluids? |
| *Eustachian tube dys.* | Do you feel that your ears 'pop' often? |
| *TMJ dysfunction* | Do you suffer from a stiff jaw or does it click? Is the pain worse on chewing foods? |
| *Perforation* | Did the pain come on suddenly on one side? Was there any trauma? Did you notice any bloody discharge or reduced hearing? |

## RED FLAGS

| | |
|---|---|
| *Otalgia* | Persistent unilateral ear pain with normal examination |
| *Cholesteatoma* | Cheesy smelling discharge or bloody discharge, unilateral tinnitus |

## PAST HISTORY

| | |
|---|---|
| *Medical* | Do you suffer from any medical problems? (otitis externa, otitis media) |
| *Surgery* | Have you had any operation or procedures? (grommets, tympanoplasty) |

## DRUG HISTORY

| | |
|---|---|
| *Medication* | Are you taking any medications (SSRIs, lamotrigine, zolpidem)? |

## SOCIAL HISTORY

| | |
|---|---|
| *Smoker* | Do you smoke? How many cigarettes do you smoke per day? |
| *Alcohol* | Do you drink alcohol? How much do you drink and how often? |
| *Occupation* | Are you working at the moment? What do you work as? |
| *Travel* | Did you travel by plane recently? Did you dive or go scuba-diving when away? |

## IDEA, CONCERNS, EXPECTATIONS

| | |
|---|---|
| *Idea* | Do you have any ideas what may be causing your symptoms? (ear wax) |
| *Concerns* | Have you had any particular worries about it? (perforated drum, hearing) |
| *Impact on life* | How has it affected you day to day? |

## CSA TIPS

Ear pain is an acutely painful and problematic symptom. It causes much discomfort in the sufferer and may give rise to anxiety if associated with hearing loss. The most common causes are benign and related to a recent URTI. In such cases, reassure the patient and manage as appropriate. Make sure that you consider extra-auricular causes such as dental or TMJ problems.

## PHYSICAL EXAMINATION

| | |
|---|---|
| *Vitals* | Temperature |
| *Face* | Look for any facial rash (herpetic blisters) or paralysis (Ramsay Hunt) |
| *Ear exam* | Hold autoscope like a pen. Pull ear upwards and backwards (only backwards in children) to straighten the external canal |
| Inspection | Inspect the pinna (and behind) for sinuses, abscesses, furuncle. Look inside the ear canal for inflammation, impacted wax, foreign bodies or debris (otitis externa). Note any discharge. Before inserting the otoscope check that the pinna is not painful (otitis externa) |
| Tympanic M. | Observe the tympanic membrane (intact, perforated), colour, shape and presence of a light reflex |

---

### Different Type of Discharge from the Ear

| | | | |
|---|---|---|---|
| *Cheesy smell* | Cholesteatoma | *Sanguineous* | Trauma |
| *Purulent* | Otitis media | *Watery* | Possible CSF fluid |

---

| | |
|---|---|
| Palpation | Palpate the mastoid process for any tenderness (mastoiditis) |
| *TMJ* | If indicated, palpate the TMJ joints whilst at rest and with jaw opened noting crepitus or restricted movement |
| *Neurology* | If referred pain consider cranial nerve assessment (V,VII,IX,X) |

## INVESTIGATIONS

| | |
|---|---|
| *MC&S* | Swab any discharge |
| *Specialist (other)* | Audiogram, TMJ X-ray (no longer performed) |

## MANAGEMENT   *treat the underlying cause*
### Conservative

| | |
|---|---|
| Cleaning | Do not use cotton buds to clear out ear as they can cause impaction. Using a pipette, drop a few drops of olive oil into the affected ear. Lie down on the opposite side, with |

| | |
|---|---|
| | your ear facing upwards for 1-2 minutes. Place some cotton wool in your ear to prevent the oil from leaking out. Do this 2-3x a day for 10 days |
| Flying | Ear pain is made worse when flying. Advise to suck a sweet or try and swallow when the plane is descending. For children, give them a dummy or bottle-feed. Consider purchasing pressure-control earplugs |
| Analgesia | Simple analgesia (paracetamol) or NSAIDs can be prescribed. Ensure no CI for NSAIDS (ulcers, gastritis or asthma). Add PPI in the elderly |
| Strong | Consider weak opioid (co-dydramol, co-codamol) if others fail. Strong opioids for short period only. Consider laxatives for constipation |
| | |
| *Otitis Media* | Most (80%) resolve <3d without abx. Self limiting, advise fluid hydration, analgesia, delayed prescription of abx (amoxicillin) if persists >72hrs |

---

**Antibiotic Prescription for Otitis Media -** *Ref: Adapted from MeReC Bulletin 2006;17(3):9-11*
- Antibiotics should not be prescribed routinely for acute otitis media in children
- May reduce pain for minority but has to be weighed against side effects (D&V) and resistance
- Consider in children if: <2yr if bilateral, ear discharge, systemically unwell, recurrent infection
- Consider delayed prescription of antibiotics

---

| | |
|---|---|
| *Otitis externa* | |
| *Conservative* | Do not poke your ear with cotton buds, towels, avoid cotton buds when cleaning ears. Clean debris and wax with olive oil |
| Swim | If swimming, keep ears dry. Consider swimming cap covering ears or special earplugs. If after bathing or swimming you have water in your ears, drain by tilting head to one side. Dry ears by using low setting on hair drier |
| Shower | Can use ear plugs when showering to prevent water or soap entering |
| *Medical* | Offer analgesia for pain. Steroid or antibiotics ear drops. Can consider oral antibiotics |
| | |
| *Perf. ear drum* | Often heals spontaneously. If persists >6wk refer for surgical repair |
| | |
| *Cholesteatoma* | Refer to specialist if suspected |
| | |
| *Furunculosis* | Consider abx (flucloxacillin), I&D if severe pain and swelling |
| | |
| *Impacted wax* | Use ear drops (olive oil, otex, almond oil, sodium bicarbonate). Avoid cotton buds. If still persists, refer for syringing |
| *TMJ dysfunction* | |
| *Conservative* | Avoid chewing gum. Eat soft diet to relax the jaw. Avoid opening jaw widely such as singing, yawning. Try ice packs over the joints. Relaxation techniques if stressed (as may clench teeth). Gently stretch ligaments in joint by opening jaw slowly and relaxing exercises |
| *Medical* | Offer analgesia (NSAIDS), muscle relaxants or TCAs. Refer for splints (dentist). Surgery last resort |
| | |
| *Refer* | |
| ENT | Refer to specialist urgently if evidence of mastoiditis (needs IV abx). Cholesteatoma should be rapidly referred for further investigations. Persistent unexplained unilateral |

|  | pain >4wks in the head or neck with otalgia but normal otoscopic examination warrants urgent referral |
|---|---|
| *Dentist* | Request the patient to see a dentist to discuss TMJ or dental caries |
| *Safety netting* | If pain in the ear persists for 4 weeks attend for review |

## DIFFERENTIAL DIAGNOSIS

| Condition | Characteristic exam feature |
|---|---|
| **Otitis media** | Infection of the middle ear. Often unilateral ear pain with fever. If ear discharge (perforation) often resolves pain. OE: bulging red ear drum |
| **Otitis externa** | Inflammation and / or infection of the outer ear canal. Often associated with eczema of canal. May be seen in swimmers, visitors to humid countries or regular cotton bud use. Often causes ear pain, itchy ear and discharge (offensive). OE: the pinna can be painful to touch or move, ear canal has debris or discharge |
| **Mastoiditis** | Rare. Can occur from spreading of infection from otitis media to mastoid bone. Causes throbbing ear pain, whitish profuse discharge with hearing loss. OE: ear sticks out, mastoid process tender |
| **TMJ dysfunction** | Causes pain and limited movement around the joint. May note crepitus as well. Multifactorial aetiology due to muscle overactivity, dental problems and underlying OA |
| **Cholesteatoma** | Skin that is trapped within the middle ear. Presents with foul smelling discharge and hearing loss. Local invasion can result in vertigo, facial nerve palsy, cerebellopontine angle syndrome. OE: an attic crust is seen (top of ear drum), conductive hearing loss |
| **Impacted wax** | Can cause irritation and ear pain, hearing loss, tinnitus in unsuspecting patients |
| **Barotrauma** | Linked to poor Eustachian tube function. Seen in air travel or diving. Presents with pain or pressure in ears with hearing loss. OE: haemorrhagic areas on TM, fluid behind drum noted. Prevented by yawning or sucking sweets during flight |

## EXPLANATIONS

*Otitis media*    The ear is separated into different parts with the ear canal known as the outer ear and the small space behind the eardrum, the middle ear. Otitis media means that you have an infection of the middle ear. This often affects the area behind the ear drum making it red and angry looking and may give rise to an ear ache.

*Otitis externa*    This is redness and infection of the outer part of the hearing system namely the ear canal. It is more common in people who swim. Infection usually gives rise to pain, itching and discharge from the ear. Although not usually serious, it is best to get treated to prevent any problems.

| | |
|---|---|
| *TMJ dysfunction* | This refers to the problem that affects the joint between the jaw and the skull. We do not know what causes it, but sometimes grinding or clenching your teeth at night can make it worse. It gives rise to pain around the jaw, ear pain as well as a clicking or popping feeling when you chew. |
| *Impacted wax* | Earwax is produced by the ear to help clean and protect the inner ear and drum from dirt. It usually does not cause any problems as the hairs inside the ear canal push it out. However, sometimes the wax can become dry and hard, and cause a blockage of the canal. This may be due to using cotton buds or because of an ear infection. |
| *Cholesteatoma* | A cholesteatoma is an abnormal collection of cells in your middle ear. It sometimes occurs because of eustachian tube dysfunction and leads to a buildup of dead skin cells. As it grows, it can put pressure on the delicate organs in your middle and inner ear causing pain, hearing loss and a ringing sensation. |
| *Perforated eardrum* | This means that the eardrum that helps convert the sounds around us has been damaged. Usually, the damage is small and the drum will heal itself by 6 weeks. It may be damaged due to putting an object in the ear, trauma, or fluid or infection buildup behind the drum. It gives rise to symptoms such as ear pain, discharge and occasionally, reduced hearing. |

# 8.2 Hearing loss/tinnitus

Hearing loss is a subjective reduction in the ability to listen or hear things. It is often objectively assessed using an audiogram (pure tone audiography). Although it may affect all ages, it is more common in the elderly. Hearing loss can be due to damage anywhere along the hearing pathway from the outer ear (auricle) through the middle and onto the inner ear. Broadly speaking, it is classified into conductive or sensorineural loss with Weber's and Rinne's tests useful to distinguish between the two types.

Tinnitus relates to the unwanted hearing of a ringing, buzzing, humming or clicking sound from within the ear. It is not audible to others and denotes a symptom rather than a diagnosis. It affects around 10% of the population, but only 1% has a severe form that is debilitating.

---

**Causes of Hearing loss**

| | |
|---|---|
| Conductive | Impaction with wax or a foreign body, eardrum perforation or infection, collection of fluid, otosclerosis, cholesteatoma |
| Sensorineural | Congenital, presbycusis, ototoxic drugs, previous meningitis, mumps or measles, acoustic neuroma, noise exposure |

---

**HISTORY**

| | |
|---|---|
| **Communication** | Read the notes and establish if the patient is deaf or hard of hearing. If they are, try and agree what the best mode of communication is. You may wish to say: I understand that you have problems with your hearing. How do you wish to communicate today? Are you able to lip read or should we communicate by writing? |
| **Open questions** | Can you tell me more about the pain in your ear? How did it start? |

**Focused questions**

| | |
|---|---|
| *Hearing loss* | When did it start? How long has it been going on for? |
| Side | Does it affect one or both ears? Which one? |
| Nature | Do you have no hearing on that side or is it just muffled? |
| Onset | Did it come on suddenly (perforation) or has it slowly been getting worse? |
| Pitch | What types of sounds can you hear in your ears? (high/low pitched) |
| Exposure | Have you been exposed to any loud noises? |

| | |
|---|---|
| *Tinnitus* | When did it start? How long has it been going on for? |
| Character | Can you describe to me what the noise sounded like? Was it a ringing, clicking, hissing or buzzing sound? |
| Nature | Does it come or go or is it there all the time? |
| Side | Does it affect both ears or just the one? |

**Associated history**

| | |
|---|---|
| *Dizziness* | Have you had any dizziness, fever or recent coughs or colds? |
| *Pain* | Did you have any ear pain? What does it feel like? |
| *Discharge* | Any liquidy discharge from the ear? (blood, purulent, waxy) |

**Differentials**

| | |
|---|---|
| *Otitis media* | Do you have ear pain, fever or sweats? Any recent coughs or colds? |

| Meniere's | Have you had any dizziness or vertigo (the whole room spinning around)? Do you feel a pressure or fullness in your ear? Do your ears ever ring? |
|---|---|
| Earwax | Do you have muffled hearing? Has it been slowly getting worse? How often do you clean your ears? |
| Head injury | Have you recently had a blow or knock to the head? |
| Cholesteatoma | Do you get a cheesy smelly discharge from your ear? Any ringing as well? |
| Perforation | Did the pain come on suddenly on one side? Was there any trauma (noise, water, cotton bud)? Did you notice any bloody discharge? |
| Otosclerosis | Does it affect both sides? Is it slowly getting worse? Is it worse during pregnancy? |
| Presbycusis | Are both ears affected? Has it been slowly getting worse? Is it mainly high-pitched sounds that you cannot hear? Do you have difficulty making out what people are saying in a crowd? |
| Acoustic neuroma | Do you feel the room is spinning around you? Do you hear ringing in your ears as well? Have you noticed any pain or numbness in your face? |

**RED FLAGS**

| ENT | Unilateral or sudden deafness, bloody discharge |
|---|---|
| Cholesteatoma | Cheesy smelling discharge or bloody discharge, unilateral tinnitus |
| Acoustic neuroma | Facial weakness, ataxia |
| Psychiatric | Depression, suicidal ideation |

**PAST HISTORY**

| Medical | Do you suffer from any medical problems? Do you wear a hearing aid? |
|---|---|
| Hearing loss | Recurrent otitis media, meningitis, neurofibromatosis (acoustic neuroma) |
| Tinnitus | DM, hypothyroidism or hyperthyroidism |
| Surgery | Have you had any ear operations? (grommet, tympanectomy) |

**DRUG HISTORY**

| Medication | Are you taking any medications? |
|---|---|
| Affects both | Gentamicin, NSAIDS, aspirin, furosemide |
| Tinnitus | Chloroquine, methotrexate, TCAs, diazepam withdrawal, erythromycin |

**SOCIAL HISTORY**

| Smoker | Do you smoke? How many cigarettes do you smoke per day? |
|---|---|
| Alcohol | Do you drink alcohol? How much do you drink and how often? |
| Travel (hearing loss) | Have you travelled by plane recently? Any recent diving? |
| Occupation | Are you working? Are you exposed to loud sounds on a daily basis? |

---

**Occupational Causes for Hearing loss**

Often causes bilateral hearing loss due to work related noise pollution. >80 decibels can lead to damage. UK law states that persons who are regularly exposed to 85 decibels daily must be offered ear protection e.g. construction, airplane workers, firearms sports, DJs

---

**FAMILY HISTORY**

| Medical | Does anyone in your family suffer from hearing problems? (otosclerosis, osteogenesis imperfecta) |
|---|---|
| Pregnancy | Did your mother ever have mumps or rubella during pregnancy? |

## IDEA, CONCERNS, EXPECTATIONS

| | |
|---|---|
| *Idea* | What did you think could have caused your symptoms? |
| *Concerns* | Have you had any particular worries about it? |
| *Impact on life* | How has it affected you? Has it stopped you from doing anything (watching TV, using telephone, talking to friends)? |

## CSA TIPS

Hearing loss is a problem that is more commonly seen in the elderly. It is categorized as mild, moderate or severe. Since hearing plays an integral part in communication and social interaction, problems with hearing can lead to a poor quality of life. Patients may isolate themselves socially, acutely embarrassed when repeatedly having to ask people to speak up. When dealing with patients with hearing problems, it is key that you establish right from the onset how they wish to communicate with you. Finding out that a patient can lip-read will save you precious time and reams of paper being passed to and fro during the consultation!

Hearing loss can present suddenly or gradually. Patients may not even realise that they are suffering with hearing problems and it is important to ask discriminatory questions that may point to a hearing deficiency. Useful questions would be to enquire whether the patient is having problems understanding people, or if they are repeatedly asking people to repeat what they are saying. Often a key indicator is from others complaining that the patient is putting the volume of the radio or TV higher affecting others around them.

## PHYSICAL EXAMINATION

*Hearing tests*

| | |
|---|---|
| Whisper test | Stand behind the patient and create a masking noise. Whisper 3 letters or numbers into the other ear e.g. '3, V, 8' and ask them to repeat back |
| Weber's | Strike the tuning fork (512Hz) and place it on their head. Ask them to state if the sound is equal in both ears or if it is louder to one side. If lateralised to one ear then suspect conductive hearing loss on that side or a sensorineural hearing loss in the other ear |
| Rinne's | Strike the tuning fork and hold stem against the mastoid process for 3sec. Ask when they no longer hear it vibrate. Next hold it 1 inch away from their ear and check if vibrations can be still heard |

---

**Interpreting the Rinne's tests**

| | |
|---|---|
| *Positive* | If vibrations heard, air conduction is greater than bone conduction (AC > BC). Represents normal finding, i.e. no conductive hearing loss, or possible nerve deafness on other side |
| *Negative* | If vibrations cannot be heard, bone conduction is greater than air conduction (BC > AC). This suggests a conductive hearing loss in that ear |

---

| | |
|---|---|
| *Auroscope* | Hold auroscope like a pen. Pull ear upwards and backwards (only backwards in children) to straighten the external canal |
| Inspection | Look inside the ear canal for impacted wax. Note any discharge. Before inserting the otoscope check that the pinna is not painful |
| Tympanic M. | Observe the tympanic membrane (intact, perforated), colour (flamingo tinge, red, dull), shape and the presence of a light reflex. Inspect for a fluid level behind the TM (glue ear) or the presence of any grommets. Look for cholesteatoma on the attic just in front of the TM |

| Neurology | Do a focused CN exam (V, VII VIII) if acoustic neuroma is considered |

## INVESTIGATIONS

| *Bloods* | FBC (anaemia), TFT, glucose |
| *MC&S* | Swab any discharge |
| *Specialist (other)* | Audiogram, MRI brain (acoustic neuroma) |

## MANAGEMENT

### Hearing loss

*Conservative*

| Sitting closer | Suggest sitting in closer proximity to the person speaking |
| Lip reading | Ask people to speak more slowly and more clearly. Consider lip reading |
| Modifications | Install a phone amplifier, doorbell alert |
| Benefits | Advise patient if benefits available such as DLA, ESA or IIDB |

*Treatment*

| Hearing aids | Electronic hearing devices are loaned to the patient for free. Refer to an audiology department for consideration and fitting |
| Cochlear implants | Considered in severe hearing loss in both ears or those who have had little or no benefit from a hearing aid |

### Tinnitus

*Conservative*

| Reassure | Reassure patient that if red flags are not present, tinnitus may not have a serious underlying cause |
| Counselling | Refer for counselling. Tinnitus can have a large negative impact on life |
| Support groups | Put the patient in contact with support groups (Tinnitus Association) |
| *Idiopathic* | Consider masking sounds that can divert patient's attention away or distract them from the tinnitus. Have background music running in house or leave TV on. Can use white noise devices from ENT department or wearable devices similar to earphones/hearing aids |

### Glue ear

| | Reassure up to 80% resolve within 3mth. Some may require grommets, surgery for drainage or adenoidectomy. Consider speech therapy particularly in young |

### Meniere's

| *Acute attack* | Patient should remain still and if open eyes, fix at a single spot. Avoid fluids as may induce vomiting. Continue stationary position until peak vertigo attack is over. Treat with prochlorperazine 5-10mg tds or cinnarizine 15-30mg tds or buccal routes if vomiting excessively |
| *Between episodes* | Suggest to stop smoking and salt and fluid restriction. Reduce amount of coffee and alcohol consumed. Can treat with betahistine 16mg tds to prevent episodes or thiazide diuretic |

### Barotrauma

| | Reassure, often heals within 3wks. Recommend to yawn or suck on boiled sweets during take off or descent when flying. Consider nasal decongestants |

### Noise induced

| | Avoid precipitants. Wear ear protectors. May need hearing aids if permanent. Eligible for compensation if occupational |

| | |
|---|---|
| IIDB | Industrial Injuries Disablement Benefit available if the patient had been exposed to noise at work over a long period of time. Patients are eligible if hearing loss degree is ≥20% and they worked in a listed occupation for ≥10yr |
| *Impacted wax* | Use ear drops (olive oil, otex, almond oil, sodium bicarbonate). Avoid cotton buds. If still persists refer for ear syringing |
| *Presbycusis* | Refer to ENT/audiology for formal assessment and hearing aids |
| *Refer* | Refer to specialist urgently if evidence of red flag symptoms |

## DIFFERENTIAL DIAGNOSIS

| Condition | Characteristic exam feature |
|---|---|
| **Otitis media** | Infection of the middle ear. Often unilateral ear pain with fever. If ear discharge (perforation) often resolves pain. OE: bulging red ear drum |
| **Glue ear** | Glue ear presents as otitis media but there is an associated effusion. It normally affects children and hearing loss is a common complaint. If it is not treated early, children may develop speech and language delay or problems with balance. OE: may have a bulging eardrum with creamy discharge or air bubbles |
| **Otitis externa** | Inflammation and/or infection of the outer ear canal. Associated with eczema of canal. Often seen in swimmers, visitors to humid countries or regular cotton bud use. Often causes ear pain, itchy ear and discharge (offensive). OE: the pinna can be painful to touch or move, ear canal has debris or discharge |
| **Cholesteatoma** | Skin that is trapped within the middle ear. Presents with foul smelling discharge and hearing loss. Local invasion can result in vertigo, facial nerve palsy, cerebellopontine angle syndrome. OE: an attic crust is seen (top of ear drum), conductive hearing loss |
| **Impacted wax** | Can cause irritation and ear pain, hearing loss, tinnitus in unsuspecting patients |
| **Presbycusis** | More common in >75yrs old. Usually bilateral and gradual. Patients may complain of not being able to hear people in noisy, crowded areas. May be associated with tinnitus. OE: nil to find. High pitched hearing loss on audiology |
| **Otosclerosis** | AD inherited condition and may have a strong FHx. Usually seen in 20-40yr olds and presents with tinnitus and deafness. Worsens in pregnancy. OE: conductive deafness |
| **Meniere's disease** | Condition affecting middle-aged. Pts complain of episodes of tinnitus, vertigo and a muffled hearing loss with a sense of fullness lasting from minutes to hours. OE: decreased hearing, nystagmus and a +ve Romberg test |

| Acoustic neuroma | Rare condition causing unilateral symptoms. May have a FHx and bilateral found in neurofibromatosis type 2. Patients complain of deafness, tinnitus and vertigo. May have headache. If is large, facial nerve palsy may also be seen. OE: unilateral sensorineural deafness (CN VIII), absent corneal reflex (V) and facial palsy (VII) |
|---|---|

## EXPLANATIONS

*Presbycusis*

This is deafness that is due to the ageing process. Once we pass the age of 40, the hearing in both ears begin to deteriorate. Over time, it worsens gradually, however, initially you may not notice it. People sometimes notice that they have problems hearing high-pitched sounds such as bird's songs and later find it more difficult to hear in crowded areas.

*Acoustic Neuroma*

An acoustic neuroma is a rare, non-cancerous growth that affects one of the nerves that controls hearing and balance. We do not know what causes it, but sometimes it is linked to an inherited condition called neurofibromatosis. As the growth gets larger, it may impede the hearing pathways so you may get problems hearing, suffer with ringing of the ears and may suffer with vertigo, where you feel the room is spinning around.

*Otosclerosis*

The middle ear has tiny bones that convert the movements of the eardrum into vibrations that are passed into the inner ear and then onto the brain as electrical signals. In otosclerosis, extra bone material forms on the tiny bones in the middle ear preventing them from moving freely. As a result, the movements from the eardrum do not pass well onto the brain and hearing can be severely affected.

*Noise damage*

When the ears are exposed to very loud noises over a period of time, the whole hearing apparatus is working at a higher activity level than normal. Over time, the increased stimulation and activity causes the small bones and the labyrinths to become gradually damaged. If the noise levels persist, the damage continues until your hearing is permanently affected.

*Hearing aid*

A hearing aid is an electronic device that helps to improve hearing. It works by increasing the surrounding sounds to make them appear louder and clearer, passing them into the ear so that hearing is improved.

*Cochlear Implant*

A cochlear implant is an advanced electronic device that helps people hear when they have severe hearing loss. It is made up of 2 parts, an internal part that sends signals to the hearing nerve and is placed in the bone behind the ear during an operation; and an external part that captures the sounds around you and converts it into electrical signals.

*Tinnitus*

Tinnitus is the medical name given for ringing or buzzing in the ear. It usually means that something is wrong with the hearing system as the noise is not from the environment around you. In most cases, we do not know what the cause is but a lot of cases are due to wax, a tear in the eardrum or due to the ageing process.

# 8.3 Vertigo

Vertigo is a debilitating symptom that is a subset of dizziness. A patient feels an abnormal sensation that everything around them or they themselves are moving or spinning, in the absence of any actual movement. It is usually accompanied with symptoms such as nausea or vomiting. Dizziness as a symptom is extremely common, however, effort should be made to confirm what the patient means by their dizziness and ensure that a patient is suffering from true vertigo and not generalised unsteadiness or pre-syncope. The majority of patients presenting in primary care with balance problems suffer from generalised unsteadiness with only 20-30% having true vertigo. Vertigo is classified into peripheral or central depending on the location of the dysfunction on the vestibular pathway.

| Causes of Vertigo | |
|---|---|
| Central | Acoustic neuroma, MS, CVA, TIA, cerebellar tumour, migraine, epilepsy |
| Peripheral | BPPV, vestibular neuronitis, Meniere's disease, labyrinthitis, eustachian tube dysfunction |

**HISTORY**

| **Open questions** | Can you tell me more about the dizziness you have been feeling? Could you tell me about what has been troubling you? |
|---|---|

**Focused questions**

| Vertigo | When you feel dizzy do you feel light-headed or do you feel everything spinning around you? |
|---|---|
| Onset | Did it come on suddenly? |
| Duration | How long do the episodes last (a few seconds or days)? Do they come and go or are they persistent? |
| Timing | Do you have periods where you have no symptoms at all? |
| Triggers | Does anything make the symptoms better (sitting still with eyes closed - motion sickness) or worse? Does anything bring it on (turning the head, anxiety, travel)? |
| Severity | How bad are the episodes? |

**Associated history**

| Nausea & vomiting | Do you feel sick or have you vomited with your dizziness? |
|---|---|
| Ear problems | Do you have any hearing loss, discharge or ringing in your ears? |
| Visual | Have you had any visual symptoms like double vision or flashing lights? |

**Differentials**

| BPPV | Did you bang your head recently? Is it worse when you move your head? |
|---|---|
| Menieres | Do you feel a pressure or fullness in your ear? Do your ears ever ring? Do you have severe vertigo? |
| Vestibular neuron. | DId you have a cold recently? Did you feel a fullness in your ear? Did you feel sick or vomited with it? Do you feel unsteady on your feet? |
| Migraine | Do you get a throbbing headache? Any visual symptoms (flickering lights, spots, zig-zag lines)? Do you feel sick or have you vomited? |
| Postural Hypoten. | Does the dizziness start first thing in the morning when you get out of bed? Or when you are standing for long periods? |

| TIA / CVA | Did you have slurred speech? Any weakness of your arms or legs? |
|---|---|
| Epilepsy | Do you get warning signs beforehand (prodromal - taste, smell)? Did your body go stiff and then fit? Did you bite your tongue or wet yourself? |
| MS | Have you had any eye problems? Have you had different symptoms over a period of time? Any urine or bowel problems? |

**RED FLAGS**  Acute onset of severe and persistent vertigo, headache, acute deafness in absence of ear symptoms

## PAST HISTORY
| Medical | Have you ever suffered from any medical conditions? (MS, BP, brain tumour, DM, meningitis) |
|---|---|

## FAMILY HISTORY
| Medical | Are there any illnesses that run in your family (Meniere's)? Do people suffer with migraine? |
|---|---|

## DRUG HISTORY
| Medication | Are you taking any medications? (gentamicin, furosemide, carbamazepine, BDZ's, aspirin, TCA's, anti-hypertensives) |
|---|---|

## SOCIAL HISTORY
| Home | Who lives with you at home? |
|---|---|
| Hobbies | Did you recently return from flying or go scuba diving? |
| Occupation | Are you currently working? Has it affected you at work? |
| Smoker | Do you smoke? How many cigarettes do you smoke per day? |
| Alcohol | Do you drink alcohol? How much do you drink and how often? |

## IDEA, CONCERNS, EXPECTATIONS
| Ideas | Have you had any thoughts what may be causing your symptoms? |
|---|---|
| Concerns | Do you have any worries about the pain you have been experiencing? |
| Expectations | How did you think I could help you today? |
| Impact | How have the symptoms affected your life? |

## CSA TIPS
Vertigo is an unpleasant sensation and attacks may besot a patient for many years. Dizziness is much more common and is usually benign. It is important to distinguish clearly between the two when taking your history and clarify what the patient means. You may need to ask clearly phrased closed questions to be ensure you can arrive at the correct diagnosis.

## PHYSICAL EXAMINATION
| Vitals | Temp (fever), lying and standing BP, pulse |
|---|---|
| Gait | Ask patient to walk to end of room and back (waddling). Consider Romberg's test (sway to ipsilateral side in neuronitis) |
| Inspection | Inspect for facial asymmetry, resting tremor |
| Neurological | Inspect eyes for nystagmus. Perform CN examination (V, VII, IX, X if acoustic neuroma). Check for power (hemiplegia) and sensation (mono/polyneuropathy) |
| Coordination | Dysdiadochokinesis, finger nose test to exclude cerebellar causes |

| | |
|---|---|
| ENT | Check ears for infection, discharge, cholesteatoma. If hearing loss consider doing whisper test and performing weber's & rinne's |
| Special tests | |
| Hallpike manoev. | (Benign positional vertigo) Keep eyes open, sit upright on couch 45 degree angle with head facing to one side. Lie down rapidly with head extended (30 degrees). +ve if signs of nystagmus. Repeat other side |
| Unterberger's test | (Labyrinthitis) Ask patient to have eyes closed and march on spot for 30sec. With labyrinthine dysfunction patient may laterally rotate to side of lesion |

**INVESTIGATIONS** — *to exclude other causes*

| | |
|---|---|
| Bloods | *Not usually performed in primary care.* FBC, ferritin (anaemia), CRP, ESR (infection) |
| ECG | Exclude cardiac causes of dizziness |
| Specialist | Hallpike maneuver, MRI (brain tumour, MS), audiometry (sensorineural hearing loss) |

**MANAGEMENT** — *treat underlying cause*

| | |
|---|---|
| **General** | During episodes avoid risks at work (ladders, heavy machinery, driving). Recommend not to drive during episodes |

**BPPV**

| | |
|---|---|
| Conservative | Reassure recovery usually over few weeks. Advise to get out of bed slowly. Avoid activities/task that require to look up (ladders) |
| Manoeuvres | |
| Epley's | Sit patient upright on cough with head turned 45 degrees to affected side. Lower head to couch (similar to hallpike) with head extended by 30 degrees. Rotate head 90 degrees to otherside. Roll the patient to their side with head fixed then ask patient to look to the ground. Sit the patient up keeping head position. before returning to central position. Each position held for 30sec |
| Brandt-Daroff | With eyes closed, lie in bed on one side. Turn head 45 degrees and look up to ceiling. Hold position for 30sec until vertigo settles. Sit upright with eyes closed and hold position for 3sec. Repeat on other side. Repeat 3-4x/d until no symptoms |

**Labyrinth/neuronitis**

| | |
|---|---|
| Conservative | Reassure recovery usually over few weeks. Avoid alcohol and advise bed rest during acute phase |
| Medication | Offer buccal/oral prochlorperazine or IM if severe. Take regularly 3d then PRN. Advised SE of dystonic reaction. Consider antihistamines (cinnarizine, cyclizine) |

**Meniere's disease**

| | |
|---|---|
| Conservative | Suggest low salt diet, avoid caffeine, alcohol and stop smoking. Recommend support groups (Meniere's society). To inform DVLA for driving. For tinnitus consider masking devices or sound therapy. If hearing loss consider hearing aids. Avoid loud sounds |
| Medication | Offer buccal/oral prochlorperazine for 7-14d or IM if severe. Consider antihistamines (cinnarizine, cyclizine) |
| Preventative | Trial betahistine 16mg tds (with food) reducing severity and frequency of attacks |

**Referral**

| | |
|---|---|
| Admit | Admit if severe vomiting and cannot keep fluids down |
| BPPV | Refer for education of Epley manoeuvres or symptoms >4wks |
| Neuronitis | Refer if symptoms persist >6wks or if not improving despite treatment for >1wk |
| Meniere's | Refer to ENT for formal diagnosis, considering diuretic or surgery |

*Follow up*                Review typically 1 week after onset of symptoms to ensure improving

## DIFFERENTIAL DIAGNOSIS

| Condition | Characteristic exam feature |
|---|---|
| **Benign Positional Vertigo** | Sudden onset of vertigo that lasts a few seconds (<30sec) and exacerbated by head movement. Often worse in mornings (turning in bed). Affects any age but common in 50yrs. Can be precipitated by virus (neuronitis) or head injury. Associated with nausea but no hearing loss or tinnitus. Can be diagnosed by the Hallpike test and treated with Epley maneuver or Brandt-Daroff exercise |
| **Meniere's Disease** | Sudden onset of severe vertigo not affected by posture often with dulled hearing of affected ear and tinnitus. Episodes last anything from 30mins to 2-3 hrs with severe nausea and vomiting. Can experience clustering of episodes (6-11/yr). Patient may feel a fullness in the ear, hearing loss and associated tinnitus. Ear symptoms often unilateral but develop bilaterally later. Hearing loss requires confirmation with audiometry |
| **Vestibular Neuronitis/labyrinthitis** | Inflammation of the vestibular nerve or labyrinth. Caused by recent onset of URTI. Often affects 20-30yr olds. Presents with severe acute onset of vertigo and nausea and vomiting that recurs for several days. Head movements can precipitate symptoms. Hearing loss only in labyrinthitis and not in neuronitis. Nystagmus fast direction to healthy side. Patients sway to ipsilateral side during Romberg's or on gait assessment |
| **Motion Sickness** | Vertigo, nausea and vomiting that only occurs when travelling in a vehicle, plane or boat |

## EXPLANATIONS

*Auditory Apparatus*    The brain captures and interprets sounds using the auditory apparatus. This is made up of three parts, the outer, middle and inner ears. The outer ear consists of the ear auricle (cartilage appendage), the ear canal and the ear drum. This captures the external sounds and transmits it to the middle ear. The middle ear has very tiny bones that convert the movements of the eardrum into vibrations that are passed into the inner ear. The inner ear is made up of fluid filled chambers that move fine hairs changing the vibrations into electrical signals that are sent to the brain.

*Benign Pos. Vertigo*    This is a problem with the inner ear. The inner ear helps control balance and posture. It does this by using fluids in chambers called vestibules. As the fluid moves, it moves tiny hairs inside that tell the brain the position of your head. In BPPV, it is thought that crystals build up in the fluid and when you move your head these touch against the fine hairs and confuse the brain giving rise to your intense dizziness.

*Epley Manoeuvre*    This is a special movement which the doctor can perform on you to try and cure your symptoms of BPPV. It involves moving your head and body to 4 positions to try and reset the fine hairs and fluid in your vestibules. The Dr may have to repeat this movement 3 times for it to be successful.

You begin sitting in an upright position with your legs outstretched in front of you. Your head should be rotated 45 degrees towards where you feel the problem is. The Dr will then quickly force you down and backwards into a lying position with your head bent backwards facing the ground. You will stay in this position for up to 2 minutes.

They will then turn your head 90 degrees to the opposite side such that your other ear faces the ground. Again you will remain here up to 2 minutes. WIth your head and neck fixed, you will turn your shoulders such that your body moves 90 degrees to the direction you are facing. You will stay here up to 2 minutes before finally being returned slowly to your initial upright sitting position and will stay here for 30 seconds.

| | |
|---|---|
| *Meniere's Disease* | This is a disorder of the inner ear where it is believed that there is increased pressure due to an increased amount of fluid in the vestibules (endolymph). It is a long term condition that may give rise to vertigo, ringing in the ears and hearing loss. |
| *Vestibular Neuritis* | This is a problem with your inner ear that is most commonly due to a viral infection. The infection can affect one of the nerves (vestibular) that controls your balance or affects the fluid filled chambers (labyrinths). The infection sends out confused signals to the brain that gives rise to your symptoms of severe dizziness, nausea and vomiting. |
| *Motion Sickness* | This is the condition that gives rise to the unpleasant symptoms of dizziness, nausea and vomiting that happens when you travel. It is thought that it occurs when the information from your eyes conflicts with the information from your inner ears. |

# 8.4 Sleep apnoea

Snoring refers to the noise made during sleep due to upper airway muscle relaxation. This results in narrowing of the airways which during breathing, causes turbulent airflow. Although most cases of snoring are mild with little impact on life, occasionally it can be so severe that it affects both the patient and their partner causing undue strain on the relationship. A common cause is obstructive sleep apnoea (OSA) where the patient suffers from periods of absent breathing in their sleep. Although these episodes can last for a few seconds a time, they may have profound effects on the patient's life and health with research showing an increased incidence of hypertension, myocardial infarction and strokes.

## HISTORY

**Open questions**     Can you tell me more about the problems you are having with your sleep?

## Focused questions

| | |
|---|---|
| *Sleep apnoea* | When did it start? How long has it been going on for? How often does it happen? |
| Sleep | Do you have disturbed sleep? Do you snore at night? |
| Partner | Are you in a relationship? Does it affect your partner's sleep as well? |
| Triggers | Does anything make it better or worse? |
| Worse | Lying on your back, drinking alcohol, caffeine, sedatives |
| Apnoea | Has your partner mentioned that they noticed that you occasionally stop breathing during your sleep? How often does this occur in a single night? How long are the episodes of pauses in breathing? |
| Daytime sleepy | When you wake up do you feel refreshed? Do you ever feel sleepy first thing in the morning? Have you had trouble concentrating during the day? |

## Associated history

| | |
|---|---|
| *Depression* | How is your mood? Have you noticed a change in your personality? |
| *Tiredness* | Do you feel tired all the time? |
| *Headaches* | Do you get headaches first thing in the morning? |

## Differentials

| | |
|---|---|
| *Tonsillitis* | Have you noticed any fever, sweats, coughs or colds? Any throat pain? |
| *Hypothyroidism* | Do you feel cold when others feel hot? Have you put on any weight? Do you suffer from dry skin? Any neck swellings (goitre)? |

## PAST HISTORY

| | |
|---|---|
| *Medical* | Do you suffer from any medical problems? (hypothyroidism, IHD, CVA, HTN, Kidney disease- water retention) |

## DRUG HISTORY

| | |
|---|---|
| *Medication* | Are you taking any medications? |
| Worsens | Sedatives – diazepam, zopiclone, TCAs |

## FAMILY HISTORY

| | |
|---|---|
| *IHD* | Anyone in the family suffer from heart problems? |
| *OSA* | Does anyone have similar problems with sleep/snoring in the family? |

## SOCIAL HISTORY

| | |
|---|---|
| *Smoker* | Do you smoke? How many cigarettes do you smoke per day? |
| *Alcohol* | Do you drink alcohol? How much do you drink and how often? |
| *Occupation* | Are you working at the moment? What do you work as? |
| *Driving* | Do you drive a car? |

## IDEA, CONCERNS, EXPECTATIONS

| | |
|---|---|
| *Idea* | What did you think may be causing your symptoms? |
| *Concerns* | Is there anything particularly worrying you about it? (relationship problems, poor focus at work) |
| *Impact on life* | How has it affected you? Has it affected your relationship/employment (partner cannot sleep, late to work, missing deadlines)? |

## CSA TIPS

Patients suffering with OSA may not realise they have a problem; making the diagnosis for the Dr a tricky affair. Classically, they may attend with a partner who is at the end of their tether due to poor sleep as a result of their partner's snoring. The relationship may even be close to termination with both partners sleeping in separate rooms. In other cases, patients may attend complaining of headache, poor sleep, lack of libido, symptoms that may suggest depression or stress.

## PHYSICAL EXAMINATION

| | |
|---|---|
| *Vitals* | BP, BMI |
| *Collar size* | Use a tape measure to measure the neck/collar size. Sizes >43cm (17 inches) is associated with OSA |
| *ENT exam* | Inspect the nasal passages for any nasal polyps, and the throat for enlarged tonsils or tonsillitis |
| *Thyroid exam* | If indicated, examine the thyroid gland for the presence of a goitre |

## INVESTIGATIONS

| | |
|---|---|
| *Bloods* | TFT, cholesterol, DM |
| *Other* | Epworth sleepiness scale, Refer for sleep studies |

---

### Epworth Sleepiness Scale (ESS) to assess Obstructive Sleep Apnoea

Assesses the likelihood of the patient dozing off or falling asleep in the following situations

| Situation | Chance of dozing |
|---|---|
| Sitting and reading | 0, 1, 2, 3 |
| Watching TV | 0, 1, 2, 3 |
| Sitting inactive in a public place (e.g a theater or a meeting) | 0, 1, 2, 3 |
| As a passenger in a car for an hour without a break | 0, 1, 2, 3 |
| Lying down to rest in the afternoon when circumstances permit | 0, 1, 2, 3 |
| Sitting and talking to someone | 0, 1, 2, 3 |
| Sitting quietly after a lunch without alcohol | 0, 1, 2, 3 |
| In a car, while stopped for a few minutes in traffic | 0, 1, 2, 3 |

Score each heading out of 3. >10 suggests obstructive sleep apnoea

0 - no chance of dozing, 1 - slight chance, 2 - moderate chance, 3 - high chance of dozing

---

## MANAGEMENT

### Conservative

| | |
|---|---|
| Lose weight | If raised BMI encourage to lose weight until BMI is <25. Consider referral to dietician or exercise programme |
| Smoking cessation | If smoker, advise to stop. Refer for smoking cessation advice/clinic |
| Alcohol | Suggest to cut down alcohol to DoH levels. Avoid evening consumption |
| Caffeine | Avoid or cut down caffeine consumption |
| Sleep position | Avoid sleeping on back. Elevate head of bed with bricks to at least a 30 degree angle. Have 1 thick or 2 thin pillows for ideal pharyngeal opening |
| Ear plugs | Suggest partner wears ear plugs |
| Sedatives | Avoid medications that induces sedation such as sleeping tablets |
| DVLA | Advise not to drive if feels sleepy in the morning. If group 2 vehicle, patient needs confirmation by specialist that symptoms controlled |

### Medical

| | |
|---|---|
| Nasal congestion | Offer beclomethasone nasal spray 2 puffs bd or ipratropium bromide nasal spray 2 puffs on to treat symptomatic nasal congestion |

### Refer

| | |
|---|---|
| Respiratory | Refer for sleep studies to confirm diagnosis and for CPAP |
| ENT | Refer if there is an ENT related problem i.e. enlarged tonsils, polyps, septal straightening or mandibular advancement device is required |

---

**When to Refer patients with Obstructive Sleep Apnoea**

If Epworth Sleepiness Scale (ESS) >10 or sleepiness in dangerous situations, normal ESS in combination with symptoms associated with OSAHS should prompt referral to a sleep service

*Ref: SIGN, Management of Obstructive Sleep Apnoea/Hypopnoea Syndrome in Adults, 2003*

## SAFETY NETTING

| | |
|---|---|
| Follow up | If symptoms persist or feels drowsy in the morning to review in 2-4wks |

| Condition | Characteristic exam feature |
|---|---|
| **OSA** | Snoring and daytime somnolence most common symptoms. Patients may be obese and have associated IHD risk factors. OE: large neck circumference, nasal polyps |
| **Tonsillitis** | Common illness mainly seen in children. May present with sore throat, painful swallowing, headache and loss of voice. Pain may radiate to ears. OE: red tonsils with exudate, tender anterior cervical lymph nodes |
| **Hypothyroidism** | Patients complain of tiredness, weight gain, cold intolerance, constipation and menstrual irregularities. OE: dry skin, thinning hair and reduced reflexes. A goitre may be present |

## EXPLANATIONS

*Sleep apnoea*    Obstructive sleep apnoea is a condition whereby you have brief spells where your breathing stops when you are sleeping. This is because the airways (throat or upper airway) may become temporarily blocked affecting the flow of air. When you sleep, the muscles in the back of the throat relax and become floppy. In some people this can cause a blockage in your airway when you sleep. Most people who have this are unaware of these episodes as they usually pass from a deep sleep state to a lighter one, helping to restore their breathing. However, during the daytime you may get severe tiredness, lack of concentration or headaches.

*CPAP*    CPAP is a device that is used to keep your airways open when you sleep. It blows air through the face mask and into your nose at a slightly raised pressure. This can dramatically improve sleep in some patients.

*Mandibular device*    The mandibular advancement device is like a gum shield that you wear at night to push the lower jaw forward a little to keep your airways open. This can be bought without prescription or you can get your dentist to fit it for you.

# 8.5 Facial pain

Facial pain describes any pain that may be experienced within the confines of the face. This can include pain originating from structures underlying the skin i.e. teeth, muscle or bone, or from deeper neurological and vascular structures. Do not overlook the fact that pain may be referred into the facial area from an external site such as the ear or throat. Although most cases of facial pain are benign, it is important to exclude serious causes such as malignancy and temporal arteritis.

## HISTORY

**Open questions**    Can you tell me more about the pain that you are having? How did it start?

## Focused questions

| | |
|---|---|
| *Facial pain* | When did it start? How long has it been going on for? How often does it happen? |
| Site | Where exactly do you feel the pain? (ear, jaw, eye, teeth, temporal area) |
| Radiation | Does it move anywhere? |
| Character | How would you describe the pain? (sharp dull ache, throbbing, lanciating) |
| Aggravating | Does anything make it worse? |
| Worsen | Touch, washing, shaving, periods, eating, yawning |

## Differentials

| | |
|---|---|
| *TMJ dysfunction* | Does the pain come on when you eat or yawn? Do you notice any clicking sounds from your jaw? |
| *Sinusitis* | Does your pain get worse when you lean forwards? Does it feel like a heaviness in your head? Any coughs, colds or fevers or runny noses? |
| *Dental* | Any pain when you eat? Is there a bitter taste in your mouth? Any fevers? |
| *Trigeminal neuralgia* | Do you experience 'electric shock like' pains in the face? Are there any areas on the face that when touched bring on the pain? Is it worse when you shave? |
| *Temporal arteritis* | Do you have pains when you chew your foods or if you comb your hair? Any stiffness or weakness in your muscles? |
| *Shingles* | Any rashes on the face? Does it burn? Have you had chickenpox in the past? |
| *Parotid stones* | Do you have pain when you are eating or producing saliva? (salivating) |
| *Otitis* | Do you have any ear pain? Any discharge or hearing problems? |
| *Cold Sores* | Do you have a rash on your face? Do they burn or tingle? Did you have a recent cold or fever? |

## RED FLAGS

| | |
|---|---|
| *Trigeminal neuralgia* | Atypical facial pain (<50yrs), failure to respond to treatment |
| *Temporal arteritis* | Blurred vision or sudden loss of vision |
| *Periorbital oedema* | Signs of infection or periorbital swelling or cellulitis |

## PAST HISTORY

| | |
|---|---|
| *Medical* | Do you suffer from any medical problems? (Polymyalgia rheumatica) |
| *Trauma* | Have you had any injuries to you face? (TMJ) |

## DRUG HISTORY

| | |
|---|---|
| *Medication* | Are you taking any medications? |

## SOCIAL HISTORY

| | |
|---|---|
| *Smoker* | Do you smoke? How many cigarettes do you smoke per day? |
| *Alcohol* | Do you drink alcohol? How much do you drink and how often? |
| *Occupation* | Are you working at the moment? What do you work as? |

## IDEA, CONCERNS, EXPECTATIONS

| | |
|---|---|
| *Idea* | What did you think was causing the pain that you are experiencing? |
| *Concerns* | Any particular worries about it? (stroke) |
| *Impact on life* | How has it affected you? (unkempt, cannot shave, depressed, insomnia) |

## CSA TIPS

The causes of facial pain are numerous and varied. The key is to facilitate the patient to describe the symptoms in their own words and for you, the Dr, to encourage them with open questions to obtain a clear and relevant history.

## PHYSICAL EXAMINATION

| | |
|---|---|
| *Skin* | Inspect for shingles (rash does not cross the midline) and cold sores. Feel over the maxillofacial sinuses for any localised tenderness |
| *Nose* | Inspect for polyps, mucosal inflammation, mucosal oedema or discharge |
| *Neurology* | |
| 5th nerve | Check sensation over the face with your finger (cotton wool) |
| 7th nerve | Inspect the facial symmetry and for evidence of weakness. Ask the patient to raise their eyebrows, screw their eyes tight and blow out their cheeks. Request them to bite and move their jaw from side to side. Palpate for crepitus |
| *Ear exam* | Inspect the skin near the ear for a rash (Ramsey Hunt). Touch the pinna for any pain (otitis externa). Look inside for any debris or infection |
| *Vascular* | Palpate the temporal artery for any tenderness or rigidity |

## INVESTIGATIONS

| | |
|---|---|
| *Bloods* | FBC, ESR (temporal arteritis), CRP (infection) |
| *Xray* | Facial X-ray (sinusitis) |
| *Other* | CT/MRI (nasopharyngeal cancer), Sialography (parotid duct stones) |

## MANAGEMENT

| | |
|---|---|
| **MANAGEMENT** | *treat underlying cause* |
| **Trigeminal neuralgia** | Offer carbamazepine or gabapentin- reduces frequency and intensity of attacks. Low dose amitriptyline alternative. Severe cases consider surgery. See trigeminal neuralgia chapter |
| *Carbamazepine* | Start 100mg od/bd increased gradually titrated to response; usual dose 200mg tds/qds, up to 1.2g daily. Perform annual FBC, LFT, UEs |
| Side effects | Dry mouth, nausea, vomiting, cerebellar signs, drowsiness, haemolytic anaemia, jaundice, peripheral neuropathy |
| Seek advice | If evidence of fever, rash, ulcers, bleeding (agranulocytosis) |
| **Post-herpetic neuralg.** | Advise to have cool baths or use ice packs for the pain. Start on amitriptyline. Titrate upwards. Alternatively try gabapentin, pregabalin |
| *Amitriptyline* | Initiate 10mg at night, increased if necessary to 75 mg od |
| Side effects | Dry mouth, constipation, stomatitis, palpitation, drowsiness, blurred vision, nausea, restlessness, fatigue, mydriasis, and increased IOP |
| Advice | May take 4-6wks before benefits are felt |

**Managing Neuropathic Pain** - *Ref: Neuropathic pain NICE 2010*

Defined as pain which occurs following damage or disruption to the nerves post-herpetic neuralgia, diabetic neuropathy, prolapsed intervertebral disc

| | |
|---|---|
| *1st line* | Amitriptyline or pregabalin. If reduction in pain with amitriptyline but cannot tolerate side effects, consider imipramine or nortriptyline |
| *2nd line* | If started on amitriptyline, change to or combine with pregabalin. If first-line was with pregabalin, switch to or combine with amitriptyline |
| *3rd line* | Tramadol, topical lidocaine for localised pain (orals not tolerated) |
| *Exceptions* | Carbamazepine (trigeminal neuralgia), duloxetine (diabetic neuropathy) |

**TMJ dysfunction**

| | |
|---|---|
| *Conservative* | Majority improve. Avoid chewing gum. Eat soft diet to relax the jaw. Avoid opening jaw widely such as singing, yawning, try ice packs over the joints. Relaxation techniques if stressed (as may clench teeth). Gently stretch ligaments in joint by opening jaw slowly and relaxing exercises |
| *Medical* | Consider bite guards at night. Offer physiotherapy or simple jaw exercises. May require TCAs or intra-articular joint injections |

**Temporal arteritis**    Initiate high dose prednisolone 40mg if suspected. Refer urgently for ESR and/or temporal artery biopsy. See temporal arteritis chapter

**Sinusitis**

| | |
|---|---|
| *Conservative* | Most are self limiting (10d). Increase fluid intake and steam inhalation |
| *Medical* | Try simple analgesia (paracetamol/NSAIDs). Consider short course of decongestant (7-10d), steroid nasal sprays, or oral antibiotics (1st line - amoxicillin, 2nd line - augmentin) if signs of infection (unilateral discharge, severe pain, fever >38) |

**Refer**

| | |
|---|---|
| *Neurologist* | Refer if atypical features of trigeminal neuralgia, <50 yrs old, treatment fails, neurological deficit between attacks |
| *Ophthalmologist* | Refer urgently if shingles like rash noted on the tip of nose (nasociliary branch of the trigeminal nerve), may indicate eye involvement |
| *Dentist* | If dental abscess, or pain refer to a dentist for further treatment |

**SAFETY NETTING**

| | |
|---|---|
| *Follow up* | Review 2-4 weeks if symptoms not improving |

**DIFFERENTIAL DIAGNOSIS**

| Condition | Characteristic exam feature |
|---|---|
| **Trigeminal neuralgia** | Unilateral, sharp intense knife like pains with sudden onset and termination with short intervals. Affects the trigeminal distribution (rare in ophthalmic), triggered by light touch (shaving, washing, brushing teeth, yawning, eating) to trigger areas. Absence of symptoms between episodes |
| **Post-herpetic** | Complication of shingles infection. Can persist despite shingles disappearing. Presents with paraesthesia, hyperalgesia or allodynia. First episode often occurs within first |

| neuralgia | month of shingles rash |
|---|---|
| **Dental abscess** | Severe, dull aching pain often from within the mouth. Worse on chewing or eating. Tooth can be sensitive to cold or sweet foods. Poor dentition. Associated with fever, sweats and foul taste in the mouth |
| **Sinusitis** | Pyrexia with throbbing headache or facial fullness, nasal obstruction, post nasal drip and cough. Pain is worse with head tilted. OE: tenderness over sinus |
| **Temporal arteritis** | Common in >60, Unilateral headache (temporal region), scalp tenderness (on combing the hair) and jaw claudication. OE: Palpation of the superficial temporal artery is painful and pulseless. Raised ESR. Associated with polymyalgia rheumatica |
| **Salivary gland stones** | Intermittent pain triggered at mealtimes. Worsened with citrus fruits. OE: focal pain over gland, hard lump, reduced saliva |

## EXPLANATIONS

*Trigeminal neuralgia*   In trigeminal neuralgia, the nerve that supplies the area of your face becomes over-active. Thus when you touch those areas you may feel a sharp stabbing pain. This can be made worse by simply touching certain trigger points or sensitive areas such as by shaving, washing your face, blowing, eating or brushing your teeth.

Carbamazepine   Carbamazepine is a drug usually used to treat epilepsy. It can also be used to treat your condition. This is because it is believed that a similar mechanism takes place in trigeminal neuralgia that of overactive nerves. Carbamazepine works by dulling nerve overactivity which is why it is effective in both conditions.

*Post herpetic n.*   Post herpetic neuralgia is a nerve pain that can remain after you have had shingles. Often the rash goes, but the pain may persist and return at unpredictable intervals. What happens is that shingles (caused by a virus) can infect the nerve and cause irritation locally.

Amitriptyline   Amitriptyline is a drug that has been used in the past to treat depression. Whilst this may be the case with high doses, recent studies have shown that using low doses is very good at treating nerve pain. This is because it acts on the nerves and reduces the number of impulses that are fired. By taking low doses of amitriptyline tablets it does not mean that you suffer from depression.

# 8.6 Rhinitis

Rhinitis refers to the feeling of congestion or blockage of the nasal passages often associated with a watery discharge. Although an allergic cause is typically found, this might not always be the case. Common allergens include glass and tree pollen, cat dander or house dust mites. Non-allergic causes include hormonal imbalance, air pollution, emotion or as a side-effect of medication.

## HISTORY

**Open questions**          Can you tell me more about your blocked nose? How did it start?

### Focused questions

| | |
|---|---|
| *Rhinitis* | When did it start? How long has it been going on for? |
| Site | Which side is affected? |
| Nature | Is it there all the time (perennial) or does it come and go? Does it occur during particular months (seasonal)? |
| Discharge | Do you suffer from a runny nose? What colour is it (clear, yellow, bloody)? |
| Post nasal drip | Do you have the feeling of liquid dripping down the back of your throat? |
| Nasal pruritus | Is your nose particularly itchy? |
| Nasal obstruction | Do you suffer from a blocked nose? Does it cause you to snore? |
| Trigger | Does anything bring it on? (stress, food, environment, fumes, trees/grass, work) |

### Associated history

| | |
|---|---|
| *Smell* | Have you noticed any change in smell? Or reduced taste? |
| *Itching* | Do you have any itchiness in the nose? Or anywhere else (eyes, ears, throat)? |

### Differentials

| | |
|---|---|
| *Allergic* | Do you have itchy eyes and throat? Do you find that you sneeze a lot? |
| *Infective (sinusitis)* | Do you have a headache (frontal)? Is it worse when you lean forwards? Is it like a heaviness in your head? |
| *Polyps* | Have you seen any fleshy lumps in your nose? Is it on one or both sides? |
| *Cold* | Have you recently had a cold? Do you have muscle aches or a headache? |
| *Vasomotor* | Do you get the discharge all the time? Is it worse when the temperature changes? Or after eating spicy food or drinking alcohol? |

## RED FLAGS

| | |
|---|---|
| *Malignancy* | Unexplained bloody or unilateral nasal discharge, nasal pain or deformity |

## PAST HISTORY

| | |
|---|---|
| *Medical* | Do you suffer from any medical (asthma, hayfever, eczema) or thyroid problems (hypothyroidism)? |
| *Trauma* | Have you had any injuries to you face? (TMJ) |

## DRUG HISTORY

| | |
|---|---|
| *Medication* | Are you taking any medications? |
| Worsen | ACE inhibitors, beta-blockers, chlorpromazine, aspirin, NSAIDs |
| *OTC* | Are you using any OTC medication such as nasal decongestants? How long have you been using them for (rebound symptoms)? |

## FAMILY HISTORY

| | |
|---|---|
| *Atopy* | Anyone in the family suffer from asthma, eczema or hay fever? |

## SOCIAL HISTORY

| | |
|---|---|
| *Smoker* | Do you smoke? How many cigarettes do you smoke per day? |
| *Illicit drugs* | Do you take any recreational drugs such as glue sniffing or cocaine? |
| *Alcohol* | Do you drink alcohol? How much do you drink and how often? |
| *Occupation* | Are you working at the moment? Do your symptoms worsen at work (cook using flour, chemicals – painter, hairdresser, carpenter)? |
| *Pets* | Do you have any pets? (cat, dog dander) |

## IDEA, CONCERNS, EXPECTATIONS

| | |
|---|---|
| *Idea* | What did you think was causing the pain that you are experiencing? |
| *Concerns* | Any particular worries about it? |
| *Impact on life* | How has it affected you? (work, sleep) |

## CSA TIPS

Nasal congestion or discharge is an uncomfortable symptom that may impact on the patient's quality of life. It may cause a change in voice, or leave the sufferer having to constantly embarrassingly use tissues at work. Patients may only get symptoms when at work and it would be useful to take a full occupational history and tease out what the offending cause could be.

## PHYSICAL EXAMINATION

| | |
|---|---|
| *Nose exam* | Perform a focused nose examination |
| Inspection | |
| External | Note any obvious deviation (stand behind) discharge. Inspect the vestibule (raise tip of nose with thumb) looking for cartilaginous collapse (cocaine use, repeated operations) |
| Inner | Inspect the nasal septum, inferior, middle turbinates and mucosa, noting for any collapse, ulceration, active bleeding, perforation, FB or nasal polyp |
| Palpation | Palpate the frontal and maxillary sinuses (sinusitis). Press over the supra and infraorbital areas and gently percuss eliciting any tenderness. Feel for the LN in the cervical and head and neck chain |

## INVESTIGATIONS

| | |
|---|---|
| *Bloods* | FBC (eosinophilia), TFT, Immunoglobulin levels, RAST tests (grass pollen, cat/dog dander, trees, house dust mites, dust) |
| *Xray* | Facial X-ray (sinusitis) |
| *Specialist (other)* | MRI sinuses/nasal passages (polyps), skin prick tests, nasal endoscopy |

## MANAGEMENT
### *Allergic Rhinitis*

*treat underlying cause*

| | |
|---|---|
| *Conservative* | Reduce allergen exposure by regularly cleaning the house, vacuuming carpets & curtains, changing of bed linen, avoid pets (keep off bed), keep windows shut and avoid cut grass. Keep aware of pollen charts on news. Avoid walking in grassland in the morning or evening |
| *Occupation* | Wear a mask or use latex free gloves. Ensure adequate air and ventilation in workplace |
| *Medical* | Offer intranasal (Na. cromoglycate) or antihistamines (azelastine) as first line. Consider intranasal steroids spray/drops (up to 2wks to work) - beconase, flixonase, |

mometasone. If persists try oral steroids. Try short course of nasal decongestants (ephedrine) or anticholinergics (ipratropium bromide)

### Non-Allergic Rhinitis

| | |
|---|---|
| *Conservative* | May resolve spontaneously if due to virus. Avoid triggers such as smokey or polluted environments. Reduce spices and alcohol. Stop any OTC nasal decongestant use |
| *Medical* | Consider changing medication that may be implicated. Offer intranasal saltwater spray (Sterimar) or solution to use as a nasal douche first thing in the morning. Consider antihistamine sprays, intranasal steroids spray or short course of nasal decongestants (ephedrine) or anticholinergics (ipratropium bromide) |

**Sinusitis** — Most are self limiting (10d). Try simple analgesia, increase fluid intake and steam inhalation. Consider short course of decongestant (7-10d), steroid nasal sprays, or oral antibiotics (poor evidence)

**Polyps** — Consider steroid nasal drops (flixonase drops) until they shrink (1mth) then maintain with steroid nasal sprays. If persists, consider oral steroids before referring for polypectomy. May recur post surgery

### Refer

| | |
|---|---|
| *ENT* | Refer unilateral polyps with irregular shape or if ulcerated and bleeding |
| *Admission* | Admit if clear fluid post trauma dripping from the nose (CSF rhinorrhoea) |

### SAFETY NETTING

| | |
|---|---|
| *Follow up* | Review 2-4 weeks if symptoms not improving |

### DIFFERENTIAL DIAGNOSIS

| Condition | Characteristic exam feature |
|---|---|
| **Allergic rhinitis** | Seasonal or perennial sneezing, bilateral nasal obstruction, nasal discharge (clear) with post-nasal drip or nasal pruritus. Can be triggered by chemicals (tar, perfumes, drugs or allergens (cats/dogs, dust mites, pollen etc). Severe case can affect sleep and daily activities. FHx atopy may be present. OE: inflamed turbinates, red conjunctiva |
| **Sinusitis** | Pyrexia with throbbing headache or facial fullness, nasal obstruction, post nasal drip and cough. Pain is worse with head tilted. OE: fever and tenderness over sinus |
| **Nasal polyps** | Common in those with atopy, CF or asthma. Patients may complain of a disfigured nose, rhinitis, or problems smelling or mouth breathing at night. OE: fleshy, yellow or grey coloured tear-dropped shape mass in the nasal antrum |
| **Nasal Carcinoma** | More common in males from Africa and SE Asia (chinese). Occupational exposure to fume, dust, nickel have been implicated. Most patients are asymptomatic. However, they may notice cervical LNs, facial pain and drooping. Consider in unilateral symptoms with bloody nasal discharge |

**EXPLANATIONS**

*Allergic rhinitis*        This is a condition where the lining of your nose is irritated by certain allergens (things that cause a sensitivity reaction). This causes swelling and inflammation to the inside of your nose resulting in blockage and a runny nose often associated with sneezing and itching.

*Sinusitis*        The sinuses are small air pockets found within the forehead and cheekbones (almost like a honey comb). These drain fluid or mucus into the nose. In sinusitis, there is swelling and inflammation to the lining of these spaces usually caused by a viral infection.

*Nasal polyps*        Nasal polyps are fleshy swellings that may be noticed in the nose. There may be some clear or coloured discharge from it. They are non-cancerous and usually harmless. However, they may affect both nostrils and may grow in size blocking the nasal passages and causing the feeling of having a constant blocked nose.

*Nasal drops*        It is important to take the nose drops correctly otherwise they will not work properly. Before you begin to use them, blow your nose gently to clear out any discharge or blockage. Either lie on your bed with your head hanging backwards over the edge, or kneel down and place your forehead on the floor with your nose pointing upwards. Drop the required amount of drops in each nostril and stay in this position for at least 2 minutes.

# 8.7 Halitosis

Halitosis is the medical term for bad breath; a common problem experienced by patients. Although usually not a sign of sinister disease, the symptom may have a significant impact upon the patient's work life and personal relationships. Of note, whilst it is common it should be distinguished from halitophobia which is the fear of bad breath in the absence of any objective presence. Family members or partner's opinion should be sought to confirm the presence of the problem.

## HISTORY

| | |
|---|---|
| **Open questions** | Can you tell me more about the symptoms you have been experiencing? How did it start? |

## Focused questions

| | |
|---|---|
| *Halitosis* | When did it start? How long has it been going on for? |
| Timing | Is it worse first thing in the morning after waking or between meals? |
| Smell | What does it smell like (fishy, sweet)? |
| Triggers | Is there anything that makes it better (mouthwash) or worse (foods)? |
| Diet | What type of foods do you eat? |
| Lifestyle | Do you smoke or drink alcohol? |
| Dental hygiene | How often do you brush your teeth? Do you floss regularly? |

## Differentials

| | |
|---|---|
| *Gingivitis* | Do your gums bleed? Does it bleed after you brush your teeth? |
| *Tonsillitis* | Do you have a sore throat or fever? Have you noticed any neck glands? |
| *Sinusitis* | Do you have a headache (frontal)? Is it worse when you lean forwards? Is it like a heaviness in your head? Any coughs, colds, fevers or runny nose? |
| *GORD* | Do you experience a burning feeling after you eat foods or when you are hungry? Any bitter taste or excessive saliva in your mouth? |
| *Pharyngeal pouch* | Have you noticed a bulge in the side of the neck? Do you bring up food? |

## PAST HISTORY

| | |
|---|---|
| *Medical* | Do you suffer from any medical problems (DM, liver disease, hiatus hernia)? |
| *Dental* | Have you seen a dentist about your problem (gum disease)? Do you wear dentures? |

## DRUG HISTORY

| | |
|---|---|
| *Medication* | Are you taking any medications? |
| Worsen | TCAs (xerostomia), isosorbide dinitrate, disulfiram, phenothiazines |

## SOCIAL HISTORY

| | |
|---|---|
| *Smoker* | Do you smoke? How many cigarettes do you smoke per day? |
| *Alcohol* | Do you drink alcohol? How much do you drink and how often? |
| *Illicit Drugs* | Are you using any recreational drugs such as amphetamines? |
| *Occupation* | Are you working at the moment? |

## IDEA, CONCERNS, EXPECTATIONS

| | |
|---|---|
| *Idea* | What did you think was causing the pain that you are experiencing? |
| *Concerns* | Any particular worries about it? |

| *Impact on life* | Has anyone else commented about your bad breath? How has it affected you (work)? |
| --- | --- |

## CSA TIPS

Halitosis is an embarrassing problem that may affect a patient's ability to make or hold down a relationship. Although common and rarely due to any significant illness, the symptom may have a profound effect on the sufferer's life leading to poor social interaction and eventual isolation. Be aware that a significant proportion of sufferers, have pseudo-halitosis and may have no objective problem. Patients working in customer service roles or in jobs that require much people interaction may be particularly affected.

## PHYSICAL EXAMINATION

| ENT | Subjectively assess for halitosis by smelling the patient's breath |
| --- | --- |
| Inspection | Ill-fitting dentures, poor dental hygiene (gum hypertrophy, bleeding gums), tonsillitis |
| Palpation | Palpate the sinuses for any tenderness (sinusitis) |

## INVESTIGATIONS

| **INVESTIGATIONS** | *Not routinely needed* |
| --- | --- |
| *Bloods* | Glucose (DM), LFTs |
| *Urine* | Dipstick for ketones |
| *Stools* | Stool for H. pylori |
| *Specialist* | OGD if no cause found, Barium swallow (pharyngeal pouch) |

## MANAGEMENT

### Conservative

| *Avoid certain foods* | Advise to avoid certain foods that may perpetuate the problem including, onions, garlic, curry/spices, radishes, cheese, fizzy drinks |
| --- | --- |
| *Smoking cessation* | Recommend to stop smoking. Refer to clinic if necessary |
| *Alcohol advice* | Advise to stop drinking alcohol |
| *Oral hygiene* | Brush teeth at least 2x day. Floss between the teeth to clear food particles |
| Tongue cleaning | Clean the back of the tongue with a scraper or toothbrush |
| Gargles | Gargle regularly using mouthwashes |
| Dentures | Keep dentures left out at night |
| Gum | Recommend to chew gum regularly to increase saliva in the mouth |

### Medical

| *Mouthwash* | Offer chlorhexidine 0.2% to reduce dental plaque formation |
| --- | --- |
| *H. Pylori* | Treat if present. See dyspepsia chapter |

### Refer

| *Dentist* | Advise to see a dentist if evidence of gum disease |
| --- | --- |
| *ENT* | Recurrent tonsillitis, sinonasal disease or recurrent sinusitis |

## EXPLANATIONS

| *Halitosis* | Bad breath is often caused by a build-up of bacteria or debris in the mouth. As the bacteria breaks down the food particles stuck between our teeth it can release foul smelling gases giving rise to bad breath. |
| --- | --- |
| *Treatments* | Regular brushing and flossing clears the bits of foods that gets stuck between the teeth. Also use the back of your toothbrush (with thistles), toothbrush dipped into mouthwash or a scraper to remove any coating at the back of the tongue where bugs may collect. |

# 8.8 Mouth ulcers

Most mouth ulcers are painful lesions located within the oral cavity. They are a great nuisance for patients as they can interfere with essential everyday tasks such as eating, drinking or brushing teeth. They are a very common problem but thankfully are usually self limiting. However, persistent mouth ulcers may be indicative of significant underlying illness such as oral cancer.

## HISTORY

**Open questions**      Can you tell me more about the problems you have had in your mouth? How did it start?

## Focused questions

| | |
|---|---|
| *Mouth ulcers* | When did it start? How long has it been going on for? |
| Site | Where in the mouth do you have the ulcer (inner cheek, lip, tongue, palate)? Do you have ulcers anywhere else in the body (anus, groin)? |
| Recurrent | Does it come and go or is it there all the time? |
| Pain | Is it painful? |
| Bleeding | Does it bleed? |

## Associated history

| | |
|---|---|
| *Stress* | Have you been suffering from any recent stress or anxiety? |
| *Trauma* | Did you hurt yourself before the ulcer came out (bite tongue or lip, toothbrush abrasion)? |
| *Diet* | Do you eat a healthy balanced diet (lack of fruit & veg)? Do eating the following strawberries, chocolate or nuts make the ulcers worse? |
| *Chew* | Do you chew tobacco, paan leaves or betel nuts? |
| *Weight loss* | Have you lost any weight recently? |

## Differentials

| | |
|---|---|
| *Herpes simplex* | Any fever or flu like symptoms? Does the ulcer blister or cause pain on drinking or eating? Did you feel a tingling feeling before they broke out? |
| *Trauma* | Any recent injuries to the mouth? Have you bitten your tongue/inner check? Do you wear dentures that can be loose? |
| *Crohn's* | Have you noticed any blood or mucus in your stools? Any ulcers in the back passage? Any tummy pain or bloody diarrhoea? |
| *Coeliac* | Do you have any pale stools that are difficult to flush away? Any rashes on your legs? Are your symptoms linked to particular foods (wheat, rye, barley)? |
| *Hand, foot, mouth* | Did you have a fever a few days before the ulcers came out? Do you have spots on your hand and feet as well? |
| *Behçet's* | Do you have eye pain (uveitis)? Do you have any ulcers on your genitals? Do you suffer with muscle or joint pains? Are you from the Middle east or Central Asia? |

## PAST HISTORY

| | |
|---|---|
| *Medical* | Do you suffer from any medical problems? (Crohns, coeliac, malabsorption) |
| *Dental* | Do you wear dentures or braces? |

**DRUG HISTORY**

| | |
|---|---|
| *Medication* | Are you taking any medications? |
| Worsen | Steroids, gold, nicotine, aspirin, NSAIDs, Nicorandil, B-blockers |

**SOCIAL HISTORY**

| | |
|---|---|
| *Smoker* | Do you smoke? How many cigarettes do you smoke per day? |
| *Alcohol* | Do you drink alcohol? How much do you drink and how often? |
| *Occupation* | Are you working at the moment? What do you work as? |

**FAMILY HISTORY**

| | |
|---|---|
| *Bowel* | Does anyone in your family suffer from any medical problems? (coeliac) |
| *Aphthous* | Do people in your close family have similar ulcers? |

**IDEA, CONCERNS, EXPECTATIONS**

| | |
|---|---|
| *Idea* | What did you think was causing your mouth ulcer? (vitamin deficiency) |
| *Concerns* | Do you have any specific worries about it? |
| *Impact on life* | Does it affect your ability to eat or swallow? How has it affected you? |

**CSA TIPS**

Mouth ulcers are extremely common and patients frequently attend with them. They cause much localised pain and suffering, particularly when eating or drinking. The majority of causes are unknown or are due to a viral infection which spontaneously resolve within 10 days. Persistent ulcers in patients who are alcoholic or smokers should be referred as a 2WW referral.

**PHYSICAL EXAMINATION**

*Mouth Exam*

| | |
|---|---|
| Inspection | inspect the ulcer for it site, size, colour, shape (irregular margins), bleeding, colour |
| Palpation | Palpate the neck for any lymph nodes |

**INVESTIGATIONS**

| | |
|---|---|
| *Bloods* | FBC (anaemia), ferritin, B12, folate, ESR, CRP, coeliac screen |
| *Specialist* | Biopsy for persistent mouth ulcers |

**MANAGEMENT** *treat underlying cause*

**Aphthous ulcer**

| | |
|---|---|
| *Conservative* | Reassure that no underlying disease and will spontaneously resolve in 10 days |
| Mouthwash | Offer chlorhexidine 0.2% or difflam to reduce pain and encourage healing |
| Barrier creams | Consider carmellose sodium (orabase) |
| Analgesics | Use analgesia such as Bonjela or benzydamine spray (Difflam) |
| Steroid lozenges | Consider for difficult to treat ulcers |
| Food | Avoid spicy food, change brand of toothpaste (use SLS free) |

| | |
|---|---|
| *Herpes Simplex* | Try acyclovir cream (x5/d - 5d) or oral if severe or immunocompromised |
| *Coeliac DIsease* | Suggest lifelong gluten free diet. Check labels on foods. See diarrhoea chapter |
| *Crohn's* | Offer elemental diet. See PR bleeding chapter |
| *Malabsorption* | Treat cause. Consider B12, folate or Fe replacement if deficient |
| *Behçet's* | High dose corticosteroid therapy. Refer to specialist for assessment |

## Refer

| | |
|---|---|
| *Maxillofacial* | Refer to specialist if persisting ulcers |
| *Dentist* | Refer to dentist if braces causing ulcers for wax treatment |

---

**Urgent Referral for mouth ulcers** - *Ref: NICE Referral Guidelines for Suspected Cancer (June 2005)*
- Ulceration of the oral mucosa persisting for more than 3 weeks
- Oral swellings persisting for more than 3 weeks
- Red or red and white patches of the oral mucosa, particularly if they are painful or swollen or bleeding
- The level of suspicion is further increased if the patient is a heavy smoker or heavy alcohol drinker and is aged over 45 years and male; other forms of tobacco use and chewing betel, gutkha, or paan should also raise suspicion

---

## SAFETY NETTING

| | |
|---|---|
| *Follow up* | Review patient if symptoms persist for more than 3wks or worsen |

## DIFFERENTIAL DIAGNOSIS

| Condition | Characteristic exam feature |
|---|---|
| **Minor Ulcers** | Aphthous ulcers more common in young adults. Affect the buccal, floor of the mouth, soft palate and lingual mucosa more commonly. Yellowish-grey in appearance and <10mm in size. Spontaneously resolve within 10 days |
| **Herpetiform** | More frequently affects women. Very painful, numerous <3mm lesions in clusters. May last many months |
| **Cancer** | >45 year old male more common. Usually heavy smokers or alcoholics. Red, painful ulcers that bleed and are friable. Persists >4wks |
| **Behçet's** | Common in Middle Eastern and Central Asia. Presents with recurrent mouth ulcers (at least 3x in 1yr), genital ulcers and visual problems including uveitis and iritis |

## EXPLANATIONS

| | |
|---|---|
| *Aphthous Ulcer* | These are small breaks or sores of the skin in the mouth. The majority of them are due to cold like illnesses and last up to 10 days before resolving themselves. They are not contagious so cannot be spread by simple touch. |
| *Herpes Simplex* | This is a viral infection that is linked with cold sores. It causes small painful blisters that can develop around the mouth or the lip. The virus is extremely contagious and can spread from you to others. It usually clears up itself but there are special creams available that can quicken the healing time. |

# 9.1 Red eye

The term 'red eye' refers to the reddish appearance of the eye that may be caused by infection, inflammation or allergy. It is an extremely common problem that presents regularly in the primary and emergency care settings. It is usually a non-life threatening condition but may represent underlying systemic disease and illness. Any of the structures of the eye may be implicated such as the conjunctiva, sclera, episclera or uvea and a clear history of symptoms and onset must be taken to make a discernible diagnosis.

**Differentials of Red Eyes**

| | |
|---|---|
| *Unilateral* | Acute glaucoma, corneal ulceration, subconjunctival haemorrhage, FB |
| *Bilateral* | Conjunctivitis, episcleritis, scleritis, anterior uveitis, FB |

**HISTORY**

| | |
|---|---|
| **Open questions** | Can you tell me about your eye problems? Could you tell me more about what has been troubling you? |

**Focused questions**

| | |
|---|---|
| *Red eye* | When did first notice it? How long has it been going on for (hours/days)? |
| Site | Which eye is affected (unilateral/bilateral)? Are the eyelids or eyelashes affected as well (blepharitis)? |
| Onset | Did it come on suddenly (glaucoma, subconjunctival haemorrhage) or gradually (uveitis, conjunctivitis)? |
| Relieving | Does anything make it better? (sleep, washing eyes, dark room) |
| Aggravating | Does anything make it worse? (watching TV, reading, pollen, dust, coughing) |

**Associated history**

| | |
|---|---|
| *Pain* | Is your eye painful (uveitis, glaucoma, ulcer, conjunctivitis)? How would you describe the pain (gritty, boring, ache)? |
| *Fever* | Have you had a fever, sweats or shakes? (rigors) |
| *Rash* | Did you have a rash? (herpes) |
| *Nausea & vomiting* | Do you feel sick or have you vomited? (glaucoma) |
| *Visual disturbances* | Have you had any visual symptoms? |
| Photophobia | Do you have problems with the light? (uveitis, glaucoma, ulcer) |
| Blurred vision | Any blurring of your vision? (uveitis, glaucoma, scleritis) |
| *Trauma* | Have you had any injuries to the eye? Did anything get into it (chemical)? |

**Differentials**

| | |
|---|---|
| *Inf. Conjunctivitis* | Do you get a sticky discharge from your eye? Did it spread from one side to the other? Have you had a cold? |
| *Allergy conjunctivitis* | Are your eyes watery or itchy? Do you get a runny nose or sneeze a lot? Does it only happen during the spring/summer seasons? Is it worse when you are in the park? |
| *Glaucoma* | Do you see halos around bright lights? Is it really painful especially when you move your eyes? Do you feel sick? Do you have problems with the light? |
| *Subconj. haem.* | Have you been coughing or straining recently? |
| *Blepharitis* | Do you have dry eyes? Are the eyelids sticky in the morning? |

| RED FLAGS | Sudden onset of severe pain, photophobia, small pupil, loss of vision, zoster skin rash, high velocity injuries |

**RED FLAGS**  Sudden onset of severe pain, photophobia, small pupil, loss of vision, zoster skin rash, high velocity injuries

**PAST HISTORY**

*Medical*  Do you suffer from any medical conditions (AS, RA, IBD, sarcoidosis)? Do you suffer from any chronic diseases (DM, BP)?

*Ophthalmological*  Have you ever had any eye operations? Did you suffer from uveitis before?

*Contact lens*  Do you wear contact lens? Did you forget to take them off (ulcer)?

*Glasses*  Do you wear glasses? When was your last eye test?

**FAMILY HISTORY**

*Glaucoma*  Does anyone in your family suffer from eye problems? (primary open angle glaucoma)

**DRUG HISTORY**

*Medication*  Are you taking any medications or eye drops? (anticoagulants - subconjunctival haemorrhage, high dose steroids - glaucoma, amiodarone - optic neuropathy)

**SOCIAL HISTORY**

*Occupation*  Are you working at the moment? (welder, builder, working with chemicals, teacher - infective conjunctivitis)

*Home*  Who is at home with you? Do they have similar symptoms (inf. conjunctivitis)?

*Smoker*  Do you smoke? How many cigarettes do you smoke per day?

*Alcohol*  Do you drink alcohol? How much do you drink and how often?

**IDEA, CONCERNS, EXPECTATIONS**

*Idea*  Have you had any thoughts around what may be causing your eye problems?

*Concerns*  Do you have any worries about it? (blindness)

*Expectations*  How were you hoping I could help you? (benefits, registering blindness)

*Impact*  How have your symptoms affected your life?

**CSA TIPS**

Eye conditions cause much angst in patients for fear of losing vision. Although most causes of the red eye are benign, occasionally more serious pathology is present that requires urgent assessment by an ophthalmologist.

**PHYSICAL EXAMINATION**

*Vitals*  BP, pulse, temp

*Inspection*  Inspect conjunctiva (injection - conjunctival, hemorrhage - subconjunctival), cornea (ciliary injection - acute glaucoma), sclera (episcleritis) and lids (conjunctivitis, blepharitis). Consider using fluorescein stain (corneal ulcer)

Pupils  Inspect the pupil size & shape (fixed semi-dilated not reactive to light - glaucoma, small irregular - anterior uveitis). Check pupil reflexes

*Palpation*  If indicated press on the eyeballs (glaucoma)

*Neurological*  Consider visual fields, acuity and CN examination (III, IV, VI)

*Systemic*  Consider systemic examination if PMHx suggests

## INVESTIGATIONS

| | |
|---|---|
| *Bloods* | *Not routinely required:* FBC, INR (subconjunctival haemorrhage), ESR & CRP with Rh factor if systemic cause suspected |
| *Swabs* | Swabs sent for MC&S (viral, bacterial, chlamydia) |
| *Specialist* | Slit-lamp fluorescein staining (FB, corneal ulcer), IOP measurements |

## MANAGEMENT *Treat underlying cause*

| | |
|---|---|
| ***Allergic conjunct.*** | Avoidance of allergens. Offer topical antihistamines (xylometazoline, azelastine, olopatadine etc). Other treatments include sodium cromoglycate, nedocromil. Avoid steroids drops (risk of glaucoma, cataracts) |
| ***Infective conjunct.*** | Often self limiting (3-5d). Suggest bathing eyes with clear water or OTC eye drops (hypromellose). Can wash eye with wet cotton wool. Avoid contact lense during illness. Infection can be contagious (wash hands, not to share towels) |
| *Treatment* | If bacterial, offer chloramphenicol or fusidic acid drops for 7-10d |
| ***Acute Glaucoma*** | Refer urgently to ophthalmologist and advise to avoid eye patch (dilated pupil worsen symptoms). Offer topical pilocarpine for pupillary constriction and acetazolamide (given by hospital) to reduce IOP |
| *Ongoing mx* | Advise to avoid using a computer or watching the TV in dim or low lit rooms. Consider beta blocker (timolol), prostaglandin analogues (latanoprost) or alpha2-adrenoceptor agonist (brimonidine) |
| ***Uveitis / Scleritis*** | Refer urgently to ophthalmologist for consideration of steroid or antibiotic drops. Not to be treated in primary care |
| ***Corneal Injury*** | |
| Foreign body | Remove if possible. Irrigate eye with water or 0.9% saline. Offer pain relief and topical abx to prevent infection. All high-velocity injuries due to hammering, grinding, glass, darts should be referred as an emergency |
| Chemical | Remove contact lens. Irrigate eye immediately with water or 0.9% saline for 15mins. Refer for emergency assessment |
| ***Corneal ulceration*** | Refer urgently to ophthalmologist to establish type and treatment (dendritic - acyclovir, bacterial - antibiotics) |
| ***Subconjunc haem.*** | Usually self limiting. Consider artificial tears to reduce mild irritation. Stop any offending medications (NSAIDs, warfarin) as appropriate |
| ***Blepharitis*** | Good lid hygiene. Use cloth warmed in hot water and apply to the closed eyelid for 10 minutes. Clean the eyelids every morning with a cleanser / cooled boiled water and cotton bud. Consider topical abx if signs of infection |

## SAFETY NETTING

| | |
|---|---|
| *Follow up* | Review 2-4 weeks if symptoms not improving. If any deterioration or loss of vision to attend emergency department |

# DIFFERENTIAL DIAGNOSIS

| Condition | Characteristic exam feature |
|-----------|------------------------------|
| **Acute closed angle glaucoma** | Occlusion to the angle of the eye resulting in sudden increased intraocular pressure. Often seen in >50yr, females with SE Asian descent (rare in blacks). Associated with FHx. Presents with acute severe pain in the orbit, reduced acuity with halos around lights, nausea and vomiting and headache. OE: fixed unreactive semi-dilated pupil, hard on palpation of the pupil, hazy cornea |
| **Conjunctivitis** | Inflammation of the conjunctiva. Commonest cause of red eye. Gritty feeling or itchy (allergic) sensation in eye. Infective cause often presents with purulent, mucoid discharge with sticking of eyelids. Allergic caused by pollen, dust, cats etc. |
| **Uveitis** | Inflammation of the iris and ciliary body. Mainly affects the young or middle-aged patients and more common in HLA B27 +ve patients (RA, AS). Present with pain worse on reading, photophobia and reduced acuity. Often seen as a patient who is unresponsive to treatment for conjunctivitis. OE: pupil may be small and irregular with redness around corneal edge (ciliary injection) |
| **Subconjunctival Haemorrhage** | Due to the rupture of a vessel between the sclera and conjunctiva. May be due to trauma such as sneezing, coughing or itching. Often associated with raised BP and warfarin use. OE: painless, unilateral red eye causing not covering the cornea |
| **Corneal ulceration** | Causes an acutely painful red eye with reduced acuity. Often feels as if a foreign body in the eye. Can experience blurred vision and photophobia. Seen with contact lense use, trauma or injection. OE: often circumcorneal injection but conjunctiva can be inflamed (keratoconjunctivitis). Keratitis of white/grey patches on cornea. Fluorescein reveals ulcer |
| **Scleritis** | Inflammation of the sclera. Presents with severe deep painful eye with eventual loss of vision. Can be bilateral or unilateral with diffuse redness. Associated with autoimmune conditions (RA, AS, SLE, IBD) or infections (HZV, TB, syphilis). More common in 40yr old and women |
| **Episcleritis** | Inflammation of the episcleritis. Often unilateral and self limiting. Patients can have only mild irritation of the eye with redness with normal acuity |

## EXPLANATIONS

*Infective Conjunctivitis* This is an extremely common problem where the eye becomes red due to an infection of the thin skin (membrane) that covers the white of the eye known as the conjunctiva. The infection may be from a virus (in which case it should go itself within 5-7 days) or a bacteria (in which case it may need abx drops to help). It usually happens when your body becomes weak from a cold or cough and can be spread quite easily to others.

Eye hygiene

In order to reduce the chance of spreading your eye infection to others you should make sure that you wash your hands everytime you touch your eyes. Ensure that each family member in your house has their own towels and do not share pillow covers.

*Allergic Conjunctivitis*

This is a red eye that is caused by an small localized allergic reaction to something (allergen). It may be seasonal in which case it may be due to pollen from grass or trees; or all year (perennial) when the likely source of irritation is house dust mite. The body directs its immune system against anything harmful and in these cases it reacts against the allergen and causes itching, watering and redness.

*Acute Glaucoma*

Glaucoma is a condition where the pressure in the pupil rises too quickly as fluid cannot be drained out of the eye due to a blockage. As fluid builds up, pressure is put on the nerve at the back of the eye (optic nerve) and causes symptoms of headaches, eye pain and blurring of vision.

*Subconjunc. Haem.*

This is when a small vessel in the thin lining between the white part of the eye and the central part bursts. We do not always know what causes it, but usually some form of trauma or irritation such as itching the eye or increase in pressure like when you sneeze or vomit is implicated. Although it looks alarming, it is not a serious condition and your vision will not be affected. It usually goes away itself within 7-10days.

# 9.2 Loss of Vision

Loss of vision describes the alarming symptom of the complete or partial loss of sight. It may occur acutely or progress gradually over time, affecting one eye or both. It is an extremely distressing and debilitating symptom, not least given vision is an integral part of our sensory perception. Visual disorders may affect the sharpness or clarity of a patient's vision, restrict their visual fields or reduce their ability to perceive colour.

In the UK, it is estimated that over 2 million people have visual problems with 360,000 registered blind or partially sighted. Most of these are elderly patients with 20% of over-75s suffering from visual impairment increasing to 50% in those over 90. Blindness is defined as a person having a visual acuity of less than 3/60 whilst partial sightedness is an acuity between 3/60 and 6/60.

---

**Differentials of Loss of Vision**

| | |
|---|---|
| *Sudden onset* | Retinal artery or retinal vein occlusion, retinal detachment, optic neuritis, acute closed angle glaucoma, vitreous haemorrhage |
| *Gradual onset* | Cataract, diabetic retinopathy, chronic glaucoma, macular degeneration |

---

**HISTORY**

**Open questions**    Can you tell me more about your eye problems? Could you tell me about what has been troubling you?

**Focused questions**

| | |
|---|---|
| *Loss of Vision* | When did you first notice it? How long has it been going on for? Can you not see anything at all or is it just blurred? |
| Site | Which eye is affected? (unilateral/bilateral) |
| Size | Did you have problems with your colour vision (red desaturation)? Did you lose sight in a small part of your vision (optic neuritis, AMD, migraine), half of it (cva) or all of it (vessel occlusion, haemorrhage, migraine)? Can you see around the peripheries of both eyes (retinitis pigmentosa, glaucoma, pituitary tumour)? |
| Onset | Did it come on suddenly (glaucoma, haemorrhage, TIA) or gradually (AMD, cataract)? |
| Timing | Is it persistent (vessel occlusion, cva) or does it come and go (migraine, TIA)? |
| Relieving | Does anything make it better? (sleep, dark room) |
| Aggravating | Does anything make it worse? (watching TV, reading, night time) |

**Associated history**

| | |
|---|---|
| *Pain* | Is your eye painful (glaucoma, optic neuritis)? How would you describe the pain (gritty, boring, ache)? Do you get pain when looking at lights (migraine, closed angle glaucoma)? |
| *Fever* | Have you had a fever, sweats or shakes? (rigors) |
| *Rash* | Did you have a rash? (herpetic keratitis) |
| *Nausea & vomiting* | Do you feel sick or have you vomited? (glaucoma) |
| *Visual disturbances* | Have you had any visual symptoms? |
| Photophobia | Do you have problems with the light? (uveitis, glaucoma, ulcer) |
| *Trauma* | Have you had any injuries to the eye? Did anything get into it? |
| *Flashing lights* | Did you see any flashing lights or floaters? Did it happen suddenly with no pain? |

**Differentials**

| | |
|---|---|
| *Age-related MD* | Does it affect both eyes? Is your central vision blurry? Are you finding it difficult to make out people's faces or having problems reading? |
| *Glaucoma* | Do you see halos around bright lights? Is it really painful especially when you move your eyes? Do you feel sick? Do you have problems with the light? |
| *Migraines* | Have you had any headaches? Do you get a warning before the symptoms come on? Do you feel sick or vomit when it starts? |
| *Temporal Arteritis* | Are your headaches worse on chewing food or combing your hair? Do you have any muscle pain? Do you get pain in your jaw when chewing? |
| *TIA* | Did you have slurred speech? Any weakness of your arms or legs? Was the loss of vision like a curtain coming down? |
| *Thyroid* | Do you have any weight loss, sweating, diarrhoea or tremor in the hands? |

**RED FLAGS**     Sudden onset of severe pain, acute loss of vision

**PAST HISTORY**

| | |
|---|---|
| *Medical* | Do you suffer from any medical conditions (DM, BP, AF)? Do you suffer from migraines? |
| *Ophthalmological* | Have you ever had any eye operations? (cataract removal - AMD) |
| *Contact lens* | Do you wear contact lens? Do you clean them often? |
| *Glasses* | Do you wear glasses? When was your last eye test? Are you short-sighted (open angle glaucoma, retinal detachment) or long-sighted (closed angle glaucoma)? |

**FAMILY HISTORY**

| | |
|---|---|
| *Glaucoma* | Does anyone in your family suffer from any eye problems? (primary open angle glaucoma, retinitis pigmentosa) |
| *Migraines* | Does anyone suffer with migraines? |

**DRUG HISTORY**

| | |
|---|---|
| *Medication* | Are you taking any medications or eye drops (high dose steroids - glaucoma, amiodarone - optic neuropathy)? Are you on the COCP (migraine)? |

**SOCIAL HISTORY**

| | |
|---|---|
| *Occupation* | Are you working at the moment? (HGV driver, welder) |
| *Home* | Who is at home with you? |
| *Hobbies* | Do you do any hobbies? (squash) |
| *Smoker* | Do you smoke (glaucoma, AMD)? How many cigarettes do you smoke per day and for how long? |
| *Alcohol* | Do you drink alcohol? How much do you drink and how often? |
| *Drive* | Are you driving at the moment? |

**IDEA, CONCERNS, EXPECTATIONS**

| | |
|---|---|
| *Idea* | Did you have any thoughts about what may be causing your eye problems? |
| *Concerns* | Do you have any worries about it? (unable to drive / read) |
| *Expectations* | How were you hoping I could help you? |
| *Impact* | How have your symptoms affected your life? |

## CSA TIPS

Patients attending with deteriorating vision may be quite anxious, worried and concerned that they will eventually go blind. Others may be confused about what is happening and may suspect that they had a stroke. It is important for you to take a clear history and advise the patient on the most likely cause for their symptoms. Patients may also present requesting a sick note to take time off work, or want a medical report to be completed for a disability application.

## PHYSICAL EXAMINATION

| | |
|---|---|
| *Vitals* | BP (raised - retinal detachment), pulse, temp |
| *Inspection* | Inspect cornea (ciliary injection - acute glaucoma). Consider using fluorescein stain (corneal ulcer) |
| Pupils | Inspect the pupil size & shape (fixed semi-dilated not reactive to light - glaucoma, small irregular - anterior uveitis). Check red reflex (cataract) and pupillary reflexes (MS). Check for scotoma and red desaturation (colour plates) |
| Fundoscopy | Examine the fundi for pale discs and the cup to disc ratio (DM & BP retinopathy, AMD, retinal detachment) |
| *Palpation* | if indicated press on the eyeballs (glaucoma) |
| *Neurological* | Consider visual fields (cva, glaucoma), acuity and CN examination (III, IV, VI) |
| *Systemic* | Consider systemic examination if PMHx suggests |
| Thyroid | Have hands outstretched for tremor. Inspect the eyes for signs of exophthalmos, loss of hair in the outer 1/3 of eyebrow, lid lag/retraction, ophthalmoplegia. Inspect and palpate the neck for presence of goitre |
| *Temporal artery* | Check for tenderness, thickening or pulselessness of artery |

## INVESTIGATIONS

| | |
|---|---|
| *Bloods* | *Not routinely required:* FBC, TFTs, ESR and CRP |
| *MRI* | Gadolinium-enhanced MRI (optic neuritis) |
| *Specialist* | Slit-lamp fluorescein staining, IOP measurements |

## MANAGEMENT   *Treat underlying cause*

| | |
|---|---|
| *Visual Aids* | |
| Reading | Advise patients to use magnifying glasses or large print books for reading. Brighter lamps may also improve readability. Consider learning Braille |
| Gadgets | Purchase large button telephones or remote controls to help |
| Talking | Consider using talking alarms, newspaper, audiobooks, phone apps to read messages and text |
| Walking | Consider using a long cane or a guide dog for mobilisation |
| *Support group* | Suggest to contact the Royal National Institute of Blind People (RNIB) for support |
| *Driving* | If registered partially sighted or blind ineligible to drive. Can only drive if VA is 6/12 (can read number plate at distance of 20m) |
| *Registering Blind* | Consultant Ophthalmologists can register a patient blind or partially sighted by completing a Certificate of Visual Impairment (CVI). Once registered, patients may be entitled to disability benefits and concessions such as half-priced TV licence, free public transport, council tax and income tax allowances. Advise to speak to the council's social services department / job centre plus for more advice |

| AMD | Stop smoking and reduced alcohol. Increase omega-3 fatty acids via oily fish and oral antioxidant intake (Vit A,C,E, Zn). Control BP and avoid direct sunlight by wearing sunglasses |
|---|---|
| *Refer* | Refer to low vision clinic in the hospital for vision rehabilitation. For wet AMD refer to an ophthalmologist to consider laser treatment, anti VEGF (vascular endothelial growth factor) injections or surgery |
| | |
| *Acute Glaucoma* | See red eye chapter |
| | |
| *Retinal Detach.* | Refer urgently to ophthalmologist. Keep BP well controlled |
| | |
| *Vessel Occlusion* | Control risk factors such as lowering BP, keeping DM controlled, lose weight, reduce cholesterol through diet and exercise, smoking cessation and reducing alcohol intake |
| Venous | Refer to an ophthalmologist to consider laser treatment, steroid injections or anti VEGF injections to the macular area |
| Arterial | No proven treatment to improve vision. However, if presents early, refer as an emergency to the ophthalmologist for immediate management. Consider commencing aspirin prophylaxis |
| | |
| *Cataract* | Keep DM under tight control. If mild cataracts, then advise simple reading aids and brighter lights. Patient may need a stronger prescription for glasses |
| *Referral* | Once mature, refer for cataract surgery. Will need to wear lifelong glasses after the operation |

**SAFETY NETTING**

| *Follow up* | Review 2-4 weeks if symptoms not improving. If any deterioration or loss of vision to attend emergency department |
|---|---|

**DIFFERENTIAL DIAGNOSIS**

| Condition | Characteristic exam feature |
|---|---|
| **Acute closed angle glaucoma** | Occlusion to the angle of the eye resulting in sudden increased intraocular pressure. Often seen in >50yr, females of SE Asian descent (rare in blacks). Associated with FHx. Presents with acute severe pain in the orbit, reduced acuity with halos around lights, nausea and vomiting and headache. OE: fixed unreactive semi-dilated pupil, hard on palpation of the pupil, hazy cornea |
| **AMD** | Most common cause of loss of vision in those >50. Two types 'wet' and 'dry'. Due to degeneration of the cells of the macula affecting the centre of vision. Dry is more common and slowly progressive giving rise to problems recognising faces or written text. Wet is more acute and is due to haemorrhage from choroidal neovascularisation that can lead to rapid visual loss. OE: drusen (yellow deposits) and increased pigment |
| **Cataract** | These are cloudings of the lens in the eye that cause a gradual reduction in the clarity of vision. Age is the most common cause but may be accelerated due to trauma, medications and diabetes. OE: Lack of red reflex in affected eye |

| | |
|---|---|
| **Vessel Occlusion** | *Retinal vein occlusions* are usually due to thrombus formation and are associated with DM, BP, raised cholesterol and obesity. Patients present with more gradual unilateral painless deterioration of vision. OE: dilated vessels and increased tortuosity with dot and blot haemorrhages <br><br> *Retinal artery occlusions* are associated with the same conditions and presents with more acute painless loss of vision. OE: disc pallor, silver wiring, cherry-red spot, optic disc oedema on fundoscopy |
| **Retinal Detachment** | Caused by detachment of the inner neurosensory retina from the retinal pigment. Causes progressive loss of vision with floaters and flashing lights. If not treated can lead to permanent vision loss. May be associated with very high BP. OE: loss of red reflex with pale, detached retinal folds on fundoscopy |

**EXPLANATIONS**

*Acute Glaucoma*  Glaucoma is a condition where the pressure in the pupil rises too quickly as fluid cannot be drained out of the eye due to a blockage. As fluid builds up, pressure is put on the nerve at the back of the eye (optic nerve) and causes symptoms of headaches, pain in your eyes and blurring of vision.

*AMD*  This is a condition where a small area at the back of your eye that controls your central vision is affected. We do not know what causes it, but we know that it is more common as we grow older and it affects women and smokers more commonly. Initially, you may notice blurriness when looking at people or the TV, and this may slowly worsen. It does not affect your peripheral vision nor lead to total blindness.

*Cataract*  This is when the lens that focuses the light and image onto the retina becomes cloudy. The most common cause for this is changes due to ageing, but sometimes diseases like diabetes can make it worse. If left, the lens becomes less clear and affects your ability to see properly in that eye. It can be corrected quite easily with a simple operation.

*Retinal Detachment*  This is a rare problem that occurs when the lining at the back of the eye known as the retina separates from the layer that gives it food, blood and nutrients. As it begins to separate, you will notice flashing lights or dark spots that appear to float in your field of vision. As it progresses, your sight may get worse. We don't always know what causes it, but sometimes an injury or very high blood pressure may make it worse.

*Vessel Occlusion*  This is when a small vessel in the retina becomes blocked and stops delivering oxygen and nutrients to light sensitive areas of the eye. If the blood supply does not continue then those area may decay and die leading to loss of vision. Usually things like high fat in the blood (cholesterol), raised sugar (DM), smoking and obesity may make this more likely.

# 10.1 Menorrhagia

Menorrhagia is the medical term for heavy periods. It is usually defined as the loss of more than 80mls of blood during the menstrual cycle. On average a woman's period lasts for between 2-5 days. Periods that last longer than 7 days are considered abnormal. In 60% of cases no abnormality can be found and this is termed dysfunctional uterine bleeding (DUB). Patients often complain of increased use of sanitary towels or tampons, and may experience floods or passing of clots. Bleeding associated with secondary dysmenorrhoea which occurs several days before the onset of menstruation may be indicative of fibroids, endometriosis, adenomyosis or ovarian tumours.

## HISTORY

**Open questions**     Tell me more about the heavy periods that you have been experiencing?

**Focused questions**

*Menorrhagia*     When did your heavy periods first start? Do they last longer than usual? On which days are they the heaviest?

    Quantity     How many tampons/pads or sanitary towels did you have to use each day? Are you using more than usual?

        Flooding     Any flooding or soiling of your underwear with blood? Were there any clots?

    Cycle     Are your periods usually regular? How many days do they last? When was the first day of the last period?

**Associated history**

*Postcoital (PCB)*     Do you experience bleeding after sex?

*Intermenstrual (IMB)*     Have you noticed any bleeding or spotting between periods?

*Pain*     Do you get pains during your periods? When does it occur in your cycle? Does it move anywhere? How long does it last for?

    Dyspareunia     Do you get pain during intercourse?

*Anaemia*     Have you been feeling tired recently? Any shortness of breath?

*Pregnant*     Any chance you are pregnant? Are you trying for a child?

**Differentials**

*Thyroid disease*     Have you felt any intolerance to hot or cold weathers? Have you put on or lost any weight? Any dry skin?

*Ovarian cancer*     Have you lost any weight or noticed any bloating recently? Any constipation or diarrhoea? Have you had any urinary symptoms?

*PID*     Have you had any recent unprotected sex? Any vaginal discharge? Have you had pain during sex or a mild fever?

*Coil*     Do you have a coil in place?

**RED FLAGS**     Poscoital bleeding, intermenstrual bleeding

## PAST MEDICAL HISTORY

*Medical*     Do you have any medical problems (fibroids, thyroid, clotting disorders)?

*Surgery*     Have you had any recent surgery (hysterectomy, hysteroscopy)?

*Smear*     Have you had a recent smear? What was the result? Have you had any abnormal smear tests in the past?

## SEXUAL HISTORY

| | |
|---|---|
| *Sexual History* | Are you sexually active? Do you have a regular or casual partner? |
| Contraception | Do you use a coil? Have you an implant or are you on POP? |
| STDs | Have you or any of your partners been diagnosed with an STI? |

## DRUG HISTORY

| | |
|---|---|
| *Medication* | Are you taking any medications? (tamoxifen, POP, coil, HRT, warfarin) |

## SOCIAL HISTORY

| | |
|---|---|
| *Smoker* | Do you smoke? How many cigarettes do you smoke per day? |
| *Alcohol* | Do you drink alcohol? How much do you drink and how often? |

## FAMILY HISTORY

| | |
|---|---|
| *Medical* | Anyone in the family suffers from any illness? (bleeding disorders, ovarian ca, endometriosis) |

## IDEA, CONCERNS, EXPECTATIONS

| | |
|---|---|
| *Ideas* | Have you had any thoughts as to what may be causing your heavy periods? |
| *Concerns* | Are you worried about them in any way? |
| *Expectations* | What were you hoping we could do for you today? |
| *Impact on life* | How have your heavy periods affected you? (off work, embarrassment) |

## CSA TIP

Heavy periods affect many women at some point in their life. The heaviness of the flow does not necessarily equate to the seriousness of the problem and in most cases no cause is found. Blood flow could be so excessive that it leaves the patient suffering from symptoms of anaemia.

## PHYSICAL EXAMINATION

| | |
|---|---|
| *Chaperone* | Request for a chaperone |
| *Vitals* | BP (hypotension), pulse (tachycardia), temperature, BMI |
| *Abdomen* | Inspect the hands for signs of koilonychia (fe def). Palpate the abdomen particularly the lower segment for any tenderness or guarding |
| *Pelvic exam* | Perform a pelvic examination as well as a speculum (cervix, polyps) |
| Inspect | Inspect the vulva for irritation, ulceration, swellings, cancers or bartholin's abscess |
| Palpate | Attempt to palpate the cervix, uterus as well as adnexae |
| Cervix | Palpate for masses or tenderness (excitation) |
| Uterus | Ballot the uterus between the opposing fingers of your two hands feeling for fibroids, or an endometrial carcinoma |
| Adnexae | Palpate both adnexae for masses (ovarian ca, cysts) or pain (salpingitis) |
| *Thyroid exam* | Perform focused thyroid exam if clinically indicated |
| *Other* | Inspect for striae, hirsutism, bruising or petechiae. Look for signs of anaemia (tongue pallor, koilonychia) |

## INVESTIGATIONS

| | |
|---|---|
| *Bloods* | FBC & ferritin (anaemia), TFTs (if symptomatic) coagulation screen (if FHx), CA-125 (ovarian cancer), hormone profile, ESR & CRP (PID) |
| *HVS* | Swab for STIs |
| *US* | Endometrial or ovarian cancer, fibroids, structural abnormality |

| Specialist | Endometrial sampling, hysteroscopy |

## MANAGEMENT

| *Conservative* | Perform a detailed menstrual diary regarding the number of pads or tampons used and symptoms. Note if there is any flooding or clots |

*Medical*

| Mirena IUS | First line if long term contraception also sought. Most effective in reducing heavy heavy periods. Can cause amenorrhoea (12mths) |
| Tranexamic acid | (1gm tds) Take for 3-5 days during heavy periods |
| NSAIDs | Naproxen or mefenamic acid (500mg tds) |
| COCP | Offers rapid reversible contraception and period control |
| Norethisterone | Taken from day 5 – 26. Offer 5mg tds |
| Depo-provera IM | Long acting progestogen given IM every 12wks |

*Other*

| Stop bleeding | Give norethisterone 5mg tds for 10 days to arrest bleeding. Works within 1-3 days but patients will experience withdrawal bleeding after stopping. Consider 10mg tds for 7d reduced to 5mg tds thereafter if flooding |

| *Refer* | Refer if heavy bleeding affecting quality of life of the patient or is considering surgery (endometrial ablation, myomectomy) or persistent iron deficiency anaemia despite treatment. Refer urgently if PCB, IMB, vulval mass/ulceration or abdominal mass (not fibroid like) or ovarian cancer |

## DIFFERENTIAL DIAGNOSIS

| Condition | Characteristic exam feature |
| --- | --- |
| **Dysfunctional Uterine Bleed** | Represents 50% of complaints. No pathology found |
| **Fibroids** | Benign uterine tumours. Often seen in African-Caribbean women in their 40ys. Presents with menorrhagia, painful colicky periods, can press on bladder causing urinary frequency or retention. Occasionally can cause infertility or dystocia. OE: firm uterine mass on examination |
| **Endometrial polyps** | Endometrial hyperplasia forming a mass of the inner lining of the uterus that often is pedunculated into uterine cavity. Presents with menorrhagia, intermenstrual bleeding or post menopausal bleeding |
| **Endometriosis** | Endometrial lining found outside the endometrial cavity. Regresses during pregnancy or menopause. It presents with menorrhagia and dysmenorrhoea, deep dyspareunia, pelvic pain or infertility |
| **Pelvic inflammatory** | Caused by an ascending STI (chlamydia, gonorrhoea) from the cervix. Risk factors include IUCD, multiple partners, lack of barrier contraception, TOP. Presents with |

| | |
|---|---|
| disease (PID) | lower abdominal pain, deep dyspareunia, purulent discharge, abnormal bleeding (PCB, IMB). OE: lower abdominal tenderness with cervical excitation and fever. Complications include infertility, ectopic pregnancy |
| Endometrial carcinoma | Often adenocarcinoma arising from the endometrium. Risk factors includes nulliparity, obesity, late menopause (>52), HNPCC, tamoxifen, HRT. Presents with postmenopausal bleeding |

**EXPLANATIONS**

*Fibroids*               These are common non-cancerous swellings found within the muscle of the womb. They vary in size from a small pea to the size of a grapefruit. They can be found within or in the outer wall of the womb or lie within the womb but attached to the wall through a narrow stalk.

*Endometrial polyps*    These are often non cancerous swellings arising from the lining of the womb. They are caused by an overgrowth of the tissue of the lining of the womb (endometrium).

*Endometriosis*      This is a common condition where the lining of the womb (endometrium) is also found outside the womb. It can affect different area including the ovaries, surrounding ligaments and vagina. It often causes pain and heavy periods.

*PID*                   Pelvic inflammatory disease is when a sexually transmitted infection (often caused by chlamydia or gonorrhoea) spreads to affect the female reproductive organs including the womb, ovaries and fallopian tubes.

# 10.2 Secondary Amenorrhoea

Amenorrhoea is the absence of a menstrual period in a woman of reproductive age. There are two types of amenorrhoea, primary and secondary. Primary refers to the complete absence of any menstrual flow in a 14 year old girl along with the absence of secondary sexual characteristics or the absence of menstruation in a 16 year old girl. Secondary amenorrhoea refers to women who have had no periods for 6 months despite previously having normal cycles in the presence of a negative pregnancy test. It is worth remembering that amenorrhoea is a normal finding in prepubescent girls, during pregnancy and lactation as well as postmenopausal.

## HISTORY

| | |
|---|---|
| **Open questions** | Tell me more about why you attended today? Tell me more about the problems you are experiencing with your periods. |

## Focused questions

| | |
|---|---|
| *Absence of periods* | When was your last menstrual period? How long have you not had a period for? |
| Cycle | Were your periods regular? How many days would they last? |
| Menarche | How old were you when you started having periods? |
| *Sexual History* | When did you last have sexual intercourse? Did you use contraception? Is there any chance you are pregnant? |

## Questions for Differentials

| | |
|---|---|
| *Thyroid disease* | Have you felt any intolerance to hot or cold temperatures? Have you put on or lost any weight? Any dry skin? |
| *PCOS* | Do you suffer from acne? Have you noticed any unusual hair growth on your face or body (chest or abdomen)? |
| *Prolactinoma* | Have you noticed any milky discharge from your nipples? Have you had any headaches or problems with your vision? |
| *Ovarian cancer* | Have you lost any weight or noticed any bloating recently? Any constipation or diarrhoea? Have you had any urinary symptoms? |
| *Early menopause* | Do you suffer with hot flushes or vaginal dryness? |
| *Asherman's synd.* | Have you ever had a termination of pregnancy? Have you ever had a surgical procedure to remove the pregnancy? |
| *Anorexia* | How is your appetite? Have you lost weight recently? |
| *Exercise* | Do you do much exercise? Do you do any gymnastics or dancing? |
| *Mood* | How is your mood recently? |

| | |
|---|---|
| **RED FLAGS** | Visual changes, galactorrhoea in absence of recent delivery, galactorrhea and amenorrhoea postpartum (Sheehan's syndrome) |

---

## Complications of Amenorrhoea

| | |
|---|---|
| *CVD* | Amenorrhoea that is due to decreased oestrogen levels may lead to an increased risk of cardiovascular disease similar to that found in postmenopausal women |
| *Osteoporosis* | Oestrogen has a protective effect on bones via decreasing bone resorption and increasing deposition of new bone. Low oestrogen levels may lead to osteoporosis and is particularly of concern in adolescent girls who are going through their growth spurt |

| Infertility | In amenorrhoea there may be a lack of ovulation and ladies will be unable to get pregnant. However, this should not be relied upon as a form of contraception. Treatment of the underlying disorder may resolve fertility issues. |
|---|---|

## PAST MEDICAL HISTORY

| Radio./chemo. | Have you ever had radio or chemotherapy? (cranium or ovaries) |
|---|---|
| Procedures | Have you ever had any operations? (D&C, endometrial curettage) |
| Surgery | Have you had any recent surgery? (oophorectomy) |

## DRUG HISTORY

| Medication | Are you taking any medications (methyldopa, cimetidine, opiates, metoclopramide, antipsychotics - hyperprolactinoma)? Have you ever taken oral steroids (Cushings)? |
|---|---|
| Contraceptive | Have you ever used any forms of contraception? What types have you used (mirena, injection, POP, implant)? |

## SOCIAL HISTORY

| Smoker | Do you smoke? How many cigarettes do you smoke per day? |
|---|---|
| Alcohol | Do you drink alcohol? How much do you drink and how often? |
| Drugs | Have you ever used illicit drugs? (cocaine) |
| Stress | Have you been experiencing any stress recently? |

## FAMILY HISTORY

| FH | Anyone in the family suffers from early menopause <40yr? |
|---|---|

## IDEA, CONCERNS, EXPECTATIONS

| ICE | Have you had any thoughts as to what may be causing your lack of periods? |
|---|---|
| Concerns | Are you worried about them in any way? |
| Expectations | What were hoping we could do for you today? Were you hoping for a particular treatment or investigation? |
| Impact on life | How has this affected your life? (lack of self-esteem, inability to conceive) |

## CSA TIPS

Women suffering from a lack of periods having had normal periods may be quite an emotional and upsetting experience. Patients may attend anxious, worried and quite concerned that something serious is amiss. The key to such cases is to take a thorough history to help exclude the wide range of differentials that could be causing the amenorrhoea. Another scenario that may be faced could be a patient attending worried about being infertile who in fact has secondary amenorrhea that needs investigating.

## PHYSICAL EXAMINATION

| Chaperone | Request for a chaperone if performing intimate examination |
|---|---|
| Vitals | BP, BMI |
| Urine | Pregnancy test |
| Inspection | Observe for 2ndry sexual characteristics, webbed neck (Turner's syndrome) |
| PCOS | Look for fat distribution, increased hair growth (Hirsutism) and acne |
| Cushings | Look for central fat obesity, striae, buffalo hump, bruising |
| Thyroid | Dry skin, midline neck swelling, tremor, sweating |
| Examination | |
| Thyroid | Perform focused thyroid exam if suspected |

| Fundoscopy | Fundoscopy and visual fields if pituitary cause suspected |
| Breast | Complete breast exam if galactorrhea (hyperprolactinaemia) suspected |
| Abdo & pelvic | Examine external genitalia for clitoromegaly, palpate uterus/ovaries, pelvic masses |

## INVESTIGATIONS

| *Urine* | Pregnancy test |
| *Bloods* | TSH, T4, CA-125 (ovarian ca) |
| Hormones | LH, FSH, Free testosterone, SHBG, prolactin |

---

**Interpreting Hormonal levels**

| *Ovarian failure* | Raised FSH (>20U/L) & raised LH (>40 U/l) twice in women <40yr |
| *PCOS* | Normal FSH & mildly raised LH (>10 U/l), testosterone (>2.5nmol) |
| *Hypothalamic cause* | Normal or low FSH (<20U/l) & normal or low LH (<40U/L) |
| *Prolactinoma* | Prolactin >1000mIU/L suspect pituitary adenoma/hypothyroidism |
| *Testosterone* | >5 nmol/l investigate for Cushings, congenital adrenal hyperplasia, androgen secreting tumour |
| FAI | Free androgen index (FAI) >5 with testosterone <5nmol/l suspect PCOS |

---

| *Imaging* | |
| Ultrasound | Polycystic appearance to ovaries, ovarian carcinoma |
| CT | Abdomen, pelvis (adrenal tumours, ovarian carcinoma) |
| MRI | Head / pituitary (adenoma) |

| *Hysteroscopy* | Under secondary care for uterine adhesions |

| **MANAGEMENT** | *depending on cause* |
| **Conservative** | |
| *Lifestyle* | Try and increase weight by eating a balanced diet. Aim for a BMI 25kg/m2. Decrease exercise, consider referral dietitian. Stop illicit drugs |

**Medical treatment**

| *Medication* | Stop the offending drug if appropriate. Change POP or remove mirena / implant. Consider psychiatric referral if on anti-psychotic |
| *Hypothyroidism* | Start thyroxine and monitor response. May take 6 months before periods are corrected |
| *Pregnant* | See Pregnancy chapter |
| *PCOS* | See PCOS chapter |
| *Prem. Menopause* | See Menopause chapter |
| *Infertility* | Treat underlying disorder. See Infertility chapter |

| *Referral* | |
| Gynae | Refer if secondary amenorrhoea >6mth with no cause established. Refer if primary ovarian failure (women <40yr), recent uterine or cervical surgery, ovarian cancer (2WW) |
| Endocrine | Hyperprolactinoma, suspected Cushing's syndrome |
| Psych | Anorexia or eating disorder |

*Follow up*              Review in 3 mths for response to treatment

**DIFFERENTIAL DIAGNOSIS**

| Condition | Characteristic exam feature |
|-----------|------------------------------|
| Anorexia | Affects young girls after the age of 16. Low BMI <17.5. Missing meals, vomiting or using laxatives. Obsessed with body image and looking in the mirror. OE: thin, yellow skin, pale conjunctiva, calluses on knuckles, pallor, low bp and bradycardia |
| PCOS | Hirsutism, obesity, acne. Irregular periods and fertility problems |
| Premature Menopause | Amenorrhoea in >40yrs old with raised FSH and FHx of premature menopause. Periods that are heavier or lighter than usual, hot flushes, vaginal dryness, irritability, mood swings, decreased libido |
| Prolactinoma | Headache, double vision, poor peripheral vision, galactorrhoea, infertility |
| Ovarian Cancer | Fifth most common cause of female cancer. Usually affects >50yrs old. Pelvic pain, bloating, decreased appetite, weight loss |
| Hypothyroidism | Increased in BMI, dry skin, thin hair, feeling cold, reduced reflexes, low BP, bradycardia, low mood, constipation, tiredness |
| Cushings | Central obesity, skin bruises easily, depression, decreased libido, red puffy face, purple striae |

**EXPLANATIONS**

*Amenorrhoea*        This simply means no periods. This can happen either in young girls around 16 years of age who have never had a period or the other type, which is when the periods stop for more than 6 months having previously had regular periods. There are a wide range of causes that may lead to your periods stopping. However, I need to ask you a few more questions and perhaps undertake a number of investigations to find out what the possible reasons could be.

*Prolactinoma*       This is a mass or swelling in the pituitary gland (located near the base of the brain) that produces a specific hormone (chemical messenger) called prolactin. It is a benign tumour and not a cancer, i.e. the cells do not become malignant and spread. Prolactin is a hormone that helps women secrete milk after a child is born. However, it has other effects on the body such as decreasing libido, increasing hair growth and stopping periods. In a prolactinoma, the cells of the pituitary gland become excessive and release more of the hormone. If the cells become too much, the gland may increase in size and cause symptoms such as headache and double vision.

| Treatment | In many cases we watch and wait. If the prolactinoma is not causing many symptoms then we will monitor it with scans and blood tests to see if it is changes. However, in such cases, you may be started on the pill to maintain your hormone levels and prevent any bone thinning due to low oestrogen levels. If you are getting a lot of symptoms, there are medical treatments that can help reduce these and may even shrink down the mass. These are called  bromocriptine, cabergoline; however, the specialist will discuss these with you in more detail. If the mass is quite large, you may opt to have surgery to remove the mass. The operation is usually done under a GA. |
| --- | --- |

# 10.3 Polycystic ovary syndrome (PCOS)

Polycystic ovarian syndrome is a common condition in the UK affecting 1 in 10 women. It is an endocrine disorder that presents with multiple cysts in the ovaries along with irregular periods (oligomenorrhoea, amenorrhoea) as well as acne and hirsutism. It is more prevalent in the SE Asian population who usually present earlier and with more prominent symptoms.

---

**Diagnosing Polycystic ovarian Syndrome (2 out of 3)** - *Ref: Rotterdam (2003)*
1. Clinical Hyperandrogenism (Ferriman-Gallwey Score >8 - e.g. hirsutism, acne, male pattern baldness, alopecia) or Elevated levels of Total/Free Testosterone) **OR**
2. Infrequent (<6-9 Menses/yr) or no ovulation **OR**
3. Polycystic Ovaries on Ultrasound (>= 12 Follicles in One Ovary or Ovarian Volume >= 10cm3)

---

**HISTORY**

**Open questions**

Tell me more about why you attended today? Tell me about the problems you have been facing?

**Focused questions**

*Menstrual*

When was your last period (LMP)? Are your periods irregular, light or absent (oligomenorrhoea, amenorrhoea)? How many days do they last? How long have these problems been going on for?

*Acne*

Do you suffer from acne? Where are the spots? Do you have white and blackheads?

*Hair*

Have you noticed any unusual hair growth on your face or body? (chest or abdomen) Have you found that the hair on your head is thinning?

**Associated History**

*Fertility*

Are you trying to get pregnant? How long have you been trying?

*Obstetric*

Have you ever fallen pregnant? Have you had any terminations or miscarriages?

*Other symptoms*

Have you had problems with your weight (obesity)? Have you suffered with problems with mood? (depression)

**PAST HISTORY**

*CVD*

Have you ever suffered with raised blood pressure? Raised cholesterol or Type 2 diabetes? Do you suffer from metabolic syndrome?

*Sleep Apnoea*

Have you ever had problems sleeping? Such as appearing to stop breathing during the night? Do you snore or feel tired during the daytime?

*Epilepsy / Bipolar*

Do you suffer from any of these conditions? Are you taking any medications for them (semi-sodium valproate)?

---

**PCOS and Diabetes** - *Ref: RCOG (2007) Long-term consequences of polycystic ovary syndrome*
PCOS patients who are obese (>30 BMI), strong FHx type 2 diabetes, or >40yrs should be recommended to have diabetic screening (e.g. OGTT) due to an increased risk of type 2 diabetes.

---

## DRUG HISTORY

| | |
|---|---|
| *Medication* | Are you taking any medications? |

## FAMILY HISTORY

| | |
|---|---|
| *PCOS* | Has any else in your family had similar problems? Has anyone been diagnosed with polycystic ovarian syndrome? |

## SOCIAL HISTORY

| | |
|---|---|
| *Smoker* | Do you smoke? How many cigarettes do you smoke per day? |
| *Alcohol* | Do you drink alcohol? How much do you drink and how often? |

## IDEA, CONCERNS, EXPECTATIONS

| | |
|---|---|
| *Ideas* | What do you know about what may be the cause of your symptoms? |
| *Concerns* | Do you have any worries about the symptoms you are suffering with? |
| *Expectations* | Was there anything specific you wanted me to help with you today? |

## CSA TIP

Given the reasonably high prevalence of PCOS in the population, it is feasible that a patient may present asking to be checked for PCOS and an explanation about what it is. However, it is more likely that a patient would present with symptoms such as acne, irregular periods or delayed pregnancy and you would have to take a comprehensive history in order to make a diagnosis. Other possible cases may include, interpreting blood and ultrasound results and explaining the findings to the patient.

## PHYSICAL EXAMINATION

| | |
|---|---|
| *Vitals* | BP, BMI (low, or high) |
| *Urine* | Pregnancy test |
| *Inspection* | Observe the general habitus of the patient and look for fat distribution |
| Skin | Observe for increased hair growth (hirsutism) on the face, chest and lower abdomen. Inspect for acne (face, back, chest). Inspect the scalp for evidence of hair thinning |

## INVESTIGATIONS

| | |
|---|---|
| *Bloods* | Hormonal blood test performed in 1st week of cycle |
| Hormones | LH (>10 IU/l), FSH (LH:FSH ratio 3:1), SHBG (low) |
| | Free testosterone (>2.5nmol/l) - >4.8nmol/l consider differentials (adrenal hyperplasia, Cushing's syndrome, androgen secreting tumour) |
| | Calculate free androgen index (FAI) - (>5 with PCOS) |
| Diabetes | Fasting glucose, cholesterol |
| *Ultrasound* | Polycystic appearance to ovaries (⅓ have polycystic ovaries on scan) |

## MANAGEMENT

### Conservative

| | |
|---|---|
| *Lifestyle* | Try and lose weight by eating a balanced diet and increase exercise (30mins 5x week). Aim for a BMI <25 kg/m2, consider referral dietitian. Stop smoking |
| *Hirsutism* | Weight loss, cosmetic: shaving, plucking, bleaching, waxing |

### Medical

| | |
|---|---|
| *Fertility* | Clomiphene (cause multi-pregnancies), refer to secondary care |
| *Periods* | COCP, POP or mirena coil if not wanting pregnancy |

*Acne*
   Topical                Benzoic acid, abx, retinoids
   Oral                   COCP (Yasmin), abx (tetracycline, erythromycin), Isotretinoin
*Hirsutism*             Vaniqa (Eflornithine) cream, Dianette, Yasmin. Secondary care: Anti-androgens; spironolactone, cyproterone acetate or finasteride
*Metformin*           Helps increase insulin sensitivity, improves frequency of menstruation and ovulation rates

**Surgical**

*LOD*                   A simple surgical procedure known as laparoscopic ovarian drilling (LOD) is sometimes used as a treatment for fertility problems. It lowers the male testosterone levels and increases FSH helping to balance the hormones and release an egg

**SAFETY NETTING**

*Follow up*           Review in 3 mths to see response to treatments. Consider referral to specialists if no response to first line treatment

**EXPLANATIONS**

*PCOS*               Polycystic ovarian syndrome is a common condition affecting 1 in 10 women in the UK. It is a condition that causes women's hormones to be out of balance leading to increased hair growth, obesity, a lack of eggs being released and problems getting pregnant. It is not 100% known why it occurs but it is thought that there is a problem with managing sugar and insulin levels in the body which leads to an increase in the male hormone testosterone produced by the ovaries.

*Ultrasound*        Often in PCOS you can have small cysts in the ovaries that is noticed on the ultrasound scan that can lead to the hormonal imbalance.

# 10.4 Hirsutism

Hirsutism describes the excessive hair growth of coarse, dark hair over an androgen dependent (male) distribution where otherwise hair would often be absent in women i.e. face, jaw, chest, nipples. It is caused by an excess of androgens or increased sensitivity to them. It commonly affects 1 in 10 women and varies upon ethnicity (asian less often, mediterranean more common). The most common cause is idiopathic or PCOS. If there are signs of virilism then consider other differentials such as ovarian or adrenal tumours.

**Causes of Hirsutism**

| | |
|---|---|
| PCOS | Most common cause (70%) |
| Idiopathic | Familial. Onset from puberty with slow development |
| Drugs | Steroids, COCP, danazol, metoclopramide, phenytoin, sodium valproate, methyldopa |
| Menopause | Facial hirsutism. Decreasing oestrogen levels with unopposed androgen effects |
| Ovarian | Ovarian cancer |
| Adrenal | Congenital adrenal hyperplasia, Cushing's syndrome (sudden weight gain, bloating around chest and stomach), androgen producing adrenal tumour |
| Endocrine | Hypothyroidism, prolactinoma, acromegaly |

**HISTORY**

| | |
|---|---|
| **Open questions** | Tell me more about why you attended today? Tell me about the problems you have been facing? |

**Focused questions**

| | |
|---|---|
| Hirsutism | Have you noticed any unusual hair growth? Where is it (face - upper lip & chin, chest, nipple, abdomen, inner thighs & buttocks)? |
| | How long have you had the problem? Did it start recently or has it been there for a long time? |
| Virilism | Have you noticed a deepening in your voice? Have you noticed a receding hair line from the side of your head? |

**Questions for Differentials**

PCOS

| | |
|---|---|
| Periods | Are your periods irregular, light or absent (oligomenorrhoea, amenorrhoea)? How many days do they last? How long have these problems been going on for? |
| Acne | Do you suffer from acne? Where are the spots? Do you have white and blackheads? |
| Weight gain | Have you noticed that you have put on any weight recently? |

| | |
|---|---|
| Menopause | When was your last period? Do you suffer from hot flushes, headaches, and excessive sweating? |
| Hypothyroid | Have you felt any intolerance to hot or cold temperatures? Have you put on or lost any weight? Any dry skin? |
| Cushing's syndrome | Have you suddenly gained any weight recently or noticed weight gain around the face? Have you noticed any stretch marks or bruising of the skin? Any bloating around the chest or stomach? |
| Ovarian cancer | Have you lost any weight or felt bloated? Any constipation or diarrhoea? Have you had any urinary symptoms? |

## PAST HISTORY

| | |
|---|---|
| *CVD* | Have you ever suffered with raised blood pressure? Raised cholesterol or Type 2 diabetes? Do you suffer from metabolic syndrome? |
| *Sleep Apnoea* | Have you ever had problems sleeping? Such as appearing to stop breathing during the night? Do you snore or feel tired during the daytime? |
| *Epilepsy / Bipolar* | Do you suffer from any of these conditions? Are you taking any medications for them (semisodium valproate)? |

## DRUG HISTORY

| | |
|---|---|
| *Medication* | Are you taking any medications such as anabolic steroids or COCP? (Phenytoin, methyldopa, metoclopramide, progestogens) |

## FAMILY HISTORY

| | |
|---|---|
| *FHx* | Has any else in your family had similar problems? |

## SOCIAL HISTORY

| | |
|---|---|
| *Smoker* | Do you smoke? How many cigarettes do you smoke per day? |
| *Alcohol* | Do you drink alcohol? How much do you drink and how often? |
| *Mood* | How has your mood been? |
| *Occupation* | Are you currently working? What do you work as? Has it affected you at work? |
| *Relationships* | Are you currently in a relationship? Has it affected it? |

## IDEA, CONCERNS, EXPECTATIONS

| | |
|---|---|
| *Ideas* | Did you have any thoughts as to what may be causing it? |
| *Concerns* | Do you have any worries about the symptoms you are suffering with? |
| *Expectations* | Was there anything specific you wanted me to help you with today? |
| *Impact on life* | How has the abnormal hair growth affected you? (confidence, depression) |

## CSA TIP

Excess hair growth in females commonly affects their confidence and may make them feel embarrassed. Although the problem may be more prevalent in patients of specific ethnicities, the most common cause is due to PCOS. However, there are also serious underlying medical conditions including cancers that can also cause hirsutism.

## PHYSICAL EXAMINATION

| | |
|---|---|
| *Vitals* | BP (Cushing's), BMI, weight (obesity) |
| *Inspection* | Observe distribution of hirsutism on the face, chest, thigh and lower abdomen using the Ferriman-Gallwey score |
| PCOS | Inspect for acne (face, back, chest). Inspect the scalp for alopecia |
| Cushings | Look for moon face, stretch marks, bruises |
| *Pelvic exam* | To exclude pelvic mass (ovarian cancer) if suspected. Look for signs of clitoromegaly (virilism) |

---

### Modified Ferriman-Gallwey score

Method to evaluate severity of hirsutism in women. Hair growth is rated from 0 to 4, 0 - no growth of hair, 4 extensive hair growth over 9 areas of the body (upper lip, chin, chest, back (upper & lower), abdomen (upper & lower), upper arms, thighs). The total number of each area is added to obtain a score. Maximum score 36. A score >15 indicates moderate/severe hirsutism.

---

## INVESTIGATIONS

| | |
|---|---|
| *Bloods* | Often not needed if mild and no other signs |
|   Hormones | Hormonal blood test performed in 1st week of cycle |
|     FSH/LH | PCOS: LH (>10 IU/l), FSH. LH:FSH ratio 3:1 with low SHBG |
|     Testosterone | Testosterone >2.5nmol/l consider PCOS. >4.8nmol/l consider differentials (adrenal hyperplasia, Cushing's syndrome, androgen secreting tumour) |
|     Other | TFT, prolactin, OGTT (acromegaly) |
| | |
| *Urine* | 24 hour urine cortisol to exclude Cushing's syndrome |
| *Imaging* | Consider US (PCOS), CT/MRI (ovarian tumour), brain MRI (pituitary tumour) |

## MANAGEMENT
### Conservative

| | |
|---|---|
| *Lifestyle* | Try and lose weight if obese |
| *Cosmetic* | Consider shaving, depilation (removal of hair through using creams that dissolve hair), plucking, bleaching, waxing, threading |
|   Electrolysis | Removal of hair through using electric current. Damages hair permanently |
|   Laser | Laser & intense pulsed light (IPL) damage hair at the root. Performed over few months, results not permanent but long lasting |

### Medical

| | |
|---|---|
| *Dianette* | Increase risk for CVD and DVT/PE (1.5-2x more than OCP). Not licenced for solely contraception. Take as per advice for COCP |
|   Contraindicated | PMHx DVT or several RF for arterial disease (smoker, obesity, etc) or DVT |
| *Yasmin* | Yasmin is alternative. Both take 6mths to work |
| | |
| *Eflornithine cream* | Consider Vaniqa if COCP is contraindicated or have not worked for facial hirsutism. Slows growth of hair making it finer. Takes 6-8wks for effects to be seen. Stop if >4mths no results. If stopped, hair returns to normal after 8wks |
|   Application | Rub into skin, do not wash treated area for 4hrs after use. Cosmetics can be applied 5min later |
|   Side effects | Acne, burning and stinging sensation |
|   Contraindicated | Pregnancy, breastfeeding, not licenced <18yr |
| | |
| *Specialist* | Spironolactone, finasteride, metformin, pioglitazone |
| *Metformin* | Unlicenced in PCOS. Treatment required for 6-12mths before benefits noticed. Initiate 500mg od 1wk, 500mg bd 1wk then 500mg tds |

## SAFETY NETTING

| | |
|---|---|
| *Follow up* | Review in 3 mths to see response to treatments |
| *Referral* | Consider referral to specialists if red flags (Cushing's syndrome, virilisation, pelvic mass) or recent rapid progression of symptoms. Refer if treatment has not been effective after 6-12mth or testosterone levels >5nmol/l |

## DIFFERENTIAL DIAGNOSIS

| Conditions | Characteristic exam feature |
|---|---|
| **PCOS** | Hirsutism, obesity, acne. Irregular periods and fertility problems |
| **Ovarian Cancer** | Fifth most common cause of female cancer. Usually affects >50yrs old. Pelvic pain, bloating, decreased appetite, weight loss |

## EXPLANATIONS

*Hirsutism*    This is when a lady has excessive hair growth on areas such as the face, neck, chest and lower back. It is usually caused by increased male hormones (chemical) or by a heightened response to their effects in the female body. Other symptoms that you may see include facial spots, oily skin and sometimes a deepening of the voice.

*Eflornithine cream*    This is a special cream that is used to reduce the excess facial hair. It works by stopping the effects of a hormone that causes hair growth. However, its effects do not last permanently, and the hair will usually return within 2 months of stopping the cream.

Infertility is the inability to conceive or fall pregnant after having regular, unprotected coitus for one year (at least twice weekly), in the absence of any known reproductive pathology. 1 in every 7 couples have difficulty conceiving. However, after 1 year, 84% of couples will conceive increasing to 92% within 2 years. Whilst there are many causes for infertility, in 25% of cases none is found. Causes of infertility include ovulatory disorders (25%), tubal damage (20%), uterine/peritoneal disorders (10%) as well as male infertility such as low sperm count or low sperm quality (30%).

## HISTORY

| | |
|---|---|
| **Open questions** | Tell me more about why you attended today? Can you tell me the problems you have been experiencing trying to get pregnant? |

**Focused questions**

| | |
|---|---|
| *Concieve* | How long have you been trying to conceive? |
| *Intercourse* | How often do you have sex? Have you noticed any problems (retrograde ejaculation, erectile dysfunction, dyspareunia)? |
| Contraception | Have you used any contraception during that time? When did you stop? |

**Associated history**

| | |
|---|---|
| *Menstrual History* | Are your periods usually regular? How many days do they last? |
| PCB, IMB | Have you noticed any bleeding after sex or between your periods? |
| *Abdominal pain* | Do you have any abdominal pain? |
| *Galactorrhoea* | Have you had any problems with milky breast discharge? |
| *Hirsutism* | Have you noticed any unusual hair growth on your face or body? |

## PAST HISTORY

| | |
|---|---|
| *Previous preg.* | Have you had any previous pregnancies, miscarriages or terminations? Does your partner have any children from previous relationships? |
| *STI* | Have you had any sexually transmitted infections? |
| *Smears* | When was your last smear? Any abnormal smears in the past? |
| *Medical* | Do you have any medical problems such as thyroid disorders, diabetes? |
| Male | Varicocele, mumps, measles, testicular trauma |
| Female | PCOS, ectopic pregnancy, endometriosis, PID |
| *Surgery* | Have you had any previous surgery? (appendectomy, pelvic surgery) |

## DRUG HISTORY

| | |
|---|---|
| *Medication* | Are you taking any medications? (NSAIDs, spironolactone, cytotoxic, neuroleptic, metoclopramide & antipsychotics - hyperprolactinoma) |

## SOCIAL HISTORY

| | |
|---|---|
| *Alcohol* | Do you drink alcohol? How much do you drink and how often? |
| *Recreational drugs* | Do you take any recreational drugs such as marijuana or cocaine? |
| *Relationships* | Are you currently in a relationship? Does your partner smoke or drink? Are they overweight? |
| *Occupation* | Are you working at the moment? Exposure to chemicals (pesticides, solvents)? |
| *Stress* | Have you been experiencing any stress recently? |

| Exercise | Have you been trying to lose weight or do lots of exercise? |
|----------|------------------------------------------------------------|

## IDEA, CONCERNS, EXPECTATIONS

| Ideas | Have you had any ideas as to why you have had difficulties conceiving? |
|-------|------------------------------------------------------------------------|
| Concerns | Do you have any particular worries about it? |
| Expectations | What were you hoping for today? |

## CSA TIPS

Patients may present with fertility problems in a number of different ways. The most common of which may simply be a lady who is settled in a relationship and keen to fall pregnant attending for general advice about the whole process. Other cases may involve a patient presenting with results indicating that the partner has azoospermia and wanting information about ways she can fall pregnant. More difficult cases may present around negotiating with a lady who has already had 3 failed IVF cycles on the NHS requesting a re-referral for another cycle.

## PHYSICAL EXAMINATION

| Vitals | BMI (obesity) |
|--------|---------------|
| Female | Inspect for acne, hirsutism, androgenisation, galactorrhoea, abnormal genitalia |
| Pelvic exam | Examine for tenderness (endometriosis, PID) |
| Bimanual | Examine for fibroids, ovarian cysts |
| Male | Presence of testicles, varicocele, abnormal genitalia, gynaecomastia |

## INVESTIGATIONS

| Criteria | Investigations are considered when couples fail to conceive after 1yr or prior if they are less likely to conceive |
|----------|-------------------------------------------------------------------------------------------------------------------|
| Female | |
| Swabs | Swab for STIs (chlamydia) |
| Blood tests | Day 21 progesterone (confirm ovulation), LH, FSH (if irregular periods) |
| | TFT, prolactin, rubella screening, testosterone |
| TV Ultrasound | To check for PCOS, fibroids |
| Male | |
| Urine | First void urine sample for chlamydia screen |
| Semen analysis | If abnormal, repeat after 3mths. If 2 abnormal results - refer to urology |
| Specialist | Anti-Mullerian Hormone (AMH) to check ovarian reserve (premature ovarian failure - very low AMH, if postmenopausal - undetectable) |
| | Check tubal patency by hysterosalpingogram (HSG), laparoscopy (endometriosis) |

---

### Producing a semen analysis

- Produce specimen within a pot provided by the surgery. Do not use a sample from a condom
- Avoid sex for at least 2 days before and no longer than 7 days should have gone since last having sex
- The sample should arrive at the lab within 1 hour of production and kept in a warm place i.e. pocket

---

## MANAGEMENT

### Conservative

| Reassure | 84% of couples will conceive within 1yr; increasing to 92% within 2 yrs |
|----------|--------------------------------------------------------------------------|
| Intercourse | Recommend having intercourse 2-3x a week |

*Lifestyle*

| | |
|---|---|
| Smoking | Advise to stop smoking or recreational drugs |
| Alcohol | Advise to cut down alcohol |
| *Men* | Reduce alcohol intake (3u/day per wk), Excess reduces sperm quality |
| *Women* | No alcohol whilst trying to conceive. If cannot, then <1-2u once or twice a week |
| Weight | Aim for BMI <25, have balanced diet. Consider referral dietitian or exercise programme. No evidence that tea or coffee consumption affects fertility |
| Men | Wear loose-fitting underpants & trousers, avoid very hot baths or saunas |
| *Counselling* | Offer counselling if mood is affected. Consider fertility support group |

**Medical**

| | |
|---|---|
| *Preconception* | Folic acid 400mcg daily pre-conception |
| *Fertility* | Clomiphene, refer to secondary care |
| *Referral* | Refer to specialist if has been trying for >1yr and no obvious cause for infertility. Consider referring earlier if woman >36yr and there is a known clinical cause for the infertility |
| IUI | Consider unstimulated intrauterine insemination as a treatment option in people who are unable to, or would find it very difficult to, have vaginal intercourse, suffer from a clinically diagnosed physical disability or psychosexual problem or in people with conditions that require specific consideration (e.g. after sperm washing in a HIV male partner) |
| IVF | Offer IVF treatment to women with unexplained infertility who have not conceived after 2 years of regular unprotected sexual intercourse |

---

**Access to fertility treatment**
- NICE recommend up to 3 cycles of IVF or intracytoplasmic sperm injection
- Should be available to women 23-39yr old, identifiable cause of infertility (azoospermia, blocked fallopian tubes), or >3yrs of fertility problems

---

| | |
|---|---|
| Sperm donor | Consider donor sperm in cases of male azoospermia if there is a high risk of an inherited genetic deformity or if there is a high risk of passing an infectious disease to the woman or child |
| Oocyte donor | Consider a donor egg when the woman suffers premature ovarian failure, failure due to chemo- or radiotherapy, gonadal dysgenesis or has had bilateral oophorectomy |

**SAFETY NETTING**

| | |
|---|---|
| *Follow up* | Review in 6mths for response to treatment |

**EXPLANATIONS**

| | |
|---|---|
| *Infertility* | This is when a couple are unable to fall pregnant despite trying regularly for over a year without any contraception. There are a number of reasons why this may be, and the problems may be either from the woman or from the man. However in a quarter of cases we never find a reason. |
| Female | In women, common problems include not producing or releasing an egg on time, blockage of the tubes that carry the egg to the womb or due to conditions such as thyroid or polycystic ovarian disease. |

| | |
|---|---|
| Male | In men, the most common causes include not being able to produce any sperm, producing poor quality sperm or due to damaged testicles. Sometimes men suffer with retrograde ejaculation which is when the sperm do not actually get released from the penis but instead pass up into the bladder |
| *Intrauterine insem.* | This is a procedure used to separate out the healthy, fast moving sperm from the poor quality sperm that your partner has produced under a microscope. The sperm are then washed and placed into your womb using a small tube around 36-40 hours after ovulation takes place during days 12-16 of your cycle. |
| *In vitro-fertilisation* | IVF is a procedure that is used when couples are having problems falling pregnant. It involves taking healthy eggs from the female and using healthy sperm samples from the male partner inserting them into the egg in a process known as fertilisation. This takes place in the lab and when the egg is ready, it is then placed (implanted) into your womb to help it grow. |
| Success | Although IVF techniques are becoming more and more advanced, only about a quarter of procedures are successful. The chances of success are increased the younger the female is. |
| Risks | Undertaking the procedure does have some risks. The procedure may leave you with some pain and there is a slight risk of infection being introduced into the womb. However, if you do fall pregnant, there is also a chance that you may have twins or multiple pregnancies. |

# 10.6 Combined oral contraceptive pill

The combined oral contraceptive pill (COCP) refers to the form of contraception that contains both oestrogen and progesterone as the main components. Although there are numerous different types of COCP, they largely differ based upon the amount of hormone contained (monophasic, biphasic, triphasic and quadriphasic), the type of progesterone and the strength of oestrogen (low or standard).

When considering a patient for the combined pill, it is important to thoroughly risk assess them to see whether they are at a higher risk of side-effects; and if they are, then to offer alternative forms of contraception. Do not forget that the pill does not protect against sexually transmitted diseases. There are also three methods in which the COCP can be taken, as a pill, a patch or as a vaginal pessary.

---

**Common Contraceptive Pills -** *Ref: BNF*

| Oestrogen | Progesterone | Brand |
|---|---|---|
| Ethinylestradiol 20mcg | Desogestrel 150mcg | Gedarel, Mercilon |
| | Gestodene 75mcg | Femodette |
| | Norethisterone 1mg | Loestrin 20 |
| Ethinylestradiol 30mcg | Desogestrel 150mcg | Gedarel, Marvelon |
| | Drospirenone 3mg | Yasmin |
| | Gestodene 75mcg | Femodene |
| | Levonorgestrel 150mcg | Levest, Microgynon, Rigevidon |
| | Norethisterone 1mg | Loestrin 30 |
| Ethinylestradiol 35mcg | Notgestimate 250mcg | Cilest |

---

**HISTORY**

**Open questions**      Tell me more about why you attended today?

**IDEA, CONCERNS, EXPECTATIONS**

*Ideas*          What do you know about the combined contraceptive pill?

*Concerns*          Do you have any particular worries about taking the pill?

*Expectations*          Did you have a specific pill you wanted me to prescribe today? Did you want to take the contraception any particular way (i.e. patch, orally or as a pessary)?

**Focused questions**

*Menstrual History*          When was your last period (LMP)? Are your periods usually regular? How many days do they last?

*Contraceptive Hx*          Have you ever used any forms of contraception? What types have you used? Why do you want to change to the combined pill now?

*Last Episode*          When did you last have sexual intercourse? Did you use contraception? If not, is there any chance you are pregnant? *If the patient had UPSI <120hrs then offer a form of emergency contraception if they do not want to fall pregnant*

*Consensual*          Are you feeling pressured into having sex?

*Fraser competence*          *If a child presents and is less than 16 years old, check if they have comprehension and understanding of the issues at hand. Respect confidentiality if they are Fraser competent. Refer to the Emergency Contraception chapter for more information*

## Associated History

*Sexual Infections*      Have you ever suffered from a sexually transmitted infection? Have you had any symptoms such as a vaginal discharge or itching? Has any of your partners been diagnosed with chlamydia or gonorrhoea?

*Obstetric*      Have you ever been pregnant? Are you currently breast feeding?

## PAST HISTORY

*DVT*      Have you ever had a blood clot in your leg or lungs?

*Breast cancer*      Have you been diagnosed with breast cancer before?

*Migraines*      Do you suffer from migraines? Do you get any visual symptoms (fortification spectra) or weakness or numbness in your arms or legs?

*IHD*      Do you suffer from heart disease, high blood pressure?

*Diabetes*      Have you been diagnosed with diabetes? Do you suffer from the complications of it such as nerve, eye or kidney damage?

## Advantages vs Disadvantages of the COCP - *Ref: FFPRHC (2007) First prescription of COCP*

| Advantages | Disadvantages |
|---|---|
| Halves risk of ovarian & endometrial cancer. Benefits last >15yrs | Small increase in risk ofbreast cancer. Risk becomes normal after 10 years of stopping meds. Small increase in risk of cervical cancer. Reduced risk of colorectal cancer (RR 0.82) |
| Effective form of contraception (99.5%) | DVT: 3-5x increased risk |
| Does not interfere with intercourse | 2 fold increase in strokes. Small increase risk for CHD |

## DRUG HISTORY

*Medication*      Are you taking any medications such as the pill? Have you had a coil fitted? Are you taking any other medications (anticonvulsants, Rifampicin, St John's Wort)? Have you ever taken the emergency contraception before?

### Hepatic enzyme inducing antiepileptic drugs (AED)

Patients taking an enzyme inducing antiepileptic drugs (AED) i.e. phenytoin, carbamazepine, should start on a 50mcg oestrogen OCP. If break-through bleeding occurs, the oestrogen content should be increased to 75-100mcg/d and tricycling (3 packs back-to-back) be considered. Condoms should be used in addition or having progesterone depot injections. Sodium valproate is not an enzyme inducer, so does not interact with COCP

*Ref: NICE (2004) The epilepsies: the Dx & Mx of the epilepsies in adults & children in primary & secondary care*

## FAMILY HISTORY

*DVT*      Have any close (first-degree) relatives suffered with a blood clot in the lungs or the legs? How old were they when they were diagnosed (<45yrs)?

## SOCIAL HISTORY

*Smoker*      Do you smoke? How many cigarettes do you smoke per day?

*Alcohol*      Do you drink alcohol? How much do you drink and how often?

**Absolute vs Relative Contraindications for the COCP**

| Absolute UKMEC4 | Relative UKMEC3 |
|---|---|
| PMHx DVT/PE | FHx DVT/arterial disease (<45yr) |
| Migraine with aura | Migraine without aura |
| Cancer breast/cervix | BRCA1 gene carrier/PMHx breast cancer |
| >=35yr & Smoker >=15/d | >=35yr & Smoker <15/d |
| BP >160/95 | BP <160/95 |
| IHD/CVA/TIA | Risk Factors for CVD |
| Major Surgery | BMI >=35 kg/m2 |
| Breastfeeding <6wk | Breastfeeding 6wk - 6mths |

*Ref: FSRH (2009c) UK medical eligibility criteria for contraceptive use. www.fsrh.org*

## CSA TIP

When offering your explanation of the oral contraceptive pill, it may appear quite daunting to explain all elements of it i.e. missed pill rule, side effects, pros and cons etc. in a 10 minute consultation. To save valuable time in the exam, ask the patient what areas they would like to discuss and check their understanding around the other areas, as often patients may already be quite well acquainted with some elements of the pill. Ensure that you risk assess them against the UKMEC criteria before deciding which type of contraception to initiate. Practice being able to explain the pill and missed-pill rules to a patient who is hard of hearing.

## PHYSICAL EXAMINATION

| | |
|---|---|
| Vitals | BP, BMI |
| Urine | If in doubt request a pregnancy test |

## MANAGEMENT / EXPLANATIONS

| | |
|---|---|
| Pill Explanation | The combined oral contraceptive pill is so called as it contains two hormones, namely oestrogen and progesterone, that are similar to those found naturally in the body. By taking the pills, your body's hormone balance is altered such that you do not release an egg each month from your ovary making it difficult to fall pregnant. The pill also works to prevent sperm from entering the womb for fertilisation by thickening the cervical mucus. It also thins the lining of the womb making it difficult for a fertilised egg to attach to. |
| How to take | To get the maximum benefit, it is best to start the pill on the first day of your period. Take the pill at the same time every day for 3 weeks (if a 21 day pack) and have a break of 7 days during which time you may notice a withdrawal bleed. At the end of the 7 days, restart a new pack immediately to continue the effects of the contraception. |
| Everyday pack | If your COCP preparation is an everyday pack then continue taking the pill daily at the same time. There are 7 placebo pills that will result in the withdrawal bleed when taking them. |
| Efficacy | The combined pill is an extremely good form of contraception. If taken correctly the chances of falling pregnant are less than 0.5%. However, with common errors and missing pills, its effectiveness is still around 95%. |
| Side effects | Headaches, nausea, vomiting, breast tenderness, low mood |
| N+V | If severe vomiting occurs <2hrs of taking OCP, take another pill. If diarrhoea or vomiting lasts >24hrs consider condoms for 7d |

| Missed pill rule | Missing a single pill (>24hr late) anytime during your pill pack should not cause any problems. Take a pill as soon as you remember and take the next one at the normal time even if it means taking 2 pills together. |
|---|---|
| 2 or more pills | Take the last pill that you missed as soon as possible. Continue taking the remainder of your pills as normal. Use condoms for next 7d. If you had UPSI in last 7d you may require emergency contraception. |
| No. of pills left | >=7: If there are =>7 pills in your pack, complete it and have the 7d break as normal<br><7: Complete the pack and start next pack without the 7d break |

## Situational Advice when using the COCP

| | |
|---|---|
| Pregnancy | When prescribing or supplying hormonal emergency contraception, women should be advised: |
| Avoid withdrawal bld | Not known to be harmful to have back to back packs |
| No withdrawal bld | Exclude pregnancy or consider lower strength COCP |
| Breakthrough bld | Can be normal for 3mths. Exclude STIs, pregnancy, cervical lesions. Consider different progesterone or higher oestrogen in COCP |
| Side effects | Consider OCP containing desogestrel (Gedarel), drospirenone (Yasmin), and gestodene (Femodette, Femodene) if patients suffer side-effects such as acne, headache, depression, breast symptoms, and breakthrough bleeding with other OCPs |
| Changing pills | |
| COCP -> COCP | Start the new COC pill on the day after the last active COC pill. There is no need to wait for the next menstrual period |
| POP -> COCP | Start the COC at any time during the menstrual cycle provided it is certain that the woman is not pregnant |
| DEPO -> COCP | Start the COC on or before the day that the injection was due |

## Other forms of contraception

| | |
|---|---|
| *Patch Explanation* | The combined oral contraceptive patch works in the same way as the pill. The hormones are absorbed into the bloodstream through the skin. |
| *How to take* | To get the maximum benefit, it is best to place the patch on the first day of your period. Change the patch every 7 days for the first 3 weeks. Then you will have a break of 7 days during which time you may notice a withdrawal bleed. At the end of the 7 days, restart a new patch immediately to continue the effects of the contraception. The patch is sticky and can be worn on the body even when showering. |
| *Efficacy* | The patch is an extremely good form of contraception. If taken correctly the chances of falling pregnant are less than 0.5%. |
| *Side effects* | Skin irritation, headaches, nausea, vomiting, breast tenderness, low mood |
| Skin Irritation | Some patients suffer with skin irritation due to the patch and by rotating the sites where it is applied may reduce this. You can place it on the upper arms, thighs or buttocks. However, 2 out of 100 women suffer quite bad irritation and will not be able to continue using it. |
| Adhesives | Bandages or adhesives should not be used to secure the patch in place. If it is no longer sticky, replace with a new patch. |
| *Missed patch rules* | |
| <48hrs | If the patch falls off <48 hours from its site then re-apply it immediately and continue as normal. The effectiveness of the contraception should not be affected. |
| >48hrs | If the patch is detached >48 hours then you should apply a new patch and start this as if it was the first week of protection. You should use barrier contraception for the next seven days as well and then using 2 further weekly patches, complete a patch cycle. |

| | |
|---|---|
| UPSI | If you have had sexual intercourse within 5 days of noticing the patch was detached then you should consider emergency contraception. |
| *Ring Explanation* | The vaginal ring, is a flexible plastic transparent ring (2 inches in size) which contains two hormones, namely oestrogen and progesterone that prevent you from becoming pregnant. The hormones are absorbed through the skin of the vagina. |
| *How to take* | Insert the ring on the first day of your period whilst squatting or lying down. Squeeze it between your forefinger and thumb to help you insert it as high up as you can. The exact position does not affect its efficacy. You can leave the ring for 3wks, but do check its position regularly. Remove the ring with your finger like a hook and replace it with a new ring exactly 1 week later |
| *Efficacy* | The ring is as effective as the COCP |
| *Side effects* | Headaches, vaginitis, vaginal discharge |
| *Missed ring rules* | |
| <3hrs | If the ring falls out less than 3hrs then rinse in water and reinsert straight away. No additional precaution is necessary. |
| >3hrs | If the ring is expelled >3hrs then addition precautions are required: |
| wk 1-2 | If expelled in week 1 or 2 then wash and reinsert and use condoms for 7d |
| wk 3 | If expelled in week 3 then insert a fresh ring and start a new cycle without a week off. Or permit a withdrawal bleed for 7d then insert a new ring. This option should only be considered if the ring was used for at least 7d prior to the expulsion. Condoms should be used in both cases for 7d. |
| 4wks in situ | If the ring has been left in for 4wks no additional precautions are required. More than 4wks pregnancy should be excluded prior to replacing |

**SAFETY NETTING**

| | |
|---|---|
| *Late period* | If the next period is later than expected do a pregnancy test |
| *Symptoms* | Review as soon as possible if patient has chest pain (pleuritic), SOB, haemoptysis, calf swelling, weakness/numbness arms or legs, unusual or worsening headaches |
| *Follow up* | Review in 3mths then 6-12 months |

# *10.7 Progesterone only contraception*

The progesterone only contraception (POP) is a type of contraception that uses the hormone progesterone to prevent pregnancy. It is used especially when the combined pill is contraindicated for the patient due to breast-feeding, risk of VTE, liver disease or migraine with aura.

Progesterone contraception comes in three different forms including orally as a pill, an intramuscular injection and via an implant. Do not forget that these forms of contraception do not protect against sexually transmitted diseases.

**Common Progesterone Contraceptives** - *Ref: BNF*

| Brand Name | Progesterone | Strength (mcg) |
|---|---|---|
| Micronor | Norethisterone | 350 |
| Norgeston | Levonorgestrel | 30 |
| Femulen | Ethynodiol diacetate | 500 |
| Noriday | Norethisterone | 350 |
| Cerazette | Desogestrel | 75 |

**HISTORY**

**Open questions** — Tell me more about why you attended today?

**IDEA, CONCERNS, EXPECTATIONS**

*Ideas* — What do you know about the progesterone only pill? Is there any reason why you wanted this type of contraception?

*Concerns* — Do you have any worries about taking the pill?

*Expectations* — Did you have a specific pill in mind that you wanted me to prescribe today?

**Focused questions**

*Menstrual History* — When was your last period (LMP)? Are your periods usually regular? How many days do they last? Are they irregular or heavy? How long has it been going on for? Do you pass clots? How many sanitary towels/pads do you use per day?

*STIs* — Have you suffered from a sexually transmitted infection? Have you had any symptoms such as a vaginal discharge or itching? Has any of your partners been diagnosed with chlamydia or gonorrhoea?

*Contraceptive History* — Have you ever used any forms of contraception? What types have you used? Why do you want to change to this pill now?

*Last Episode* — When did you last have sexual intercourse? Did you use contraception? If not, is there any chance you are pregnant? *If the patient had UPSI <120hrs then offer a form of emergency contraception if they do not want to fall pregnant*

**Associated History**

*Obstetric* — Have you ever been pregnant? Are you currently breast feeding?

## PAST HISTORY

| | |
|---|---|
| *Ectopics* | Have you ever suffered from an ectopic pregnancy before? |
| *Breast cancer* | Have you been diagnosed with breast cancer within the past 5 years? |
| *Liver* | Have you ever suffered any liver diseases including cirrhosis or hepatitis? |
| *Other* | Do you have any other medical conditions? (SLE, acute porphyria) |

## Risks of Breast cancer taking the POP

There is a small increase in breast cancer associated with women using the POP. The most important risk factor is the age at which the POP is stopped. The risk disappears after 10yrs after stopping i.e. a comparison of 10,000 women who never used the POP compared to those on it for 5yrs then stopped aged 40 showed an estimated extra 10 cases of breast cancer.

## DRUG HISTORY

| | |
|---|---|
| *Medication* | Are you taking any medications such as carbamazepine, phenytoin, itraconazole or St. John's Wort? Have you had a coil fitted? |
| | Have you taken the emergency contraception before? |

## Hepatic enzyme inducing antiepileptic drugs (AED)

POPs are not recommended as a reliable form of contraception in women taking enzyme-inducing AEDs. Their efficacy (POP, implants) are reduced by these drugs and alternative methods should be sought. Women on POP/implant whilst starting a short course of AED (2mths) could be given a single injection of DMPA. They should also consider additional contraceptive precautions during AED use and for 1mth after stopping.

*Ref: NICE (2004) The epilepsies: the Dx and Mx of epilepsies in adults & children in primary & secondary care*

## SOCIAL HISTORY

| | |
|---|---|
| *Smoker* | Do you smoke? How many cigarettes do you smoke per day? |
| *Alcohol* | Do you drink alcohol? How much do you drink and how often? |

## CSA TIP

Patients rarely would attend requesting specifically for the progesterone only pill. Rather, it is more likely that a patient will attend for the COCP but have a condition falling within the UKMEC 3/4 criteria that makes it unsafe to prescribe. Hence, you would have to consider an alternative contraception. In addition, it is important to be aware how to explain the other forms of progesterone contraception such as injection or implant.

## PHYSICAL EXAMINATION

| | |
|---|---|
| *Vitals* | BP, BMI |
| *Urine* | If in doubt, request a pregnancy test |

## MANAGEMENT

| | |
|---|---|
| *Pill Explanation* | The progesterone only pill is so called as it contains the hormone progesterone that is similar to the one found naturally in the body. By taking the pill, your body's hormone balance is altered creating a thicker mucus in the womb preventing sperm from entering it. In some women it also works to prevent the release of an egg |
| *How to take* | To get the maximum benefit, it is best to start the pill on the first day of your period. Take the pill at the same time every day continuously with no break. When you finish a pack it is important to start the next pack immediately the next day. If you have just |

| | given birth and start the pill within 3 weeks of delivery, then the pill will work straight away |
|---|---|
| *Efficacy* | The pill is a good form of contraception. If taken correctly the chances of falling pregnant are <1%. However, with common errors and missing pills, its effectiveness is still over 92% |
| *Side effects* | Change in weight, transient breast pain and menstrual irregularities |
| Period | The main side effect of the progesterone pill is causing irregular menstrual bleeding. 4 out of 10 women will have no problems with their periods; a further 4 out of 10 will experience irregular bleeding and 2 out of 10 women will have no periods at all |

---

**Situational Advice when using the POP**

| *After childbirth* | POP can be initiated from day 21 postpartum without any further precautions |
|---|---|
| *Changing from COCP* | Start the POP the day after completing the COCP pills without a break |

---

| *Missed pill rule* | If you forget a pill, take it as soon as you remember and carry on with the next pill at the right time. If the pill was more than 3 hours overdue you are not protected. Continue normal pill-taking but you must also use another method, such as the condom, for the next 2 days. (Ref: FSRH) |
|---|---|
| Emerg. contra. | Emergency contraception should be considered if POP is >3hrs late and unprotected intercourse occurred recently |
| Cerazette | The missed pill window can be upto 12hrs without further measures |
| D+V | Vomiting and severe diarrhoea can affect the absorption of the POP. If you vomit within 2hrs of taking the POP consider taking a replacement pill. With persistent vomiting or severe diarrhoea continue taking the POP but consider other forms of contraception (condoms) for the period of the illness as well as 2d after recovery |
| *Injection Explanation* | The progesterone injection contains the hormone progesterone that is similar to the one found naturally in the body. By taking an injection, your body's hormone balance is altered creating a thicker mucus in the womb preventing sperm from entering it. In some women it also works to prevent the release of an egg. It is usually given by a health professional into the buttock at regular intervals |
| *How to take* | To get the maximum benefit, it is best to start the injection during the first 5 days of your period. You can take the injection outside this time, but your should make sure you are not pregnant and use barrier contraception for the next 7 days. Ensure that you take the next injection after 12wks (if depot medroxyprogesterone acetate) or 13wks (if depot medroxyprogesterone acetate) |
| *Efficacy* | The pill is a good form of contraception. If taken correctly the chances of falling pregnant are less than 1%. However, with common errors and missing pills, its effectiveness is still over 97% |
| *Side effects* | Increase in weight, transient breast pain and menstrual irregularities |
| *Period* | The main side effect of the progesterone injection is causing irregular menstrual bleeding and it can delay return to fertility up to 1 year after stopping the injections. |
| *Implant Explanation* | The Implanon is a rod shaped implant that is inserted into the upper arm that prevents pregnancy by releasing a progesterone hormone just under the skin. It works primarily by preventing ovulation but also increases the thickness of the mucus in the womb preventing sperm from passing through the cervix |
| *How to take* | If inserted within the first 5 days of your cycle it provides immediate protection. However, on any other day of your cycle, you will require extra protection for 7 days |

319

| | |
|---|---|
| | with barrier methods, such as condoms. It works effectively for up to 3 years. However, if you wish to fall pregnant then the device can only be removed by a trained health professional |
| *Efficacy* | The implant is an excellent form of contraception as it provides over 99% of protection against pregnancy and one does not have to be reminded to take it |
| *Side effects* | Increase in weight, transient breast pain and menstrual irregularities. There is also a small risk (1 in 100) of scarring or infection at the site where the implant is inserted |
| *STI risk* | Advise the patient that unprotected intercourse can expose them to the risk of contracting an STI. If the patient is engaging in risky sexual practices then advise to use condoms |
| *Alternative Contracep.* | Give advice about alternative forms of contraception if the progesterone contraception is unsuitable such as, barrier or long term contraception advice i.e. coil |

---

**Expected bleeding patterns after starting hormonal contraception and in the longer term**

| Contraception | Bleeding pattern in longer term |
|---|---|
| COCP | 20% have irregular bleeding for first 3mth before settling |
| POP | <15% have no periods. 30-40% will have irregular periods |
| Implant | 50% have irregular bleeding (infrequent, frequent or prolonged) which may not improve |
| Injectables | 70% have no periods at 1yr |
| Hormonal-IUS | 65% have no periods or light periods at 1yr. 90% reduction in period volume after 1yr of use |

*Ref: FSRH (2009). Management of Unscheduled Bleeding in Women Using Hormonal Contraception*

---

**SAFETY NETTING**

| | |
|---|---|
| *Late period* | If the next period is later than expected do a pregnancy test |
| *Follow up* | Review in 3 mths then 12 monthly |

# 10.8 Emergency Contraception

Emergency contraception (EC) is a form of contraception that is taken to prevent unwanted pregnancies in those cases where either no contraception was used during sexual intercourse or in the event of contraception failure such as a split condom or a missed tablet.

There are currently three forms of EC, two tablets and an intrauterine device. EC are only effective if taken within a defined window period post-coitus and it is important that patients understand the risk of failure.

## HISTORY

**Open questions**          Tell me more about why you attended today?

**Focused questions**

*History PC*              Why do you need the emergency contraception?

    Contra. Failure     Why did it fail? Did the condom split? Did you forget to take your pills? How many pills did you miss?

---

**Contraception Failure: When EC is indicated** - *Ref: FSRH Guidance Emergency Contraception (August 2011)*

*Condom*                 If the condom splits

*Progesterone pill*        If the woman has a late or missed pill (>27hrs)

*Combined pill*           If the woman misses 2 consecutive pills in week 1

*Progesterone injection*  If there is a gap more than 14wks since the last injection

---

*Last Episode*            When did you last have sexual intercourse? Was it several hours ago or a few days? With whom? Was it a regular partner or a one-night stand?

*Consensual*             Did you feel pressured into having sex?

*Fraser competence*      *If the child attends and is less than 16 years old, check if they have comprehension and understanding about the issues at hand. Respect confidentiality if they are Fraser competent.*
Have you spoken to your parents about it? Is there a reason why you have not?

---

## Fraser Guidelines

In 1985, Lord Fraser set out a guidance during his judgement of the Gillick case in the House of Lords, specifically relating to contraception in the under 16's:

*"...a doctor could proceed to give advice and treatment provided they are satisfied in the following criteria:*

- That the girl (although under the age of 16 years of age) will understand their advice;
- That they cannot persuade her to inform her parents or to allow the Dr to inform the parents that she is seeking contraceptive advice;
- That she is very likely to continue having sexual intercourse with or without contraceptive treatment;
- That unless she receives contraceptive advice or treatment her physical or mental health or both are likely to suffer;
- That her best interests require him to give her contraceptive advice, treatment or both without the parental consent."

## Associated History

| | |
|---|---|
| STI | Do you have any discharge, pain or itchiness in your vagina? |
| Cycle | Are your periods usually regular? How many days do they last? When was the first day of the last period? |
| Obstetric | Have you ever been pregnant? Have you missed your period? |

## RED FLAGS

| | |
|---|---|
| Rape | If non-consensual, consider referring to sexual assault referral centre (SARC). Do not perform an internal examination |
| Vulnerable child | If the child is under 13 years, make a referral to the Child Protection team. If the partner is significantly older than the child then consider contacting the police / child protection services |
| Pregnancy | Are you pregnant? Have you done a pregnancy test? |

## PAST HISTORY

| | |
|---|---|
| Medical | Do you suffer with any liver problems? Have you ever been diagnosed with Porphyria? |

## DRUG HISTORY

| | |
|---|---|
| Medication | Are you taking any medications such as the pill? Have you had a coil fitted? Are you taking any other medication (warfarin, Rifampicin)? Have you ever taken the emergency contraception before? |

## SOCIAL HISTORY

| | |
|---|---|
| Smoker | Do you smoke? How many cigarettes do you smoke per day? |
| Alcohol | Do you drink alcohol? How much do you drink and how often? |

## IDEA, CONCERNS, EXPECTATIONS

| | |
|---|---|
| Ideas | What do you know about the emergency contraception? |
| Concerns | Do you have any particular worries about falling pregnant? |

## CSA TIP

Cases involving the emergency contraception often present themselves as young adults or teenagers attending requesting the pill following an episode of unprotected sexual intercourse. In such cases it is important to ensure that you have correctly asked the age of the partner and whether the episode was consensual. Do not forget to establish Fraser competence and educate patients about the risk of STIs and offer long-term contraception for future use.

## PHYSICAL EXAMINATION

| | |
|---|---|
| Vitals | BP, weight, BMI |
| Urine | If in doubt, request for a pregnancy test |

## MANAGEMENT

| | |
|---|---|
| Levonorgestrel | Also known as Levonelle, 1.5mg stat dose of progesterone hormone. It is effective up to 72 hours after unprotected sexual intercourse with efficacy reducing with time (24hrs - 95%, 72hrs - 58%) |
| Explanation | This pill contains a higher dose of a hormone called Progesterone similar to what the body naturally produces. It works by altering the balance of hormones in the body, |

| | |
|---|---|
| | preventing or delaying an egg from being released (ovulation). It also makes if difficult for the fertilised egg from settling and implanting in the womb |
| Side effects | Nausea, vomiting. If the patient vomits within 2 hours of taking, they should take a replacement dose. Occasionally causes spotting or light bleeding |
| *Ulipristal acetate* | Also known as ellaOne. It is effective up to 120 hours after an episode of unprotected sex with an efficacy rate of around 98%. Contraindicated for repeated use in a menstrual cycle |
| Explanation | This pill contains the active ingredient ulipristal acetate, which is a selective progesterone receptor modulator. This works in a similar way to the progesterone pill inhibiting or delaying ovulation and making it difficult for a fertilized egg to implant in the womb |
| Side effects | Headaches, nausea and vomiting. If the patient vomits within 3 hours of taking, they should take a replacement dose |

**Advise after using emergency hormonal therapy -** *Ref: BNF*

When prescribing or supplying hormonal emergency contraception, women should be advised:

- That their next period may be early or late;
- That a barrier method of contraception needs to be used until the next period;
- To seek medical attention promptly if any lower abdominal pain occurs because this could signify an ectopic pregnancy;
- To return in 3 to 4wks if the subsequent menstrual bleed is abnormally light, heavy or brief, or is absent, or if she is otherwise concerned (if there is any doubt as to whether menstruation has occurred, a pregnancy test should be performed at least 3 weeks after unprotected intercourse)

| | |
|---|---|
| *Copper IUCD* | This is a small copper based device that is inserted into the womb. It can be used up to 120 hours after an episode of unprotected sex with an efficacy rate of almost 100% if used correctly |
| Explanation | The coil is a small metal device that is inserted into the womb by a doctor or nurse. It works by acting as a barrier and preventing the fertilised egg from settling into the womb. Once inserted, the coil may remain in place for up to 5 years acting as an effective form of ongoing contraception |
| Side effects | The coil may make your periods feel heavier, longer or more painful but these may settle down after a few months of use |
| Contraindication | Pregnancy, STI, unexplained PV bleeding, copper allergy |
| *STI risk* | Advise the patient that unprotected intercourse can expose them to the risk of contracting an STI. Refer to GUM clinic or nurse for swabs |
| *LARC* | Give long term contraception advice i.e. implanon, coil, injections |

**SAFETY NETTING**

| | |
|---|---|
| *Ectopic pregnancy* | If the patient experiences lower abdominal pains or abnormal PV bleeding to review as soon as possible |
| *Late period* | If the next period is later than expected do a pregnancy test |

# 10.9 Menopause & HRT

The menopause is the period when the female menstrual cycle ceases due to the permanent loss of ovarian activity. The average age this takes place in the UK is between 51 and 52 years old. It is diagnosed when a year has passed since the last period in women of this age group. Although it usually occurs in women >50yrs, it can occur in women much younger and is known as premature menopause (if <40yrs) and early (if <45yrs) usually due to ovarian failure.

Prior to the periods stopping completely, women usually have a period of 2yrs whereby they suffer with a number of symptoms due to the altering level of hormones. This is known as the climacteric phase (or perimenopause) and is characterised by hot flushes, dry vagina, night sweats, mood swings and problems sleeping.

**HISTORY**

**Open questions**    Tell me more about why you attended today? Can you tell me more about the menopausal symptoms you have experienced?

**Focused questions**

*Menstrual History*    When was your last period (LMP)? Were your periods usually regular? How have your periods been over the past year? Have you noticed them becoming shorter? or longer? or more erratic?

*Hot flushes*    Have you noticed any hot flushes recently? Where abouts do you notice these (chest, face and neck)? How long do they usually last for (1min)?

*Night Sweats*    Have you also begun feeling hot and sweaty at night? How often does this happen? Do you have to change the bedding in the morning?

*Vaginal atrophy*    Have you noticed any symptoms in your vagina? Is it more dry? Do you have an itch? Do you get pain when having sexual intercourse (dyspareunia)?

*Other symptoms*    How has your mood been recently? Do you have difficulty sleeping (insomnia)? Has your interest in sex (libido) reduced of late?

**Associated History**

*Obstetric*    Any chance you are pregnant?

**RED FLAGS**

*PMB*    Have you experienced any vaginal bleeding?

---

**NICE guidelines for Postmenopausal bleeding (PMB)** - *Ref:NICE (2005) cancer referrals*
*If bleeding following 12mth of amenorrhoea. All patients require full pelvic exam & speculum exam of cervix*
*Not on HRT*    Refer all patients with PMB under 2 week wait rule (2WW) including patients on tamoxifen with PMB or endometrial thickness >4mm on US
*HRT related bleeding*    Stop HRT for 6wks and refer if ongoing bleeding

---

## PAST HISTORY

| | |
|---|---|
| *DVT / PE* | Have you ever had a blood clot in your leg or lungs? |
| *Cancer* | Have you been diagnosed with cancer (breast/endometrial)? |
| *IHD/CVA* | Have you suffered with angina? or had an MI? or suffered a stroke? |
| *Liver* | Have you ever had any problems with your liver or any abnormal liver blood tests? |
| *Radio./chemo.* | Have you ever had radio or chemotherapy on the pelvis or ovaries? |
| *Surgery* | Have you had any recent surgery (oophorectomy/hysterectomy)? |

## Advantages vs Disadvantages of HRT

| Advantages | Disadvantages |
|---|---|
| Controls symptoms (stops flushing, headaches, insomnia, vaginal atrophy) | Small increase in breast, endometrial & ovarian cancer. Breast: Risk of breast cancer if >5yrs on HRT postmenopausal (6 per 1000 extra cases/yr). Risk normalises after 5yrs of stopping. No increased risk of breast cancer if <50yrs |
| Improves psychological symptoms (confidence, mood) | Small increased risk DVT and PE |
| Reduces osteoporosis and fracture rates | Small increase risk of CVA. No increased risk if <60yrs |

## DRUG HISTORY

| | |
|---|---|
| *Medication* | Are you taking any medications? |

## FAMILY HISTORY

| | |
|---|---|
| *DVT* | Have any close relatives suffered with a blood clot in the lungs or the legs? |

## SOCIAL HISTORY

| | |
|---|---|
| *Smoker* | Do you smoke? How many cigarettes do you smoke per day? |
| *Alcohol* | Do you drink alcohol? How much do you drink and how often? |

## IDEA, CONCERNS, EXPECTATIONS

| | |
|---|---|
| *Ideas* | What do you know about what may be causing your symptoms? |
| *Concerns* | Do you have any specific worries about what you are facing (symptoms, HRT)? |
| *Expectations* | Were you hoping for anything in particular e.g. medication - HRT? |
| *Impact on life* | How has it affected your life? |

## CSA TIPS

Patients entering their 50's may begin to start noticing odd symptoms that they never had before and may worry that a serious process may be taken place. They are likely to attend the GP with numerous complaints that on the surface may not appear related. They may be worried or anxious as a result and will need reassurance and convincing that they are entering the menopause. Others may be well aware that they are in the menopause, but would like your expert opinion as to whether their choice of HRT is safe or whether there is a risk between HRT and getting breast cancer.

## PHYSICAL EXAMINATION

| | |
|---|---|
| *Vitals* | BP, BMI |
| *Urine* | If in doubt, request for a pregnancy test |
| *Blood test* | FSH (>40 mIU/L is diagnostic) |
| *Ultrasound* | In PMB looking for thickening of the endometrial lining (>4mm) |

## MANAGEMENT
### Lifestyle

| | |
|---|---|
| Exercise | Take regular exercise and lose weight to reduce hot flushes (50%) |
| Foods | Avoid trigger foods i.e. spicy foods, caffeine, alcohol to reduce night sweats |
| Others | Wear light clothes, sleep in a cool room and stop smoking |
| Vag. atrophy | Use lubricant gel if having painful SI. Stop using soap and use clean water instead. Avoid using lotions and perfumed products on the vulval area |

### Medical
*Medical Non-HRT*

| | |
|---|---|
| Topical oestrog. | Vaginal cream, rings, tablet to reduce atrophy |
| Hot flushes | Low dose SSRI (fluoxetine 20mg, unlicensed), gabapentin (unlicensed), norethisterone 5mg od, clonidine 50mcg bd |
| Mood | Consider counselling, CBT, psychotherapy, SSRI |

*Medical HRT*

| | |
|---|---|
| Without uterus | Oestrogen alone for continuous use except in endometriosis |
| With uterus | |
|     Cyclical | Consider if periods have just stopped or erratic; offer oestrogen daily and progesterone added to last 12-14d of cycle. Will experience monthly periods |
|     Continuous | Consider if patients has no periods for 1yr. Offer combination of oestrogen and progesterone daily. No monthly periods experienced |
| Side effects | Nausea, headaches, migraines, cramps, fluid retention, breast enlargement, weight gain, spotting for first 3 months |

| | |
|---|---|
| *Contraception* | Consider adding contraception if patient still having periods as HRT does not act as contraceptive. No need for contraception if periods stopped >1yr in >50yrs or >2yrs in <50yrs |
| *Tibolone* | Contains oestrogen, progesterone and androgen properties. Useful for sweats, hot flushes and vaginal dryness. Consider in patients without periods for 1yr. Use in similar way as continuous HRT. Has less breast cancer risk |

## SAFETY NETTING

| | |
|---|---|
| *PMB* | If the patient has any abnormal bleeding to return ASAP |
| *Symptoms* | Consider stopping HRT if patient has chest pain (pleuritic), SOB, calf swelling, weakness / numbness arms or legs, unusual or worsening headaches |
| *Follow up* | Review in 3mths to assess response |

## EXPLANATIONS

| | |
|---|---|
| *Menopause* | This is when the body responds to the declining hormone levels as a lady gets older by ceasing periods. The average age in the UK for this to happen is 52 years however it may happen before or after this date. Women whose periods stop before 40 years of |

age are known as having premature menopause and those who stop at 45 are known as having early menopause.

Symptoms      Just before the periods stop for good, sometimes the change in hormonal levels give rise to symptoms such as irregular periods, hot flushes, night sweats, changes in your mood or sleep. These are quite common and can be treated in a number of ways.

HRT      Hormone replacement therapy or HRT is a form of treatment that is effective in reducing the symptoms that a lady experiences once she has reached the menopause. It usually consists of the same two hormones, oestrogen and progesterone, that have reduced in level due to the menopause. It comes in different packs and preparations, but they all generally use the same hormones but in different doses. You can also take the HRT as a tablet, patch or vaginal ring. It is important to be aware that if you have had a hysterectomy then you can only take a type of HRT that contains a single hormone, oestrogen.

Risks      There have been many studies that have looked at the risks of taking HRT. There is some evidence that taking HRT for more than 5 years may slightly increase the risk of developing breast, endometrial or ovarian cancer, as well as there being a slight increase in stroke and blood clot risk.

# 10.10 Premenstrual syndrome

Premenstrual syndrome (PMS) is a condition that affects women in the luteal phase of their cycle prior to their menstrual period. It is defined as, *'distressing physical, psychological and behavioural symptoms not caused by organic disease which regularly recur during the luteal phase of the menstrual cycle, and significantly regress or disappear during the remainder of the cycle'.*

It usually affects middle-aged woman between the ages of 30 and 40 and causes physical (fluid retention, breast fullness, bloatedness), psychological symptoms (irritability, depression, loss of libido) and behavioural symptoms (aggression). In most cases symptoms are bearable but in a significant minority (5%), symptoms may affect day to day functioning.

## HISTORY

**Open questions**  Tell me more about why you attended today? Tell me more about the symptoms you have been experiencing. Can you describe the symptoms you have been getting before your period?

**Focused questions**

*Physical symptoms*

| | |
|---|---|
| Bloatedness | Do you suffer from a bloated feeling in your tummy? |
| Breast tenderness | Have you noticed any pain or fullness of the breast? |
| Headaches | Do you suffer from headaches? |
| Weight gain | Have you put on any weight recently? How much? |
| Bowel habits | Have you noticed any change in your bowel habits? |

*Psych. symptoms*

| | |
|---|---|
| Mood changes | Tell me about your mood? Have you noticed that you are suffering with low mood? How has your concentration been? Do you find yourself suffering with mood swings? |
| Irritability | Have you become more irritable these days? |
| Loss of libido | Are you currently in a sexual relationship? Do you still enjoy having sex? Have you noticed that your interest for sex has lessened? |

| | |
|---|---|
| *Duration* | How long have you been experiencing these symptoms? |
| *Cyclic* | Are they related to your menstrual cycle? |

## PAST HISTORY

| | |
|---|---|
| *Depression* | Do you suffer from low mood or depression? |
| *Other* | Any other medical conditions? |

## DRUG HISTORY

| | |
|---|---|
| *Medication* | Are you taking any medications such as the pill? Did this help the symptoms? |

## FAMILY HISTORY

| | |
|---|---|
| *PMS* | Has anyone in your family suffered with similar symptoms? Has anyone been diagnosed with premenstrual syndrome? |

### Types of Premenstrual syndrome - *Ref: RCOG 2007. Mx of premenstrual syndrome*

| | |
|---|---|
| *Mild* | When symptoms do not interfere with personal, social, and professional life |
| *Moderate* | When symptoms partially interfere with personal, social and professional life resulting in daily functions able to be performed, but suboptimally |
| *Severe* | Patient withdraws from social and professional activities and cannot perform daily functions adequately |

## SOCIAL HISTORY

| | |
|---|---|
| *Diet* | Do you drink tea or coffee? How many cups a day do you drink? Do you have a balanced diet? |
| *Smoker* | Do you smoke? How many cigarettes do you smoke per day? |
| *Alcohol* | Do you drink alcohol? How much do you drink and how often? |

## IDEA, CONCERNS, EXPECTATIONS

| | |
|---|---|
| *Ideas* | What do you think may be causing your symptoms? |
| *Concerns* | Do you have any worries about the problems you have been experiencing? |
| *Impact* | How have the symptoms affected and impacted upon your life? |

## CSA TIP

Patients presenting with a myriad of different symptoms that appear to be unrelated may lead the heart to sink. However, with a clear structure, valid questions and a good history you should be able to gain the information you require to make a diagnosis. If you ever get stuck and are unclear about a diagnosis, pause and summarise you key findings back to the patient and then proceed to take a more comprehensive systems review. Simply asking the patient if they have any other symptoms may lead to the response, *'like what doctor?!'*

## PHYSICAL EXAMINATION

| | |
|---|---|
| *Vitals* | BMI |
| *Examination* | Although examination is not necessary to make a diagnosis of PMS, it may be helpful to exclude other potential diagnoses. Offer to examine the relevant areas where the patient presents with symptoms i.e. breast exam for breast pain, abdominal exam for bloating and/or bowel changes |

## MANAGEMENT

### Conservative

| | |
|---|---|
| *Menstrual diary* | Advise to keep a symptom diary to check if it correlates with their periods (premenstrually). Record weight as well through period |
| *Lifestyle* | Recommend exercise, diet advice (small, regular portions, reduce caffeine, increase fibre), regular sleep and weight loss. Advice to stop smoking and reduce alcohol intake |
| *Psychological* | Advise counselling (CBT) or relaxation techniques if appropriate |
| *Vitamins* | Consider Evening primrose oil (breast tenderness). Vitamin B6 (evidence) or calcium/vitamin D, magnesium or vitamin A supplements 2wk before periods start (limited evidence) |

### Medical

| | |
|---|---|
| *Pain* | Offer simple analgesics such as paracetamol or an NSAID to help treat breast or abdominal pains |
| *COCP* | In patients with moderate PMS, consider commencing the COCP especially if the lady requires contraception (Yasmin, Cilest) |

| | |
|---|---|
| *SSRI* | Consider in unresponsive severe PMS e.g. SSRIs (fluoxetine, citalopram, sertraline) can be prescribed continuously or solely during days 15-28 of the period. Trial for at least 3 months before continuing for 1yr |
| *Diuretic* | Spironolactone 25mg od (d18-26) to treat fluid retention or breast tenderness |

## SAFETY NETTING

| | |
|---|---|
| *Follow up* | Review in 3mths for response to treatment |
| *Referral* | Refer to specialist if poor response or if there is underlying psychiatric illness |

## DIFFERENTIAL DIAGNOSIS

| Conditions | Characteristic exam feature |
|---|---|
| **Affective disorder** | Prolonged low mood, poor concentration, insomnia, anxiety, decreased libido, hopeless, helpless, worthless |
| **Diabetes mellitus** | Thirst, weight loss, malaise, increase urinary frequency |
| **Hypothyroidism** | Weight gain, tiredness, oedema, malaise, cold intolerance, dry skin |
| **SE of COCP** | Headaches, low mood, breast tenderness, breakthrough bleeding |
| **Perimenopause** | Irregular periods, hot flushes, breast tenderness, tiredness, mood swings, insomnia, decreased libido |

## EXPLANATIONS

| | |
|---|---|
| *PMS* | PMS is a common condition that affects women particularly around their periods causing interference with daily life. It is thought that the time of the egg being released (ovulation) is a trigger for the symptoms, making them more sensitive to hormonal changes. |

# 10.11 Antenatal counselling

In 2012 there were more than 700,000 live births in the UK with the highest number of children being born to women aged 30-34. Once a woman falls pregnant, it is important that they have an early booking (<10wks) as this will give them the greatest chance to participate in screening programs and help develop a planned package of care. Women who are thought to have an uncomplicated and low risk pregnancy can be managed via shared care protocols between the midwifes and the GP. Whereas those who have complex needs (mental health, multiple miscarriages, previous still-birth) or are at high risk (BP, DM, epilepsy) should be overseen by a named consultant obstetrician and have access to relevant specialist consultant input as needed.

**HISTORY**

**Open questions**     We have your results back and the urine test is positive. This means that you are pregnant. How do you feel about that?

**Focused questions**

*LMP*     When was your last menstrual period?
Calculate the gestation and EDD using an obstetric wheel

---

**Calculating Estimated Date of Delivery (EDD)**
EDD = LMP − 3 months + 1 year and 7 days + [cycle length − 28]

---

*Pregnancy*
  Moving     Have you felt the baby move or kick recently? (18wks+)
  Oedema     Have you noticed any leg swelling or breast tenderness?
  Morning sickness  Have you felt nauseous or actually vomited? Is it worse in the morning?
  Heartburn     Do you suffer from burning or an indigestion feeling in your stomach?

*PV bleeding*     Have you had any vaginal bleeding? When did it begin? How long for?
  Volume     Any spotting on your clothes? Have you had to use any tampons, pads or sanitary towels? Were your clothes soaked? Any clots?

---

**Causes of Vaginal bleeding in Pregnancy**
Early (<24wks)     Miscarriage, ectopic pregnancy, hydatidiform mole
Late (>24wks)     (Antepartum haemorrhage) Placental abruption, placenta praevia, uterine rupture

---

*Abdominal pain*     Have you experienced any abdominal pain?
*Mood*     How is your mood? During the past month, have you often been bothered by feeling down, depressed or hopeless? During the past month, have you often been bothered by having little interest or pleasure in doing things?

---

**Causes of Abdominal Pain during Pregnancy**
*First trimester*     Ectopic pregnancy (amenorrhoea, colicky & shoulder tip pain)
Miscarriage (passage of products of conception, uterus normal size)
*Second trimester*     Miscarriage
*Third trimester*     Labour (contractions between 5-10min, water breaks)

|  | False labour (irregular non-persistent contractions) |
|  | Preterm labour (labour <37 weeks) |
|  | Placental abruption (dark painful blood, woody hard uterus) |
|  | Uterine rupture (scarred uterus) |
| *Other causes* | Appendicitis, cholecystitis, GORD, UTI, gastroenteritis |

## PAST HISTORY

| *Obstetric* | Have you been pregnant before? What type of delivery did you have (spontaneous / induced, caesarian, ventouse/forceps)? |
|  | Did you had any miscarriages or stillbirths in the past? |
| *Medical* | Do you suffer from any medical problems such as raised blood pressure, diabetes, epilepsy or blood clots in your leg? Do you suffer from anaemia or sickle cell anaemia? |
| *Psychiatric* | Have you suffered from depression, bipolar disorder or schizophrenia? |

## FAMILY HISTORY

| *FHx* | Does anyone in your family suffer from diabetes or raised blood pressure? Is there any history of twins or blood disorders (sickle cell)? Are there any inherited conditions that run through the family? Has anyone suffered with pre-eclampsia before? |

## DRUG HISTORY

| *Medication* | Are you taking any prescribed medications or OTC treatments such as folic acid? |

---

**Medication Contraindicated in Pregnancy**

Tetracycline, gentamicin, trimethoprim, ciprofloxacin, ACEI, statin, warfarin, sulphonylurea, retinoids, NSAIDS (3rd trimester), lithium, chloramphenicol, methotrexate, antiepileptics

---

## SOCIAL HISTORY

| *Relationships* | Are you currently in a relationship? |
| *Home* | Who lives at home with you? |
| *Support networks* | Will there be any help at home when the baby is born? |
| *Occupation* | Are you working or studying at the moment? |
| *Smoker* | Do you smoke? How many cigarettes do you smoke per day? |
| *Alcohol* | Do you drink alcohol? How much do you drink and how often? |
| *Drugs* | Have you taken any illicit drugs at all? |

## IDEA, CONCERNS, EXPECTATIONS

| *Concerns* | Do you have any concerns regarding the current pregnancy? |

## CSA TIPS

Patients may present with a urinary test result that shows they are pregnancy. It is important to inform the patient of the results and then ask them how they feel. If they are happy and wish to keep the pregnancy, then you should congratulate them and explain what will happen next. In those women who are unsure about what to do, ensure that you explain to them the different options available and share a management plan that is the most appropriate for their situation and circumstances. Patients may present at any stage of the pregnancy and may also present with reduced fetal movements. It is essential that you know how to perform a routine antenatal examination as you may be requested to do this in the examinations.

## PHYSICAL EXAMINATION

| | |
|---|---|
| *Vitals* | BP, BMI |
| *Urine* | Dipstick urine (protein, ketones - hyperemesis, glucose - gestational DM) |
| *Obstetric exam* | Lie the patient flat on the couch |
| Inspection | Previous caesarian scar, skin changes (linea nigra or striae) |
| Palpation | |
| SFH (24wks+) | Establish the fundus using the ulnar border of your hand. Measure the SFH with the tape measure blindside up from fundus to pubic symphysis. Turn the tape measure to reveal SFH |
| Lie | Place one hand on either side of the uterus and palpate. Locate your foetus's back and limbs and determine if lie is longitudinal, oblique or transverse |
| Presentation (36wks+) | Press firmly over the symphysis pubic and establish presentation. Check if cephalic or breech |
| Auscultation | Use a sonicaid to listen to the heartbeat (normal HR 110-160) |

---

## Care for Scheduled appointments - *Ref: NICE (2008) antenatal care (modified 2010)*

| | |
|---|---|
| *25 Weeks* | *(For nulliparous women)* Measure SFH, BP, urine (proteinuria) |
| *28 – 34 weeks* | Measure SFH, BP, urine (proteinuria). Offer 2nd screening for anaemia. Offer anti-D for rhesus negative |
| Info (34wks) | Offer labour and birth plan |
| *36 – 38 weeks* | Measure SFH, BP, urine (proteinuria). Check position of baby. Offer external cephalic version for breech presentation. Review US (placenta previa) |
| Info (36wks) | Discuss breastfeeding and postnatal care (postnatal depression, care of baby, Vit K for baby) |
| *40 weeks* | *(For nulliparous women)* Measure SFH, BP, urine (proteinuria) |
| *41 weeks* | If not given birth offer membrane sweep or/and induction of labour. Measure SFH, BP, urine (proteinuria) |

---

## INVESTIGATIONS

| | |
|---|---|
| *Urine* | Pregnancy test |
| *Bloods* | FBC, Haemoglobinopathies, Blood group & RH status, Hepatitis B status, HIV, rubella immunity, syphilis |
| OGTT | For at risk patients to exclude gestational dm (BMI>30, PMHx gestation DM, previous baby >4.5kg, FHx DM, ethnicity) |
| Down's | Offer/refer for Down's screening (triple test + nuchal translucency scan) |
| *Ultrasound* | Dating scan (10-14 weeks), anomaly scan (18-21 weeks) |

---

## Complications from lifestyle

| | |
|---|---|
| *Alcohol* | Fetal alcohol syndrome, growth & mental retardation, facial anomalies |
| *Smoking* | intrauterine growth retardation, miscarriage, premature delivery, stillbirth |
| *Illicit drugs* | |
| Cocaine | Spontaneous abortion, premature delivery, low birthweight, sudden infant death, placental abruption |
| Heroin | IUGR, premature delivery, low birthweight, perinatal mortality |

# MANANGEMENT

*ref: NICE (2008) antenatal care (modified 2010)*

## Medication

| | |
|---|---|
| *Folic acid* | Initiate on folic acid 400mcg (reduce incidence of neural tube defects). Give 5mg folic acid if history of NTD or on anticonvulsants |
| *Ferrous* | Do not offer routine iron supplementation |
| *Vitamin D* | Offer vitamin D 10mcg for at risk groups (ethnic, poor diet, BMI>30) |
| *Immunisation* | Consider rubella immunisation if warranted |

## Lifestyle

| | |
|---|---|
| *Diet* | Avoid food-acquired infections |
| Listeriosis | Avoid soft cheese, uncooked ready meals, pate, unpasteurized milk |
| Salmonella | Avoid uncooked/partially cooked eggs (mayonnaise), meat |
| Toxoplasmosis | Wash all fruits and veg. Avoid cleaning cat litter |
| Caffeine | Avoid more than 200mg a day (>2 mugs of coffee) |
| Other | 5x fruit and veg/d. Drink plenty of milk (calcium + vit d), avoid liver (excess vitamin A) |
| *Smoking* | Offer cessation advice. NRT is safe, champix is contraindicated |
| *Alcohol* | Avoid drinking especially in first 3mths (miscarriage). If continues to drink, suggest a maximum of 1-2units once or twice a week. Binging (7.5units) may be harmful |

## Complications from lifestyle

| | |
|---|---|
| *Alcohol* | Fetal alcohol syndrome, growth & mental retardation, facial anomalies |
| *Smoking* | Intrauterine growth retardation, miscarriage, premature delivery, stillbirth |
| *Illicit drugs* | |
| Cocaine | Spontaneous abortion, premature delivery, low birthweight, sudden infant death, placental abruption |
| Heroin | IUGR, premature delivery, low birthweight, perinatal mortality |

| | |
|---|---|
| *Exercise* | Moderate regular exercise, avoid contact/high impact sports, scuba diving |
| *Intercourse* | Not known to cause any adverse outcome |
| *Travel* | *Fly-* Advise increase risk of DVT. Consider compression hosiery |
| | *Car-* Have belts above and below bump not over it |
| *Prescription* | Offer exemption to prescription costs |

## Financial Benefits during Pregnancy

| | |
|---|---|
| *Maternity Leave* | All employed pregnant women are entitled to 1 year of maternity leave consisting of 26wks ordinary maternity leave and 26wks of additional |
| *Maternity Allowance* | If post 26wks pregnant and not eligible for SMP |
| *SMP* | Statutory Maternity Pay eligible if you have worked for your employer continuously for at least 26 weeks up to the 15th week before the expected week of childbirth. Statutory Maternity Pay (SMP) is paid for up to 39 weeks. 90% of your average weekly earnings (before tax) for the first 6 weeks then £138.18 or 90% of your average weekly earnings (whichever is lower) for the next 33 weeks |

## Other

| | |
|---|---|
| *Morning sickness* | Resolves by 16-20wks. Consider, ginger/P6 wrist acupressure or antihistamines |
| *Heartburn* | Lifestyle advice (small regular meals, increase pillows) or antacids |
| *Constipation* | Diet modification (bran or wheat) |

| | |
|---|---|
| *Illicit drug use* | Refer to MDT. Require detoxification programme prior to conception. to be stable on methadone during pregnancy. Consider Hep B/C, HIV screen |
| *Down's syndrome* | Offer combined test and advice regarding risk score |

## Screening for Down's Syndrome

| | |
|---|---|
| *Maternal age* | Risk increases with age: 20yr - 1:1500, 30yr - 1:800, 40yr - 1:100, any age 1:800. Risk increase with PMHx of Down's syndrome baby |
| *Combined test* | Blood test (B-HCG, PAPP-A) performed with nuchal translucency scan |
| Results | Results expressed as risk score low risk (e.g. 1:>150), high risk (e.g. 1:<150). If high risk will be offered screening test |
| Amniocentesis | Performed 15-18 wks. 1% risk of miscarriage, later TOP then CVS |
| CVS | Performed 10wks. Permits earlier TOP if required. 2% risk of miscarriage |

| | |
|---|---|
| *Refer* | Refer to midwife services early for booking |
| miscarriage | If <16 weeks refer to EPAU for assessment |

| | |
|---|---|
| *Follow up* | |
| Nulliparous | In uncomplicated pregnancies, schedule 10 appointments until delivery |
| Parous | In uncomplicated pregnancies, schedule of 7 appointments until delivery should suffice |
| Future visits | BP and urine dipstick should be carried out on all future antenatal visits |

| | |
|---|---|
| *Safety net* | If experiences abdominal pain or PV bleed to seek medical advice (ectopic, miscarriage) |
| | Seek emergency advise if experiences severe headache, blurred vision, vomiting (preeclampsia) |

## EXPLANATIONS

| | |
|---|---|
| *Miscarriage* | This is when the pregnancy stops growing and occurs in 20% of pregnancies. We do not always know the reason for it, but there is nothing you could have done to prevent it. Usually the miscarriage will pass naturally without any need for us to do anything. You may take some painkillers to reduce the pain which may feel like a heavy period. The whole process should be completed within a week; however if you do not think that you have fully passed it or are having heavy periods then you should seek medical advice. |
| *Ectopic* | This is when the pregnancy is growing outside of the womb and usually in one of your tubes. This is known as an ectopic pregnancy and may be the reason why you are suffering from pain and bleeding. I'm sorry to have to tell you that your pregnancy is not viable and will have to be removed to protect your health. |
| *Amniocentesis / Chorionic Villus samp.* | Chorionic villus sampling or amniocentesis are techniques that allow us to take a sample from the womb of the baby's cells. This is done by passing a fine needle through the wall of your tummy under ultrasound guidance so that no harm comes to your baby. It is performed in early pregnancy (10wks CVS, 15-18wks - amniocentesis) and will help give us a clearer picture whether your child has any inherited illnesses. |

However, the test is not 100 percent accurate and even though we have the scan to guide us, there is a slight risk of causing a miscarriage.

Gestational DM

This is a type of diabetes caused by a temporary increase of sugar during pregnancy. It is more likely in women with risk factors (obesity, ethnicity, FHx). It is normally treated by diet advice alone; however, if the sugar levels remain high we may need to give insulin injections to keep it controlled. If we do not keep on top of it, it may affect your pregnancy with increased risk of abnormalities, increased birth weight and premature delivery.

Pre-eclampsia

This is a common condition affecting 1 in 20 women occurring after 20wks of pregnancy. It is when your BP is raised and we find some protein in your urine. In the early stages it is unlikely that you may even notice it; however, we will routinely look for it during your antenatal visits. If detected, it should be treated, as if left alone it may lead to you having a fit and the child coming to harm. If you ever suffer from any signs of severe headaches and vomiting, visual problems or swelling of feet, hands and face you should immediately seek medical advice.

# 10.12 Termination of pregnancy

In the UK approximately 1 in 5 pregnancies are terminated in the UK with most carried out within 13wks of gestation (84%). Most (60%) are performed on women aged <24yrs old. It involves either taking medication or a simple surgical procedure to remove the pregnancy depending on the gestation of the pregnancy. It is currently legal in the UK up to 24 weeks of pregnancy if certain conditions are met, but can be extended if there is evidence of more serious sequelae to the mother or child such as permanent harm or death.

### The UK Abortion Act of 1967

Termination of Pregnancy (TOP) was legalised in the UK under the 1967 Abortion Act. It can be artificially induced up to 24 weeks of pregnancy. In the UK 90% of abortions take place before 12 weeks. Two doctors (e.g. GP & gynaecologist) must give consent stating that to continue with the pregnancy it would:
- Endanger the life of the mother
- Endanger the physical or mental health of the mother
- Be a risk to the physical or mental health of the siblings
- The foetus would have a high chance of being handicapped

The majority of abortions in the UK (98%) fall under the second category. Patients must be referred for a termination of pregnancy by their GP, family planning centre or private centres. No doctor is obliged to consent or participate in an abortion, but have a duty of care to refer the individual to the correct department.

### HISTORY

**Open questions**      Why would you like to have a termination? How did you find out you were pregnant?

**Focused questions**

| | |
|---|---|
| *Contraception* | Were you using any contraception at the time? What went wrong (split condom/missed pill/lost patch)? |
| *LMP* | When was your last menstrual period? Were they regular? |
| *Partner* | Did you have unprotected sex with your regular partner or a casual partner? Does your partner know about your pregnancy? |
| Consensual | Was it consensual? |
| *Fraiser* | Have you spoken to your parents about it? Why not? |

### Fraser's Guidelines for <16 years old

It is legally acceptable for doctors to consent patients for abortions without parental consent provided that:
- The young individual understands the advice
- Cannot be persuaded to inform their parents
- Unless they receive treatment, their physical or mental health, or both, are likely to suffer

In such situations an effort should be made to encourage patient to speak to their parents.

### RED FLAGS

| | |
|---|---|
| *Symptoms* | Do you have any abdominal pain or a fever? |
| *Risk factors* | Physically abusive relationship (domestic violence), socially isolated, young child or vulnerable adult |

## PAST HISTORY

| | |
|---|---|
| *Obstetric* | Have you ever fallen pregnant? Have you had any terminations or miscarriages? |
| *Surgery* | Have you had any previous operations? (pelvic surgery) |
| *Psychiatry* | Have you ever been diagnosed with depression? |

## DRUG HISTORY

| | |
|---|---|
| *Medication* | Are you taking any medications? |

## SOCIAL HISTORY

| | |
|---|---|
| *Relationships* | Are you currently in a relationship? |
| *Home* | Who lives with you at home? |
| *Support networks* | Have you spoken to anyone about it? |
| *Occupation* | Are you working or studying at the moment? |
| *Smoker* | Do you smoke? How many cigarettes do you smoke per day? |
| *Alcohol* | Do you drink alcohol? How much do you drink and how often? |

## IDEA, CONCERNS, EXPECTATIONS

| | |
|---|---|
| *Reason* | Tell me why would you like to have a termination? |
| *Conviction* | How sure are you that you want it? |
| *Idea* | Do you have any ideas about what a termination involves? What do you know about it already? |
| *Concerns* | Do you have any worries about it? |
| *Expectations* | How were you hoping I could help you with your situation? |
| Options | Have you considered other alternatives such as keeping the baby or adoption? |

## CSA TIPS

Discussing termination of pregnancies with patients can be a challenging task. It is important to establish the reason for the request whilst discussing all alternative options available to the patient other than the termination (adoption, keeping the pregnancy) to allow them to make a fully informed decision. If they choose to have a termination then counsel the patient about the different methods available and about the need for future contraception if they do not wish to fall pregnant again.

## PHYSICAL EXAMINATION

| | |
|---|---|
| *Vitals* | BP, BMI |

## INVESTIGATIONS

| | |
|---|---|
| *Urine* | Pregnancy test |
| *Bloods* | Hb level, HB screen, Blood group & RH status (usually performed by provider) |
| *Ultrasound* | Viability and dating scan prior to TOP |

## MANAGEMENT

| | |
|---|---|
| *Counsel* | Counsel the patient to make sure that they are certain of their decision. Offer alternatives such as keeping the baby or adoption |
| *Explanation* | Offer appropriate termination advice depending on number of weeks of pregnancy |
| 5 - 24 weeks | Medical termination – taking 2 medications, 48 hours apart at clinic. Patient offered oral mifepristone that *'stops the pregnancy hormones from working'* and then returns 2 days later for prostaglandin pessary (or orally), *'which makes the womb contract and expels the pregnancy.'* It should feel, *'like a natural miscarriage'* – patient can |

| | experience pain, vaginal bleeding and expulsion of products of pregnancy. Patient may require analgesia and may have repeat doses depending on the gestation to help induce the abortion. They may also have to proceed to surgical procedure if unsuccessful |
|---|---|
| 7 - 14 weeks | Conventional vacuum aspiration – *'A small plastic tube will be passed through the neck of the womb and the contents of pregnancy is removed by gentle suction'* |
| >15 weeks | Dilatation and evacuation (D&E) where surgical procedure is required – *'You will be put to sleep under general anaesthetics. The neck of the womb will be gently stretched. The pregnancy will be removed using forceps and a suction tube'* |
| Risks | The risks of complications are low (1%) particularly if done in early pregnancy (<12wks). Common complications includes bleeding, damage to the neck and body of the womb |

**Potential complications of terminations**

*Common*

| Infection | Genital tract infection (1:20) – However risk reduced by pre-procedural screening for chlamydia and treating with antibiotics |
|---|---|
| Cervix | Cervical trauma (1:100) |
| Bleeding | Post op haemorrhage (1:1000) |

*Uncommon*

| Uterine | Uterine perforation (2:1000), uterine rupture (<1:1000) |
|---|---|
| Failed TOP | Medical (7:1000) surgical (2.5:1000) |
| Miscarriage | Debatable evidence of small increase in middle trimester miscarriages via cervical incompetence |

| *Refer* | Refer to termination services (e.g. BPAS, Marie Stopes clinic) |
|---|---|
| Counselling | Offer psychological or emotional support / counselling |
| *Follow up* | |
| LARC | Discuss about long term contraception (pill / implanon / mirena coil) |
| STI | Offer an STI screen (chlamydia) |

**SAFETY NETTING**

| *Follow up* | If experiences abdominal pain or fever to seek medical advice (exclude ectopic) |
|---|---|

Vaginal discharge that is clear or white is often a normal physiological finding that may occur at any time during the monthly cycle. However, the discharge usually becomes clearer and wetter when the egg is ready to ovulate. Any change in the colour, smell, amount or consistency may mean that the discharge is abnormal, particularly if it is associated with other symptoms such as itch, pain, intermenstrual or post-coital bleeding. There are a number of different causes that may lead to these changes including infection, inflammation, ectopy or polyps and it is important to take a thorough history and examine the patient to make a clear diagnosis.

## HISTORY

| | |
|---|---|
| **Open questions** | I can see that you seem a little embarrassed to talk about your problem. Genital problems are conditions that we see and treat everyday, so please do not feel embarrassed at all. Tell me more about why you attended today? Tell me about the symptoms you have been experiencing? |

## Focused questions

| | |
|---|---|
| *Discharge* | Have you noticed any discharge? Can you describe it? |
| Nature | Is it thick, thin or frothy? |
| Colour | What colour is it? (clear, white, purulent, bloodstained) |
| Odour | Is there any smell associated with it? (fishy) |
| Pruritus | Do you experience an itch or soreness in the groin area with it? |
| Timing | Is the discharge related to your menstrual cycle? |

---

**Different Colours of Discharge**

| | |
|---|---|
| *Clear* | Physiological |
| *Yellow/white* | Atrophic vaginitis, chlamydia |
| *Greyish/white* | Bacterial vaginosis |
| *Cottage cheese* | Candidiasis |
| *Green* | Trichomonas (green/grey), Gonorrhoea (green/yellow) |
| *Reddish/brown* | Cervical / endometrial carcinoma |

---

| | |
|---|---|
| *Pain* | Do suffer from any abdominal pain with it? Where abouts is it? |
| Dyspareunia | Have you experienced any pain during intercourse? |
| Dysuria | Do you have any discomfort or a burning feeling when you pass urine? |
| Fever | Have you had any fevers or temperatures? |

| | |
|---|---|
| *PV Bleeding* | |
| IMB | Have you had any bleeding between your periods? |
| PCB | Do you suffer bleeding after intercourse? |

| | |
|---|---|
| **RED FLAGS** | Weight loss, Intermenstrual menstrual bleeding (IMB), Post-coital bleeding (PCB) |

| | |
|---|---|
| *Sexual History* | Are you sexually active? Do you have a regular or casual partner? |
| Partner | Was your partner male or female? |
| Type | Did you have vaginal, oral or anal sex? |

| Contraception | Do you use any condoms/diaphragm? |
| STDs | Have you or any of your partners been diagnosed with an STI? |

## Associated History

| Menstrual History | When was your last period (LMP)? Are your periods irregular, light or absent (oligomenorrhoea, amenorrhoea)? How many days do they last? |
| Obstetric History | Are you pregnant? Do you have any children? |

## PAST HISTORY

| Medical | Have you ever suffered with diabetes? Do you suffer from any weaknesses of your immunity (HIV, leukaemia)? |

## DRUG HISTORY

| Medication | Are you taking any medications? Are you on the Pill? Have you taken antibiotics recently? Have you been on oral steroids? |

## SOCIAL HISTORY

| Smoker | Do you smoke? How many cigarettes do you smoke per day? |
| Alcohol | Do you drink alcohol? How much do you drink and how often? |
| Travel | Have you been abroad recently? Did you have unprotected sexual intercourse when abroad? |

## IDEA, CONCERNS, EXPECTATIONS

| Ideas | What do you think may be the cause of your symptoms? |
| Concerns | Do you have any worries about the symptoms you are suffering? |
| Expectations | Was there anything specific you wanted me to help you with today? |

## CSA TIPS

Patients presenting with vaginal discharge may feel embarrassed or awkward when speaking to the doctor. It is unlikely that they will be forthcoming with their problem unless they feel comfortable with you. It is important to reassure them that everything you will discuss will be confidential and that you regularly deal with patients who present with a whole range of different symptoms and problems. Assure them that there is no need to feel embarrassed.

## PHYSICAL EXAMINATION

| Vitals | Pulse, temperature |
| Urine | Isolated 2++ leucocytes - suggestive of chlamydia |

*Gynaecological exam*

| Abdominal | Palpate abdomen for iliac fossa or suprapubic tenderness |
| Vaginal | Inspect for redness, ulceration or irritation. Palpate for adnexal or cervical tenderness |
| Speculum | Inspect cervix (lesions, polyps, strawberry cervix) |

## INVESTIGATIONS

| Urine | Pregnancy test, MSU for NAATs (chlamydia, gonorrhoea) |
| pH & Whiff Testing | pH <4.5 candida, pH >4.5 TV, BV |
| Vaginal Swabs | Endocervical (chlamydia, gonorrhoea), high vaginal (candida, bacterial vaginosis) |
| Bloods | HIV, syphilis serology (VDRL), Hepatitis |
| Specialist | Ultrasound / laparoscopy |

## MANAGEMENT
### Conservative

| | |
|---|---|
| *Barrier Contraception* | The patient needs to be educated around using condoms or diaphragms that reduce the risk of STI transmission |
| *Candida* | Wear loose fitting undergarments from natural materials (cotton) |
| | Avoid using perfumed soaps, bubble baths. Do not excessively douche the vaginal area; use unscented soaps and water to clean |
| | Advise 'natural' remedies such as natural live yoghurt placed inside the vagina, tampons with tea tree oil or measures to change the acidity of the vagina such as using bicarbonate of soda or vinegar in baths |

### Medical

| | |
|---|---|
| *Contact Tracing* | Offer contract tracing - often performed at the GUM clinic |
| *Atrophic vaginitis* | Vaginal oestrogen for 6mths |
| *Antibiotics* | |
| PID | Olfloxacin 400mg bd + oral metronidazole 400mg bd for 14d. Consider IV abx if severe |
| Candida | Clotrimazole cream or pessary. Oral fluconazole 150mg stat, itraconazole 200mg bd for 1d |
| Recurrent | Oral fluconazole 150mg od for 3d, then wkly for 6mths, topical imidazole for 2wks then clotrimazole pessary wkly for 6mths |
| BV | Oral metronidazole 400-500mg bd for 5-7 days or 2gm stat. Alternatives; metronidazole gel or clindamycin 2% cream |
| TV | Oral metronidazole 400-500mg bd for 5-7 days or tinidazole 2gm stat |
| Chlamydia | Doxycycline 100mg bd 7d or azithromycin 1gm stat. Alternatives; erythromycin 500mg bd 14d or olfloxacin 200mg bd 7d |
| Gonorrhoea | Ceftriaxone 500 mg IM stat + azithromycin 1g PO stat |

## SAFETY NETTING

| | |
|---|---|
| *Follow up* | Consider reviewing the patient in a few weeks after they have had all their test results back or if their symptoms persist |
| *Secondary care* | Consider referral to specialists (GUM) if no response to first line treatments |

| Conditions | Characteristic exam feature |
|---|---|
| **Candida** | Yeast like fungal infection due to *Candida albicans* and is not an STI. Most common cause of vaginitis. Thick, white, cottage cheese-like discharge with severe pruritus, vulval redness and irritation. Can affect vulva, groin. Occasionally there is superficial dyspareunia and dysuria. pH<4.5 |
| **Bacterial Vaginosis** | Caused by *Gardnerella vaginalis* and is also not an STI. Most common cause of vaginal infection in women. Thin greyish white discharge with distinct fishy odour. No pruritus but occasionally dysuria. pH<4.5 |
| **Gonorrhoea** | STD caused by *Neisseria gonorrhoea* bacteria. Asymptomatic in 50%. Urethritis (pain and frequency), cervicitis and greeny-yellow discharge |

| Chlamydia | Gram negative organism and most common STI. Common cause of PID and can cause ectopic pregnancy and infertility. Often asymptomatic (70%). Yellowy discharge often with lower abdominal pain and urethritis |
|---|---|
| Trichomoniasis | Caused by the flagellate parasite *Trichomonas vaginalis.* May lead to preterm labour. Asymptomatic (70%). Profuse, frothy greeny yellow discharge with an offensive odour. May also have superficial dyspareunia, itchiness and dysuria. Strawberry cervix |
| PID | Usually caused by STIs including chlamydia and gonorrhea. Pain on sexual intercourse, vaginal discharge and intermenstrual bleeding are common symptoms |

## EXPLANATIONS

*Chlamydia*

Chlamydia is one of the most common sexually transmitted infections which is passed from person to person through unprotected sex. Often it has no symptoms but if you are diagnosed with it, it is important to treat it to prevent risk of spreading to other parts of your body including your ovaries and tubes (PID) and causing infertility.

*Gonorrhoea*

Gonorrhoea is a bacterial sexually transmitted infection that is otherwise known as *'the clap.'* It can affect the neck of the womb in women or the urethra (tube) of the penis.

*Candida*

Candidiasis is a very common cause of vaginal discharge in women. Candida is a yeast which is found naturally on most people's skin and is not sexually transmitted. In your case there is an overgrowth of the bug in your vagina causing the symptoms you have been complaining of.

*PID*

Pelvic inflammatory disease refers to a disorder where the ovaries, womb and/or fallopian tubes become irritated and inflamed, often due to a sexually transmitted infection that has spread from the vagina. It is essential that we treat it early to prevent scarring or damage to the fallopian tubes, increasing the chance of ectopic pregnancies or reducing your chance of falling pregnant in the future.

# *10.14 Breast pain & lumps*

Breast pain in an extremely common problem that women of all ages will experience sometime in their life. The most common cause is cyclical breast pain that is related to the periods and may occur a few days prior. It is usually associated with mild pain and lumpiness of the breasts that eases once the period starts. Around one third of cases are non-cyclical and usually affect those aged 40 and above. It is important to note that breast pain is NOT an early sign of breast cancer and patients should be reassured accordingly.

### HISTORY
**Open questions** — Tell me more about why you attended today? Tell me more about the problems you are having with your breasts

**Focused questions**

*Pain* — Is there any pain or tenderness in your breasts (mastalgia)? When did it start? Is it only in one breast or is it in both breasts? Is it always there or does it come and go? Does anything make the pain better or worse?

**Causes and features of Breast Pain (Mastalgia)**

| | |
|---|---|
| *Cyclical* | Cyclic premenstrual breast pain, young (35yrs), tender upper outer breast. Increase size of breast, lumpiness. Symptoms relieved by menstruation |
| *Non-cyclical* | Not linked to periods, older (40+yrs), can be chest wall or referred |
| Breast pain | Mastitis/abscess, fibroadenosis, carcinoma (rare) |
| Other | Costochondritis, thoracic spondylosis, bornholm disease, lung disease, gallstone |

*Discharge* — Is there any discharge from the nipples? Is it from one or both nipples? How much discharge is there?

Colour — What colour is the discharge? (clear, milky, yellow, green, bloody)

*Lump* — When did you first notice the lump? Has the lump changed in size since then? How many lumps have you noticed? Are the lumps only in one breast or are they in both breasts?

*Duration* — How long have you been experiencing these symptoms?

*Cyclic* — Are they related to your menstrual cycle?

**Associated history**

*Menstrual history* — When was your last period (LMP)? Are they regular? Are they painful?

Age — At what age did you start your periods? At what age was your menopause?

*Obstetric history* — Do you have any children? How many children do you have? Did you breastfeed your children? Are you pregnant?

### PAST HISTORY

*Breast disease* — Have you previously had any breast problems?

*Investigations* — Have you had any previous investigations of your breasts (ultrasound, mammography, biopsy)?

## DRUG HISTORY

*Medication*  Are you taking any medications such as the pill or HRT? Are you taking any other medication? (Worsens breast pain: sertraline, venlafaxine, spironolactone, metronidazole)

## FAMILY HISTORY

*Breast cancer*  Has anyone in your family suffered from breast disease (parents, grandparents, siblings, children)? For each member ask the age it was diagnosed, whether it was unilateral or bilateral and establish what degree relative they are (first, second or third)

*Prostate cancer*  Has anyone been diagnosed with prostate cancer?

---

### Referral from Primary Care for Familial breast cancer

People without a PMHx of breast ca who meet the following criteria should be offered referral to secondary care:

- 1st degree female relative with breast cancer < 40yrs
- 1st degree male relative with breast cancer at any age
- 1st degree relative with bilateral breast cancer diagnosed <50yrs
- 2x 1st degree relative or 1st degree + 2nd degree relative diagnosed breast cancer at any age
- 1st degree or 2nd degree relative with breast cancer at any age AND 1st degree or 2nd degree relative diagnosed with ovarian cancer at any age (one of these should be a first-degree relative)
- 3x 1st degree or 2nd degree relatives diagnosed with breast cancer at any age

---

## SOCIAL HISTORY

*Smoker*  Do you smoke? How many cigarettes do you smoke per day?

*Alcohol*  Do you drink alcohol? How much do you drink and how often?

## IDEA, CONCERNS, EXPECTATIONS

*Ideas*  What do you think may be causing your symptoms (cancer)?

*Concerns*  Do you have any worries about the problems you have been experiencing?

*Impact*  How have the symptoms affected and impacted upon your life?

## CSA TIPS

Women presenting with breast pain are a fairly common occurrence in day-to-day general practice. Most are concerned that this may be an early indicator that there may be an underlying condition, particularly that of breast cancer. It is important to reassure them that if following examination all is in order and manage accordingly. Other patients may present asymptomatically but with concerns about a family history of breast cancer. In such cases you should take a detailed history about who has been affected with cancer and their relationship to the patient. Management will depend on the presence or absence of a lump and the ages when the first or second degree relatives were diagnosed.

## PHYSICAL EXAMINATION

*Chaperone*  Request a chaperone

*Inspect*  With the patient's arms by their side then elevated. Look for any skin changes (peau d'orange, eczema), tethered lumps or nipple changes

*Palpate*  Have the patient lying on the couch (45 degree angle). Ask the patient to place the ipsilateral hand behind their head before examining

Examination  Palpate the breast using the flats of the fingers in a rotary motion from the nipple outwards in a concentric ring. Feel for any lumps noting its location compared to the areola (e.g. 3 o'clock position), size, consistency (rubbery, firm, soft) and mobility (mobile, fixed, tethered)

| | |
|---|---|
| Nipple Discharge | Request the patient to express their nipples if there is any discharge |
| Axillary Nodes | With the arm slightly abducted (e.g. right), support the patient's wrist with your hand (e.g. right). Use your other hand (e.g. left) to examine the axilla for any lymph nodes. Check both sides |

## INVESTIGATIONS  *often performed by secondary care*

| | |
|---|---|
| *Swab* | Swab any discharge for microbiology and cytology |
| *Imaging* | Mammogram, US, MRI scan (younger women) |
| *Biopsy* | Biopsy of lump, fine needle aspiration for cytology |

## MANAGEMENT
### Conservative
*Breast pain*

| | |
|---|---|
| Cyclic | Wear better fitting bra during day, soft supporting bra at night. Keep pain chart/diary |
| Non-cyclic | Firm support bra. Resolves 50% of women's problems. Consider acupuncture |
| Mastitis | If breast feeding continue to do so. No harm to baby |
| | If too tender to feed, express milk via pump or hand. Helps stop the breast becoming engorged and painful. Use cold packs |

---

**Measures not routinely recommended for cyclic breast pain** - *Ref: Cyclic breast pain CKS NICE 2012*
Stopping or changing COCP, POP, evening primrose oil, diets (low in fat, high in carbohydrate, low caffeine), antibiotics, diuretics, pyridoxine, tibolone, vitamin E

---

| | |
|---|---|
| *Lifestyle* | Recommend exercise, diet advice (small, regular portions, reduce caffeine, increase fibre), regular sleep and weight loss. Advice to stop smoking and reduce alcohol intake |
| *Psychological* | Advise counselling (CBT) or relaxation techniques if appropriate |
| *Vitamins* | Consider Evening primrose oil (breast tenderness) |
| | Vitamin B6 (evidence) or calcium/vitamin D, magnesium or vitamin A supplements 2wks before periods start (limited evidence) |

### Medical
*Breast pain*

| | |
|---|---|
| Cyclic | Topical NSAIDs or oral paracetamol/NSAIDs PRN. 2nd line treatment refer to specialist |
| Non-cyclic | Treat cause. Investigate referred pain. If pain from chest wall consider local anaesthetic or steroid injection |
| Mastitis | Offer paracetamol/ibuprofen for analgesia. Antibiotics - Flucloxacillin 500mg qds 14d or erythromycin 500mg qds 14d (if penicillin allergy) |

## SAFETY NETTING

| | |
|---|---|
| *Follow up* | Review in 3 mths for response to treatment |
| *Referral* | Refer to specialist if poor response or according to guidelines below |

---

**Urgent referral for suspected breast cancer** - *Ref: NICE (June 2005). Referral Guidelines for Suspected Cancer*
- Discrete, hard lump with fixation, +/- tethering irrespective of age
- >=30yr with discrete lump that persists through next period, or presents after menopause
- <30yr with either enlarging lump, fixed and hard, or FHx
- PMHx breast cancer who presents with suspicious symptoms or further lump

- Unilateral eczematous skin or nipple changes not responding to topical treatment
- Nipple distortion of recent onset or spontaneous unilateral blood discharge
- Male, >=50yr with unilateral, firm subareolar mass +/- nipple distortion or skin changes

**Non-urgent referral**
- Female <30yr with a lump
- Breast pain with no lump after treatment fails or unexplained symptoms persist (mammography not recommended)

---

**DIFFERENTIAL DIAGNOSIS**

| Conditions | Characteristic exam feature |
|---|---|
| Fat necrosis | Hard irregular lump, can be tethered with history of trauma. Evidence of shrinkage |
| Breast abscess | Tender lump with pus caused by blocked duct. Fever, hot to touch, red inflamed skin, flu like symptoms |
| Fibroadenosis | Most common lump (cystic) in reproductive age. Peak 35-50yr. Can be single or multiple, painful, bilateral with lumpiness of breast. Size and pain associated with cycle |
| Fibroadenoma | Benign tumour occurring in women common <35yr. Discrete, non-tender, firm, mobile lump described as 'breast mice'. Can grow in pregnancy and shrink in menopause. Can spontaneously resolve |
| Carcinoma | Lump (upper outer quadrant), hard, tethered, peau d'orange, dimpling, nipple inversion, blood stained discharge, non-cyclic breast pain (uncommon). Risk factors: PMHx (breast, endometrial, ovarian ca), FHx, age, early menarche, late menopause, nulliparity, OCP/HRT, obesity alcohol |

**EXPLANATIONS**

*Investigations*    The specialist doctor will first organise some scans (US, MRI) or special X-ray (mammogram) to find out what the lump could be.

Biopsy    They may also organise a biopsy whereby they take a small sample of tissue from the lump using a needle with the help of an ultrasound or mammogram. The sample is then looked under the microscope for any abnormal (cancer) cells.

*Fibroadenoma*    Fibroadenomas are common, non-cancerous, smooth breast lumps that are often caused by overgrowth of glands and connective tissue in the breast. They are believed to occur due to increased sensitivity to female hormones (oestrogen).

*Fibroadenosis*    Fibroadenosis are common cysts or fluid filled lumps in the breast. They are particularly common as you approach the menopause. They are believed to be caused by the breast responding abnormally to hormonal fluctuations within the menstrual cycle.

| | |
|---|---|
| *Fat necrosis* | Fat necrosis are non-cancerous breast lumps caused by an injury or trauma to the fatty tissue of the breast. They usually go away on their own but persistent lumps can be surgically removed. |
| *Breast abscess* | Breast abscesses are painful collections of pus within the breast caused by bacterial infection. They usually affect women who are breastfeeding as the ducts that carry the breast milk become blocked. Bacteria then enter the cracks in the nipple developing an abscess. |
| *Mastitis* | Mastitis is when the breast becomes inflamed usually caused by an infection. These get into the milk ducts often through a crack or sore nipple. It is common in breast feeding mothers. |
| Treatment | Continue to breastfeed as this will help unblock the ducts and stops the breast from becoming engorged. Your baby will not be harmed from the breast milk as the bacteria will be killed by the acid in your baby's stomach. |

# 10.15 Cervical Smear

The cervical screening programme in the UK was established to pick up early signs of changes in the cells of the womb that may lead to cancer. All women aged between 25 and 64 years of age are invited into a regular, rolling programme of cervical smear testing. Those aged between 25 and 49 are recalled every 3 years, whereas those between 50 and 64 have smear tests every five years. As a result of the programme, 3,000 people are diagnosed with cervical cancer each year.

### 20-24 Year Olds

The programme no longer tests for changes in women less than 25 years of age as in this cohort the prevalence of cervical cancer is <50 cases as year. It is hoped that the prevalence of cancer in this age group will drop greatly as a result of the HPV vaccination programme. In addition, it was found that the percentage of patients found with abnormal cells was far greater than those who went on to develop cervical cancer.

### HPV

More recently, the programme now detects for the presence or absence of HPV. HPV is an extremely common virus with over 100 different types. Of the types, HPV-16 and HPV-18 are deemed to be high-risk and are implicated in most cases of cervical cancer. If HPV is detected in low-grade or borderline dyskaryosis then a patient should automatically be referred for colposcopy.

### HISTORY

**Open questions**       Tell me how I can help you today?

### IDEA, CONCERNS, EXPECTATIONS

| | |
|---|---|
| *Ideas* | I understand that you received your smear results by post. What do you understand by them? |
| *Concerns* | Do you have any worries about the results? |

### Focused questions

| | |
|---|---|
| *Sexual History* | Are you sexually active? Do you have a regular partner? |
| *Gynae History* | |
| LMP | When was your last period? (LMP) |
| Irregular | Are your periods irregular or heavy? How many days do they last? Do you pass clots? How many sanitary towels/pads do you use per day? |
| IMB | Have you noticed any spotting or bleeding between periods? |
| PCB | Or bleeding after sexual intercourse? |
| Dyspareunia | Do you have any pain during sex? |
| *STIs* | Have you noticed any abnormal discharge or itching? Have you suffered from a sexually transmitted infection in the past? Has any of your partners been diagnosed with chlamydia or gonorrhoea? |
| *Weight loss* | Have you noticed any loss of weight? |

### PAST HISTORY

| | |
|---|---|
| *Smears* | Have you ever had any abnormal smears in the past? How were they treated (colposcopy)? |

## FAMILY HISTORY

*Cervical cancer*  Have any of your family members been diagnosed with cervical cancer?

## DRUG HISTORY

*Medication*  Are you taking any medications such as the COCP or tamoxifen?
Have you ever taken the emergency contraception before (breast tenderness)?

## SOCIAL HISTORY

*Smoker*  Do you smoke? How many cigarettes do you smoke per day?
*Alcohol*  Do you drink alcohol? How much do you drink and how often?

## CSA TIPS

It is unlikely that you will be requested to carry out a smear test on a manikin, but you may have to explain the procedure to a patient who has just turned 25 years of age and is anxious of entering the smear programme. Other cases may involve patients presenting having received the results of a recent cervical smear and requesting some explanation and clarity around what they mean. Patients may have worries around HPV infection and whether there is a treatment available for them or whether they are eligible for the HPV vaccination programme.

## PHYSICAL EXAMINATION

*Smear*  Perform a liquid cervical smear test via speculum examination if not already done

---

### How to take a smear test

*Explanation*  The smear test is carried out on women aged between 25 and 49 years every three years and on women aged between 50 and 64, every five years. It involves taking a sample of cells using a cervical brush from the neck of the womb. The cells are transferred to a slide and sent to the hospital where they are checked under a microscope to make sure there are no changes
*Chaperone*  Inform the patient that you would like to request a chaperone
*Mid-cycle*  Establish if the patient is approximately mid-cycle through her period
*Position*  Have the patient lie flat on the couch with heels brought back and knees flopped apart
*Inspection*  Examine the cervix and vulva for irritation, lesions
*Spatula*  Apply jelly to the speculum and insert into the vagina. Introduce the brush into the external os and rotate 5x 360 degrees in an anticlockwise manner
*LBC*  Check expiry date of the vial before inserting the brush into the liquid based cytology for 20 seconds to ensure transfer

---

## INVESTIGATIONS

*Smear results*  Refer for colposcopy if abnormal smear (moderate, severe dyskaryosis or 2 consecutive mild)

## MANAGEMENT

---

### Interpreting Smear Results

*Negative*  Normal smear with normal endocervical cells and negative HPV - normal recall. However, normal cells with HPV +ve requires a repeat smear in 12 months time
*Inadequate*  Insufficient smear was taken - repeat sample as soon as possible. If 3 inadequate samples found, patient should be referred for colposcopy

| | |
|---|---|
| *Borderline* | Abnormal nuclei found but could not confirm dyskaryosis. Results can revert to normal over time. Repeat smear in 6 months time |
| 3x | If 3 consecutive borderline changes, recommend colposcopy. 3 consecutive normal results are required 6 months apart before patient can revert back to normal routine recall |
| *Dyskaryosis* | Can be mild, moderate or severe. Mild dyskaryosis with no HPV can be called back as per routine recall. However mild dyskaryosis with HPV will require colposcopy. Both moderate and severe dyskaryosis warrants referral for colposcopy |

---

| | |
|---|---|
| *Dyskaryosis Expl.* | In your case there were some abnormal changes seen in the cells known as dyskaryosis. These changes are not cervical cancer or cancerous. In most cases dyskaryotic cells do not develop into cancer and most will change back into normal cells. However, in a few cases, if left untreated, these abnormal cells may change into cancer in the future |
| *HPV Explanation* | HPV stands for Human Papilloma Virus. It is a very common virus that is spread by sexual intercourse. Once it is caught, it does not usually cause any symptoms so most people with it would not know that they even had it. However, the virus has been found to lead to a few problems including warts and may even lead to cervical cancer. |
| Treatment | In patients who have the HPV virus, there is currently no treatment available to make it go away. However, the body sometimes can clear it by itself through its normal defence mechanisms |
| Prevention | Although there is no treatment for HPV, we can reduce the risk of transmission by using barrier contraceptives (condom, diaphragm) this can also help prevent you from getting other sexual diseases including infections and warts. In girls aged 12-13 years, there is a national vaccination program to prevent them from catching the virus given at schools. Unfortunately, such injections do not treat HPV once it has been caught and at the present time, the vaccines are not available on the NHS for people outside this age group. However, you can get them privately if you wish to have them |
| *Colposcopy* | Colposcopy is when a doctor has a closer look at the neck of the womb. It is similar to when having a smear test in that you have a speculum inserted into your vagina. The doctor will then use a colposcope or a magnifier to get a more detailed view. They will use a special liquid and paint the neck of the womb. This will help highlight the abnormal cells. They may take a small sample of cells, or a biopsy, to look at even closer under the microscope |
| Treatment | The doctor may decide to offer you treatment at the same time depending on what they see. They may wish to treat the abnormal cells using a heat probe (loop diathermy), laser treatment, or a cold probe (cryotherapy). A small anaesthetic is given locally before any treatment is undertaken so that you do not feel any pain |

**SAFETY NETTING**

| | |
|---|---|
| *Follow up* | Review as above depending on the results offering follow-up or repeat smear accordingly |

**EXPLANATIONS**

| | |
|---|---|
| *Cervical Cancer* | Cervical carcinoma refers to the malignant changes that occur at the cervix. Despite being the second most common female malignancy in the UK, its incidence has been falling since the introduction of the cervical screening programme. Risk factors for |

cervical cancer include the presence of HPV, sex at a young age, multiple sexual partners, promiscuous male partners, smoking and chlamydia infection.

Symptoms of early disease are usually not noticed. However, established disease often causes post-coital bleeding and an offensive vaginal discharge. Inter-menstrual and post-menopausal bleeding may also be seen.

# 11.1 Chronic fatigue syndrome

Chronic fatigue syndrome, also termed myalgic encephalomyelitis (ME), is a clinical condition that is diagnosed when a patient suffers from new onset, persistent (>4mths) fatigue, to the exclusion of other medical conditions. Patients may also suffer with post-exertional malaise causing them to have a substantial reduction in activity levels. Patients may also present with accompanying problems such as joint pain, headaches, insomnia, sore throat and general flu-like symptoms.

## HISTORY

**Open questions**         How can I help you today? Tell me more about the problems you are having

## Focused questions
*Fatigue*

| | |
|---|---|
| Onset | When did your tiredness start? |
| Frequency | How often do you get tired? Is it there all the time or does it come and go? |
| Post exertional | Do you suffer from tiredness or fatigue after carrying out any activity? When does it usually start (>24hrs) and how long does it last (several days)? |
| *Function* | Has it affected your ability to do things? (walking, cooking, climbing stairs, dressing) |

## Associated history

| | |
|---|---|
| *Sleep Disturbance* | How is your sleep pattern? (insomnia, early morning waking) |
| *Joint Pain* | Do you have any pain or stiffness in your joints? Which ones are affected? |
| *Flu-like* | Do you suffer with any headaches, sore throat or flu like symptoms? |
| *Dizziness* | Do you feel dizzy or faint? Do you feel sick as well? Have you vomited? |
| *Cognitive* | Are you able to concentrate? Do you get distracted easily? Do you feel it more difficult to make decisions or complete everyday task? |
| *Lumps* | Have you noticed any swollen lumps anywhere in your body? (neck, underarm, groin) |

**Differentials**         See tiredness chapter

**RED FLAGS**         Weight loss, night sweats, persistent fevers, haemoptysis, PR bleeding, postmenopausal PV bleeding, dysphagia, swollen LN

## FAMILY HISTORY
*CFS / ME*         Does anyone in your family suffer from similar symptoms?

## SOCIAL HISTORY

| | |
|---|---|
| *Mood* | How is your mood? Any changes recently? |
| *Relationships* | Are you currently in a relationship? How are things? |
| *Support network* | Who lives with you at home? Do you have any close friends or family? |
| *Occupation* | Are you working or studying at the moment? Have you had to miss these activities due to your symptoms? |
| *Diet* | Tell me about your diet? |
| *Smoker* | Do you smoke? How many cigarettes do you smoke per day? |
| *Alcohol* | Do you drink alcohol? How much do you drink and how often? |
| *Recreational drugs* | Have you ever used any recreational drugs? |

## IDEA, CONCERNS, EXPECTATIONS

| | |
|---|---|
| *Ideas* | Have you had any thoughts what may be causing your symptoms? |
| *Concerns* | Do you have any worries about the tiredness you have been feeling? |
| *Expectations* | How did you think I could help you today? |
| *Impact* | How have the symptoms affected your life? |

## CSA TIPS

Chronic fatigue is a difficult symptom to manage. Patients may suffer enormously and have had to leave their jobs or relationships due to the problem. Although there may be an underlying chronic cause, in many cases no discernible diagnosis is found. Patients may be unhappy with this and instead insist they are suffering with chronic fatigue or ME and want a referral to a specialist service. You will have to negotiate with such patients and determine together what the best course of action should be.

## PHYSICAL EXAMINATION

| | |
|---|---|
| *Vitals* | Temp, BP, weight, pulse |
| *Examination* | Do a complete physical examination focussing on systems where symptoms may be present |
| Inspect | Look for general health, any lumps. Inspect throat |
| Palpate | Palpate any lumps, examine for LN in the cervical region, axillary, epitrochlear, para-aortic, inguinal and popliteal. Palpate for hepatomegaly or splenomegaly |

## INVESTIGATIONS

| | |
|---|---|
| **INVESTIGATIONS** | *to exclude common differentials* |
| *Urine* | Dipstick for blood, ketones or glucose |
| *Bloods* | FBC, ESR & CRP, LFTs, U&Es (electrolyte abnormalities), glucose, TFT coeliac screen, CK |
| Other | *Request only if clinically indicated:* B12, folate (only if FBC/MCV shows macrocytosis). Request ferritin (only if FBC suggests Fe deficiency) |
| Rheum. | Rh factor, ANA |
| Viral screen | HIV, Hep B and C, EBV, CMV, toxoplasmosis, monospot test |
| Myeloma | Consider urine Bence Jones protein and protein electrophoresis |

## MANAGEMENT

### Conservative

| | |
|---|---|
| *Lifestyle* | |
| Diet | Cut down alcohol. Eat a balanced diet and regularly |
| Nausea | Eat little and often, snack on dry starchy foods, sip fluids |
| Exclusion | Exclusion diet only if supported by dietician |
| Sleep | Relax in a dark room with minimal distraction. Go to sleep at the same time every night and have a light snack. No sleeping during the day |
| Exercise | Take low level regular exercise and try and get out even for a walk |
| Rest | Ensure any rest periods are <30min. Use breathing techniques or guided visualisation to help relax during rest period |
| Relaxation | Use relaxation techniques |
| Avoid | Advising to go to the gym or undertake unsupervised, vigorous exercise |

| | |
|---|---|
| *Sick Certificate* | Offer short fit-note if severe symptoms. Consider amended duties or altered hours if finding it difficult to carry out certain tasks or attend. Advise to attend the Jobcentre for advice around benefits, income support and disability |

*Talking therapies*

| | |
|---|---|
| CBT | Consider cognitive behavioural therapy for mild / moderate depression |
| Graded exercise | Consider referring for graded exercise therapies or activity management programs (slowly increased intensity of physical activity) |
| Groups | Suggest contact support groups i.e. ME support society |

**Medical**

| | |
|---|---|
| *Antiemetic* | Only consider if nausea severe |
| *TCA* | Consider low dose amitriptyline with poor sleep or pain. Avoid if taking SSR already due to potential SE |

**Referral**

| | |
|---|---|
| *OT* | Speak to an OT about adaptations that can be made or regarding changes at work to maintain ability to stay in employment |
| *Pain Clinic* | Consider referring to pain clinic to maximise treatment |
| *Rheumatologist* | Refer to a rheumatologist or specialist CFS service if available locally |

**SAFETY NETTING**

| | |
|---|---|
| *Follow up* | Review in 4-6wks for response to treatment or to check the diagnosis |

**EXPLANATIONS**

| | |
|---|---|
| *CFS/ME* | Chronic fatigue syndrome (CFS), as the name suggests, is a condition that presents with marked tiredness over a long period of time. It is also known as ME, or myalgic encephalomyelitis, that means muscle aches with inflammation of the brain. However, unlike the name suggests, there is no evidence of inflammation of the brain in this condition. Often these names are used interchangeably to describe the same condition. Whilst there is no known cause for CFS/ME, there are theories that the symptoms are triggered by a viral infection. |
| Treatment | Unfortunately, there is no single cure for CFS but there are a number of treatment options that may help. We can consider referring you to see a CBT psychologist who can work with you to try and modify your thoughts and make you feel more positive. There are graded exercises that your therapist will work with you to try and slowly increase your ability to exercise every day. They will also help you to pace your activity depending how you feel so that if on one day you feel tired, you may wish to do less activity that day, but when you feel good you can do more. |

# 11.2 Polymyalgia Rheumatica

Polymyalgia rheumatica is an inflammatory disease that presents with at least 2 weeks of pain and morning stiffness affecting the neck, shoulders and pelvic girdle. It often affects elderly (>50yr) women more than men (3:1) and is seen in Caucasians (northern European) more frequently than other ethnic groups. Other symptoms include a mild fever, fatigability and weight loss. It is important to diagnose in order to initiate long term (1-3yrs) steroid treatment to prevent complications such as Giant cell arteritis (15%) and potential blindness.

## HISTORY

**Open questions**   How can I help you today? Tell me more about the problems you are having with your shoulders

### Focused questions

| | |
|---|---|
| *PMR* | Is there any pain or tenderness in both of your shoulders? When did it start? |
| Onset | Did it come on quickly? |
| Character | What does the pain feel like? Are your muscles painful to touch? |
| Frequency | Is it always there or does it come and go? Does anything make the pain better (>45min being active, steroids) or worse (rest)? |
| Radiate | Does the pain move anywhere? (elbows) |
| Stiffness | Have you had any stiffness of the joint? Is it worse in the morning? |
| | Do you struggle to turn over in bed or get up to go toilet in the mornings? |
| Other joints | Does it affect any other joints? (hips, pelvis) |

| | |
|---|---|
| *Giant Cell Arteritis* | |
| Headaches | Do you suffer from headaches? (temporal) |
| Scalp tenderness | Does it hurt when you comb your hair? |
| Jaw claudication | Is it painful when you chew food or brush your teeth? |
| Vision | Have you ever had any vision disturbances? (loss, diplopia) |

### Associated history

| | |
|---|---|
| *Fatigue* | Do you feel extremely tired all the time? |
| *Fever* | Have you noticed any fever or night sweats? |
| *Weight loss* | Has it affected your appetite or caused any weight loss? |
| *Oedema* | Have you noticed any swellings of the feet or hands? |

### Differentials

| | |
|---|---|
| *Viral infection* | Have you had any flu like symptoms (cough, sore throat, coryzal)? |
| *Spondylosis* | Do you have any neck pain? |
| *Osteoarthritis* | Does it get better with rest or improve by the end of the day? What joints does it affect (hands, knee, back)? |
| *Thyroid* | Have you put on any weight recently? Do you feel intolerant to cold weather? |
| *Statins* | Are you taking any cholesterol lowering medication? |

**RED FLAGS**   Temporal arteritis (visual - diplopia or loss, temporal headaches)

## PAST HISTORY

*Medical*          Have you ever suffered from any medical conditions? (RA, OA)

## FAMILY HISTORY

*PMR*          Does anyone else in your family have similar symptoms? (HLA-DR4)

## DRUG HISTORY

*Medication*          Are you taking any medications (steroids)? Are you taking any painkillers? (NSAIDs, paracetamol, topical gels)?

## SOCIAL HISTORY

*Home*          Who lives with you at home?

*Occupation*          Are you currently working? Has the pain affected you at work?

Drive          Do you drive?

*Smoker*          Do you smoke? How many cigarettes do you smoke per day?

*Alcohol*          Do you drink alcohol? How much do you drink and how often?

## IDEA, CONCERNS, EXPECTATIONS

*Ideas*          Have you had any thoughts what may be causing your symptoms?

*Concerns*          Do you have any worries about the pain you have been experiencing?

*Expectations*          How did you think I could help you today?

*Impact*          How have the symptoms affected your life?

## CSA TIPS

PMR is a condition that relies mainly on a thorough history and functional analysis. If diagnosed, patients should be treated with steroids and be admitted if any visual symptoms or if temporal arteritis is suspected.

## PHYSICAL EXAMINATION

*Vitals*          Temp, BP, pulse

*Inspection*          Look for any muscle swelling, muscle wasting

*Palpation*          Feel for tenderness across the shoulders and pelvic girdles (if indicated). Note reduction in ROM from pain and stiffness

    Shoulders          Check abduction, adduction, flexion, extension of shoulders

    Hips          Check abduction, flexion, extension (if indicated)

*Temporal arteritis*

    Pulse          Check for tenderness, thickening or pulselessness of artery

*Neurology*          Check power against resistance. Note for absence of true weakness

## INVESTIGATIONS

*Bloods*          Request for urgent ESR and CRP

    Other          Consider Hb (WCC), U&E, LFT, CK and TFT, Rh factor, for differentials

    Myeloma screen          Consider urine Bence Jones protein and protein electrophoresis

*US*          Occasionally performed but can establish evidence of synovitis, bursitis within the shoulder and/or hip supporting diagnosis

## MANAGEMENT

**Conservative**

*Support groups*          Offer details for patient support groups (PMRGCAuk)

*Medical*

| | |
|---|---|
| Steroids | Offer low dose prednisolone initiating at 15mg od with 1wk follow up. If symptomatically controlled offer tapering dose reducing slowly over a year. Typical treatment requires 1-3yrs |
| Side effects | Advise SE of medication (weight gain, dyspepsia, bruising & thinning of skin, muscle weakness). Inform not to stop abruptly |
| Card | Recommend to carry steroid card |

---

**Guidance for steroid therapy in stable PMR**
- Initiate with prednisolone 15mg od for 3wks
- Reduce dose to 12.5mg for 3wks, then 10mg for 4-6wks
- Reduce by 1mg thereafter every 4-8wks

---

*Ref: British Society for Rheumatology (BSR) and British Health Professionals in Rheumatology (BHPR)*

| | |
|---|---|
| *Bone protection* | Consider bone protection against osteoporosis when prescribing long term steroids |

*Referral*

| | |
|---|---|
| Rheumatology | Early referral if atypical symptoms of PMR (young, lack of stiffness or shoulder involvement, normal or high ESR >100 & CRP) or advice regarding steroid use (prolonged used >2yrs, poor response, contraindicated) |

**SAFETY NETTING**

| | |
|---|---|
| Ophthalmology | Refer urgently if red flag symptoms (temporal arteritis) |
| Follow up | If initiated on steroids organise follow up after 1wk to assess response. Review in 3-4wks thereafter to consider lowering dose and recheck inflammatory markers. Check BP and BM at 3mthly reviews. Warn patient if has any headaches, jaw pain, sudden loss of vision then to seek emergency medical advise |

**DIFFERENTIAL DIAGNOSIS**

| Conditions | Characteristic exam feature |
|---|---|
| **PMR** | Seen in elderly. Causes pain (aching) and morning stiffness (cannot turn over in bed) to bilateral shoulders, pelvic girdle. Has abrupt onset and can last >2wks. Muscles are tender with no true weakness (only pain). Have raised inflammatory markers (ESR,CRP). Associated with giant cell arteritis |
| **Polymyositis** | More common in middle-aged women. Connective tissue disease that causes muscular inflammation. Leads to symptoms such as proximal muscle weakness, dysphagia and pain. Often presents with a dermatomyositis. May have raised CK 50x normal |
| **Multiple Myeloma** | Bone marrow cancer affecting plasma cells. Causes tiredness, weight loss, infections, bone pain and multiple fractures in the spine, skull, pelvis, shoulders and rib cage. May have bence jones proteins in urine |
| **Adhesive** | Also known as frozen shoulder and causes pain, stiffness and reduced movements. |

| | |
|---|---|
| **Capsulitis** | More common in women between 40-60 and diabetics. Leads to restriction of all shoulder movements (particularly ext rotation) whether active or passive. Tends to severely affect ADLs such as dressing or washing |
| **Thyroid Disease** | Underactive thyroid gland. Presents with cold intolerance, hair loss, dry skin, fatigability, heavy periods, increased weight, low mood |
| **Chronic Fatigue Syndrome** | Persistent tiredness and fatigue unrelated to activity and persisting for at least 4 months. Sufferers experience myalgia, unrefreshing sleep, malaise and arthralgia |

**EXPLANATIONS**

*PMR* — Polymyalgia rheumatica is a condition that causes pain (myalgia), stiffness and inflammation of the large muscles (poly) of the body. It typically affects the shoulders, neck and hip. It can cause tenderness and stiffness making it hard for you to get out of bed in the morning.

Steroids — Often we treat it with a medium dose of steroid medication that reduces the swelling or inflammation. This is a different steroid than that which bodybuilders may use. Often after taking it you should feel much better quite quickly (2-3d). We hope to reduce the medication over a few months once your symptoms get better.

*Temporal arteritis* — This is a condition where there is swelling or inflammation of a blood vessel that supplies the scalp of the head known as the temporal artery. This leads to tenderness over the area and headache. If it is left untreated for a long time it may cause damage to your vision and eventually can lead to blindness.

# *11.3 Osteoporosis*

Osteoporosis is a progressive disease of the bone causing a decrease in bone density with a subsequent increase in fragility and an increased risk of fracturing. It is painless and sufferers may not realise they have it until they experience a fracture. Common sites of fragility fractures including the wrist, spine and hip if sustained when falling from standing height or less. Osteoporosis is defined by the WHO as bone density that is -2.5 standard deviations below the mean peak bone mass and is usually diagnosed on a DEXA scan.

---

**Risk Factors for Osteoporosis**

| | |
|---|---|
| *Epidemiology* | Females, increase with age, ethnicity (caucasians, asians) |
| *Fracture* | Colles, hip or vertebral fracture (loss of height, kyphosis), recurrent falls |
| *PMHx* | *Endocrine:* Hyperthyroidism, hyperparathyroidism, DM1, Cushing syndrome, hypogonadism (orchidectomy, oophorectomy, premature menopause), *Rheum:* RA, AS *GI:* IBD, coeliac disease |
| *FHx* | Osteoporosis, kyphosis or hip fractures <50yrs |
| *DHx* | Steroids, anticonvulsants, thyroxine (high dose) |
| *SHx* | |
| Smoking | Increases risk |
| Alcohol | >4 units/day |
| Diet | Low calcium & vitamin D intake, excess caffeine |
| Exercise | Immobility (housebound), sedentary lifestyle, low BMI (<20 F, <25 M) |

---

**HISTORY**

| | |
|---|---|
| **Open questions** | How can I help you today? What is your understanding about your (DEXA) results? |

**Focused questions**

*Osteoporosis symptoms*

| | |
|---|---|
| Falls | Have you had a fall recently? |
| Fractures | Have you ever fractured your bones before? (spine, wrist, hip) |
| Height | Have you noticed a loss in your height or that you are stooping (bent forward) more than before? |
| Back pain | Do you have any persistent back pain? |

*Risk factors*

| | |
|---|---|
| Hyperthyroid | Do you feel intolerant to warm weather? Have you lost any weight? How is your appetite? |
| Bowels | How are your bowels? Do you feel bloated (coeliac)? Any diarrhoea (IBD)? |
| Menopause | How are your periods? What age were you when you entered the menopause (<45yr)? |

| | |
|---|---|
| **RED FLAGS** | Anorexia, fragility fracture in <50yr, recurrent falls, chronic disease (hyperthyroidism, hyperparathyroidism), steroids |

**PAST HISTORY**

| | |
|---|---|
| *Osteoporosis* | Do you have a history of any bone problems? (osteoporosis, RA) |
| *Bowel disease* | Have you been diagnosed with any bowel problems? (IBD, coeliac, RA) |
| *Other* | Do you suffer from any other medical problems? (DM type 1, CKD, hyperthyroidism) |

## FAMILY HISTORY

| | |
|---|---|
| *Osteoporosis* | Does anyone in your family suffer from osteoporosis? |
| *Fractures* | Does anyone in your family suffer have any fractures? (parental hip) |

## DRUG HISTORY

| | |
|---|---|
| *Steroids* | Are you taking any long term steroid medication? (>3mths) |
| *Medications* | Have you ever taken pioglitazone for diabetes? Or taken methotrexate or lithium? |

## SOCIAL HISTORY

| | |
|---|---|
| *Smoker* | Do you smoke? How many cigarettes do you smoke per day? |
| *Alcohol* | Do you drink alcohol? How much do you drink and how often? (=>4u/d) |
| *Exercise* | Do you do any exercise? Do you live a sedentary lifestyle? |
| *Diet* | How is your diet? (lack of calcium/Vitamin D) |
| *Occupation* | Are you currently working? |
| *Support network* | Who lives with you at home? Do you have any close friends or family? |

## IDEA, CONCERNS, EXPECTATIONS

| | |
|---|---|
| *Concerns* | What worries do you have about your bones? |
| *Expectations* | How did you think I could help you today? |
| *Impact* | How have the symptoms affected your life? |

## CSA TIPS

Asymptomatic patients with a recent DEXA scan may present for discussions about the diagnosis and what the results mean. Patients who are on long term steroids should have a discussion about the possibility of developing osteoporosis and what can be done to reduce their risk.

## PHYSICAL EXAMINATION

| | |
|---|---|
| *Vitals* | Weight, height (loss), BMI (<19 kg/m2) |
| *Examination* | Examine the joints (wrist - colles, vertebrae, hip) for any fractures. Examine the back for kyphosis/kyphos |

## INVESTIGATIONS

| | |
|---|---|
| *Risk Calculator* | Request for QFracture (UK) score or FRAX (WHO) thats reports the 10 year probability of a major osteoporotic fracture |
| FRAX | High risk for women >11.1%, men >2.6% |
| *Bloods* | FBC, U&Es, TFT, calcium, PO4, PTH, Vit D, LFTs, ALP, LH & FSH, testosterone (hypogonadism) |
| *Urine* | Bence jones proteins if myeloma considered |
| *Imaging* | |
| X-ray | Thoracic/lumbar spine can identify osteopenia |
| Bone scan | DEXA scan for osteoporosis |

---

**Interpreting DEXA scans -** *Ref: WHO & International Osteoporosis Foundation (IOF) & NICE*

| | |
|---|---|
| *Normal* | DEXA scan T-score between 0 and -1 |
| *Osteopenia* | DEXA scan T-score between -1 and -2.5 |
| *Osteoporosis* | DEXA scan T-score less than or equal to -2.5 |
| Severe | T-score <-2.5 + fracture |

### Indications for DEXA scan

| | |
|---|---|
| *Fragility fracture* | If <75yr with fragility fracture |
| *Risk factors* | If <75yr with risks factors for osteoporosis |
| *Osteopenia* | If <75yr with X-ray suggesting osteopenia |
| *LT steroids* | If <65yr on steroids for at least 3mths (prednisolone 7.5mg od) |

## MANAGEMENT
### *Conservative*
*Lifestyle*

| | |
|---|---|
| Diet advice | Supplement diet with calcium (milk, cheese, yoghurt) & vitamin D (salmon, mackerel, tuna, sardine, sunlight) |
| Exercise | Recommend weight bearing exercises (aerobic, dancing, running) |
| Smoking | Advice to stop smoking |
| Alcohol | Cut down alcohol to recommended levels (3u/d male, 2u/d female) |

*Aids*

| | |
|---|---|
| Walking stick | Offer walking stick to reduce load on contralateral joint (hip). Consider heel raise to correct unequal leg lengths |
| Assisted devices | Include tap turners, enlarged grips for writing, non-slip mats, electric can openers, long hand reachers |

| | |
|---|---|
| *Falls prevention* | Remove hazards e.g. uneven rugs, slippery floor, loose wires |
| Hip protectors | Recommend hip protectors for those with risk of falls |

### *Medical*

| | |
|---|---|
| *Supplements* | Offer calcium (0.5-1g/d) and Vitamin D (800u/d) for immobile or at risk groups (Asian) i.e. Adcal D3 1 bd |
| *Analgesia* | Offer analgesia (paracetamol/NSAIDs) for vertebral fractures. Add PPI with NSAIDs |
| *Bisphosphonates* | Offer as first line therapy alendronate (70mg wkly, 10mg od) or risedronate (35mg wkly, 5mg od) if alendronate not tolerated. Avoid with NSAIDs/aspirin (GI) |
| How to take | Taken >30min before breakfast, medications or other drink (milk). Swallow whole with cup of water. Taken in upright position, remain sitting up for 30mins |
| SE | GI symptoms (nausea, oesophagitis), pain (bone, joint, muscle), atypical stress fractures (femur) |
| CI | Hypocalcaemia, pregnancy/breastfeeding, low eGFR (<35), ulcer |

### Treat with Bisphosphonates

| | |
|---|---|
| *Fragility fracture* | If >75yr initiate medication. If 65-75yr then perform DEXA scan first |
| *LT (>3mths) steroids* | If >65yr initiate medication. If <65yr request for DEXA scan |
| *Age* | >75yr treat without DEXA scan. If 65-75yr treat if DEXA shows osteoporosis (<= -2.5). If <65yr treat if DEXA <=-3 or <=2.5 and >=1 risk factor |

| | |
|---|---|
| *HRT* | Used to treat premature menopause (<45yr). Use until the age of 50yr |

## Referral

**Rheumatologist**      If cannot tolerate bisphosphonates. Treatment includes strontium, raloxifene, teriparatide. Refer all men or premenopausal women with osteoporosis / fragility fracture to investigate the cause

**OT**      Speak to an OT about adaptations that can be made to minimise risk of falls at home (bath aids, chair, raised toilet sets, stair rails or removal of rubs and raised carpet edges)

**Falls Clinic**      In patients with 2 or more falls in the last year refer for falls management

## SAFETY NETTING

**Follow up**      Review in 4-6wks for response to treatment

## EXPLANATIONS

**Osteoporosis**      This is a condition where your bones are more thin, weak and more likely to break if you were to fall. After the age of around 40, the body's bone mass begins to lessen naturally but there are other factors that may make this process accelerate such as excessive alcohol and smoking, early menopause or even some medications like steroids.

**DEXA scan**      DEXA stands for Dual-Energy X-ray Absorptiometry which uses special X-rays to check the density of your bones. It tests to see how much of the X-rays pass through your bones. The less X-ray that pass through, the thicker or denser your bones are therefore the less likely they are to break. Conversely, the same is true, the more X-rays that pass through, the thinner the bones and the more likely they are to break.

**Bisphosphonates**      This is a type of drug that is used in patients who have weaker bones or osteoporosis. They work on the cells that make bone in the body to help lay down more bone and strengthen them. As the bone gains mass and weight it becomes harder to break thereby protecting it. However, the medicines take between 6-12 months to work and once you start you should take them for at least 5 years.

    **How to take**      The tablets are usually taken once a week. You should take them on an empty stomach to make sure enough of the medicine is taken up into the body. Take the tablets first thing in the morning with plenty of water. You should take the medicines when upright and then continue to sit up for at least half an hour to prevent the tablets irritating your food pipe and giving you a burning sensation. Eat your normal breakfast 2 hours after the tablet has been taken.

Gout is a condition that is due to raised serum uric acid levels leading to deposition of urate crystals in the joints and allied tissues. As the crystals build up and solidify they irritate the joint and cause inflammation giving rise to severe pain and swelling. Gout is commoner in men and the elderly with only 5% having the disease before 25 years of age. Although the single main cause of gout is hyperuricaemia, gout may present with normal serum uric acid levels and those with raised levels do not always get symptoms.

**HISTORY**

**Open questions** — How can I help you today? Tell me more about the problems you are having with your foot

**Focused questions**

*Foot pain* — Is there any pain or swelling in your foot? When did it start?
- Site — Does it affect one or both feet? Can you point to it?
- *Other* — Do you have a similar problem in other joints? (ankle, knee, elbow, hand)
- Character — What does the pain feel like? (burning, aching, sharp, stinging)
- Frequency — Is it always there or does it come and go? Does anything make the pain better (medications, rest) or worse (movements i.e. walking, standing)?
- Swelling — Has you noticed any swelling or redness of a toe?
- Severe — How strong is the pain? ('worst ever')

**Associated history**

*Injury* — Did you have a fall? Have you ever injured your foot recently? (OA)
*Tophi* — Do you have any fleshy swellings on the fingers, elbows or the ears?

**Differentials**

*Septic arthritis* — Have you had a very high swinging fever?
*Sciatica* — Do you have any shooting pain that starts from your back and go down your foot?
*Periph. Vasc. Dis.* — How far can you walk before you get the pain? Does your foot feel cold? Do you have an ulcer?

**RED FLAGS** — Fever or sweats (septic arthritis), significant deformity

**PAST HISTORY**

*Medical* — Have you ever suffered from any medical conditions? (DM, CKD, Raised Trigs, BP, IHD) Have you ever had kidney stones?

**DIET HISTORY**

*Alcohol* — Do you drink alcohol? How often? What do you drink (beer, port wines)?
*Fluids* — How much fluid do you drink everyday?
*Diet* — What foods do you eat?
- Meat — Do you eat red meat (pork, beef, lamb)? Do you eat offal (liver, heart)?
- Fish — Do you eat fish? (crab, anchovies, mackerel, sardines or shrimps)
- Veg — Are you vegan or vegetarian? (pulses, asparagus or spinach)

## FAMILY HISTORY
*Medical*               Do you have any foot problems that run in the family? (gout)

## DRUG HISTORY
*Medication*            Are you taking any medications (NSAIDs, paracetamol, topical gels)? Are you taking any diuretics (thiazide), ACE-I or aspirin?

## SOCIAL HISTORY
*Occupation*            Are you currently in employment? (barman)
*Smoker*                Do you smoke? How many cigarettes do you smoke per day?

## IDEA, CONCERNS, EXPECTATIONS
*Ideas*                 Have you had any thoughts what may be causing your foot pain?
*Concerns*              Do you have any worries about the pain you have been experiencing?
*Expectations*          How did you think I could help you today?
*Impact*                How have the symptoms affected your life?

## CSA TIPS
Gout is a common complaint. Patients may attend describing excruciating pain in a single joint (most commonly the big toe). It is important to treat the pain and offer treatment to prevent its reoccurrence. However, you should ensure that you take a clear diet history to help advise the patient against foods and beverages that may cause an increased chance of reoccurence.

## PHYSICAL EXAMINATION
*Vitals*                Temp, BMI, BP, pulse
*Look*                  Inspect the affected joint for swelling and redness
*Feel*                  For warmth and tenderness. Check for tophi on the elbow, fingers and helix of the ear
*Move*                  Check active and passive movement of the joint (usually reduced due to pain)

## INVESTIGATIONS
*Bloods*                *Not routinely needed:* Uric acid (gout but can be normal), U&Es (dehydration), lipids (raised TGs)
    Other               Hb, WCC, ESR, CRP (osteomyelitis, inflammatory arthritis)
*Xray*                  Consider to exclude fracture or chondrocalcinosis (calcification of the cartilage)
*Aspiration*            Usually performed in secondary care if diagnosis in doubt. Joint aspiration if suspecting septic arthritis or for presence of urate crystals

## MANAGEMENT
### Conservative
*Rest*                  Elevate and rest the limb. Keep the affected area open and uncovered
*Cold*                  Apply cold / ice pack to the area (frozen peas)
*Alcohol*               Avoid binging and conform to the DoH recommended amounts for female 14u weekly, men 21u weekly. Cut down on beer and stout
*Diet*                  Cut down purine foods i.e. offal, liver, kidney and yeast extract. Avoid herring and sardines. Consider food diary
*Fluids*                To keep well hydrated >2L water a day. Cut down fizzy and sugary drinks
*Weight*                Recommend losing weight if BMI >25
*Sick Certificate*      Offer short fit-note if unable to work. Consider amended duties or altered hours if finding it difficult to carry out certain tasks

| Medical | Acute Attack |
|---|---|
| NSAIDS | Oral NSAIDs (naproxen, indomethacin, diclofenac). Ensure that the patient has no contraindications for NSAIDS (ulcers, gastritis or asthma, <30 eGFR) |
| Colchicine | Use if CI to NSAIDs or no response to treatment. Start with 500mcg bd-qds until pain relief (max. 6mg per tx, do not rept for 3d). In elderly or mild renal failure do not exceed 500mcg bd |
| Steroids | Oral steroids (or intra articular) considered if above medications are CI (prednisolone 20-40mg for 5d). Can be taken with paracetamol |

| Medical | Prevention |
|---|---|
| Indications | Consider prophylaxis treatment if >1 attacks/yr, tophi, arthropathy, urate renal stones. Aim for urate levels below <6mg/dl. Treatment often lifelong |
| Flare up | Prophylaxis treatment should not be initiated during acute attack (prolong symptoms). Starting prophylaxis treatment can cause an acute attack. Co-prescribe with colchicine (6mths) or NSAIDs (6wks) |
| Stop | Stop aspirin or thiazide diuretics |
| Allopurinol | Reduces synthesis of uric acid. Start 1-2wks after gout has settled. Start at 100mg daily and increase by 50mcg fortnightly until taking 300mg daily. Can give up to 900mg in divided doses |
| Bloods | Check serum urate and renal function at 3mths |
| Febuxostat | 2nd line only if intolerant or CI to allopurinol. Start 1-2wks after gout has settled. Start at 80mg daily and increase by to 120mg until symptoms settled |
| Bloods | Do LFTs before initiating and regularly whilst on it. Check serum urate and renal function at 3mths |

| Referral | |
|---|---|
| Admission | Admit if signs of septic arthritis |
| Dietician | Refer to dietician for more advice regarding low purine diet |
| Rheumatology | If suspicion of RA, gout in pregnancy or young pt (<25yr). If on maximum anti-inflammatory dose or complications (stones, tophi) |
| Injection | Persistent pain may warrant steroid or local anaesthetic injections to reduce the pain and inflammation in the joint in the short term. |

**SAFETY NETTING**

| CVD | Patients with gout have risk of metabolic syndrome. Offer CVD risk assessment and management |
|---|---|
| Follow up | Review in 2wks for response to treatment |

**DIFFERENTIAL DIAGNOSIS**

| Conditions | Characteristic exam feature |
|---|---|
| **Gout** | Unilateral (often early morning) joint pain usually due to raised uric acid levels. May be as a result of diet rich in purines (kidney, offal, scrimp, quorn) or poor hydration or fluid intake. Often affects 1st MTP or ankle, fingers. Presents with 'worse ever pain' in joint with difficulty to put socks on, which peaks in 6hrs and resolves after few days. OE: hot, swollen joint, red skin |

| Septic Arthritis | Often affects extremes age (children, elderly). Localised hot, painful and swollen joint (monoarticular) often knee (adults) or hip (child). Associated with systemic illness such as temp and malaise. OE: tachycardia, high pyrexia, tender to touch, painful and swollen joint with pain on movement |
| --- | --- |

**EXPLANATIONS**

*Gout*

Gout is a condition caused by a buildup of crystals within the joint space. These crystals irritate the joint causing pain and discomfort. They are usually made up of a chemical known as uric acid that is normally found in your blood. However, certain foods and drinks can cause these levels to rise and cause painful flare ups.

*Septic arthritis*

Septic arthritis is when germs (septic) have infected the joint. If left untreated it can cause permanent damage to the joint (arthritis) unless antibiotics or drainage of the infected fluid is carried out. The bacteria often gets into the joint and multiplies through the bloodstream from elsewhere or from a local injury from a cut or wound.

# 11.5 Joint Pain (RA/OA)

Joint pain and musculoskeletal symptoms are very common presentations that patients may attend the surgery with. The key symptoms associated with joint pain include swelling, stiffness and numbness. When taking a history and examining, it is important to take a clear history from the patient to distinguish between whether there is an inflammatory or a degenerative process at play.

## HISTORY

**Open questions**    How can I help you today? Tell me more about the problems you are having

## Focused questions

*Joints*    Which joints are affected?
    Number    Is it one joint (OA, gout) or more (OA/RA)? Is it on both sides (RA/OA) or only one side (OA)?

*Pain*    Do you have pain or tenderness in your joints? When did it first start?
    Site    Can you point to the areas of pain?
    Character    What does the pain feel like? (burning, sharp, aching)
    Frequency    Is it always there or does it come and go? Does anything make the pain better (medications, rest) or worse (bending, walking)?
    Timing    Is it worse during the day (RA) or at night (OA)?
    Radiate    Does the pain move anywhere?
    Injury    Have you had a fall or injured yourself recently?

*Stiffness*    Do you suffer with stiffness of your joints? When did it first start?
    Site    Which joints does it affect?
    Timing    How long does it last? (>45mins RA)
    Exacerbation    Does anything make the stiffness worse (activity - OA) or better (activity - RA)?
    Frequency    Is it worse during the day (RA) or at night (OA)?

*Swelling*    When did it first start?
    Site    Where is the swelling?
    Frequency    Is it always there (OA) or does it come and go (RA)?

## Associated history

*Numbness*    Have you also suffered from any pins and needles or numbness? (OA)
*Raynauds*    Do your fingers change colour in the cold?
*Dry eyes*    Do you suffer with dry eyes? (Sjorgen's)
*Fever*    Have you noticed any fever or sweats?
*Rash*    Have you had an associated face rash? (SLE)
*Crepitus*    Do you feel any grating or noise when moving the joint? (OA)
*Mood*    How has your mood been recently?
*Function*    Do you have problems when walking up and down stairs? Are you able to comb or do your hair? How far can you walk before you experience pain? Are you able to dress yourself or put your shoes or socks on without pain?

**RED FLAGS**    Severe pain, trauma, fever, weight loss

## PAST HISTORY

*Medical*            Have you ever suffered from any medical conditions? (IBD, psoriasis)

*Surgery*            Have you had any previous joint operations?

## DRUG HISTORY

*Medication*            Are you taking any medications (steroids)? Are you taking any painkillers (NSAIDs, paracetamol, topical gels)? Have you ever been on diuretics, statins, PPIs or olanzapine that can cause joint pains?

## FAMILY HISTORY

*Rheumatoid*            Does anyone in your family suffer from arthritis (psoriasis, rheumatoid)?

## SOCIAL HISTORY

*Support network*        Who lives with you at home? Do you have any close friends or family?

Carers            Do you have any carers? Are they helping you doing day to day tasks?

*Occupation*            Are you currently working? Has the pain affected you at work?

*Smoker*            Do you smoke? How many cigarettes do you smoke per day?

*Alcohol*            Do you drink alcohol? How much do you drink and how often?

## IDEA, CONCERNS, EXPECTATIONS

*Ideas*            Have you had any thoughts what may be causing your symptoms?

*Concerns*            Do you have any worries about the pain or stiffness you have been experiencing?

*Expectations*            How did you think I could help you today?

*Impact*            How have the symptoms affected your life?

## CSA TIPS

Patients presenting with generalised joint pains should be examined to exclude a rheumatological cause for their symptoms. Picking up such conditions early will help reduce destructive joint disease and the need for an operation in the future. Patients with joint pains may suffer with significant dysfunction and have a much reduced quality of life. It is important to work with the patient and if relevant, their carers to help improve their life.

## PHYSICAL EXAMINATION

*Vitals*            Temp, BP, pulse

*Examination*            Look, feel and move appropriate joints

## INVESTIGATIONS

Bloods            FBC (anaemia), ESR & CRP (active disease), ANA, CCP (80%), Rh. factor (80%) to exclude inflammatory arthritis

Other            Bone profile, PSA (elderly), Vit D (low, worsens pain), urate (gout)

                      HLA B27, IgA for AS, performed in secondary care

*Imaging*

X-ray            OA of joint, fractures

MRI            Consider for, infection, fracture

Bone scan            DEXA scan for osteoporosis

## MANAGEMENT

### Osteoarthritis - Conservative

*Rest*            If pain is to due to repetitive movements advise to rest for up to 12 wks

| Ice / Heat | Apply an ice or heat pack if worsened after activity |
|---|---|
| Support | Considering purchasing support bandages, appropriate footwear (shock-absorbing), insoles |
| Exercise | Continue simple exercises (aerobic/muscle strengthening) as the pain eases to help maintain and improve your ROM and prevent stiffness |
| Weight | If BMI>25 suggest losing weight |
| Aids | |
|    Walking stick | Offer walking stick to reduce load on contralateral joint (hip). Consider heel raise to correct unequal leg lengths |
|    Assisted devices | Include tap turners, enlarged grips for writing, non-slip mats, electric can openers, long hand reachers |

## Medical

*Pain*

| Simple | Simple analgesia (paracetamol) or NSAIDs can be prescribed as topical creams or oral Ensure no CI for NSAIDS (ulcers, gastritis or asthma) |
|---|---|
|    PPI | Add PPI with NSAIDs |
|      Topical | Topical capsaicin as adjunct for knee or hand OA |
| Strong | Consider weak opioid (co-dydramol, co-codamol) or tramadol. Strong opioids for short period only. Consider laxatives for constipation |
|    TENS | Consider TENS as adjunct to pain relief |
| *Avoid* | Glucosamine, chondroitin, acupuncture, topical rubefacients not recommended |

## Referral

| Physio | Physiotherapy helpful in strengthening the muscles. Can recommend on strapping and splints |
|---|---|
| OT | Speak to an OT about adaptations that can be made (bath aids, chair or bed raisers, raised toilet sets, stair rails) |
| Chiropodist | To assist with foot-care or insoles |
| Pain Clinic | Consider referring to MSK or pain clinic to maximise treatment |
| Injections | Offer intra-articular steroid injection for OA of large joints with moderate to severe pain |
| Surgery | Refer if symptoms have rapidly deteriorated or is causing disability |

## Rheumatoid Arthritis - Medical

*Pain*

| Simple | Offer paracetamol with or without codeine (co-dydramol) |
|---|---|
|    NSAIDs | Consider NSAIDs (e.g. ibuprofen, naproxen, indomethacin, Coxib (celecoxib, etoricoxib)). Ensure no CI for NSAIDS (ulcers, gastritis, asthma) |
|      PPI | Add PPI with NSAIDs |
|      CVD | If IHD offer ibuprofen (400mg tds) or naproxen (500mg bd) |

| Steroids | Do not initiate steroids unless reviewed by specialist |
|---|---|

| DMARDs | Disease modifying drugs help slow the progression of RA and reduces permanent damage e.g. methotrexate, hydroxychloroquine, leflunomide |
|---|---|
|    Methotrexate | Once a wk treatment given with folic acid |
|      Bloods | Every 2wks unless stable then 2-3mths. Check FBC, LFTs, U&Es |

| Toxicity | Advised if rash, oral, ulcer, N&V or diarrhoea or SOB, cough to withhold medication and review. If severe sore throat of bruising to withhold medication and for urgent FBC |
| Biological | Newer drugs that prevent immune system from attacking the lining of the joints. Examples include infliximab, rituximab and tocilizumab |

| *Flare up* | If flare up consider intra-articular or IM steroid injection. Tapering oral steroid if not give IM i.e. 2wks course of 10mg 7d, 5mg 7d |

### *Referral*

| *Rheumatologist* | Refer urgently within 2wks if signs of synovitis affecting hands, >1 joint. Normal blood tests do not exclude diagnosis of RA |
| *Physio* | Physiotherapy can offer night time splints for joints when inflamed to rest joints. Can demonstrate passive movements when joints inflamed and active when improves |
| *OT* | Speak to an OT about adaptations that can be made |
| *Surgery* | Refer for joint replacement if causing disability |

### SAFETY NETTING

| *Follow up* | Review in 4-6wks for response to treatment or urgently if red flag symptoms |

### DIFFERENTIAL DIAGNOSIS

| Conditions | Characteristic exam feature |
|---|---|
| **Rheumatoid Arthritis** | Mainly affects middle-aged women more than men. Bilateral symmetrical swelling and pain of the small joints of the hands, wrists and feet. Swelling and stiffness is worse in the morning and may improve after exercise. Usually associated with systemic problems such as fever, malaise and weight loss. Patients may have extra-articular symptoms including eye redness or pain, skin nodules or fibrosis of the lungs. May have a FHx of disease and raised ESR, CRP and +ve Rh Factor |
| **SLE** | Autoimmune connective tissue disease that causes inflammation in multiple organs including the skin, kidneys, heart, vessels and liver. 10x more common in women than men. Characteristically patients have a butterfly facial rash, tiredness and muscle pain |
| **Osteoarthritis** | Progressive unilateral or bilateral pain and degeneration usually in the weight bearing joints of the body (knee, hip) but may also affect the hand, feet, ankles and spine. Pain increased with activity and reduced with rest. Patient may be obese and are usually in their middle-ages. Previous falls or trauma may accelerate the development of OA. OE: patients may have crepitus and knobbly joints |
| **Gout** | Unilateral joint pain usually due to raised uric acid levels. May be as a result of diet rich in purines (kidney, offal, scrimp, quorn) or poor hydration or fluid intake |

**EXPLANATIONS**

*Rheumatoid Arthritis*   RA refers to a chronic condition that causes pain and swelling mainly of the hands and feet. It is a disease whereby the body's defense system attacks the lining of the joints causing swelling, pain and stiffness.

*Osteoarthritis*   This refers to the wear and tear of the joint(s) over time. We do not always know what triggers it, but it seems that with increased usage and perhaps previous falls or injury, this leads to localized stiffness and inflammation that slowly wears away the shock absorbing pads that helps the joints move freely. The weaker and thinner the cartilage get, the more pain you feel and the more restricted the movement.

*SLE*   Systemic Lupus Erythematosus is a condition where the body's defense system attacks some of the tissues of the body causing swelling (inflammation) and pain. We don't always know what starts it, but when it begins it usually causes inflammation in the skin giving rise to a face rash, joint swelling and pain and in the kidney.

*Gout*   Gout is a condition caused by a buildup of crystals within the joint space. These crystals irritate the joint causing pain and discomfort. They are usually made up of a chemical known as uric acid that is normally found in your blood. However, certain foods and drinks can cause these levels to rise and cause painful flare ups.

Back pain is a common complaint that affects 8 out of 10 people at some point in their life. Most cases of back pain are fairly innocuous, mainly caused due to muscle sprain or poor posture. However, a minority of cases may have a serious underlying cause and require immediate intervention to prevent permanent nerve damage (cauda equina).

## HISTORY

| | |
|---|---|
| **Open questions** | How can I help you today? Tell me more about the problems you are having with your back |

**Focused questions**

| | |
|---|---|
| *Back pain* | Is there any pain or tenderness in your back? When did it first start? |
| Site | Can you point to it? |
| Character | What does the pain feel like? (burning, sharp, aching) |
| Frequency | Is it always there or does it come and go? Does anything make the pain better (medications, rest) or worse (bending, walking)? Is it worse during the day or at night? |
| Radiate | Does the pain move anywhere? (hip, foot) |
| Stiffness | Have you had any stiffness of the joints? Is it worse in the morning (RA) or evening (OA)? |
| Injury | Have you had a fall or injured your back recently? |
| Trigger | Were you carrying or lifting anything heavy at the time? Were you involved in an RTA? |

| | |
|---|---|
| **RED FLAGS** | Severe night pain, thoracic pain, <20yrs or >50yrs, PMHx cancer, fever, saddle paraesthesia, urinary retention or incontinence, faecal incontinence, leg weakness (cauda equina) |

| | |
|---|---|
| **YELLOW FLAGS** | Psychological causes that turn acute back pain into a chronic disability financial / relationship problems, anxieties, stress, social withdrawal |

**Associated history**

| | |
|---|---|
| *Neurology* | Do you get any weakness, numbness or pins & needles affecting your legs? |
| *Fever* | Have you noticed any fever or sweats? Have you felt any rigors? |
| *Function* | Do you have problems when walking up and down stairs? How far can you walk before you experience pain? Are you able to dress yourself or put your shoes or socks on without pain? |

**Differentials**

| | |
|---|---|
| *Reactive Arthritis* | Have you had any eye pain (conjunctivitis, iritis) or discharge (urethral)? Are there any other joints affected (ankle, feet)? |
| *Ankylosing Spond.* | Have you had any neck pain? Do you have pain over your hips? Do you have stiffness in the morning? Any eye symptoms (uveitis)? |
| *Metastasis* | Have you lost any weight? Have you had night sweats? Have you had prostatic cancer or breast cancer before? |
| *Cauda equina* | Have you lost any feeling around the groin area (buttock, back of thighs)? Have you lost control of your bladder or bowels? |

## PAST HISTORY

| | |
|---|---|
| *Medical* | Have you ever suffered from any medical conditions? Have you had any cancers in the past? |
| *Surgery* | Have you had any previous operations? |

## DRUG HISTORY

| | |
|---|---|
| *Medication* | Are you taking any medications (steroids)? Are you taking any OTC painkillers (NSAIDs, paracetamol, topical gels)? |

## SOCIAL HISTORY

| | |
|---|---|
| *Support network* | Who lives with you at home? |
| *Occupation* | Are you currently working? Has the pain affected you at work? (delivery, builder, IT) |
| *Smoker* | Do you smoke? How many cigarettes do you smoke per day? |
| *Alcohol* | Do you drink alcohol? How much do you drink and how often? |

## IDEA, CONCERNS, EXPECTATIONS

| | |
|---|---|
| *Ideas* | Have you had any thoughts what may be causing your back pain? |
| *Concerns* | Do you have any worries about the pain you have been experiencing? (time off work) |
| *Expectations* | How did you think I could help you today? (MRI) |
| *Impact* | How have the symptoms affected your life? |

## CSA TIPS

Back pain can be a worrying symptom for patients. They may be seriously affected as a result and subsequently have taken long periods off work. Patients should be examined to ensure that there are no red flags symptoms and then a clear management plan developed. Back pain is the single most common cause for time off work and it is essential to discuss the prognosis with the patient.

## PHYSICAL EXAMINATION

| | |
|---|---|
| *Vitals* | Temp, BP, pulse |
| *Look* | Request patient to undress to their undergarments (chaperone). Observe gait (antalgic). Inspect for deformity (kyphos, kyphosis, scoliosis, loss of lumbar lordosis), asymmetry (shoulder, pelvis), wasting (paravertebral, gluteal) |
| *Feel* | Check temperature and for tenderness. Palpate the spine over the spinous processes, paraspinal muscles and sacro iliac joints |
| *Move* | |
|    Extension | Request patient to lean backwards as far as they can |
|    Flexion | Advise to touch their toes while keeping their knees straight |
|    Lat. flexion | Ask to slide their hand down their leg |
|    Rotation | Hold firm the pelvis and ask patient to rotate thorax |
| *Special tests* | |
|    SLR | Have patient lying supine, lift foot off the couch keeping the leg straight. Note the angle when pain starts (sciatica 30 - 70 degrees) |
| *Neurology* | |
|    Power | Ask the patient to 'walk on their heels' – foot dorsiflexion, (L4/5) |
| | Ask the patient to 'walk on their toes' – foot plantar flexion, (L5/S1) |
|    Sensation | Perform a sensory examination if reports altered or loss of sensation |

| Reflexes | Focused reflex assessment depending on history. Sciatic pain radiating to foot perform ankle reflex (S1). If pain only radiates to thigh perform knee reflex (L3/L4). PR only indicated if cauda equina suspected |
|---|---|

## Neurological Signs of Back Pain based on Nerve Root

| Root | Sensory loss | Weakness | Reflex loss | Special test |
|---|---|---|---|---|
| L3 | Inner thigh | Knee extension | Knee | +ve femoral stretch test |
| L4 | Ant. knee | Knee ext. + foot dorsiflexion | Knee | +ve femoral stretch test |
| L5 | Dorsum foot | Foot + big toe dorsiflexion | None | +ve sciatic stretch test |
| S1 | Lateral foot | Foot plantarflexion | Ankle | +ve sciatic stretch test |

## INVESTIGATIONS

| Bloods | FBC, ESR, ANA, Rh. factor to exclude inflammatory arthritis (AS), bone profile, PSA (elderly), Vit D (low, worsens pain) |
|---|---|
| Other | HLA B27, IgA for AS, performed in secondary care |
| X-ray | Not routinely done in non-specific back pain. Young (sacroiliac joints – AS), elderly (vertebral collapse), trauma |
| MRI | Consider for malignancy, infection, cauda equina, fracture |
| Bone scan | DEXA scan for osteoporosis |

## MANAGEMENT
### Conservative

| Avoid rest | Avoid prolonged bed rest and return to normal activities (including work) as soon as possible. Avoid unsupported sitting or heavy lifting. Increase physical activities over a few days or weeks |
|---|---|
| Ice / Heat | Apply an ice or heat pack if worsened after activity |
| Daily activities | Sit down for chores (ironing, cooking), avoid lifting and carrying heavy objects, place a pillow in between the knees when sleeping on one side, prop up the legs and knees when lying in bed |
| Self help | Can contact self help groups: 'Backcare - The National Back Pain Association' |
| Exercises | If not returned to normal activities structured exercise programmes should be considered |

### Medical
Pain

| Simple | Simple analgesia (paracetamol) or NSAIDs can be prescribed as topical creams or oral. Ensure no CI for NSAIDS (ulcers, gastritis or asthma). Add PPI in the elderly |
|---|---|
| Strong | Consider weak opioid (co-dydramol, co-codamol) or tramadol, TCA (amitriptyline) if others fail. Strong opioids for short period only. Consider laxatives for constipation |
| Muscle relaxant | Consider diazepam if back muscles spasm for short period only |
| Sick Certificate | Offer short fit-note if unable to work. Consider amended duties or altered hours if finding it difficult to carry out certain tasks (bending, lifting) |

### Referral

| Manipulation | Considered within first 6 weeks for those requiring not returning to normal activities (chiropractor, osteopath) |
|---|---|
| Physio | Physiotherapy helpful in strengthening the muscles around the back. Can prescribe walking-aids, ZF, wheelchair if severe dysfunction |

| | |
|---|---|
| OT | Speak to an OT about adaptations that can be made for occupational induced back pain (ergonomic chairs) |
| CBT | If associated with stress or low mood |
| Acupuncture | Limited availability on NHS (chronic back pain) |
| Pain Clinic | Consider referring to MSK or pain clinic to maximise treatment or offer epidural / facet-joint injections |
| Orthopaedics | Refer if symptoms have rapidly deteriorated or is causing disability |
| Rheumatology | If suspecting AS refer for assessment and ophthalmologist urgently if anterior uveitis becomes painful, photophobia |
| 2WW | If suspecting back secondaries from cancer |
| Admit | Cauda equina symptoms refer immediately |

## SAFETY NETTING

| | |
|---|---|
| Follow up | Review in 4-6wks for response to treatment or urgently if red flag symptoms |

## DIFFERENTIAL DIAGNOSIS

| Conditions | Characteristic exam feature |
|---|---|
| Spondylosis | OA of the spine, and damage to the discs. Causes hypertrophy of the superior articular processes of the spinal bodies and may cause osteophyte formation. Gives rise to lower back pain that may radiate to the buttocks |
| Sciatica | Disc pressing on the sciatic nerve due to degeneration and bulging. Can be caused by strenuous activity (lifting). Causes electric shock like pain from the lower back to the ipsilateral leg. May be bilateral. May also cause numbness in affected dermatomes and foot drop and loss of reflexes if chronic. Reduced SLR |
| Ankylosing spondylitis | Chronic inflammatory rheumatic disease commonly affecting caucasian young males. Associated with FHx (HLA B27). Presents with insidious onset of morning back pain & stiffness worsened with inactivity, fatigue. OE: reduced ROM back, tender sacroiliac joints, loss of lumbar lordosis, kyphosis, achilles tendonitis, atlantoaxial subluxation. Extra articular involvement include aortic regurgitation, pulmonary fibrosis, anterior uveitis, amyloidosis |
| Spinal cord compression from mets | Can present in cancer patients often affects thoracic region. Presents with back pain worse on movement, weakness of legs. If lesion above L1 may have UMN signs (increase tone, reflexes) with sensory level. If below L1 presents with LMN signs (reduce tone, reflexes) and perianal numbness (cauda equina) |
| Spinal Stenosis | Narrowing of the spinal canal may be congenital or due to acquired spondylolisthesis. Causes bilateral calf pain, tingling and numbness in the legs when walking |
| Cauda Equina | Emergency condition that requires urgent admission to prevent permanent damage. Compression of spinal nerve roots causing lower back pain, bladder and bowel incontinence with saddle anaesthesia |

| Discitis | Infection of a spinal disc. Causes fever, severe back pain and focal tenderness |
|---|---|

**EXPLANATIONS**

*Mechanical Back pain*  Most causes of back pain are not due to a serious problem and are usually due to muscle or stretched ligaments. We do not always find out the reason for this type of pain, but they usually improve within 6 weeks with simple pain relief and stretches.

*Spondylosis*  This refers to the wear and tear of the spine joint over time. We do not always know what triggers it, but it seems that with increased usage and perhaps previous falls or injury, this causes localized stiffness and inflammation that slowly wears away the shock absorbing discs that helps the spine move freely. The weaker and thinner the disc gets, the more pain you feel and the more restricted the movement.

*Sciatica*  This is caused when a disc that lies in between the bony spine is loosened and catches on one of the nerves that comes out. The disc causes irritation and pressure on a nerve called the sciatic nerve that runs down from your lower back down to the foot.

*Cauda Equina*  This is when there is compression or continuous pressure on the lower spinal nerves that leads to symptoms such as having problems passing urine or bowel motions and causes severe back pain. This is sometimes due to a slipped disc and we will need to send you urgently to hospital to ensure that no permanent damage takes place.

*Ankylosing spondylitis*  Ankylosing spondylitis is a type of arthritis that causes inflammation of the rubber bands (ligaments) of the spine. Over time these harden and encourage bony growths that form bridges between the bones of the spine (vertebrae) that later fuse together and reduces movement making your back straighter.

# 11.7 Hip pain

Hip pain is a common complaint that usually worsens with ageing. The most common cause is due to osteoarthritis which may be exacerbated due to a previous fall or trauma. However, when examining a patient other serious causes must be excluded such as hip fracture or avascular necrosis of the head of the femur. Pain felt in the hip joint may not necessarily be as a result of the structures of the hip; back pain and psoas abscess problems may radiate to the hip and cause diagnostic confusion if you are not careful. Similarly, problems with the hip do not necessarily present with symptoms in the hip, rather hip pain may radiate to the knee, groin, thigh or buttocks.

## HISTORY

| | |
|---|---|
| **Open questions** | How can I help you today? Tell me more about the problems you are having with your hip |

## Focused questions

| | |
|---|---|
| *Hip pain* | Is there any pain or tenderness in your hip? When did it start? |
| Site | Does it affect one or both hips? Can you point to it? |
| Character | What does the pain feel like? (burning, stinging, sharp, aching, boring) |
| Frequency | Is it always there (malignancy) or does it come and go? Does anything make the pain better (medications, rest) or worse (movements, walking)? |
| Radiate | Does the pain move anywhere (anterolateral thigh, buttock, knee) or does it stay in one place? |
| Swelling | Has you noticed any swelling? |
| Stiffness | Have you had any stiffness of the joint? Is it worse in the morning (RA) or evening (OA)? |
| Other | Do you have any back pain (referred)? Do you feel a grinding noise when walking (hip crepitus)? |

## RED FLAGS

Fever or sweats (septic arthritis), trauma (fracture), weight loss (malignancy), acute & sudden onset night pain (AVN of femoral head)

## Associated history

| | |
|---|---|
| *Movements* | Do you have problems when standing from a seated position? Or when walking up and down stairs? Do you get pain when bending down to put your shoes and socks on? Do you get pain when turning? |
| *Fall* | Have you had a fall recently? |
| *Weight loss* | Have you lost any weight? |
| *Fever* | Have you noticed any fever, temperature or sweats? Have you felt any rigors? |

## Differentials

| | |
|---|---|
| *Back Pain* | Do you have any back pain? Does the pain move down the leg? Do you have numbness or tingling in your thigh or legs? |
| *Abdominal* | Do you have any abdominal pain? Any nausea, vomiting or diarrhoea? Have you had any change in bowel habits? |
| *Periph. Vasc. Dis.* | How far can you walk before you get the pain? |

## PAST HISTORY

| | |
|---|---|
| *Medical* | Have you ever suffered from any medical conditions (RA, SLE)? Are you currently pregnant (pubic symphysis dysfunction)? |
| *Hip* | Did you ever suffer a dislocation or fracture to your hip before (AVN)? Have you ever had joint surgery or a hip replacement? |

## DRUG HISTORY

| | |
|---|---|
| *Medication* | Are you taking any medications (steroids)? Are you taking any painkillers (NSAIDs, paracetamol, topical gels)? |

## SOCIAL HISTORY

| | |
|---|---|
| *Support network* | Who lives with you at home? Do you have any close friends or family? |
| Carers | Do you have any carers? Are they helping you doing day-to-day tasks? |
| *Occupation* | Are you currently working? Has the pain affected you at work? |
| *Leisure* | Is your hip pain affecting you from performing hobbies or leisure activities you are usually accustomed to? |
| *Smoker* | Do you smoke? How many cigarettes do you smoke per day? |
| *Alcohol* | Do you drink alcohol? How much do you drink and how often? |

## IDEA, CONCERNS, EXPECTATIONS

| | |
|---|---|
| *Ideas* | Have you had any thoughts what may be causing your hip pain? |
| *Concerns* | Do you have any worries about the pain you have been experiencing? |
| *Expectations* | How did you think I could help you today? |
| *Impact* | How have the symptoms affected your life? |

## CSA TIPS

Patients with hip pain may present with severe disability and dysfunction as a result. If they are living alone in a 3rd floor flat with no lift access, they may be struggling with their daily activities such as shopping, cooking or transferring to and from the toilet. Although addressing the pain would be an important component, the patient's social circumstances may cause a deterioration in their health and may actually be the nub of the consultation.

## PHYSICAL EXAMINATION

| | |
|---|---|
| *Vitals* | Temp, BP, pulse |
| *Look (gait)* | Ask the patient to walk from one end of the room to other. Inspect for antalgic gait (limp), Trendelenburg's gait (pelvis tilts down to opposite side), short leg gait |
| *Measure* | Have patient lying flat on couch. Square hips then measure from umbilicus to both medial malleolus (apparent) then from ASIS to medial malleolus (true). Inequality suggest limb shortening (fracture) |
| *Feel* | Locate the pain before starting. Palpate for tenderness over greater trochanter (bursitis) and for joint tenderness (distal to midpoint of inguinal ligament) |
| *Move* | |
| Flexion | Flex the patient's knees as far as possible (130 degrees) |
| Rotation | Have the hip and knee flexed at 90 degrees whilst steering the foot laterally for internal rotation of the hip and medially for external rotation |
| Abd/adduction | Place one hand on the opposite iliac crest to monitor for pelvic movement. Hold patient's calf in other hand and abduct hip. Adduct hip by crossing the leg over |

| | |
|---|---|
| *Special tests* | Consider if indicated by the history |
| Thomas's test | Have one hand under the patient's lumbar spine. Flex one knee as far as possible and observe the contralateral leg. If the leg is elevated and cannot be fully extended this is positive for fixed flexion deformity of the affected side (OA) |
| Trendelenburg's | Ask the patient to stand on one foot whilst raising the opposite foot off the ground. Place your hands on the ASIS and check for pelvic tilting/saging on unsupported side (positive sign). Common cause is hip pain and weakness to gluteus medius |

## INVESTIGATIONS

| | |
|---|---|
| *Bloods* | Not routinely needed unless suspect septic arthritis / psoas abscess. Hb, WCC, CRP, ESR, Rh Factor |
| *Hip / Pelvic Xray* | To exclude fracture, AVN of the femoral head. To check for position of previous hip replacements |
| *US / MRI* | To look for micro-fractures, tendonitis, bursitis, psoas abscess |

## MANAGEMENT
### Conservative

| | |
|---|---|
| *Diet* | Advise a healthy diet rich in omega-3 fatty acids with fresh fish, fruit and veg |
| *Rest* | If pain is due to repetitive movements advise to rest for up to 12wks |
| *Ice / Heat* | Apply an ice or heat pack if worsened after activity |
| *Splint* | Consider purchasing a splint or clasp to reduce the pressure on the joint / tendon |
| *Exercise* | Continue simple exercises (aerobic/muscle strengthening) as the pain eases to help maintain and improve your ROM and prevent stiffness |
| *OA* | If BMI>25 suggest losing weight as put less pressure on joints. Suggest heel raise for unequal leg lengths. Consider TENS |
| *Other* | *Meralgia paraesthetica:* Avoid corsets & tight belts, TEN<br>*Pubic Symphysis dysfunc:* Sit down for chores (ironing, cooking), avoid lifting and carrying, place a pillow in between the legs when in bed, try and avoid twisting or straddling movements |

### Medical

| | |
|---|---|
| *Pain* | Simple analgesia (paracetamol, codeine) or NSAIDs can be prescribed as topical creams or oral. Ensure no CI for NSAIDS (ulcers, gastritis or asthma). Add PPI in the elderly. Avoid glucosamine for pain relief (OA: poor evidence) |
| *Infection* | In septic arthritis needs orthopaedic admission for IV Abx and drainage |
| *Sick Certificate* | Offer short fit-note if unable to work. Consider amended duties or altered hours if finding it difficult to carry out certain tasks |

### Referral

| | |
|---|---|
| *Physio* | Physiotherapy helpful in strengthening the muscles around the hip. Can prescribe walking-aids, ZF, wheelchair if severe dysfunction |
| *OT* | Speak to an OT about adaptations that can be made to house such as sock aids, walk-in showers, raised chairs, stair lift or rails |
| *Injection* | Persistent pain may warrant steroid or local anaesthetic injections to reduce the pain and inflammation in the joint for the short term |
| SE | Pain on injecting, atrophy or liponecrosis, loss of colour of the skin or damage to the tendons |
| *Orthopaedics* | Refer if symptoms have rapidly deteriorated or is causing disability impacting on QoL. Often total hip replacement recommended for end stage osteoarthritis |

| | |
|---|---|
| Other | *Pubic Symphysis Dysfunction:* Epidurals considered during pregnancy. *Avascular Necrosis:* Arthroplasty, osteotomy or arthrodesis |

**SAFETY NETTING**

| | |
|---|---|
| *Follow up* | Review in 4-6wks for response to treatment |

**DIFFERENTIAL DIAGNOSIS**

| Conditions | Characteristic exam feature |
|---|---|
| **Osteoarthritis** | Progressive unilateral or bilateral pain in the groin or buttocks with radiation to the knee. Pain increased with activity and reduced with rest. Patient may be obese. Patient may have a limp and find problems getting out of a chair / car. OE: antalgic gait, +ve trendelenburg sign, apparent limb shortening, reduction of internal rotation noted (early) and fixed flexion of hip |
| **Greater Trochanteric Pain Syndrome** | Common, self-limiting causing lateral hip pain and more common in women and >40yrs. Sharp, intense, outer thigh pain, worse on lying on affected side, prolonged standing, running. OE: pain on the greater trochanter and a +ve Trendelenberg test |
| **Meralgia paraesthetica** | Caused by compression of lateral cutaneous nerve of thigh through inguinal ligament or fascia lata. Presents with burning, stinging sensation over (antero-lateral) thigh made worse by standing or walking. OE: pain on hip extensions and paraesthesia over lateral aspect of thigh. Risk factors include surgery, pregnancy, obesity, DM & others (sports, tight trousers, seat belts) |
| **Pubic Symphysis Dysfunction** | Occurs in late pregnancy or post childbirth. Pain in the pelvic region usually at the front of the pelvis but can radiate to groin, and medial aspect of thighs. Can worsen through pregnancy and with movement. Causes waddling gait and problems walking up stairs |
| **Avascular Necrosis** | Hip pain usually sudden onset and unilateral. May be severe enough to cause night time pain. Patient walks with a limp and may have continuous pain. Risk factors include steroids, SLE, Sickle cell disease, excess alcohol |
| **Psoas Abscess** | Unilateral pain and swelling associated with fever and malaise |

**EXPLANATIONS**

| | |
|---|---|
| *Osteoarthritis* | This refers to the wear and tear of the hip joint over time. We do not always know what triggers it, but it seems that with increased usage and perhaps previous falls or injury, this causes localized stiffness and inflammation that slowly wears away the shock absorbing cartilage that helps the joint move freely. The weaker and thinner the cartilage get, the more pain you feel and the more restricted the movement. |
| *Trochanteric Pain* | Greater trochanteric pain syndrome is a musculoskeletal condition that causes a burning pain that affects the side of your thigh. It is often caused by an injury you |

previously had or some irritation over the bony prominence at the top of the thigh bone, surrounding tendons, muscles or joint.

*Meralgia paraesth.*   Meralgia paraesthetica is a condition that is caused by trapped or pressure of one of the nerves of the thigh which supplies feeling to the outer part of it. As a result it gives you burning or tingling feeling over that area.

*Pubic Symphysis Dys.*   Symphysis pubic pain is pain felt over the groin area often in late pregnancy. It is believed to be caused by softening of the rubber bands (ligament) around the pubic bone in front of the bladder caused by the hormonal changes in pregnancy. As a result the bones can separate a little and rub together giving rise to pain.

*Avascular Necrosis*   Avascular necrosis of the femur is a medical term that describes the process by which the bony head of the leg bone gets reduced blood supply and begins to breakdown and eventually die. There are a number of causes, but sometimes it is due to medicines you take like steroids. It could also be due to excess alcohol use and may also occur in a fracture or dislocation of the thigh bone.

# 11.8 Knee pain

Knee pain is a common symptom that patients may present with. It may be acute or more commonly, as a chronic worsening condition in the middle-aged. Acute causes include sprain or trauma and chronic causes include osteoarthritis. The knee joint is a hinge joint between three bones, the femur, tibia and fibula with the patella also providing an articulation point. The joint also consists of 2 menisci, 2 cruciate ligaments and 2 collateral ligaments. Damage or overuse of any of these components may cause pain and stiffness.

## HISTORY

| | |
|---|---|
| **Open questions** | How can I help you today? Tell me more about the problems you are having with your knee |

### Focused questions

| | |
|---|---|
| *Knee pain* | Is there any pain or tenderness in your knee? When did it start? |
| Site | Does it affect one or both knee? Can you point to it? |
| Character | What does the pain feel like? (burning, sharp, aching) |
| Frequency | Is it always there or does it come and go? Does anything make the pain better (medications, rest) or worse (movements, walking)? |
| Radiate | Does the pain move anywhere (hip) or does it stay in one place? |
| Injury | Have you injured your knee recently? Were you playing sports when it started? What happened (snap)? Are you always bending down on your knees at work (carpenter)? |
| Swelling | Has you noticed any swelling? Did it occur after an injury? How long after did it occur (rapidly - lig. rupture, hours after - torn meniscus/lig. sprain)? |
| Stiffness | Have you had any stiffness of the joint? Is it worse in the morning (RA) or evening (OA)? |
| Locking | Does it ever lock whereby you cannot fully straighten it? (meniscal tear) |
| Give way | Does it ever give way when you are walking? (meniscal tear, patella dislocation, torn ligament) |

---

### Causes of knee pain by location

| | |
|---|---|
| *Anterior knee* | |
| Patella tendon | Osgood-Schlatter, patella tendonitis or rupture |
| Patella | Chondromalacia, OA, Bipartite patella, osteochondritis dissecans, stress fracture |
| Intra-articular | Meniscal tear, prepatellar bursitis |
| *Medial knee* | Collateral ligament sprain, medial meniscal tear |
| *Lateral knee* | Collateral ligament sprain, lateral meniscal tear, iliotibial band tendonitis |
| *Posterior knee* | Baker's cyst (popliteal), posterior cruciate ligament tear/injury |

---

| **RED FLAGS** | Fever or sweats (septic arthritis), trauma (fracture) |
|---|---|

### Associated history

| | |
|---|---|
| *Function* | Do you have problems when walking up and down stairs? How far can you walk before you experience pain? |
| *Fever* | Have you noticed any fever or sweats? Have you felt any rigors? |

## Differentials

*Reactive Arthritis*    Have you had any eye pain (conjunctivitis, iritis) or discharge (urethral)? Are there any other joints affected (ankle, feet)?

## PAST HISTORY

*Medical*    Have you ever suffered from any medical conditions?

*Knee*    Did you ever suffer a patella dislocation or fracture before? Have you ever had joint surgery or a knee replacement?

## DRUG HISTORY

*Medication*    Are you taking any medications (steroids)? Are you taking any painkillers (NSAIDs, paracetamol, topical gels)?

## SOCIAL HISTORY

*Support network*    Who lives with you at home? Do you have any close friends or family?

Carers    Do you have any carers? Are they helping you doing day to day tasks?

*Occupation*    Are you currently working? Has the pain affected you at work (carpet layer, roofer)?

*Leisure*    Is your knee pain preventing you from performing hobbies or leisure activities you are usually accustomed to (football, rugby, running)?

*Smoker*    Do you smoke? How many cigarettes do you smoke per day?

*Alcohol*    Do you drink alcohol? How much do you drink and how often?

## IDEA, CONCERNS, EXPECTATIONS

*Ideas*    Have you had any thoughts what may be causing your knee pain?

*Concerns*    Do you have any worries about the pain you have been experiencing?

*Expectations*    How did you think I could help you today?

*Impact*    How have the symptoms affected your life?

## CSA TIPS

Patients suffering with knee pain may attend the surgery to seek a diagnosis and prognosis about when things will return to normality. Patients who are young and athletic should be asked about recent trauma or sporting accidents. A clear mechanism of how the injury was resulted may point to the affected part of the knee (meniscal or ligamental damage). In the elderly, knee pain is usually due to severe OA and may be causing significant functional problems. You may need to broach the subject about a referral for surgical replacement in such cases.

## PHYSICAL EXAMINATION

*Vitals*    Temp, BP, pulse

*Look*    Observe the patient standing for deformity (valgus/varus, fixed flexion), muscle wasting (quadriceps), scars or effusion. Ask patient to walk from one end of the room to other (antalgic gait)

*Feel*    Check temperature and for tenderness. Palpate the joint line with knee flexed (ligaments, bony landmarks, tibial tuberosity, femoral condyles). With knee extended, feel the patella and popliteal fossa (Baker's cyst)

Patella tap test    Palpate for effusions by sliding your hand over the suprapatellar pouch forcing the effusion below the patella. Tap the patella with your index finger (contralateral hand). With a moderate effusion, the patella bounces up

*Move*

    Flexion/Ext           Check for active and passive flexion & extension of the knee

*Special tests*         Consider if indicated by the history

    Collateral           Hold the ankle in one hand and knee with the other. Apply valgus force by steering leg medially (medial ligament) then varus pressure by moving leg laterally (lat. ligament)

    Cruciate            Perform Drawer's test by sitting on side of foot. Hold knee with thumbs over tibial tuberosity and fingers within the popliteal fossa. Check for lag by pulling forward (ACL tear) or push backwards (PCL tear)

    Meniscal           *McMurray's test:* Warn the patient that it may cause pain. Flex the knee as far as possible. Externally rotate the foot and slowly extend knee with lateral force (medial meniscus). Repeat but internally rotate foot, extend with medial force (lateral meniscus)

## INVESTIGATIONS

*Bloods*              Not routinely needed

    Other              Hb, WCC, CRP, ESR, Uric Acid (gout), blood & joint cultures if infection

*Knee Xray*          Do AP/Lat and Skyline views to exclude fracture and look for OA or haemarthrosis

---

**Ottawa Rules regarding Knee X-rays**

Consider X-ray of the knee to exclude a fracture if 1 or more:

- Aged =>55
- Tenderness at the head of the fibula or isolated tenderness to patella
- Inability to flex knee to 90 degrees or inability to walk 4 steps at time of injury

---

*MRI*               To look for meniscal and tendon injuries, bursitis

*Aspiration*        Often done in secondary care. Joint aspiration & send for serology if swelling present

## MANAGEMENT

**Conservative**

*Rest*               If pain is to due to repetitive movements advise to rest for up to 12 wks

*Ice / Heat*         Apply an ice or heat pack if worsened after activity

*Support*          Consider purchasing a knee support

*Exercise*         Continue simple exercises (aerobic/muscle strengthening) as the pain eases to help maintain and improve your ROM and prevent stiffness

*Weight*           If BMI>25 suggest losing weight

*Insole*            Suggest purchasing insoles

*Housemaid's Knee*  Use cushions or knee pads if kneeling down

**Medical**

*Pain*               Simple analgesia (paracetamol, codeine) or NSAIDs can be prescribed as topical creams or oral. Ensure no CI for NSAIDS (ulcers, gastritis or asthma). Add PPI in the elderly. Avoid glucosamine for pain relief (OA)

*Infection*        In septic arthritis needs orthopaedic admission for IV Abx and drainage

*Sick Certificate*    Offer short fit-note if unable to work. Consider amended duties or altered hours if finding it difficult to carry out certain tasks

## Referral

| | |
|---|---|
| Physio | Physiotherapy helpful in strengthening the muscles around the knee. Can prescribe walking-aids, ZF, wheelchair if severe dysfunction |
| OT | Speak to an OT about adaptations that can be made to house such as stair lift or rails |
| Injection | Persistent pain may warrant steroid or local anaesthetic injections to reduce the pain and inflammation in the joint for the short term |
| SE | Pain on injecting, atrophy, liponecrosis, skin colour loss or damage to the tendons |
| Orthopaedics | Refer if symptoms have rapidly deteriorated or is causing disability impacting on QoL. Often total knee replacement recommended for end stage osteoarthritis |

## SAFETY NETTING

| | |
|---|---|
| Follow up | Review in 4-6wks for response to treatment |

## DIFFERENTIAL DIAGNOSIS

| Conditions | Characteristic exam feature |
|---|---|
| Osteoarthritis | Progressive worsening of knee pain, may be unilateral or bilateral. Pain increased with activity and reduced with rest. Patient may be obese and have slight stiffness in the morning. OE: crepitus, anterior knee effusion and joint line tenderness |
| Meniscal Tear | Damage to the menisci which stabilises joint. Often caused by twisting sprain whilst flexed (sports) causing knee pain, locking of the knee (particularly extension), giving way with effusion several hours later. OE: localised joint pain (medial/lateral), limited extension, +ve McMurrays or Apley's test |
| Osgood-Schlatters Syndrome | Inflammation of the tibial tubercle due to overuse. Common in teenager boys doing sports. Experience pain below the patella worse during exercise and improves with rest. Settles after 2-3 mth. OE: tender bony lump below patella |
| Housemaid's Knee | Prepatellar bursitis caused by chronic friction (bending on knees) seen in carpet fitters. Presents with knee swelling and pain worse on extreme flexion. |
| Patellofemoral Pain | Common cause of knee pain affecting young adults. Anterior dull and aching pain that is gradual in onset. Usually bilateral and may have swelling and crepitus. Patients notice worsening of symptoms when descending the stairs along with a feeling of instability or giving way |
| Ligament Injury | Damage to ligaments that support the knee from injury (sports). Causes pain, effusions and knee joint instability and snapping sound at time of injury. *ACL:* Due to sudden change in direction. Lachman +ve and anterior drawer test +ve. *PCL:* Due to blow to tibia after a fall on flexed knee or RTA. Posterior knee pain. Posterior Drawer test +ve *Medial Collateral:* Twisting injury or lateral blow to knee. Tender medial joint line. Valgus stress test +ve. *Lateral Collateral:* Twisting injury or medial blow to knee. Tender lateral joint line. Varus stress test +ve |

| | |
|---|---|
| **Chondromalacia patella** | Overuse of the knee (sports) can result in softening of the articular cartilage of the patella. Common in teenage girls. Retropatellar pain worse on standing from prolonged sitting or using stairs. OE: patella tenderness, effusion and crepitus |
| **Baker's cyst** | Fluid filled sac that can cause posterior knee pain and swelling. Is more common in females and may be caused post trauma or due to existing OA. May rupture causing fluid to leak into the calf. OE: tender, transilluminate, smooth swelling is noted in the popliteal area which is present on extension of the knee and can disappear on flexion |

**EXPLANATIONS**

*Osteoarthritis*  This refers to the wear and tear of the knee joint over time. We do not always know what triggers it, but it seems with increased usage and perhaps previous falls or injury, this gives rise to localized stiffness and inflammation that slowly wears away the shock absorbing cartilage that helps the joint move freely. The weaker and thinner the cartilage gets, the more pain you feel and the more restricted the movement.

*Meniscal Tear*  You have 2 menisci made out of cartilage in the knee joint. They act as shock absorbers for the knee and aid in cushioning and supporting the joint. They can be damaged during a violent turning motion particularly when playing sports or they may become more brittle and weak with everyday use. As a result you may get pain, swelling and the feeling of locking whereby you cannot fully open your knee due to an obstruction.

*Ligament injuries*  There are 4 strong ligaments or rubber bands that connect the bones of the knees together and keep it stable. After a serious injury these can be stretched (sprain) or torn (ruptured) and give you pain and instability of the joint.

*Patellar tendinitis*  This is where there is inflammation of the rubber-band (tendon) that connects the muscle to the knee cap itself.

*Osgood-Schlatter's*  This is where the bony protrusion of the upper part of the shin bone become inflamed. It can cause pain and swelling that settles with time.

*Chondromalacia p.*  Chondromalacia patella is a condition where there is softening and wear & tear to the lining (cartilage) of the undersurface of the knee cap.

*Housemaid's Knee*  This is due to the inflammation of a small sac that lies just over the knee cap at the front of your knee. Its job is to help the joint move well; however, because of repetitive friction or irritation it can become inflammed and irritated, particularly if you are constantly kneeling due to work.

*Baker's cyst*  This is a fluid filled swelling that is noticed behind the knee joint. It may come up for no reason, but may be because of an injury or due to wear and tear of the joint.

# 11.9 Ankle & foot pain

Foot pain is a common problem that patients may present with. The foot carries the body's weight and is put through enormous stresses on a daily basis. It is important to consider the different structures that are in the foot that may give rise to pain such as bone, tendons, plantar fascia and ligaments. But also not to forget pain radiating in from outside of the foot such as from the back (sciatica) or the ankle. You should also consider a systemic or metabolic illness that may give rise to foot symptoms such as RA, gout and even causes of a swollen foot such as CCF, CKD, HF. Do not forget that foot problems may be due to poorly fitting shoes or a flattened foot arch.

## HISTORY

**Open questions**

How can I help you today? Tell me more about the problems you are having with your foot

## Focused questions

*Foot pain*  Is there any pain or tenderness in your foot? When did it start?

Site  Does it affect one or both feet? Can you point to it?

Character  What does the pain feel like? (burning, aching, sharp, stinging)

Frequency  Is it always there or does it come and go? Does anything make the pain better (medications, rest) or worse (movements i.e. walking, standing)? Is it worse in the morning (fasciitis) or evening (stress fracture, nerve entrapment)?

Radiate  Does the pain move anywhere? (morton neuroma)

Swelling  Has you noticed any swelling or redness of a toe (gout)? Have you noticed any swelling of the ankle or foot (HF, CKD, postural oedema)?

Stiffness  Have you had any stiffness of the joint?

## RED FLAGS

Fever or sweats (septic arthritis), significant deformity

## Associated history

*Injury*  Did you have a fall? Have you ever injured your foot? (OA)

*Neurology*  Have you had any weakness, numbness or pins & needles in your foot?

*Foot drop*  Have you noticed that your foot drags along the floor?

## Differentials

*Gout*  How severe is the pain ('worse ever')? Have you had any recent injuries? How is your diet (red meat, oily fish)? *See gout chapter*

*Sciatica*  Do you have any shooting pain that starts from your back moving down to your foot?

*Periph. Vasc. Dis.*  How far can you walk before you get the pain? Does your foot feel cold? Do you have an ulcer? *See claudication chapter*

## PAST HISTORY

*Medical*  Have you ever suffered from any medical conditions? (DM, RA, OA, gout)

*Fracture*  Have you had any recent fracture of the foot? (stress)

## FAMILY HISTORY

*Medical*  Do you have any foot problems that run in the family? (pes cavus, toe deformity)

## DRUG HISTORY

| | |
|---|---|
| Medication | Are you taking any medications (NSAIDs, paracetamol, topical gels)? |
| Gout | Are you taking any diuretics (thiazide) or aspirin? |

## SOCIAL HISTORY

| | |
|---|---|
| Occupation | Are you currently in employment (postman, security guards, policeman)? |
| Hobbies | Do you do any hobbies (runner)? |
| Smoker | Do you smoke? How many cigarettes do you smoke per day? |
| Alcohol | Do you drink alcohol? How much do you drink and how often? |
| Drive | Do you drive? |

## IDEA, CONCERNS, EXPECTATIONS

| | |
|---|---|
| Ideas | Have you had any thoughts what may be causing your foot pain? |
| Concerns | Do you have any worries about the pain you have been experiencing? |
| Expectations | How did you think I could help you today? |
| Impact | How have the symptoms affected your life? |

## CSA TIPS

The foot is an extremely important limb. It may show signs of systemic disease or more usually have localised problems causing symptoms such as pain, swelling and numbness. Always enquire about activity (sports, occupation) and examine the footwear the patient presents in. Cases may present with a specific diagnosis (morton neuroma or plantar fasciitis) with your management plan being scrutinised to see whether it is shared and if you offer conservative treatment options.

## PHYSICAL EXAMINATION

| | |
|---|---|
| Look | Examine gait by walking normally then on tip toes. Inspect the shoes for asymmetrical wear. Check for any deformity (pes cavus, planus, hammer or mallet toes, genu valgum or varum). Inspect for any bunions (1st MTP), corns, callosities or skin & nail changes (ingrowing). Look for signs of ulceration around the ankle (PVD) |
| Feel | Squeeze the MTP, midfoot, ankle and subtalar joints and achilles tendon. Feel for temperature and tenderness |
| Pulses | Palpate the peripheral pulses i.e. dorsalis pedis, posterior tibial |
| Move | Check active and passive movement of the ankle, subtalar (inversion, eversion of ankle), midtarsal (fix ankle and move forefoot) and toes |
| Neurological | Check sensation if patients reports any numbness or paraesthesia |
| | |
| Special tests | Perform if clinically indicated from history |
| Mulder's click | *Morton neuroma:* Grip neuroma between forefinger and thumb (plantar surface), squeeze metatarsal heads with other hand. Click can be heard/felt with pressure |
| Windlass test | *Plantar fasciitis:* Reproduced heel pain on extension (passive dorsiflexion) of 1st MTP |

---

### Common Causes of foot pain by location

| | |
|---|---|
| Heel | Sever's disease (young), plantar fasciitis (older), pes cavus, achilles tendonitis |
| Mid foot | Kohler's disease (young), navicular bone), OA (adults), stress fracture |
| Forefoot | Morton neuroma, pes cavus/planus, RA, gout, Freiberg's disease (2nd, 3rd metatarsal heads), March fracture |
| Big toe | Gout (1st MTP) |

---

## INVESTIGATIONS

| | |
|---|---|
| *Bloods* | Not routinely needed unless suspect osteomyelitis, inflammatory arthritis (Hb, WCC, ESR, CRP) or gout (uric acid) |
| *X-ray* | Consider to exclude fracture or arthropathy (e.g. calcaneal spur) |
| *US / MRI* | To look for Morton neuroma |

## MANAGEMENT

### Conservative

| | |
|---|---|
| *Rest* | Have foot elevated where possible |
| *Weight* | Recommend losing weight if BMI >25 |
| *Shoes* | Ensure well fitted, low heeled, wide toed footwear with thick soles |
| *Pad* | *Morton neuroma:* Suggest OTC metatarsal pads or orthotic inserts for shoes which reduces pressure on metatarsal heads |
| *Exercise* | Continue simple exercises as the pain eases to help maintain and improve your range movements and prevent stiffness |
| *Fasciitis* | Avoid walking barefoot or on hard surfaces or prolonged standing. Use ice packs for 15 minutes for pain relief |
| *Orthoses* | Use shoes with cushioned heels and arch supports. Cut a small hole in the pad where heel most tender |
| *Exercise* | Roll a drinks can or tennis ball under the arch of your foot. Tiptoe several times a day. Stand on the edge of the step with heels off the edge. Lower heels down and hold position for 1min then elevate |

### Medical

| | |
|---|---|
| *Pain* | Simple analgesia (paracetamol) or NSAIDs can be prescribed as topical creams or oral. Ensure that the patient has no CI for NSAIDS (ulcers, gastritis or asthma) |
| *Sick Certificate* | Offer short fit-note if unable to work. Consider amended duties or altered hours if finding it difficult to carry out certain tasks |

### Referral

| | |
|---|---|
| *Physio* | Physiotherapy may be helpful in strengthening the muscles and stretch Achilles tendon or plantar fascia. Can reduce stiffness in foot and ankle |
| *OT* | Speak to an OT about adaptations that can be made for occupational induced foot pain (postman, security guards - shoes) |
| *Injection* | Persistent pain may warrant steroid or local anaesthetic injections to reduce the pain and inflammation in the joint for the short term |
| *Surgery* | Neurectomy or decompression of interdigital nerve considered in morton neuromas. Consider plantar fascia release and release of calcaneal spur in plantar fasciitis |

## SAFETY NETTING

| | |
|---|---|
| *Follow up* | Review in 4-6wks for response to treatment |

## DIFFERENTIAL DIAGNOSIS

| Conditions | Characteristic exam feature |
|---|---|
| **Morton Neuroma** | Benign thickening of the plantar interdigital nerve caused by compression. Common in 50yr old women. Presents with forefoot pain (between 3rd/4th MTP) described as |

| | |
|---|---|
| | having a pebble in shoe. Associated with burning or electric shock pain when walking along nerve. OE: pain with pressure over neuroma, mulder's click, loss of sensation of affected toes |
| **Plantar Fasciitis** | Inflammation of the ligamentous insertion of the plantar fascia to the heel. Gradual pain, worse in the morning, in the sole of heel when standing or walking and relieved upon resting. Common in >40yr, sedentary lifestyle, flat shoes, hard surfaces. OE: tenderness over anteromedial aspect of heel, +ve Windlass test |
| **Calcaneal Spur** | Small osteophyte formed on the calcaneus. Associated with plantar fasciitis or Ankylosing Spondylitis. Heel pain worsens after period of prolonged rest with exacerbations from walking or weightbearing |
| **Pes Planus** | Obliteration of the medial arch of the foot. Common in childhood. Often asymptomatic but can present with foot pain after prolonged walking. OE: loss of medial arches with warned out shoes (medial border, outer heel) |
| **Achilles Tendonitis** | Inflammation to the achilles tendon. Often caused by overuse, Ankylosing spondylitis or medication (ciprofloxacin, steroids). Presents with tender and swelling of tendon. Can cause rupture (sudden pain, gap in tendon) with foot drop |
| **Tarsal Tunnel Syndrome** | Known as posterior tibial neuralgia where the tibial nerve is compressed in the tarsal tunnel. Causes pain & numbness in the foot especially of the big toe & adjacent 3 toes |

## EXPLANATIONS

*Morton neuroma*

Morton's neuroma is a condition that affects one of the nerves between your 3rd and 4th toes. Often after standing or walking for a long period of time, the nerve can thicken (fibrosis) and form a swelling (neuroma) that gets irritated and causes your symptoms.

*Plantar fasciitis*

Plantar fasciitis is caused by inflammation of the strong rubber band (ligament) that runs along the sole of the foot and stretches from your heel to your middle foot bones. It acts like a shock absorber when you are walking and supports the arch of the foot. Once irritated, it gives rise to a sharp, needle like pain that is made worse when standing for long periods.

*Calcaneal spur*

This is caused by bony growth or spur coming from the heel bone and is often caused by plantar fasciitis.

*Tarsal Tunnel Synd.*

Tarsal tunnel syndrome is a condition where one of the nerves supplying parts of the foot is trapped and squashed inside a tunnel that travels through the bones of the foot. It often causes electricity like pain and pins and needles affecting the big toe and adjacent 3 toes.

Shoulder problems affects up to 30% of adults at any given time. Although, pain and stiffness are the most common complaints that patients present with, a large number may attend due to a severe reduction in their quality of life. Shoulder pain may be due to problems affecting the joints (ACJ), the muscles (rotator cuff tears) or the capsule (adhesive capsulitis). Pain may also be referred to the shoulder from the neck or be due to abdominal pathology (gallstones).

## HISTORY

**Open questions** — How can I help you today? Tell me more about the problems you are having with your shoulder

## Focused questions

| | |
|---|---|
| *Shoulder pain* | Is there any pain or tenderness in your shoulder? When did it start? |
| Site | Does it affect one or both shoulders? Can you point to it (ACJ)? |
| R/L Handed | Are you right or left handed? |
| Injury | Did you injure your shoulder recently? |
| Character | What does the pain feel like? (burning, stinging, sharp, aching) |
| Frequency | Is it always there or does it come and go? Does anything make the pain better (medications, rest) or worse (movements, night)? |
| Radiate | Does the pain move anywhere (neck) or does it stay in one place? |
| Swelling | Has you noticed any swelling? (dislocation) |
| Stiffness | Have you had any stiffness of the joint? Is it worse in the evening? (OA) |

**RED FLAGS** — Dislocation, cardiac chest pain, gallbladder disease

## Associated history

| | |
|---|---|
| *Movements* | Has it restricted your shoulder range of movements? (combing hair, reaching out) |
| *QoL* | Has it stopped you from doing things? (cleaning, dressing, writing) |
| *Fever* | Have you noticed any fever or sweats? Have you felt any rigors? |
| *Numbness* | Have you had any pins and needles or numbness around the shoulder? |
| *Stiffness* | Do you have stiffness and pain in both shoulders? |

## Differentials

| | |
|---|---|
| *Neck pain* | Do you have any neck pain? |
| *PMR* | Is the stiffness worse in the morning? Are your muscles painful to touch? Do you suffer from headaches (worse on eating)? |
| *Abdominal* | Do you have any abdominal pain? (cholecystitis, pancreatitis) |
| *CVD* | Do you experience any crushing chest pain? Does it go down your left arm? |

## PAST HISTORY

| | |
|---|---|
| *Medical* | Have you ever suffered from any medical conditions? (DM, IHD, epilepsy) |
| *Shoulder* | Did you ever suffer a dislocation, fracture or surgery to your shoulder? |

## DRUG HISTORY

| | |
|---|---|
| *Medication* | Are you taking any medications (steroids)? Are you taking any painkillers? (NSAIDs, paracetamol, topical gels)? |

## SOCIAL HISTORY

| | |
|---|---|
| *Home* | Who lives with you at home? |
| *Occupation* | Has the pain affected you at work? (builders, welders, hairdressers, IT) |
| *Drive* | Do you drive? |
| *Hobbies* | Do you do any sports or hobbies? (cricket, rugby, swimming, shot-putting, javelin) |
| *Smoker* | Do you smoke? How many cigarettes do you smoke per day? |
| *Alcohol* | Do you drink alcohol? How much do you drink and how often? |

## IDEA, CONCERNS, EXPECTATIONS

| | |
|---|---|
| *Ideas* | Have you had any thoughts what may be causing your shoulder pain? |
| *Concerns* | Do you have any worries about the pain you have been experiencing? |
| *Expectations* | How did you think I could help you today? |
| *Impact* | How have the symptoms affected your life? |

## CSA TIPS

The conditions that give rise to shoulder pain and stiffness may have quite non-specific histories with no clear trigger factor. It is important to carry out a full shoulder examination to be able to distinguish between them and then share a management plan with the patient to help resolve their complaint.

## PHYSICAL EXAMINATION

| | |
|---|---|
| *Vitals* | Temp, BP, pulse |
| *Look* | Inspect shoulder from front, back and sides. Look for abnormal posture, asymmetry, deformity (winging scapula, prominent AC joint), swelling, muscle wasting |
| *Feel* | Feel temperature, palpate along shoulder joint lines (sternoclavicular joint, AC joint, acromion, greater & lesser tuberosity, glenohumeral joint) for tenderness, effusion, crepitus |
| *Move* | |
| Abduction | Ask the patient to raise both arms to the ceiling from their sides. Notice if painful arc (60-120 degrees - supraspinatus tendonitis/partial rotator cuff tear) or at the end of the arc (acromioclavicular joint OA). If pain in painful arc passively abduct arm further if possible (rotator cuff tear) |
| Adduction | Ask the patient to move their arm across their midline and chest |
| Flexion/ext | Ask the patient to lift their arms forwards then backwards |
| Int/ext rotation | Have elbows flexed at 90 degrees by their sides then ask patient to bend arms away from body (external) then towards midline (internal) |
| *Special tests* | |
| Scratch test | Ask the patient to scratch the opposite scapular in 3 ways (hand behind neck, arm across chest or behind back) |
| Neer's test | *For impingement disorder:* Ask patient to internally rotate arms with thumb facing downwards and slowly abduct and flex the arm up. Apply downward pressure on the patient's arms (resistance) |
| *Neurology* | Check power against resistance. Ask patient to raise their arms like wings (deltoid) and arms held like a boxer (biceps/triceps). Ask to push against a wall (serratus anterior muscle). Check sensation over deltoid muscle (ant. dislocation of shoulder) |

## INVESTIGATIONS

| | |
|---|---|
| *Bloods* | Not routinely needed |
| Other | Hb, WCC, CRP, ESR if suspects PMR or LFTs if suspecting gallbladder disease |

| | |
|---|---|
| *Shoulder Xray* | To exclude fracture, calcified tendonitis, OA ACJ |
| *US / MRI* | To look for micro-fractures, rotator cuff tears, tendonitis, bursitis |

## MANAGEMENT
### *Conservative*

| | |
|---|---|
| *Posture* | Do not sit forwards with arms held by your side. Support your lower back with a cushion when seated. Maintain good posture when using a laptop or computer. When talking on the phone avoid holding it between the shoulder and head |
| *Rest* | If pain is due to repetitive movements, advise to rest for 8-12 weeks. Avoid heavy lifting |
| *Ice / Heat* | Apply an ice or heat pack if worsened after activity |
| *Sling* | Considering wearing a sling to reduce the pressure on the joint / tendon in ACJ disorders |
| *Sick Certificate* | Offer short fit-note if unable to work. Consider amended duties or altered hours if finding it difficult to carry out certain tasks |
| *Exercise* | Continue simple exercises (aerobic/muscle strengthening) as the pain eases to help maintain and improve your ROM and prevent stiffness |
| *ADLs* | |
| Shopping | Use a trolley or rucksack to avoid carrying heavy bags |
| Hoovering | When vacuuming, ensure that you do not bend over and instead, stand up straight. Try not to over stretch and use short sweeping movements |
| Ironing | Avoid only essential ironing. Ensure the board is a good height |

### *Medical*

| | |
|---|---|
| *Pain* | Simple analgesia (paracetamol, codeine) or NSAIDs can be prescribed as topical creams or oral. Ensure no CI for NSAIDS (ulcers, gastritis or asthma). Consider prescribing a PPI in the elderly or those at risk. Avoid glucosamine for pain relief (OA: poor evidence) |
| *Infection* | If you suspect septic arthritis then may need orthopaedic admission for IV Abx and drainage |
| *PMR* | Offer low tapering dose of prednisolone. Consider bone protection with steroids |

### *Referral*

| | |
|---|---|
| *Physio* | Physiotherapy helpful in strengthening the muscles around the shoulder joint and reduce stiffness |
| *OT* | Speak to an OT about adaptations that can be made to house |
| *Injection* | Persistent pain may warrant steroid or local anaesthetic injections to reduce the pain and inflammation in the joint in the short term |
| *ESWT* | Extracorporeal shock wave lithotripsy has been recommended by NICE for calcified tendonitis |
| *Orthopaedics* | Refer if symptoms have rapidly deteriorated, nerve damage or is causing disability impacting on QoL. If recurrent shoulder dislocation may need surgical correction |
| *Rheumatology* | Refer if suspecting RA or PMR |

## SAFETY NETTING

| | |
|---|---|
| *Follow up* | Review in 4-6wks for response to treatment |

## DIFFERENTIAL DIAGNOSIS

| Conditions | Characteristic exam feature |
|---|---|
| **Impingement Disorders** | Impingement disorders affecting the rotator cuff muscles gives rise to pain and shoulder weakness. Usually due to repetitive overhead activities such as skiing, tennis, swimming or those who stack shelves. Pain is usually worse at night affecting sleep. OE: painful arc between 60° and 120° of abduction. +ve Neer's test |
| **Rotator Cuff Tears** | Usually acute following a fall but may be chronic due to tendonitis. Tears can be full length or partial and give rise to a painful arc. OE: unable to actively abduct beyond 60° but can abduct to 90° passively. May have positive drop arm test (have arms fully abducted, advise patient to slowly adduct, after 90 degrees arms drop) |
| **Adhesive Capsulitis** | Also known as frozen shoulder and causes pain, stiffness and reduced movements. More common in women between 40-60 and diabetics. Leads to restriction of all shoulder movements (particularly ext rotation) whether active or passive. Tends to severely affect ADLs such as dressing or washing. Recovery 6mths to 2yrs |
| **ACJ Disorders** | Condition affecting the acromio-clavicular joint usually in young males due to high impact sports (rugby) or because of osteoarthritis. May be secondary to subacromial impingement syndrome. Pain is usually restricted to the ACJ joint but may radiate to the base of the neck. OE: a painful arc between 90° and 120° of abduction and elevation |
| **Cervical Radiculopathy** | Caused by nerve root compression in the cervical spine. May be due to disc herniation, OA or injury. Symptoms include pain, numbness and weakness in the affected nerve root distribution and may radiate to the scapula on bilaterally or unilaterally |
| **Shoulder Dislocation** | Majority of dislocations are anterior with a small minority (5%) being posterior. Occurs in young males and infrequently as a result of a sporting injury or RTA. Recurrent dislocation may lead to axillary nerve injury with tingling and numbness over the ipsilateral lateral deltoid muscle |
| **Polymyalgia rheumatica** | Seen in elderly (>65yrs), causes pain (aching) and morning stiffness (cannot turn over in bed) to bilateral shoulders, pelvic girdle. Has abrupt onset and can last >2wks. Muscles are tender with no true weakness (only pain). Have raised inflammatory markers (ESR,CRP). Associated with giant cell arteritis |

## EXPLANATIONS

*Frozen Shoulder*    Frozen shoulder describes a condition where the tissues around the shoulder (capsule) becomes stiff and inflamed occasionally forming scar like tissue that thickens and hardens restricting your range of movement.

| | |
|---|---|
| *ACJ Disorder* | Usually due to wear and tear (degeneration) at the joint between the shoulder and the collar bone. May happen due to an injury after a sporting accident or following a fall. Gives rise to localised pain over the joint. |
| *Rotator Cuff tendinitis* | The shoulder joint is supported by 4 muscles (rotator cuff). The tendons, or rubber bands that connect the muscles to the bone, become inflamed. It the most common cause of shoulder pain and normally caused by overuse. |
| *Impingement synd.* | One of the rotator cuff tendons (rubber-bands) can get trapped in the gap between the bones of the shoulder and rub against the shoulder blade which causes inflammation and eventual weakness. |
| *Rotator Cuff tear* | This is where one of the rotator cuff tendons (or rubber bands) has a small tear within it. It is often caused by a fall or accident and causes pain in the shoulder with difficulty combing your hair. It can be a minor (partial) or full (complete) tear depending on the severity of damage. |
| *Polymyalgia Rheu.* | Polymyalgia rheumatica is a condition where there is pain (myalgia) and stiffness affecting several (poly) muscles. However, it is not clear as to what causes it. It commonly affects the large muscles around the shoulder and upper arms. |

# 11.11 Elbow pain

Elbow pain is an extremely common condition. It is usually due to strains or sprains that occur after heavy activity or after a fall. However, the structures of elbow joint mean that other causes could also be at play including epicondylitis, bursitis or tendonitis. The elbow is the hinge joint created between the humerus (upper arm) and the 2 bones of the forearm, the radius and ulna. The outer part of the lower humerus is known as the lateral epicondyle and the extensor muscles attach via tendons here. The inner humeral bony prominence is known as the medial epicondyle and the muscles that flex the wrist and fingers attach here via tendons. At the back of the elbow joint is a bursa that allows for the free movement at the joint.

## HISTORY

**Open questions**     How can I help you today? Tell me more about the problems you are having with your elbow

**Focused questions**

*Elbow pain*          Is there any pain or tenderness in your elbow? When did it start?

  Site                Does it affect one or both elbows? Can you point to it?

  Character           What does the pain feel like? (burning, sharp, stinging)

  Frequency           Is it always there or does it come and go? Does anything make the pain better (medications, rest) or worse (movements i.e. pouring tea, shaking hand)?

  Radiate             Does the pain move anywhere or does it stay in one place?

  Swelling            Has you noticed any swelling or a lump?

  Stiffness           Have you had any stiffness of the joint? Is it worse in the morning or evening?

  Other               Have you noticed any weakness in your grip or difficulty carrying objects?

  Trigger (ideas)     What were you doing at the time (plumbing, painting, fishing, racket sports)? Were you lifting any heavy weights (distal biceps rupture)?

**RED FLAGS**         Fever or sweats (septic arthritis), trauma (fracture), weakness in hand

**Associated history**

*Fall*                Did you have a fall? Have you ever had any trauma or damage to the elbow (OA)?

*Strain*              Were you doing any repeated movements (washing, screwing, carrying luggage)? Do you regularly rest your elbows on the desk or chair (bursitis)?

*Fever*               Have you noticed any fever or temperature?

## PAST HISTORY

*Medical*             Have you ever suffered from any medical conditions? (RA)

## DRUG HISTORY

*Medication*          Are you taking any medications? (NSAIDs, paracetamol, topical gels)

## SOCIAL HISTORY

*Occupation*          Are you currently in employment? (carpenter, plasterer, IT)

*Hobbies*             Do you do any hobbies? (tennis, golf, rowing, javelin throwing)

*Smoker*              Do you smoke? How many cigarettes do you smoke per day?

*Alcohol*             Do you drink alcohol? How much do you drink and how often?

*Drive*               Do you drive?

## IDEA, CONCERNS, EXPECTATIONS

| | |
|---|---|
| *Ideas* | Have you had any thoughts what may be causing your elbow pain? |
| *Concerns* | Do you have any worries about the pain you have been experiencing? |
| *Expectations* | How did you think I could help you today? |
| *Impact* | How have the symptoms affected your life? |

## CSA TIPS

Elbow pain is a common presentation. Patients may attend to see a GP as the symptoms are affecting their day to day functioning. It is important to find out what the cause of the pain is and give relevant advice regarding rest and modifying activities. Do not forget to share the management plan with the patient and seek their ideas about how they wish to proceed with treatment.

## PHYSICAL EXAMINATION

| | |
|---|---|
| *Inspect* | Inspect carrying angle with elbows by their side. Look for deformity, bursitis, nodules |
| *Palpate* | Locate the pain before starting. Palpate the epicondyles (epicondylitis), olecranon process (bursitis) and joint margin for tenderness (OA), effusion or temperature. Feel for rheumatoid tophi |
| Movement | Assess both active and passive movements for flexion (flexion deformity) and extension. Assess pronation (palms facing downwards) and supination (palms facing upwards) with elbows fixed at the waist and elbow at 90 degrees |
| *Special Tests* | |
| Tennis elbow | Have the patient's forearm pronated whilst actively flexing their wrist (resisted ext.) |
| Golfer's elbow | Have the patient's forearm supinated whilst actively extending the elbow and wrist (resisted flexion). Pain noted over medial epicondyle |
| *Neurological* | Check sensation over the hand and forearm (ulnar nerve impairment) and check power at the wrist for extension and flexion |

## INVESTIGATIONS

| | |
|---|---|
| *Bloods* | Not routinely needed unless suspect septic arthritis. Hb, WCC, CRP |
| *Elbow Xray* | To exclude fracture, calcified tendonitis |
| *US / MRI* | To look for micro-fractures, tendonitis, bursitis |
| *EMG* | Exclude cubital tunnel syndrome |

## MANAGEMENT
### Conservative

| | |
|---|---|
| *Rest* | If pain is to due to repetitive movements advise to rest for up to 12 wks |
| *Ice / Heat* | Apply an ice or heat pack if worsened after activity |
| *Splint* | Considering purchasing a splint or clasp to reduce the pressure on the joint / tendon |
| *Exercise* | Continue simple exercises as the pain eases to help maintain and improve your range of movements and prevent stiffness |
| *Modifying activities* | Avoid lifting, gripping or screwing motions. Take regular breaks |
| Sports | Speak to a sports doctor or coach on how to modify sporting activity to reduce symptoms |

### Medical

| | |
|---|---|
| *Pain* | Simple analgesia (paracetamol) or NSAIDs can be prescribed as topical creams or oral. Ensure that the patient has no contraindications for NSAIDS (ulcers, gastritis, asthma) |
| *Infection* | If signs of local infection (bursitis) then may need a course of antibiotics. If you suspect septic arthritis then may need orthopaedic admission for IV Abx and drainage |

| Sick Certificate | Offer short fit-note if unable to work. Consider amended duties or altered hours if finding it difficult to carry out certain tasks |
|---|---|

**Referral**

| Physio | Physiotherapy may be helpful in strengthening the muscles around the elbow. Other treatments they may be offered include massage or manipulation to help improve the blood flow to the joint. They may also strap the joint to help reduce the pressure over the area that induces pain |
|---|---|
| OT | Speak to an OT about adaptations that can be made for occupational induced elbow pain (carpenter, plumber) |
| Injection | Persistent pain may warrant steroid or local anaesthetic injections to reduce the pain and inflammation in the joint in the short term. Maximum of 3 injections are offered |
| SE | Pain on injecting, atrophy or liponecrosis, loss of colour of the skin or damage to the tendons. |
| Other | Shockwave therapy, autologous platelet rich plasma injections, topical GTN patches, botulinum toxin A injections |
| Surgery | Small minority who do not respond will need keyhole surgery to remove adhesions or damaged tissue or surgical decompression if evidence of trapped nerve |

**SAFETY NETTING**

| Follow up | Review in 4-6wks for response to treatment |
|---|---|

**DIFFERENTIAL DIAGNOSIS**

| Conditions | Characteristic exam feature |
|---|---|
| **Tennis Elbow** | Often occurs in 40+ after history of minor injury or repetitive movements. Worse when straightening the elbow against resistance. Risk factors include hobbies and occupation (painting, racket sports, plumbing, using screwdriver or hammers, lifting baby, gardening) |
| **Golfer's Elbow** | Focal pain over medial epicondyle from repetitive movements (using hammer, ball thrower). Pain can radiate down flexor surface of arm. Pain on resisted pronation. Occasional ulnar nerve involvement (paresthesia affecting 4th & 5th finger) |
| **Olecranon Bursitis** | Swollen, painful and red bursa over the olecranon process. Usually due to repetitive movements or minor trauma (miners, gardeners, carpet layers) but occasionally due to bacterial infection. Often affects middle aged male patients or patients with RA or gout |
| **Osteoarthritis** | Progressive worsening of elbow pain and reduced movements particularly flexion and extension. May have history of previous fall or fracture. May get a grating (crepitus) sensation when testing range of movements |
| **Cubital Tunnel Syndrome** | Trapped ulnar nerve in cubital tunnel. Worsened when elbow rested on firm surface. Presents with medial elbow pain and hand weakness. Positive Tinel's test (paraesthesia over 4th & 5th digits) when tapping over cubital tunnel (funny bone) |

## EXPLANATIONS

*Tennis Elbow*

Tennis elbow is the pain that is felt on the outside of your elbow caused by soft tissue swelling usually due to overuse or repetitive movement. It is called 'tennis elbow' because it is commonly seen in tennis players due to the repetitive action of hitting the balls so often. However, it can affect almost anyone particularly those doing DIY, typing or household chores.

*Golfer's Elbow*

Golfers elbow is the pain that is felt on the inside of your elbow caused by soft tissue swelling usually due to overuse or repetitive movement. It is called 'golfer's elbow' because it is commonly seen in golf players due to the repetitive action of hitting the balls so often. However, it can affect almost anyone particularly those doing DIY, typing or household chores.

*Olecranon Bursitis*

This is due to the inflammations of a small sac that lies at the back of your elbow joint called the olecranon bursa. Its job is to help the joint move well however, because of repetitive strain it can become inflamed and irritated. Rarely, it may get infected and would require antibiotics to get better.

*Sprain*

A sprain is a stretch or small tear that happens to a ligament because of excessive movement. It usually heals itself but this depends on the severity and whether there is more than one ligament is affected and whether there is a full or partial tear.

# 11.12 Hand pain

Hand pain is an important symptom as it usually causes functional problems in the patient. The hand consists of numerous small muscles, nerves, bones and tendons that all may be implicit in the symptoms. A patient presenting following a fall onto an outstretched hand may have simply sustained a sprain or more importantly may have fractured a bone in the hand or the wrist. Repeated and repetitive movements as a result of occupation may result in tenosynovitis or tendinitis causing focal pain in the hand. Systemic conditions such as rheumatoid arthritis and hypothyroidism may also present with hand symptoms.

## HISTORY

| | |
|---|---|
| **Open questions** | How can I help you today? Tell me more about the problems you are having with your hand |

### Focused questions

| | |
|---|---|
| *Hand pain* | Is there any pain or tenderness in your hand? |
| Site | Does it affect one or both hands? Can you point to it? |
| Onset | When did it start? |
| Character | What does the pain feel like? (burning, sharp, aching) |
| Agg/relieve | Does anything make the pain better (medications, rest) or worse (movements, walking)? |
| Stiffness | Any stiffness of the joints? Is it worse in the morning (RA) or evening (OA)? |
| Swelling | Have you noticed any swelling of your joints? |
| Strength | Do you feel that you have less power in your hand, fingers or grip? |
| Injury | Have you injured your hand or had a fall recently? |

| | |
|---|---|
| **RED FLAGS** | Wasting (thenar) of muscles |

### Associated history

| | |
|---|---|
| *Function* | Do you have problems with doing fine movements (holding pen, writing, doing buttons up)? Do have problems with day to day tasks (combing, feeding, bathing)? |
| *Sensation* | Have you had any numbness or pins and needles in your hand? |

### Differentials

| | |
|---|---|
| *Psoriatic Arthritis* | Have you noticed any skin changes on your elbows or knees? Have you noticed excessive dandruff on your scalp? |
| *Carpal Tunnel* | Does your hand feel better after shaking it? Does the pain awake you at night? |
| *De Quervain's* | Do you have any wrist pain? Do you have any problems gripping? |
| *Trigger Finger* | Does your finger ever lock suddenly when making a fist? |

## PAST HISTORY

| | |
|---|---|
| *Medical* | Have you ever suffered from any medical conditions? (OA, RA) |
| *Carpal Tunnel* | Are you pregnant? Do you suffer from an underactive thyroid? |
| *Fracture* | Had you had a previous fracture of the hand? (scaphoid) |

## DRUG HISTORY

| | |
|---|---|
| *Medication* | Are you taking any medications? Are you taking any painkillers (NSAIDs, paracetamol, topical gels)? |

## SOCIAL HISTORY

| | |
|---|---|
| *Support network* | Who lives with you at home? |
| Carers | Do you have any carers? Are they helping you doing day to day tasks? |
| *Occupation* | Are you currently working? Has the pain affected you at work (musician, manual work with vibrating tools, IT)? |
| *Smoker* | Do you smoke? How many cigarettes do you smoke per day? |
| *Alcohol* | Do you drink alcohol? How much do you drink and how often? |

## FAMILY HISTORY

| | |
|---|---|
| *Carpal Tunnel* | Does anyone in your immediate family have similar problems? |

## IDEA, CONCERNS, EXPECTATIONS

| | |
|---|---|
| *Ideas* | Have you had any thoughts what may be causing your knee pain? |
| *Concerns* | Do you have any worries about the pain you have been experiencing? |
| *Expectations* | How did you think I could help you today? |
| *Impact* | How have the symptoms affected your life? |

## CSA TIPS

Hand pain can significantly affect a person's ability to function. It may affect their ability to perform hobbies or even impact on their employment. Hand symptoms may be due to overuse and arthritis, but may also be a sign of underlying inflammation.

## PHYSICAL EXAMINATION

| | |
|---|---|
| *Vitals* | Temp, BP, pulse |
| *Look* | Inspect for swellings, nail changes, scars, muscle wasting or deformity |
| Nails | Psoriatic changes (pitting, onycholysis), clubbing |
| Deformity | |
| OA changes | Heberden's nodes (DIPJ), Bouchard's nodes (PIPJ) |
| RA changes | Swan-neck & boutonniere deformity, Z-shaped thumb, ulnar deviation |
| Other | Ganglion, mallet finger, tophi |
| *Feel* | Check temperature and muscle bulk (thenar & hypothenar) |
| Joints | Squeeze the radio-ulnar joint, radial & ulnar styloid, anatomical snuffbox (scaphoid fracture), carpal bones, MCPs, IP joints for tenderness |
| Tendons | Palpate the radial styloid (de Quervain's) & ulnar styloid |
| *Move* | Also move the wrist joint (pronation, supination, flex/extension, radial & ulnar deviation). Ask the patient to make a fist then spread their fingers out. Move each joint individually |
| *Special tests* | Consider if indicated by the history |
| Phalen's test | Ask the patient to hold the reverse prayer sign for 1 minute. Pain or paresthesia in medial distribution is positive |
| Tinel's test | Tap the medial nerve at the carpal tunnel produces paresthesia |
| Finkelstein's test | Ask the patient to have thumb in their fist then tilt it into ulnar deviation |
| *Function* | If indicated, ask the patient to carry out everyday tasks such as undo buttons, write a sentence using a pen or hold a cup |

| Neurological | If indicated, test the sensation of the ulnar nerve (little finger), median nerve (index finger) and radial nerve (anatomical snuff box) |

## INVESTIGATIONS

| | |
|---|---|
| Bloods | Not routinely needed |
| Other | Hb, WCC, CRP, ESR, if suspecting infection. Rh factor if suspect RA. Request TFT and fasting glucose for carpal tunnel |
| Hand Xray | If suspect OA or fracture. If suspect scaphoid fracture repeat scaphoid views in 10 days |
| Specialist | Nerve conduction tests, US wrist |

## MANAGEMENT

### Conservative

| | |
|---|---|
| Rest | If pain is due to repetitive movements advise to rest for up to 12 wks |
| Ice / Heat | Apply an ice or heat pack if worsened after activity. Place hands in warm water for 10-20 minutes. Apply moisturising cream and massage into the hands |
| Splint | Considering purchasing a wrist splint to wear at night for carpal tunnel. A splint with a thumb strap may help reduce de Quervain's |
| Exercise | Continue simple exercises (aerobic/muscle strengthening) as the pain eases to help maintain and improve your ROM and prevent stiffness |
| Weight | If BMI>25 suggest losing weight |

### Medical

| | |
|---|---|
| Pain | Simple analgesia (paracetamol, codeine) or NSAIDs can be prescribed as topical creams or oral. Ensure no CI for NSAIDS (ulcers, gastritis or asthma). Add PPI in the elderly |
| Sick Certificate | Offer short fit-note if unable to work. Consider amended duties or altered hours if finding it difficult to carry out certain tasks |

### Referral

| | |
|---|---|
| Physio | Physiotherapy helpful in strengthening the muscles |
| OT | Speak to an OT about adaptations that can be made (minimize wrist extension, modification of tools, increased handle diameter of spoons or toothbrush) |
| Injection | Persistent pain may warrant steroid or local anaesthetic injections to reduce the pain and inflammation in the joint in the short term. Often useful to release trigger finger |
| SE | Pain on injecting, atrophy or liponecrosis, loss of colour of the skin or damage to the tendons |
| Orthopaedics | Refer if thenar eminence wasting for surgical release of carpal tunnel or trigger finger |

## SAFETY NETTING

| | |
|---|---|
| Follow up | Review in 4-6wks for response to treatment |

## DIFFERENTIAL DIAGNOSIS

| Conditions | Characteristic exam feature |
|---|---|
| **Carpal Tunnel Syndrome** | Entrapment of the median nerve in the carpal tunnel. Common in 40+ women. Burning pain, tingling and numbness in the distribution of the medial nerve (radial 3.5 fingers). Worse at night and may cause the patient to awaken, pain may improve with shaking the hand. Chronic symptoms may lead to wasting of thenar muscle. OE: |

| | |
|---|---|
| | weakness to thumb abduction, +ve Phalen's and +ve Tinel's sign. Risk factors: DM, hypothyroidism, RA, obesity, pregnancy |
| **De Quervain's Tenosynovitis** | Common in 30-50yr old women and during pregnancy. Causes pain, swelling and tenderness over the thumb. Due to repetitive strain or repeated movements such as using a mouse or certain manual jobs (carpenter, gardening). OE: radial styloid tenderness, +ve Finkelstein's test |
| **Trigger Finger** | Flexor tendon becomes trapped in the sheath resulting in difficulty extending the flexed finger (locking) often released suddenly by a snap with assistance from the other hand. Can be associated with DM, RA. Seen in carpenters (screwdriver). Commonly affects ring and middle fingers and seen in >40yr women. OE: occasionally a nodule is palpable |

**EXPLANATIONS**

*Carpal Tunnel*    Carpal tunnel syndrome is a condition whereby the nerve supplying parts of the hand gets trapped and squashed inside a tunnel that travels through the bones of the hand (carpal bones). It often causes pain and pins and needles affecting the index and middle fingers.

*Wrist splint*    The splint holds the wrist in a neutral position thereby reducing the pressure over the carpal tunnel and resting the nerve.

*De Quervain's*    De Quervain's tenosynovitis is a common condition where the tendons or cords that connect the muscle to the bone becomes inflamed. As a result it is painful to straighten your thumb.

*Trigger Finger*    This is a condition that affects the tendons of the hand. As the finger is bent towards the palm (like when making a fist) the tendon (rubber bands that connect the bone to muscle) gets stuck within the tendon sheath (tunnel), due to a thickening (nodule) and stops the finger from being straightened.

*Ganglion*    A ganglion is a small swelling often found at the back of the wrist. It often contains jelly like fluid that makes a smooth often harmless lump. They often go away by themselves with time.

# 11.13 Raynaud's Phenomenon

Raynaud's phenomenon is episodic attacks of vasospasm of the distal arteries causing ischaemia (pallor, cyanosis, redness). It is precipitated by cold or a person's emotions. It is often seen in 20-30yr old women with 90% having no underlying cause. Secondary causes include connective tissue disorder (SLE, scleroderma, RA, Sjogren's syndrome). It is often characterised by distinctive colour changes of the fingers i.e. white (ischaemia), blue (deoxygenation), red (reperfusion) with throbbing pain from rapid reactive hyperaemia.

**HISTORY**

**Open questions** | How can I help you today? Tell me more about the problems you are having with your fingers/toes

**Focused questions**

*Colour change* | Have you noticed a change in colour of your fingers or toes?
Site | Which fingers or toes are affected?
Symmetry | Does it affect one side or both?
Onset | When did it start?
Character | Describe the colour change you have noticed? (white, blue, crimson)
Triggers | Have you noticed anything that makes it worse? (cold, stress)
Pain & swelling | Do you get any pain or swelling in your fingers? (reperfusion)

**RED FLAGS** | Underlying connective tissue disorders, digital ulceration

**Associated history**

*Areas* | Have you noticed it affects other areas? (earlobe, nose, tongue, nipple)

**Differentials**

*Chilblains* | Are your fingers intensely itchy or painful (burning)? Are they linked to the seasons (winter)? How long do they last (weeks)?
*Sjogren's syndrome* | Do you suffer from dry eyes and mouth? Do you get dryness anywhere else? (dyspareunia, dry skin, dry cough)
*Rheumatoid arthritis* | Do you get pain & stiffness in the morning? Which joints are affected?
*Dermatomyositis* | Do you get pain or weakness affecting your muscles? Do you struggle to get out of a chair or climb stairs? Any skin rashes? (heliotrope)
*SLE* | Have you had a fever? Any rashes on the face? (butterfly)
*Hypothyroidism* | Any weight gain? Are you intolerant to cold weather?

**PAST HISTORY**

*Connective tissue* | Have you ever suffered from any medical conditions? (SLE, RA, Scleroderma)

**FAMILY HISTORY**

*Connective tissue* | Does anyone in your family suffer from any medical conditions? (SLE, RA, Scleroderma)

**DRUG HISTORY**

*Medication* | Are you taking any medications (B-blockers, COCP, ergotamine, clonidine)?

## SOCIAL HISTORY

| | |
|---|---|
| *Occupation* | Are you currently working? Are you exposed to cold environments (cold storage, fish industry)? Do you work with vibration tools (road digger, mine)? |
| *Smoker* | Do you smoke? How many cigarettes do you smoke per day? |
| *Diet* | Do you drink tea or coffee? |
| *Recreational drugs* | Are you taking any recreational drugs? (cocaine, amphetamines) |

## IDEA, CONCERNS, EXPECTATIONS

| | |
|---|---|
| *Ideas* | Have you had any thoughts what may be causing your symptoms? |
| *Concerns* | Do you have any worries about the pain you have been experiencing? |
| *Expectations* | How did you think I could help you today? |
| *Impact* | How have the symptoms affected your life? |

## CSA TIPS

Suffering with Raynaud's may lead to much anxiety and worry in patients. The change in colour may cause a patient to think that they have a serious underlying disorder. It is important that you take the time to elicit the patient's concerns and worries and not be dismissive of them. You should take a history and ensure that there is no associated connective tissue disorder.

## PHYSICAL EXAMINATION

| | |
|---|---|
| *Vitals* | Temp, BP (in both arms), pulse |
| *Inspection* | Inspect for colour change (pallor, cyanosis), nail changes (abnormal nail-fold capillary), digital ulcers, rashes (SLE, heliotrope) |
| *Palpation* | Check temperature or joint tenderness (RA) |
| Pulses | Check peripheral pulses |

## INVESTIGATIONS

| | |
|---|---|
| *Bloods* | FBC, ESR, ANA |
| Other | U&Es, LFTs, TFTs, Rh factor |
| *Specialist* | Capillary microscope to examine nailfold capillaries |

## MANAGEMENT   *for primary Raynaud's Phenomenon*
### Conservative

| | |
|---|---|
| *Keep warm* | Wear gloves, socks, fur lined boots, thermal underwear in cold weather. Keep whole body warm with layers. Consider warming device (battery powered gloves/socks) |
| *Coffee* | Avoid caffeine (tea/coffee) where possible |
| *Smoking* | Avoid or stop smoking |
| *Exercise* | Exercise hands and feet regularly to improve circulation |
| *Stress* | Minimise stress. Consider relaxation techniques |
| *Occupation* | Consider change of occupation or fit note for amended duties |
| *Other* | Avoid touching cold objects. Avoid handle carrying bags (impair circulation). Stop recreational drugs (amphetamines, cocaine) |

### Medical

| | |
|---|---|
| *Avoid* | Avoid beta blockers, COCP, ergotamine |
| *Vitamins* | Some evidence of using evening primrose oil and fish oils |
| *Nifedipine* | Offer immediate release, 5mg tds to 20mg tds depending on response. Offer MR preparation if side effects (20mg od increasing to 60mg od). Intermittent prophylactic |

use, prior to cold exposure, can be adequate). Other calcium channel blockers can be
considered (nicardipine, felodipine, amlodipine)

SE                     Flushing, headaches, palpitations, dizziness. Avoid grapefruit

*Other*                *Can be considered but not recommended in primary care:* Naftidrofuryl oxalate (100mg
tds increasing to 200mg tds), topical 2% GTN on affected areas, ACE inhibitors
(enalapril) or alpha blockers (prazosin), inositol nicotinate, SSRI (fluoxetine, vasodilator
effect)

*Surgery*              Sympathectomy for severe pain or ulcers (digital - hand, lumbar - feet). Debridement
amputations for ischaemia

**Referral**
*OT*                   Speak to an OT about adaptations to work
*Rheumatology*         Refer for uncontrolled symptoms

**SAFETY NETTING**
*Follow up*            Refer if evidence of secondary causes. Suspect if onset >30yr, assymetrical & intensely
painful, digital ulcers, abnormal nail capillaries +ve ANA/high ESR

**DIFFERENTIAL DIAGNOSIS**

| Conditions | Characteristic exam feature |
| --- | --- |
| **Raynaud's phenomenon** | Vasospasm of the distal arteries. Commonly affects teenage girls. Can resolve by menopause. Attacks last minutes to hours. Causes colour change (white>blue>red) with throbbing pain and swelling on reperfusion. Fingers can be cold. Occasionally it can affect other extremities (nose, earlobe). Secondary causes include CREST syndrome, dermatomyositis, SLE, RA |
| **Chilblains** | Skin inflammation of peripheral digits caused by cold or damp. Common in young women. Appear 12-24hrs after exposure lasting upto 2wks. Characterized by intense itch, burning sensation and tenderness typically in winter with resolution in summer. Can form papules, patches that appear symmetrically and bilateral |
| **Hypothyroidism** | Underactive thyroid presents with fatigue, weight gain, cold intolerance, with skin changes (dry, cold, pale complexion, alopecia), hoarse voice and arthralgia |
| **SLE** | Connective tissue disorder that is characterised by vasculitis and presents with relapsing, remitting pattern. Non-specific features include fever, oral ulcer, myalgia/myositis, Raynaud's phenomenon, lymphadenopathy. Other features include malar (butterfly) or discoid rash, photosensitivity, with arthritis of large (knee, wrist) and small bone (PIP, MCP) |
| **Sjogren's syndrome** | Associated with keratoconjunctivitis sicca (dry eyes), xerostomia (dry mouth), parotid enlargement and fatigue, myalgia, arthralgia. Often involves other secretory glands (dyspareunia, dysphagia, dry skin, dry cough & chest infections, otitis media) |

| Dermatomyositis | Acute & chronic inflammation of striated muscle fibres with dermatitis. Can cause muscle tenderness with weakness affecting proximal (symmetrical, limb girdle) muscles with preservation of muscle bulk. As a result, presents with difficulty rising from a chair or climbing up stairs. Dermatitis features include heliotrope rash, papules (Gottron's) with telangiectasias (perungal) |
|---|---|

## EXPLANATIONS

*Primary Raynaud's*

Raynaud's phenomenon is a condition that can cause the small vessel blood supply to the fingers or toes to be narrowed (constrict). This is often due to temporary spasm of the blood vessels triggered by cold weather or anxiety and stress. It can present with colour change of your fingers followed by throbbing pain that lasts from a few minutes to several hours.

*Nifedipine*

The medication works by opening up and widening the blood vessels therefore improving the blood supply to your fingers.

*Chilblains*

Chilblains are small, itchy swellings that can develop on the skin, particularly over the finger and toes. They are an abnormal reaction to cold temperatures. The small blood vessels under the skin become narrowed and change colour. If this happens too quickly, some of blood can leak out from the vessel to the surrounding tissues causing swelling and itchiness of your finger or toes.

# 12.1 Eczema

Atopic eczema is characterised by red, flaky and itchy skin following exposure to triggers such as foods, allergens and irritants. It is increasing in prevalence, currently affecting about 15-20% of school children. There is also a strong association with a family history of atopy, asthma and hay fever. The condition has a fluctuating course and resolves in about 50% of children by the age of 2. Treatment involves avoidance of all soaps and usage of emollients and ointments instead. Other agents used during a flare up include topical steroids, antihistamines and antibacterial creams.

## HISTORY

**Open questions**          Can you tell me more about the problems you have been experiencing with your skin? How did it start?

## Focused questions

| | |
|---|---|
| *Eczema* | When did it start? How long has it been going on for? Has it changed over time? |
| Distribution | Which areas of your skin are affected? |
| Children | Flexor surfaces – creases of elbows, elbows, neck wrist, ankles |
| Infants | Extensor surfaces, face or cheeks (babies) |
| Dry / itchy | Is the skin dry or itchy? |
| Chronic | Due you have thickened patches? (lichenification) |
| Aggravating | Have you noticed anything that triggers it on? |
| Worsen | Food allergy, stress, pets, irritants (soaps/detergents/perfumes), clothing (wool) |

## Associated history

| | |
|---|---|
| *Herpeticum* | Have you noticed any blisters or painful areas or ulcers? |
| *Bleed* | Do you find it itches so much that it bleeds? |
| *Infections* | Have you had any fever or sweats recently? |
| *Child* | Do you have concerns about your child's growth and development? |

## RED FLAGS          Eczema herpeticum, bleeding, secondary infections

## Differentials

| | |
|---|---|
| *Contact dermatitis* | Have you noticed the rash worsen after being in contact with something? (detergents/chemicals/oils) |
| *Scabies* | Do you have an intense itch that is worse after a bath? Does it affect the wrists, between the finger or toes? Are other members of the house affected? |
| *Seb. Dermatitis* | Have you noticed any flakiness of the skin? Does it mainly affect the face or behind the ears? Do you suffer from bad dandruff? |
| *Psoriasis* | Do you have any silvery scaly patches? Any joint pains or nails changes? |

## PAST HISTORY

| | |
|---|---|
| *Atopy* | Do you suffer from any medical problems? (hay fever, eczema, asthma, urticaria) |

## DRUG HISTORY

| | |
|---|---|
| *Medication* | Have you tried any treatments for it already? (dietary restrictions) |

## SOCIAL HISTORY

| | |
|---|---|
| *Smoker* | Do you smoke? How many cigarettes do you smoke per day? |
| *Alcohol* | Do you drink alcohol? How much do you drink and how often? |
| *Occupation* | Are you working at the moment (chemicals, animals, dyes)? Do you feel that your symptoms improve when you are away from work? |
| *Pets* | Do you have any pets? (dogs, cats) |

## FAMILY HISTORY

| | |
|---|---|
| *Atopy* | Does anyone in your family suffer from eczema, hayfever or asthma? |

## IDEA, CONCERNS, EXPECTATIONS

| | |
|---|---|
| *Idea* | What did you think was causing spots? (poor hygiene, food allergies, contact dermatitis) |
| *Concerns* | Have you had any particular worried about it? (unsightliness, disfigurement) |
| *Expectations* | Was there any specific treatment that you were hoping for today? (steroids) |
| *Impact on life* | How has your skin problem affected you? (bullying, off work, relationships, social life) |
| Mood | Has it affected your mood or self esteem? |

## CSA TIPS

Eczema can be a chronic relapsing condition that may cause significant distress to the sufferer and carers alike. Patients may suffer from recurrent infections that require titrating of their steroid dose in addition to topical or oral antibiotics. It is important to explain clearly the diagnosis to the patient, but more so how to use the creams that you wish to prescribe. A large proportion of treatment failure is due to the incorrect application of creams/ointments.

## PHYSICAL EXAMINATION

| | |
|---|---|
| *Skin* | Examine the body for signs of eczema |
| Distribution | Examine the flexural surfaces including antecubital and popliteal fossae, neck wrists and ankles area (Asian / African-caribbean can have extensor or discoid forms). Look at the face, hands and infra-orbital folds |
| Wrists | Look at the wrists and neck area for contact dermatitis (watch, necklace, bracelet) |
| Scalp | Check scalp area, behind the ears for signs of Seborrhoeic dermatitis |
| Web spaces | Look at finger and toe web spaces for any evidence of burrows (scabies) |
| Skin changes | Look for dry skin, papules, vesicles, crusting, weeping, lichenification, excoriations or scarring. Look for signs of infections (crusting, weeping rash) |

---

**Severity of Eczema** - *Ref: NICE (2007) Atopic eczema in children*

| | |
|---|---|
| *Mild* | Dry skin areas, infrequent itching (+/- small areas of redness) |
| *Moderate* | Dry skin areas, frequent itch, redness (+/- excoriation, skin thickening) |
| *Severe* | Widespread dry skin, incessant itching, redness (+/- excoriation, extensive skin thickening, bleeding, oozing, cracking, altered pigmentation) |

---

## INVESTIGATIONS

| | |
|---|---|
| *Blood tests* | *Not routinely performed:* FBC (raised eosinophils, raised WCC – infection), CRP (infection) |
| Other | RAST IgE blood tests for specific allergens |
| *Skin prick test* | Confirm contact dermatitis or for unknown allergen (secondary care) |

## MANAGEMENT
### Conservative

| | |
|---|---|
| *Avoid allergens* | Avoid irritants or allergens that are suspected. Wear cotton clothes avoid wool. Avoid excessive heat |
| Dust mites | Reduce the number of dust mites by regular hovering, remove carpets, ventilate the room, use mite proof covers for mattress and pillows, have toy in plastic bags and freeze for 24hr. However limited evidence |
| *Avoids soaps* | Avoid soaps or bubble baths including perfumes or shower gels |
| *Scratching* | Have nails cut short, avoid scratching skin. Consider gloves in bed or mitten for babies |
| *Diet* | Limited evidence, <10% may benefit. Egg and milk common allergens. Refer to dietician before recommending omitting foods in toddlers |

### Medical

| | |
|---|---|
| *Emollients* | Keep skin moist using generous amounts of emollients/moisturisers particularly when washing and bathing. Avoid perfumed products. Apply to whole body. Avoid aqueous cream. Consider applying at least 4x/day e.g. emulsifying ointment, hydrous ointment, liquid paraffin 50:50, E45. Liberal emollient use should reduce the need for more potent steroid use (250-500g wk) |
| *Topical steroids* | Use weakest cream to control symptoms. For normal skin (except face, genitals, axillae) use steroids for 7-14d. The face, genitals, axillae use for <5 days. Avoid using very potent steroids in children unless directed by specialist. Ointments most suitable for dry scaly eczema, creams best for weepy exudative eczema |
| Mild | Hydrocortisone 0.5-2.5% |
| Moderate | Betamethasone valerate 0.025% (Betnovate RD), Clobetasone butyrate 0.05% (Eumovate) |
| Potent | Fluticasone propionate 0.05% (Cutivate), Betamethasone valerate 0.1% (Betnovate) |
| Very potent | Clobetasol propionate 0.05% (Dermovate) |

**Topical Steroid Volumes** - *Ref: BNF*

| Area | Cream quantity | Area | Cream quantity |
|---|---|---|---|
| Face and neck | 15–30 g | Both arms | 30–60 g |
| Both hands | 15–30 g | Both legs | 100 g |
| Scalp | 15–30 g | Trunk | 100 g |
| Groin and genitalia | 15–30 g | | |

| | |
|---|---|
| *Finger Tip Unit* | This equates to 0.5g of steroid, sufficient to cover two palms of an adult hand |

**Area of skin and Fingertip units per Dose of Steroids**

| Area | TFU / dose | Area | TFU / dose |
|---|---|---|---|
| Hand and fingers (front and back) | 1.0 | Face and neck | 2.5 |
| One hand or foot (all over) | 2.0 | One leg (excl foot) | 6.0 |
| One arm (excl hand) | 3.0 | | |

| | |
|---|---|
| *Antihistamines* | Try sedative antihistamines to break the itch cycle (piriton, promethazine, hydroxyzine) |

| Antibiotics | If infected, try short course (7d) topical (fusidic acid cream) or oral (flucloxacillin/erythromycin). Consider swab if not resolving. Acyclovir for herpeticum |
|---|---|
| Immunosuppressant | Tacrolimus should be initiated by specialist. Used in moderate or severe eczema. Can be used as a steroid sparing agent |
| Wet wrapping | Useful in exudative eczema. Use tubigrip bandage with liberal amounts of emollient. Applications is taught by specialist |

### Refer

| Dermatologist | Refer if evidence of severe eczema that is resistant to treatment or if patient is for immunosuppressant or phototherapy. Refer for same day admission for eczema herpeticum |
|---|---|
| Counsellor | Refer to counsellor if eczema is affecting their psychological state |
| Dietician | Refer to dietician if diet modification is considered |

---

**Referral for atopic eczema in children** - *Ref: NICE Atopic Eczema in Children (2007)*
- Urgent referral (<2wks) if has not responded to optimal topical therapy after 1wk
- No response of bacterial infected eczema to treatment
- Facial atopic eczema no response to treatment
- Recurrent severe infections
- Advice on bandaging techniques

---

### SAFETY NETTING

| Follow up | Review in 6-8wks to see response to treatment |
|---|---|

### DIFFERENTIAL DIAGNOSIS

| Causes | Characteristic exam feature |
|---|---|
| **Seborrheic dermatitis** | Relapsing, remitting condition that affects the face, torso, behind the ears and scalp. Presents with red, scaly, itchy flaky skin and dandruff. |
| **Contact dermatitis** | Localised red eczematous lesions that come about post contact with an allergen. May include allergy to cements, soaps, detergents (hands), jewellry (ears, fingers, neck, wrist), nickel (buttons - waist area), hair dye (scalp, hands) etc. |
| **Scabies** | Intensely itchy rash over the hands, feet or genital areas. Patients present with a red chronic rash that is itchy and spares the face. May affect a number of people in the same household.There may be a history of travel or stay in youth hostels. OE: burrows in the web spaces of the hands or toes. |

### EXPLANATIONS

| Eczema | Eczema, simply refers to dry and inflamed skin. It may be described as 'atopic' eczema which means that it is largely due to allergies. This means that there is a greater chance that you could suffer from one of the atopic conditions such as hayfever or asthma. In eczema the fatty layer on top of the skin becomes less and water is lost, drying the skin. |
|---|---|

*Emollients*

Emollients are a lubricating cream or ointment that helps trap water onto the skin. The skin is like a balloon filled with water. In eczema unfortunately there are holes in the balloon allowing water to seep out. Emollients work by blocking those holes and help trap the water back in keeping the skin moist.

*Steroids*

Steroids are effective creams that help reduce the inflammation of the skin that can take place in eczema.

Finger tip unit

To know how much to use, you should apply a 'toothpaste amount' whereby you squeeze out some cream over the tip of your finger up to the first crease and apply this to the skin. You should gently rub the cream until it disappears into the skin.

Side effects

Steroids are potent medications and may cause side effects including thinning of the skin, bruising, bleeding or discolouration. As a result they should be used sparingly.

# 12.2 Psoriasis

Psoriasis is a chronic skin condition characterised by inflamed, red, raised lesions that develop as silvery scales on the scalp, elbows, knees and lower back. Around 2% of the population have psoriasis. Alcohol, beta blockers, lithium, NSAIDS and antimalarials can exacerbate the condition. The most common form is called discoid or plaque psoriasis. Symptoms include salmon coloured plaques with silver white scales on the extensor surfaces as well as the scalp area that are often itchy in nature. Other types include guttate and pustular psoriasis. Psoriasis can also involve the nails (in 50%) as well as the joints (7%). Nail features include, pitting, ridging, onycholysis (separation of distal nail from nail bed) and hyperkeratosis (build up of keratin below nail bed).

## HISTORY
**Open questions**        Can you tell me more about your skin problem? How did it start?

## Focused questions
*Psoriasis*              When did it start? How long has it been going on for? Has it change over time?
   Distribution          Which areas of your skin are affected? (scalp, elbows, knees, palms, soles of feet)
   Dry / itchy           Is the skin dry or itchy?
   Aggravating           Have you noticed anything that triggers it?
     Worsen          Stress, sunlight, trauma, infections, medication, alcohol

## Associated history
*Nails changes*          Have you noticed any changes to your nails?
*Arthropathy*            Do you have any joint pains?
*Strep. infection*       Did you have a sore throat recently?

## Differentials
*Eczema*                 Do you have dry inflamed skin? Do you suffer from hayfever or asthma?
*Tinea infection*        Have you seen any circular itchy rashes? Anyone else in your family had it?

## PAST HISTORY
*Medical*                Do you suffer from any medical problems? (IHD, DM, BP, Chol, CVA)

## DRUG HISTORY
*Medication*             Are you taking any medications? Have you tried any treatments for it? (dietary restrictions)
   Worsen              Lithium ACEI, beta-blockers, antimalarials, NSAIDs

## SOCIAL HISTORY
*Smoker*                 Do you smoke? How many cigarettes do you smoke per day?
*Alcohol*                Do you drink alcohol? How much do you drink and how often?
*Occupation*             Are you working at the moment?
*Stress*                 Are you feeling stressed? Any stress in your relationship or work?

## FAMILY HISTORY
*Psoriasis*              Does anyone in your family suffer from psoriasis?

## IDEA, CONCERNS, EXPECTATIONS

| | |
|---|---|
| *Idea* | What did you think was causing the rash? (food allergies, contact dermatitis) |
| *Concerns* | Have you had any particular worries about it? (relationship problems, sleep – excessive rubbing) |
| *Expectations* | How were you hoping I could help you with your skin? |
| *Impact* | How has your skin problem affected you? (relationships, cannot sunbathe, loss of job) |
| Mood | Has it affected your mood or self esteem? |

## CSA TIPS

Psoriasis is a chronic relapsing condition that has no cure. The excess turnover of skin cells leads to scaly, dry patches that in severe cases may affect a large percentage of a persons body. It can causes joint damage and has been associated with an increase in cardiovascular problems if left untreated. Patients may attend for diagnosis, or treatment advice. In many cases, patients may be left with psychological disturbances if their symptoms are not controlled properly.

## PHYSICAL EXAMINATION

| | |
|---|---|
| *Skin* | Examine the body for signs of psoriasis |
| Distribution | Examine the extensor surfaces including the knees, elbows, scalp, sacrum and hair margin. Examine the axillae (flexural psoriasis), palms and sole of the feet (palmoplantar pustulosis). Look for koebner phenomenon |
| Skin changes | Look for salmon pink waxy plaques or raindrop lesions on the chest/limbs (guttate) |
| *Nails* | Inspect the nails for pitting, onycholysis, oily patch discolouration |
| *Joints* | Inspect and palpate the hands for arthropathy |

## INVESTIGATIONS

| | |
|---|---|
| *Specialist* | Rarely performed but specialist may perform a skin biopsy |

## MANAGEMENT

### Conservative

| | |
|---|---|
| *Avoids triggers* | Avoid triggers such as sunlight and certain medications |
| *Smoking* | Try and quit smoking |
| *Alcohol* | Attempt to reduce alcohol intake to a minimum |
| *Obesity* | Try and lose weight to BMI <25 |
| *Stress* | Try and mitigate any stress or use relaxation or self-help techniques |
| *Support groups* | Contact support groups for patients with psoriasis |

### Medical

| | |
|---|---|
| *Emollients* | Offer liberal amounts of emollient to keep the skin soft and moist avoiding irritation. Helps reduce itching, scaling as well as cracking (see eczema chapter) |

**Treatment of Psoriasis** - *Ref: BNF*

| Medication | *Scalp* | *Chronic stable plaques* |
|---|---|---|
| Steroids | Betnovate scalp | Eumovate |
| Vitamin D | Dovonex (scalp) | Dovonex (ointment) |
| Coal tar | T/Gel, coal tar, Polytar | Cocois, Sebco, Psoriderm |
| Dithranol | Scalp gel | Ointment |

| Topical steroids | Use short term to help reduce inflammation. Consider moderately potent type. Short course may avoid rebound exacerbation when treatment is stopped. Topical and scalp applications available (Betnesol) |
| --- | --- |
| Vitamin D | Vitamin D analogues (Dovonex) reduces the speed of epithelial cell turnover. Cause less irritation, suitable for face or flexures. Combined forms available (Dovobet) |
| Coal tar | Leased preferred due to messiness, smell. Have anti-inflammatory properties. Useful in removing thicken plaques. Different strengths available |

## Combined Treatments for Psoriasis - *Ref: BNF*

| | Steroid | Vitamin D | Coal tar | Dithranol | Salicylic |
| --- | --- | --- | --- | --- | --- |
| Steroids | Eumovate | Dovobet | | Alphosyl HC | Diprosalic |
| Vitamin D | Dovobet | Dovonex | | | |
| Coal tar | Alphosyl HC | | | Psorin | Cocois |
| Dithranol | Scalp gel | | Psorin | | |
| Salicylic | Diprosalic | | Sebco | | Lassar's Paste |

| Dithranol | Rarely used as stains clothing (purple) can irritate skin. Apply to chronic extensor plaques only. Avoid face or flexure areas |
| --- | --- |
| Salicylic Acid | Useful as an adjunct to remove scales. Safe for long term use. Can cause irritation to normal skin |

## Location Based Treatment of Psoriasis - *Ref: BNF*

| Flexure | Can be managed with short-term use of a mild or moderate potency topical corticosteroid. Calcitriol or tacalcitol can be used in the longer-term; calcipotriol is more likely to cause irritation in flexures and should be avoided. Low strength tar preparations can also be used |
| --- | --- |
| Facial | Can be treated with short-term use of a mild potency topical corticosteroid; if this is ineffective, a corticosteroid of moderate potency, calcitriol, tacalcitol, or a low strength tar preparation can be used |
| Unstable | Widespread unstable psoriasis of erythrodermic or generalised pustular type requires urgent specialist assessment. Initial topical treatment should be limited to using emollients frequently and generously. More localised acute or subacute inflammatory psoriasis with hot, spreading or itchy lesions, should be treated topically with emollients or with a corticosteroid of moderate potency |

## Refer

| Dermatologist | Refer for phototherapy (UVB) or photochemotherapy (PUVA & UVA), oral retinoids or immunosuppressive drugs (methotrexate). Refer in extensive disease or unresponsive to treatments or affecting genitalia, generalised erythrodermic rash or pustular psoriasis |
| --- | --- |
| Rheumatologist | Refer to rheumatology if evidence of arthropathy |

| Causes | Characteristic exam feature |
|---|---|
| Erythroderma | Generalised redness to the skin (>90%). Refer urgently |
| Pustular | Small pustules that can appear all over the body or just on or just on the palms, soles and other small areas |
| Guttate | Mostly teens and presents with multiple drop-like lesions that is usually preceded by a streptococcal throat infection |
| Flexural | Common in elderly. Smooth, glazed plaque affecting axilla or submammary areas. |
| Scalp | Common. Well outlined scaly plaques with thickened scales. Differential – dandruff |

## EXPLANATIONS

*Psoriasis*

Psoriasis is an inflammatory skin condition where the top layer of the skin replaces itself too quickly. It normally takes a few months for skin to replace itself, however, this process is accelerated to often less than a week. This can cause excessive skin build up giving the appearance of thick scaly plaques. The rash is not contagious but may run in families.

*Triggers*

We are not entirely sure what causes it but we do know that there are a number of triggers that can worsen it. These include smoking, alcohol, sunlight, infection, damage to the skin, stress and certain medications.

# 12.3 Acne

Acne is a common skin condition that affects male and females alike. Peak incidence is at 18 years of age, however, it usually begins prior to the onset of puberty when the adrenal gland begins to produce and release increasing amounts of androgen hormones. It is characterised by papules, open and closed comedones (black and whiteheads), pustules, nodules and scars in the sebaceous distribution (face, neck, back and chest). The blockage and colonisation of the pilosebaceous ducts with Propionibacterium causes a hypersensitive response that gives rise to inflammatory acne.

## HISTORY

**Open questions**          Can you tell me more about your skin problem? How did it start?

**Focused questions**

*Acne*                      When did it start? How long has it been going on for? Has it changed over time?

   Distribution          Where have you experienced the spots/rash? (face, shoulders, chest, upper back)

   Rash                  What have you noticed? Black or white spots? Redness or pus filled pimples? Do you have scarring or cysts?

   Aggravating           Does anything make it better or worse?

   Worsen                Squeezing, puberty, pregnancy, periods, oily products/cosmetics

**Differentials**

*PCOS*                      Do you have any problems with your periods? Have you noticed any weight gain? Have you noticed any excess hair growth on the face or body?

*Acne Rosacea*             Do you experience flushing of the face? Is it triggered by anything (sun, alcohol, stress)? Have you noticed any change in the appearance of your nose (rhinophyma)?

## PAST HISTORY

*Medical*                   Do you suffer from any medical problems? (PCOS, Cushings)

## DRUG HISTORY

*Medication*                Have you tried any treatments for it already? (OTC/special diets)

   Worsens               Steroids (oral/topical), POP, mirena coil, lithium, phenytoin

## SOCIAL HISTORY

*Smoker*                    Do you smoke? How many cigarettes do you smoke per day?

*Alcohol*                   Do you drink alcohol? How much do you drink and how often?

*Occupation*                Are you working at the moment? (hot environment- chef)

## FAMILY HISTORY

*Acne*                      Does anyone in your family suffer from acne?

## IDEA, CONCERNS, EXPECTATIONS

*Idea*                      What did you think was causing spots? (poor hygiene, chocolate/fried food, stress)

*Concerns*                  Have you had any particular worried about it? (not going away)

*Expectations*              Was there any specific treatment that you were hoping for today?

*Impact on life*            How has your skin problem affected you? (bullying, time off, relationships, social life)

   Mood                  Has it affected your mood or self esteem?

## CSA TIPS

Despite being a common problem, a lot of patients with acne worry about possible scarring and permanent facial disfigurement. The acne may make its sufferer feel embarrassed and cause social avoidance. When assessing the patient, it is important to check the previous treatments the patient has tried and the lengths they have been used. Acne may cause psychological issues such as anxiety or depression in the adolescent or teenager, who may be victim to stigmatisation or taunting by their peers.

## PHYSICAL EXAMINATION

| | |
|---|---|
| Skin | Examine the face, back, chest area for signs of acne. Look for erythema, open (blackheads) or closed (whiteheads) comedones, papules, pustules, or cysts |

## Severity of Acne

| | |
|---|---|
| Mild | Open or closed comedones, some papules |
| Moderate | Papules, pustules, mild scarring |
| Severe | Abscess, nodules, widespread scarring |
| Conglobate | Burrowing abscesses with scarring |

## INVESTIGATIONS

| | |
|---|---|
| Bloods | *Not routinely performed:* LH, FSH, testosterone if PCOS |
| US | US ovaries if suspect PCOS |

## MANAGEMENT

### Conservative

| | |
|---|---|
| General advice | Wash your face at least twice a day with mild soap and water particularly when sweaty. Avoid greasy oils. Use a water based moisturiser cream |
| Scratching | Avoid scratching, picking or scrubbing spots (acne excoriee) |
| Cosmetics | Avoid excessive cosmetics. If used, use water based products then remove at night |
| Other | Not caused by poor hygiene, diet (chocolates, fatty food), stress. Acne is not infectious and sunlight does not improve it |

### Medical

| | |
|---|---|
| General | All treatment require 3mth use before considering changing it |
| Topical | Apply to whole face, not only spotty areas |
| Benzoyl peroxide | Initiate twice a day for 30min after washing with soap and water. Low strength works as well as strongest (Panoxyl 2.5%, 5%, 10%) |
| SE | Skin irritation, bleaches hair, clothing, avoid excessive sun exposure. If causes irritation, reduce frequency or strength and reapply |
| Topical retinoid | Apply on/bd. Spots may worsens before improving (isotretinoin, adapalene) |
| SE | Burning, erythema, skin peeling, skin dryness. Photosensitivity – apply at night, wash off in morning, wear sun cream if necessary |
| CI | Pregnancy (teratogenic) or breastfeeding |
| Azelaic acid | Available as cream (Skinoren) or gel (Finacea). Causes less skin irritation than other topical agents. Can occasionally lighten skin, photosensitivity |
| Topical abx | Resistance increasing so use with benzoyl peroxide (Dalacin T, Zineryt) |
| Combination | Benzoyl peroxide with antimicrobials (Duac, quinoderm) |
| | Benzoyl peroxide with topical retinoid (Epiduo) |
| | Topical retinoid with antimicrobials (isotrexin, aknemycin plus) |

*Oral*

| | | |
|---|---|---|
| Antibiotics | Combine topical (except antibiotics) cream with an oral antibiotic | |
| Tetracycline | Use tetracycline or oxytetracycline 500mg bd before food for 3mth. Lymecycline can be used as 2nd line | |
| SE | N&V, diarrhoea, photosensitivity (doxycycline), oesophagitis, thrush | |
| CI | Avoid in pregnancy and breastfeeding or <12yr | |
| Erythromycin | Erythromycin 500mg bd if tetracycline contraindicated | |
| SE | N&V and diarrhoea, indigestion | |
| Other | Specialist may use trimethoprim, clindamycin, clarithromycin, dapsone | |
| COC | Consider co-cyprindiol (Dianette - increase risk of DVT) or yasmin | |

***Refer***   Refer patient with severe acne (nodular, cyst, scarring) or non-responding moderate acne for consideration of Roaccutane (oral isotretinoin). Advise about side effects e.g. mucosal dryness, nose bleeding, myalgia, hypercholesterolaemia, teratogenic, headaches, depression

## DIFFERENTIAL DIAGNOSIS

| Causes | Characteristic exam feature |
|---|---|
| **Acne** | Bimodal distribution (teenagers and 30-40yrs). Typically occurs over face (periorbital sparing), upper chest, back and neck area. Presents with comedones (back/whiteheads), papules, pustules, cysts, scarring on a background of greasy skin |
| **Acne Rosacea** | Affects 40yr particularly women but often more severe in men. Presents with facial flushing of nose, cheeks and forehead, erythema, papules and pustules. Rash can be sore or itchy in nature. Associated with conjunctivitis or blepharitis and rhinophyma |
| **PCOS** | Endocrine disorder that presents with multiple cysts in the ovaries along with irregular periods (oligomenorrhoea, amenorrhoea) as well as acne and hirsutism |

## EXPLANATIONS

*Acne*   This is where the pores in your skin become blocked. As a result, excessive amounts of oil build up in the pores producing blackheads (darkened plugs) and whiteheads. The acne bug (Propionibacterium acnes), which is naturally found on the skin, grows and multiplies in these oily pores causing inflammation and pus filled spots.

Benzoyl peroxide   It works by killing bacteria, reduces inflammation, and helps to unplug blocked pores.

Topical retinoid   It works well at unplugging the blocked pores.

Topical antibiotics   Works well at killing off bacteria that causes the acne, but not in unplugging the pores.

Dianette   Helps control hormonal changes that are seen to cause acne.

Roaccutane   This works well at reducing the amount of oil produced from within the hair follicles therefore helping to clear up acne in the most severe cases.

# 12.4 Fungal infection

Fungal infections are a common presentation in GP surgeries. They are usually caused by dermatophytes which may lead to tinea corporis (body), tinea cruris (groin), tinea capitis (scalp), tinea pedis (athlete's foot) and tinea unguium (nails). It can spread through a number of different routes including via human to human contact, animal to human, and less commonly from the soil. Risk factors include DM, HIV, obesity, humid environments, skin folds, pregnancy and post antibiotics (broad spectrum) usage.

## HISTORY
**Open questions**          Can you tell me more about your skin problem? How did it start?

## Focused questions
*Fungal infection*          When did it start? How long has it been going on for? Has it changed over time?
    Distribution          Which areas of your skin are affected? (scalp, feet, web spaces, nails, groin, axillae)
    Dry / itchy          Is the skin dry or itchy? Does it bleed?
    Contact          Do you go swimming regularly? Do you use a public or shared shower after doing sports? Have you been in a changing room?

## Associated history
*Nails changes*          Have you noticed any changes to your nails? (discolouration, brittleness)
*Scalp*          Any dandruff or hair loss? Have you noticed any boggy swellings on the scalp (kerion)? Do you share combs? Anyone else in your family have it?
*Recurrent infection*          Do you get recurrent infections? Has the rash spread to the whole body?
*HIV*          Any persistent sore throats or whitish discoloration to the back of your throat?
*Diabetes*          Do you feel thirsty? Have you lost weight? Do you pass urine more often?

## Differentials
*Eczema*          Do you have dry inflamed skin? Do you suffer from hayfever or asthma?
*Psoriasis*          Is it mainly on the elbows, knee or scalp areas? Is it worsened by stress or sunlight?

## RED FLAGS          HIV, recurrent fungal infections, rapidly spreading

## PAST HISTORY
*Medical*          Do you suffer from any medical problems? (DM, HIV, obesity)

## DRUG HISTORY
*Medication*          Are you on any medications at the moment? (broad spectrum antibiotics)

## SOCIAL HISTORY
*Smoker*          Do you smoke? How many cigarettes do you smoke per day?
*Alcohol*          Do you drink alcohol? How much do you drink and how often?
*Occupation*          Are you working at the moment? Are you in contact with any animals (cattle) or do you do lots of gardening?
*Stress*          Are you feeling stressed? Any stress in your relationship or work?
*Pets*          Do you have any pets, such as cats or dogs?
*Travel*          Have you travel abroad to any humid climates?
*Sports (feet)*          Do you do doing sports or swimming? Do you wear occlusive footwear?

## FAMILY HISTORY
| | |
|---|---|
| Contact | Does anyone else have a similar rash? |

## IDEA, CONCERNS, EXPECTATIONS
| | |
|---|---|
| Idea | What did you think was causing the rash? (eczema, contagious from school) |
| Concerns | Have you had any particular worried about it? (STI, HIV) |
| Expectations | How were you hoping I could help you with your skin? |
| Impact on life | How has your skin problem affected you? (bullying, days off school) |

## CSA TIPS

Fungal infection can affect any part of the body. Commonly they are seen on the face, torso, feet and in the hair. However, they may also present on the genitals. They are usually caught from others and it is important to take a history of exposure to swimming or showers. In addition, you should give advice on how to minimise spread in the household if others are present. Be aware that treatment for fungal nail infections is considered a cosmetic procedure in some areas, and may not attract NHS funding.

## PHYSICAL EXAMINATION
*Skin*
| | |
|---|---|
| Distribution | Inspect rash area. Look at the trunk, axillae, scalp, groin, nails and feet. Check under skin folds (neck, submammary). Check digit web spaces |
| Skin changes | Look for scaling or erythema plaques with central clearing |
| Nails | Inspect nails for discolouration (yellow), hyperkeratosis or brittleness |
| Scalp | Inspect the scalp for dandruff, scaly plaques, alopecia. Look for a kerion |
| Lymph nodes | Consider examining regional lymph nodes if rash appears to be infected |

## INVESTIGATIONS
| | |
|---|---|
| MC&S | Swab if signs of secondary bacterial infections. Perform skin scrapings, nail clippings or plucked hair |
| UV wood light | Examine using UV Wood's light (brilliant green – microsporum (animals), dull green - Trichophyton schoenlenii). Rarely performed in GP setting |
| Bloods | Glucose, FBC, HIV tests (recurrent infections), LFTS (if considering oral therapy) |

## MANAGEMENT
*Conservative*
| | |
|---|---|
| General advice | Keep skin clean and dry (particularly skin folds). Wear loose garments (cotton clothes) and avoid humid conditions. Avoid sharing towel |
| Athletes foot | Wear non-occlusive footwear (open sandals). Wash feet and dry daily including between toes. Change socks daily and alternate between shoes. Wear cotton socks or leather footwear. Wear plastic sandals in changing rooms or showers. Use talcum powder to help dry the feet |
| Tinea cruris | Change underwear regularly. Wash and keep the groin area clean and dry. Wear loose fitting cotton undergarments |
| Tinea capitis | Dispose or disinfect (with bleach) contaminated objects (pillows, scissors, combs, hats) |
| Nail infection | Cut your nails short and file down. Use separate scissor to shorten infected nail only. Wear wide toe box shoes. Replace old shoes (fungal reservoir). Avoid injuries to toes. Treat athletes foot early to prevent spread |
| School | Children with fungal infections can attend school but should use precautions to prevent spread to other children |

**Medical**

Topical       Use for skin fungal infections. Try imidazoles/terbinafine or steroid adjuvant if skin is inflamed

---

**Generic and Trade name for Fungal creams** - *ref: BNF*

| Generic | Trade name | Generic | Trade name |
|---|---|---|---|
| Miconazole | Daktarin | Ketoconazole | Nizoral cream |
| Clotrimazole | Canesten | Terbinafine | Lamisil |

---

Versicolor     Try ketoconazole shampoo or selenium sulphide shampoo, dilute with small amount of water to reduce irritation. Apply to skin and leave for 10min before washing off

Oral antifungal    Use in recurrent, persistent fungal or scalp infections (terbinafine, fluconazole, itraconazole, griseofulvin)

 Tinea cruris    Consider single dose of oral antibiotic (fluconazole 200mg)

 Tinea capitis    Use oral rather than topical eg. Terbinafine 250mg od for 4wks. Can treat with ketoconazole shampoo

Nail infections    Consider amorolfine nail lacquer (Loceryl) if affects <=2 nails twice weekly. Use for up to 3-6 months for fingernails and 6-12 months for toenails. Oral antifungals for resistant or >2 nails. Offer terbinafine for 6wks for fingernails and 3mth for toenails

---

**Griseofulvin and Pregnancy** - *ref BNF*

Risk of fetotoxicity and teratogenicity; effective contraception required during and for <1mth after administration to women (important: effectiveness of oral contraceptives may be reduced, additional contraceptive precautions e.g. barrier method, required); also men should avoid fathering a child during and for <6mth after administration

---

**Refer**

Dermatologist    Refer to specialist if not improving despite treatment, widespread recurrent or severe infection or if patient is immunocompromised

## DIFFERENTIAL PRESENTATIONS

| Causes | Characteristic exam feature |
|---|---|
| **Tinea corporis** | Raised plaques on skin with scaling or erythema of outer border. Ring shaped with central clearing |
| **Tinea capitis** | Scaly area with erythema and possible alopecia |
| **Tinea pedis** | Affects webs between toes (3$^{rd}$ – 4$^{th}$ toe). Scaly crusting white rash |
| **Tinea cruris** | Affects upper thigh and occasionally scrotum. Red and scaly and itchy |

| Unguium | Affects toenails more than fingers. Brittle nails with yellow discolouration and thickening of distal edge |
| --- | --- |

## EXPLANATIONS

*Ringworm*

Ringworm is a fungal infection where there is an overgrowth of fungus found naturally on your skin. It is not in any way related to worm infestations rather the name comes from the shape of the rash. It is contagious and can be spread from person to person if you are not careful.

*Nail infections*

Fungal infections can also cause discolouration and irregular shaped nails. We can treat them with a long course of nail lacquer or tablets. However, you need to be aware that it may take several months for you to notice a difference as a new fresh nail needs to grow in its place.

Nail Lacquer

A nail lacquer is a treatment we can give to help the fungal infection that is affecting your nail. However, it is important that you apply it properly for it to work well. You should file down you nail before applying the lacquer. Coat the nail with the lacquer completely and leave to dry for 5mins. Do this once - two times a week. You may have to try for at least three months before you notice any improvement.

# *12.5 Head lice*

Head lice, otherwise known as Pediculus humanus capitis, refers to an infestation of parasitic insects on the human head. Although anyone can catch these head lice they usually affect preschool or primary school children. Head lice refers to the parasite whilst nits refer to the hatched eggs. Head lice appear as small greyish brown insects often described as being the size of a 'sesame seed'. They spread via close head-to-head contact and do not jump or fly like fleas contrary to popular belief. They are not as a result of poor hygiene or dirty hair.

**HISTORY**

| | |
|---|---|
| **Open questions** | Can you tell me more about the problems you are having? How did it start? |

**Focused questions**

| | |
|---|---|
| *Head lice* | When did it start? How long has it been going on for? |
| Scalp | Does your head itch a lot? is it itchier in a particular area? (occipital/post auricular) How intense is the itch? |
| Rash | Have you noticed a rash on your scalp? (nape area) |
| Nits/lice | Have you seen any nits (white eggs) or lice (grey-brown insect) in your hair? |

**Differentials**

| | |
|---|---|
| *Eczema* | Do you have any dry skin on the body? Do you suffer from hayfever or asthma? |
| *Psoriasis* | Do you have any rashes on the elbows or knees? Any joint pains? |
| *Tinea capitis* | Have you noticed any rashes on the head? |

**PAST HISTORY**

| | |
|---|---|
| *Head lice* | Have you had this problem before? |

**DRUG HISTORY**

| | |
|---|---|
| *Medication* | Have you tried any medication or treatments for it? |

**SOCIAL HISTORY**

| | |
|---|---|
| *School* | Are you aware of any outbreaks of head lice at your school? |
| *Occupation* | Are you working at the moment? What do you work as? |

**FAMILY HISTORY**

| | |
|---|---|
| *Head lice* | Does any one at home have head lice as well? |

**IDEA, CONCERNS, EXPECTATIONS**

| | |
|---|---|
| *Idea* | What did you think was causing the symptoms (head lice)? Did you have any idea how you may have got them? |
| *Concerns* | Any particular worries about it? (will they go away, treatments, resistance) |
| *Impact on life* | How has it affected you? (bullying, time off school, stigma) |

**CSA TIPS**

Head lice are common parasites that live off people's hair and in their scalps. They are found routinely in children, commonly from outbreaks at school. Parents may worry about their child catching lice and it spreading throughout the household. It is important to explain to the parent or carer about the problem and methods to detect and treat the condition. The scalp may become very itchy and affect their sleep.

## PHYSICAL EXAMINATION

| | |
|---|---|
| Scalp | Inspect the hair for any evidence of nits (white specks at hair roots), faecal matter (black specks) or live moving lice. Witnessing a moving louse is required for diagnosis (not nits). Inspect the nape area for a rash |

## INVESTIGATIONS

| | |
|---|---|
| Combing | Wet or dry combing used to visualise the lice and confirm diagnosis. Nits are not proof of active infection as they can remain for several weeks after death. It is nearly impossible to tell apart live and dead eggs |

### Detection Combing

- Spend 5 minutes combing the hair untangling and straightening using a normal comb
- Use specialised combs (Bug buster, hedrin detection combs) to fine comb the hair
- Comb from the scalp downwards to the ends of their hair
- Repeat each area three times before moving to an adjacent area
- Observe for lice caught within the comb as it is passed through the hair
- If a louse is visualised, catch it between comb and thumb
- Continue combing through the remainder of the hair for lice

## MANAGEMENT

### Conservative

| | |
|---|---|
| Prevention | Plait the hair to prevent the head lice from attaching to it. Regularly comb the hair. Avoid sharing pillows or brushes or combs. Recommend school have whole school 'bug busting' days. Regularly check the hair and check if any eggs or insect are noted |
| Wet combing | Use specialised combs (Bug buster). Comb can be shared with family. Methodically comb hair to remove lice. Perform at least 4 sessions (4 day intervals) over a 2wk period. Continue until no head lice is seen for 3 consecutive periods to confirm eradication |
| Contact tracing | Consider contract tracing over past months |

### Medical

| | |
|---|---|
| Principles | Ensure you treat all affected members of the household. All treatments need to be repeated more than once and none is 100% guaranteed of success. Check the hair 2 and 3 days after treatment for live lice. If none detected, check again 9 days after and if clear then the treatment has been successful |
| Dimeticone | (Hedrin) Available as lotion/spray. Apply and rub in the scalp. Leave overnight for 8hrs. And wash out using normal shampoo. |
| Malathion | (Derbac-M liquid) Apply Malathion 0.5% to the scalp and dry hair extending to the neck area and behind the ears. Allow to dry naturally. Leave for 12hrs before rinsing out. Repeat application in 1wk time. |

| Permethrin | (Lyclear crème rinse 1%) Not licensed for head lice despite being widely used. Used as a final rinse after using normal shampoo. Hair is dried first with towel prior to applying cream rinse to scalp and hair. Leave for 10min before rinsing. Repeat after 7d. Avoid in pregnancy. |
| --- | --- |
| Pregnancy | Recommend wet combing or dimeticone lotion. Malathion not contraindicated but used with caution. Avoid permethrin |
| Unsuccessful tx | Household members be assessed for head lice. Consider resistance to insecticide and try alternative. Itching may persist for 2-3wks despite successful treatment. Nits on hair alone do not represent failure of treatments |

## EXPLANATIONS

| Head lice | Head lice are small insects that can live on the head and are very common in children. They normally pass from person to person by close head contact. The bugs do not jump or fly from person to person and having them does not necessarily mean your hair is dirty. They often cause no symptoms but occasionally cause an itch to the scalp. This is caused by an allergy to the lice itself rather than from their bites. |
| --- | --- |
| Detection Combing | In order to prevent head lice it is important to keep checking your children's hair regularly. This process is known as detection combing. You should buy a special fine toothed lice comb from the pharmacist that will help catch even the smallest nits. Either do this with the hair wet or dry. Use a normal comb to straighten out the hair. Use the lice comb to file through the hair from the scalp to the end and watch the combs for any lice or nits. |

# *12.6 Scabies*

Scabies is a skin disorder that is caused by the human parasite called Sarcoptes scabiei. The scabies mite is highly contagious and is usually spread by close skin to skin contact and less often by sharing clothes or bedding. Predominant symptoms including an highly intense itch affecting the body. Whilst classically in adults there is head and face sparing, in children or in immunocompromised patients this may not be the case. Often symptoms may start 4-6 weeks post infestation, and despite treatment reinfestation is quite common.

## HISTORY
**Open questions**      Can you tell me more about the skin rash/itching you are experiencing? How did it start?

## Focused questions
| | |
|---|---|
| *Scabies* | When did it start? How long has it been going on for? |
|   Rash | What part of the body is affected (feet, fingers, web spaces, wrist, elbow, axilla, umbilicus, areolae)? Have you noticed any lumps or tracks in the skin? |
|     Itch | How intense is the itch? Is it worse at night or after a bath? |
|     Facial sparing | Does it affect the face or neck area? |

## Differentials
| | |
|---|---|
| *Eczema* | Do you have any dry skin on the body? Do you suffer from hayfever or asthma? |
| *Contact dermatitis* | Have you had a reaction to any products such as perfumes, soaps, lotions, creams? |

## PAST HISTORY
*Scabies*      Have you had this problem before?

## DRUG HISTORY
*Medication*      Have you tried any medication or treatments for it?

## SOCIAL HISTORY
| | |
|---|---|
| *School* | Are you aware of any outbreaks of scabies at your school? |
| *Accommodation* | Have you recently moved into a new home? Any stays at hostels or hotels? |
| *Occupation* | Are you working at the moment? What do you work as? |

## FAMILY HISTORY
*Scabies*      Does anyone else in the home have similar symptoms?

## IDEA, CONCERNS, EXPECTATIONS
| | |
|---|---|
| *Idea* | What did you think was causing symptoms? (allergy) |
| *Concerns* | Any particular worries about it? (family household members affected) |
| *Impact on life* | How has it affected you? (persistent itching, stigma – unhygienic, embarrassment) |

## CSA TIPS
Scabies can be quite challenging to diagnose. Often the patient reports an intense itch that is particularly worse after a hot bath or at night and there can be signs of burrows at the wrist or feet areas. If the patient is a child remember to inform them of how long they should be off school.

## PHYSICAL EXAMINATION

Skin | Inspect the interdigital web spaces of the hands, wrists and feet. Observe the fingers for any burrows or S shape tracks. Inspect the torso for rashes, papules, pustules or evidence of secondary infections. Also look behind the ears, neck and scalp areas

## INVESTIGATIONS

Extraction | Isolate and extract mite from a burrow using a sharp tipped needle

Ink test | Use special ink to reveal burrows

Skin scraping | Take skin scraping using blade or needle and observe through microscope. Diagnosis assisted with visualisation of faecal matter, eggs

STI | Consider STI screen if transmitted by sexual contact

Immunocompromise | HIV test, FBC if immunocompromised

## MANAGEMENT

### Conservative

Prevention | Avoid contact with affected individuals and those being treated

Contacts | Treat all close contacts simultaneously (household) even if asymptomatic

Machine wash | Machine wash >50° all clothes, bed linen, towel on first day of starting treatment. Clothes that cannot be washed keep in plastic bag for 3 days to kill mites

School | Avoid school until successfully treated

### Medical

Permethrin | Use as first line. Apply to whole body from neck and ears below. Cover all creases of body. Careful applications to toes and fingers. Do not apply after hot bath rather to cold dry skin. Leave on for 8 -12hrs before rinsing off. Re-apply to selected area if hands are washed. Repeat after 1wk (Lyclear Dermal Cream 5%)

Malathion | Apply Malathion 0.5% to body similar to permethrin. Instead leave on body for 24 hours. Repeat application in 1 week's time (Derbac-M liquid)

Itch treatment | Offer sedating antihistamines at night if itch is intense. Consider topical crotamiton to control itch post treatment or mild steroid (hydrocortisone 1%). Pruritus may persist for up to 6wks despite successful treatment

Pregnancy | Start with Permethrin 5%, use malathion if allergy. Mums should clear cream from nipple before breastfeeding but re-apply thereafter

### Refer

Refer to dermatologist if diagnosis is in doubt or unsuccessful despite 2 treatment. Refer to HPA if outbreak confirmed at school or institution (nursing home)

## EXPLANATIONS

Scabies | Scabies are small insects (parasites) that can be passed from person to person by close skin contact. They may have no symptoms but some are very sensitive to the bug that they have a very intense itch over the body. This is caused by an allergy to the parasite itself rather than from their bites.

Alopecia refers to hair loss. Although most people complain of hair loss affecting their scalp, it may occur anywhere around the body. It usually starts suddenly and may present with patchy hair loss initially. It is often a distressing symptom as it can affect one's self esteem. There are a number of causes with the most unpredictable and difficult to treat being alopecia areata.

## HISTORY
**Open questions**   Can you tell me more about your skin problem? How did it start?

## Focused questions
*Alopecia*          When did it start? How long has it been going on for?
   Distribution    Which areas of your skin are affected? (scalp, beard, eyebrows, male/female pattern baldness)
   Nature          Did it come on suddenly or gradually over a period of time? Is it patchy hair loss or do you find it affects the whole area?
   Nails           Have you noticed any changes to your nails? (areata)
   Scarring        Have you had any scarring to the skin?

## Gender Related Pattern Baldness
*Male Pattern*      This is the most common type of baldness. Initially presents as a receding hairline and then thinning around the crown and the temple areas. As it progresses, a horse-shoe like appearance results, before eventually going totally bald. It is more prevalent as a man ages
*Female Pattern*    In females, they may first notice increased shedding of hair before it eventually thins affecting the top then side of the head. It is more common after the menopause

## Associated history
*Stress*            Have you had any recent stress or worries?
*Diet*              Have you changed your diet recently? Are you on any diets?

## Differentials
*Thyroid (hypo/hyper)*  Do you find it difficult to tolerate hot or cold weathers? Do you have dry or oily skin? Have you noticed any change in your weight?
*Tinea infection*   Have you noticed any circular itchy rashes?
*Iron deficiency*   Do you feel tired all the time? Do you have heavy periods?
*Telogen effluvium* Are you stressed? How is work? Any problems with relationships?
*Trichotillomania*  Do you find that you have a tendency to play or pull on your hair?
*Seb. dermatitis*   Do you have an itchy scalp? Have you noticed any white flakes fall?

## PAST HISTORY
*Previous*          Have you had any hair loss like this before?
*Medical*           Do you suffer from any medical illnesses? (thyroid, pernicious anemia, Down's, SLE)
*Chemotherapy*      Did you have any chemotherapy recently?
*Post pregnancy*    Have you recently given birth?

## DRUG HISTORY

| | |
|---|---|
| *Medication* | Are you on any medication? Have you tried any treatments for it already? |
| Improves | Minoxidil (temporary), steroids, finasteride |
| Worsens | Chemotherapy, ACEI, sodium valproate, warfarin, COCP, HRT |

## SOCIAL HISTORY

| | |
|---|---|
| *Alcohol* | Do you drink alcohol? How much do you drink and how often? |
| *Smoker* | Do you smoke? How many cigarettes do you smoke per day? |
| *Occupation* | Are you working at the moment? What type of work are you doing? |
| *Mood* | Has it affected your mood or self esteem? |

## FAMILY HISTORY

| | |
|---|---|
| *Hair loss* | Does anyone in your family suffer from hair loss? (areata) |

## IDEA, CONCERNS, EXPECTATIONS

| | |
|---|---|
| *Idea* | What did you think was causing the rash? (food allergies, contact dermatitis) |
| *Concerns* | Have you had any particular worries about it? (disfigurement, scarring, relationship problems, sleep – excessive rubbing) |
| *Expectations* | How were you hoping I could help you with your skin? (specialist referral) |
| *Impact on life* | How has your skin problem affected you? (relationships, cannot sunbathe, loss of job) |

## CSA TIPS

Hair loss can be an embarrassing problem particularly if it affects women. Patients may have struggled with OTC medications or spent £100's on potions, creams and shampoos looking for a magic cure before speaking to the doctor. Patient's may attend the clinic requesting minoxidil or finasteride as a possible solution. However, it is important to discuss with them the possible causes and then consider the treatment options that are available on the NHS.

## PHYSICAL EXAMINATION

| | |
|---|---|
| *Skin* | Inspect the hair for signs of scaling, kerion, erythema, pustules. Observe for its distribution and whether symmetrical hair loss. Look for signs of exclamation mark hairs |

## INVESTIGATIONS

| | |
|---|---|
| *Bloods* | If male pattern baldness in women consider LH/FSH, testosterone (PCOS) |
| *Skin biopsy* | Rarely performed but specialist may perform skin biopsy |

## MANAGEMENT  *treat underlying cause*

| | |
|---|---|
| *Conservative* | |
| Diet | Ensure that the patient eats a healthy balance diet. Advise to reduce fast-food (animal fats) and excessive vitamin A |
| Hair | Do not pull hair tightly back into ponytails. Avoid excess brushing or heat styling as this damages the hairs |

### *Alopecia*

| | |
|---|---|
| *Conservative* | Reassure and watch and wait as most regrow within 1yr, but can be difficult to predict. Wear hats or sun cream to protect areas from sun. Consider counselling |

| Medical | Consider trial of potent steroids (betnovate 0.1%, dermovate scalp solution) for 3mth for non-facial areas. May take 3mth to work and hair growth initially fine and depigmented |
| Specialist | May consider intralesional steroid injections, topical immunotherapy, light therapy, oral steroid, minoxidil, wigs |

### Androgenetic alopecia

| Conservative | Recommend concealment by allowing lateral hair to grow and combing over area. Consider wigs or toupee. If >50% hair loss refer to dermatologist |
| Medical | |
| Minoxidil | Consider minoxidil (2%, 5%) bd (private). Used over period of time (9mths) to see benefits. Hair loss seen once stop using. 5% only for men |
| Finasteride | Consider finasteride 1mg od (private). Improvement seen after 3-6mth of use. Hair loss seen within 6-12mths once stop using. Side effects include loss of libido, erectile dysfunction |

| Telogen effluvium | Reassure, hair growth often takes 6mth. Treat underlying cause of trigger. Minoxidil can be trialled |

| Trichotillomania | Refer for behavioural therapy or CBT. Consider cropping hair. Specialist may consider olanzapine or Methylphenidate |

## DIFFERENTIAL DIAGNOSIS

| Causes | Characteristic exam feature |
| --- | --- |
| Alopecia areata | Unknown aetiology. Peak incidence 15-30yr. Associated with DM, vitiligo, thyroid disease, pernicious anaemia. Presents with round, oval patchy hair loss, with pathognomonic exclamation mark hairs around margins. Can affect any area but scalp and beard more common. Associated with pitting nails, Beau's lines |
| Androgenic alopecia (baldness) | Genetic component. Balding over crown and temples as the hairs become finer. Women have more diffuse hair loss over crown and frontal scalp with preservation of frontal hairline. Often seen in postmenopausal women |
| Telogen effluvium | Diffuse pattern hair loss upto 3mth after a stressful event (stress, illness, fever, etc). Can affect bi-temporal region in women |
| Tinea capitis | Fungal infection typically affecting children with pruritus patchy hair loss and scaling. Can presents with kerion |
| Trichotillomania | Obsessive-compulsive disorder with patients pulling out their hair. Can affect eyelashes and eyebrows. Pattern asymmetrical with unusual pattern of hair loss. Complication include trichobezoar (swallowing hair) |

## EXPLANATIONS

*Alopecia areata*

Alopecia is a form of hair loss that can come and go. It often affects the scalp and causes a round coin shape patchy hair loss. Whilst it is not entirely clear, it is believed to be caused by a problem with the immune system mistakenly thinking the hair is a foreign target.

*Baldness*

This is the most common type of hair loss. It often affects men but can affect women. Often there is a receding hairline with thinning of the hair on top as well as temples. Women typically have thinning of the hair affecting the crown only. This may run in families or may be something that happens due to the changes in hormones as we get older.

*Telogen effluvium*

This is a condition that is often caused by significant amounts of stress. It causes widespread hair loss over a period of time (3mth). Often it stops falling and regrows within 6 months.

*Tinea capitis*

This is a fungal infection where there is an overgrowth of fungus found naturally on your skin.

# 13.1 Approach to Paediatric History

Taking a history from a parent and child is a key skill that all GP's have to master. Not least, are we dealing with a history that, depending on the age of the child, is based on another person's perception and intuition but also, the child may not be old enough to describe their own problems and symptoms in a clear and meaningful way. In addition, the Dr has to deal with 2 (or possibly more participants) in the consultation which will definitely impact on the dynamics of the conversation.

Be aware then when dealing with parents of young children they may be tired, anxious or fearful. In the case of teenage children, the parents may be intrusive and over-controlling. In all situations it is important to you establish and maintain rapport and try and be empathic to their plight.

## HISTORY
### Principles

| | |
|---|---|
| *Listen to mum* | If the child is of a young age and attends with a parent, i.e. the mother, listen carefully and acknowledge what they they say. The mother should be considered correct until proven otherwise |
| *Address by name* | When talking to the parents about the child avoid addressing them as 'he' or 'she' rather call them by their first names especially if they are in the room. e.g. *Does Johnny have any tummy pain?* |
| *Rapport* | Greet the child as well as the parents when they come in the room. Maintain good eye contact with them when talking to them |
| Young | Develop rapport by talking about topics which the child may find interesting to them *Johnny...Which school do you go to? Who is your favourite teacher? Do you have a favourite friend? Why are they your favourite?* |
| Older | If the child is a little bit older talk about their hobbies. *Johnny do you have any hobbies or things that you enjoy? Do you watch football? Who is your favourite team? What is your favourite computer game?* |
| *Interaction* | Observe the interaction between the child and the parent |
| Positive | Is the parent concerned and appropriately caring for the child? Do they show love and affection to the child? |
| Negative | Does the parent scold or smack the child or is condescending towards them? Is the parent over controlling? |
| *History* | Take a history from the parent as well as the child |
| Permission | When speaking to the parents seek permission from the child or inform them that you are going to do so e.g. *Johnny, I am just going to speak to mum about you. Is that ok?* |
| Open questions | Ensure that you use open questions and avoid too many closed questions to allow the child to use their own vocabulary to describe their symptoms e.g. *Tell me how did it start? How did it begin?* |

| Tailor | Use appropriate language and vocabulary when questioning the child and avoid medical jargon e.g. *Where does it hurt? Does your tummy/belly hurt? Do you feel hot? Did you bump your nose?* |
| --- | --- |
| Props | If the child is very young consider using props such as toys or teddy bears i.e. trying to locate pain |
| Verify | Verify and corroborate their history with their parents if necessary. Avoid being dismissive to what the child says |

## Focused history

| *Detailed* | Establish in a chronological order how their symptoms developed |
| --- | --- |
| Onset | How did it begin/start? |
| Last well | When was the child last well? |
| Triggers | Anything makes it better or worse? |
| Similar episodes | Any similar episodes/illnesses in the past? |
| Contact | Have they been in contact with anyone with similar symptoms i.e. home/school |
| Days off school | Have they been off school or nursery? |

| *Infant* | If taking a history about an infant ensure that you ask questions pertinent to their age |
| --- | --- |
| Bowels | How are their bowel movements? Any wet nappies? |
| Weight | Have they lost or gained any weight recently? |
| Feeds | How often do they feed? Has it changed? |
| Type fed | Are they breast or bottle fed? |

| *Behaviour* | How is the child's usual mood or demeanour? Has there been any change? Do they have temper tantrums? Do they hit themselves or carry out any repetitive behaviours (autism)? Are they hyperactive (ADHD)? How is their sleep? |
| --- | --- |

## IDEA, CONCERNS, EXPECTATIONS

| *Ideas & concerns* | What were you worried about your child's illness? Did you have any thoughts as to what is causing your child's illness? |
| --- | --- |
| *Expectations* | How were you hoping we could address this problem? |
| *Impact on life* | How has the illness affected the family? (illness affected other, difficulty with child care, postnatal depression) |

## PAST HISTORY

| *Medical* | Enquire whether the child suffers from any medical condition (asthma, DM, epilepsy, atopy)? Do they have a learning disability? |
| --- | --- |
| *Immunisations* | Check if they are up-to-date with their childhood immunisations. Have they taking any travel vaccines? |

## BIRTH HISTORY

| *Pregnancy* | Enquire whether the mother had any problems during pregnancy? (epilepsy, DM, BP, viral illnesses - hep B, HIV, varicella) |
| --- | --- |
| *Delivery* | Ask how the child was delivered, was it via a c-section or naturally? Where there any problems in childbirth (prolonged labour)? Where forceps or ventouse required? Was the child born prematurely or at term? |
| *Treatment* | Were they admitted to the SCBU? Did they have jaundice and require light treatment? |

| | |
|---|---|
| *Feeding* | Did they breast or bottle feed? Any problems with weaning? |
| *Development* | Have there been any problems with the child's development or achieving milestones? (walking, eating, speaking, potty training) |

## FAMILY HISTORY

| | |
|---|---|
| *Genetic* | Establish if there are any genetic conditions that run in the family (CF, sickle cell) |
| *Medical* | Do any medical conditions affect other family members? (asthma, allergy) |

## DRUG HISTORY

| | |
|---|---|
| *Medication* | Is the child taking any medications? Any OTC preparations? |

## SOCIAL HISTORY

| | |
|---|---|
| *Home* | Who lives with them at home? Are parents consanguineous? |
| Siblings | Do they have brothers or sisters? How is the relationship between them? Do they have any illnesses? |
| Social services | Are they known to social services? |
| *School* | Do they go to nursery or school? Any bullying? How are they performing? Any unauthorised days off? |
| *Smoking* | Does anyone smoke at home? |
| *Pets* | Are there any pets at home? (allergies) |
| *Diet* | Does the child eat a balanced diet? Do they avoid any foods (dairy, meat)? Do they have any allergies to food (seafood, peanuts)? |

## EXAMINATION

| | |
|---|---|
| *Vitals* | Check centiles (compare to red book). If <2yr check head circumference |
| *Examination* | Examine appropriate system to physical complaint |

## RED FLAGS

Poor growth on centiles, child protection concerns, developmental delay

## CSA TIPS

In the CSA exam, children are more frequently being used who can play roles aged 6 years and above. However, cases may not actually involve the presence of a child, but may be a discussion between a dr and a concerned parent about a child, infant or neonate. In both cases the medical information will be obtained from the parents, but in the case of a child who is able to speak, you will have to tailor the consultation to include the child's own views about their problem as well.

## MANAGEMENT PLAN

| | |
|---|---|
| *Explaining* | In your explanation incorporate vocabulary that the parent used to describe their child's illness. e.g. You mentioned Johnny was 'wheezy' and 'croupy' |
| *Prognosis* | Explain the natural course of the illness and what to expect within a time line |

## SAFETY NETTING

| | |
|---|---|
| *Red flags* | Ensure that explain to the parents red flags symptoms to look out for and to seek medical advice if they encounter them |
| *Follow up* | Offer the patient a convenient follow-up appointment if relevant. If a complaint is being made explain when the patient will expect to get a response |

# 13.2 Asthma

Asthma is a chronic inflammatory disorder of the airways that is characterised by variable airway obstruction and hyper-reactivity. Exposure of the airway to environmental allergens causes bronchospasm, excessive mucus secretions and oedema. Over time, continued exposure leads to airway narrowing and gives rise to symptoms including wheeze, breathlessness, chest tightness and coughing. Its severity can be assessed using a peak flow meter which also helps in diagnosis confirmed with reversibility and improvement in PEFR following admission of a short course of bronchodilator (salbutamol).

## HISTORY

**Open questions**

Can you tell me more about your child's cough/problems with their breathing? Could you tell me about what has been troubling them?

## Focused questions

| | |
|---|---|
| *Asthma* | Have they had a cough? When did it first start? How long does it last for? |
| Diurnal variation | Is it worse at night or in the mornings? |
| Triggers | Does anything makes their symptoms better (inhalers, seasons) or worse (exercise, pets, going to park, cold weather)? |
| SOB | Are they short of breath? Have they had any noisy breathing or wheeze? |
| Chest tightness | Do they report any chest pain in the morning? |

## Associated history

| | |
|---|---|
| *Exacerbation* | Have they had a fever? Have they brought up any phlegm? Any runny nose? |
| *Vomiting* | Do they vomit after coughing? |

## DIFFERENTIALS

| | |
|---|---|
| *Foreign body* | Did the wheeze, noisy breathing or shortness of breath come on suddenly? Have they been eating peanuts? |

## RED FLAGS

Severe SOB, incomplete sentences, exhaustion, fast breathing, confusion

## PAST HISTORY

| | |
|---|---|
| *Atopy* | Do you suffer from hayfever, eczema or urticaria? |
| *Bronchiolitis* | Did they suffer from bronchiolitis or wheeze when they were an infant? How old were they when they started wheezing? |
| *Asthma attacks* | In the last year have they had any asthma attacks? How many? |
| *A&E* | Have you ever attended A&E with asthma? |

## BIRTH HISTORY

| | |
|---|---|
| *Pregnancy* | Were they born prematurely? |

## DRUG HISTORY

| | |
|---|---|
| *Medication* | Is your child taking any medications or inhalers? Do they use a face mask? How often do you use them? Do you know how to use them properly? |
| Exacerbation | Have you used oral steroids in the last year for your asthma? How many times? |
| *Immunisations* | Check if they are up-to-date with their childhood immunisations? |

## SOCIAL HISTORY

| | |
|---|---|
| *Home* | Who is at home with them? Any siblings? |
| *Smoker* | Does anyone in the family smoke at home? |
| *Pets* | Do you have any pets? (cat, dogs) |
| *Toys* | Do they have fluffy toys? (allergen) |
| *School* | Do they go to school? Have they missed school because of it? How often? |
| *Sport* | Does your child play sports? Has it interfered with their ability to compete? |

## FAMILY HISTORY

| | |
|---|---|
| *Medical* | Anyone in the family suffer from asthma, eczema or hayfever? |

## IDEA, CONCERNS, EXPECTATIONS

| | |
|---|---|
| *Idea* | What do you think may be causing your child's illness? |
| *Concerns* | Is there anything that is worrying you specifically? (asthma) |
| *Expectations* | How were you hoping we could address this problem? |
| *Impact on life* | How has the illness affected your child? (unable to compete in tournaments) |

## CSA TIPS

Children presenting with chronic cough is a common occurrence in the primary care setting. Parents often struggle with young children who awake from sleep from coughing, or whose playground activities are restricted due to breathlessness or a cough. Although most parents would appreciate a diagnosis for their child's problem, most are fearful of a diagnosis of Asthma for it conjures up pictures or repeated A&E attendances and possible ITU spells. A clear and simple explanation about asthma, its causes and treatment should help in allaying any misplaced parental fears. You may also be faced with an anxious parent who is worried about the effects of steroids upon their child's growth and overall health. It is important to acknowledge their fears and concerns and give the appropriate advice.

---

### Effects of Inhaled/oral Steroids on Growth

Children who have a total of 400 mcg of inhaled steroids do not display any stunting of growth or growth spurts. Whereas children on higher doses of inhaled steroids or regular short courses of oral steroids may experience a slow down of growth in the short term. However, it has been shown that most do in fact reach their expected height or be reach it at a slower interval. Anecdotally poorly controlled or untreated asthmatics also have poor growth

---

## PHYSICAL EXAMINATION

| | |
|---|---|
| *Vitals* | Pulse (tachycardia), respiratory rate (tachyopnea), temp, height, weight (growth charts), O2 sats |
| *Respiratory* | |
|    Inspection | Respiratory distress, accessory muscles, barrel chest, Harrison's sulcus, unable to complete sentences |
|    Auscultation | Listen to the chest for prolonged expiratory phase, wheeze, silent chest |

## INVESTIGATIONS

| | |
|---|---|
| *CXR* | Overinflated chest or unclear diagnosis |
| *Peak flow* | Unreliable in young children due to poor technique: reversibility with B-agonist/inhaled steroids |
| *Specialist* | Spirometry if >5yr if diagnosis uncertain |

## MANAGEMENT

*Diagnosis*   Diagnosis based on Hx & examination. Consider prescribing peak flow in older children

---

## High Probability of Diagnosis of Asthma
- *Symptoms:* Wheeze, SOB, chest tightness, and cough (night, early morning, after exercise, cold, allergens)
- *PMH:* Atopy or FH of atopy, asthma
- *Examination:* Widespread wheeze (expiratory, bilateral), prolonged expiration, increase RR

## Low Probability of Diagnosis of Asthma
- *Symptoms:* Associated with colds only. History of moist cough
- *Examination:* Repeated normal chest when symptomatic
- *Investigations:* Normal PEFR or spirometry when symptomatic

---

## Conservative
*Lifestyle*

| | |
|---|---|
| Allergen avoid | Although many recommend avoid, SIGN suggest no evidence of any improvement |
| Dust mite | Remove carpets, curtains, soft toys. Cover pillows, mattress, regular hovering (get someone else to hoover and return after 20min) |
| Pets | Avoid pets (cats or dogs) |
| Breastfeeding | Protective against asthma |
| Smoking | Stop passive smoking where possible |
| Exercise | Reduce weight can recommend exercise programmes |

## Medical

| | |
|---|---|
| Immunisation | If patients are on inhaled/oral steroids they should be offered annual flu vaccinations |
| Medication | Treatment should be stepped up to maintain good control and stepped down if control is good. If the patient is unable to use the inhaler, consider prescribing a spacer device to aid delivery |

*Management >5-12yr*

| | |
|---|---|
| Step 1 | Inhaled short-acting B2 agonist as required. Step up if required oral steroids for exacerbation in last 2yrs, using blue inhaler or still symptomatic >2x/wk, waking up 1 night/wk |
| Step 2 | Add inhaled steroid 200–400 mcg/d (e.g. beclomethasone). Start at appropriate steroid dose for severity (e.g. 200mcg) |
| Step 3 | Add inhaled long-acting agonist (LABA – e.g. salmeterol). Assess control: |
| Good | Good response to LABA – continue LABA |
| Inadequate | Benefit from LABA but control still inadequate – continue LABA and increase inhaled steroid dose to 400 mcg/d |
| No response | No response to LABA – stop LABA and increase inhaled steroid to 400 mcg/d. If control still inadequate, institute trial of other therapies, e.g. leukotriene, SR Theophylline |
| Step 4 | Increase inhaled steroid up to 800 mcg/d |
| Step 5 | Maintain high-dose inhaled steroid at 800 mcg/d and refer to specialist |

*Management <5yr*

| | |
|---|---|
| Step 1 | Inhaled short-acting B2 agonist as required. Step up if required oral steroids for exacerbation in last 2yrs, using blue inhaler or still symptomatic >2x/wk, waking up 1 night/wk |

| Step 2 | |
| --- | --- |
| Steroid | Add inhaled steroid 200–400 mcg/d (e.g. beclomethasone). Start at appropriate steroid dose for severity (e.g. 200mcg) |
| Leuk. antag. | Consider leukotriene receptor antagonist if inhaled steroid cannot be used |
| Step 3 | If taking steroid inhaler add leukotriene receptor antagonist or vis versa |
| Step 4 | Refer to specialist |
| | |
| QoF | Patient needs yearly QoF screening with the RCP questions |

---

### RCP Questions to Assess Asthma

*In the last month...*

- Have you had difficulty sleeping because of your asthma symptoms (including cough)?
- Have you had your usual asthma symptoms during the day (cough, wheeze, chest tightness or SOB)?
- Has your asthma interfered with your usual activities e.g. housework, work/school etc?

*Ref: Measuring Clinical Outcome in Asthma: a patient-focused approach. London: RCP, 1999*

---

| *Refer* | Refer as per BTS guidelines. Refer urgently if signs of severe or life threatening asthma |
| --- | --- |
| *Follow up* | Follow up every 3mths to consider stepping down or change to the lowest inhaled steroid dose if symptoms are controlled |

### SAFETY NETTING

| *Admission* | If patients are acute short of breath, chest tightness, wheezing, unable to complete sentences, exhausted, confused or drowsy they should seek medical advice |
| --- | --- |

### EXPLANATIONS     *see asthma chapter*

*Reassurance*   Asthma is very common and is something your child may have to live with for the rest of their life. If we took three children suffering with asthma, one child will grow out of it, the other may improve during their teen years only for the asthma to return in adulthood, and the last will continue to be asthmatic. Even if they were to suffer with asthma for the rest of their life, they should be able to maintain a normal lifestyle.

I understand that you have particular concerns about your son competing competitively in sporting tournaments. However, I would like to reassure you that there are a number of famous sport personalities who suffer with asthma, such as Paula Radcliffe and Paul Scholes, who continue to lead successful and fruitful lives.

*Spacer*   I will prescribe a device known as a volumatic spacer to help deliver the medicine to the lungs easily. It consists of two ends; on one end is the mouthpiece/mask (sticking out) and other end is where the inhaler is to be attached. Shake your inhaler well and connect it to the far end. Release two puffs into the device. As the spacer has a valve, the medicine will stay inside. Place your child's mouth over the mask ensuring you make a tight seal. Ask them to breathe in and out deeply and at a slow pace; do this around three to four times. This will ensure that your child's lungs have taken enough of the medication.

Autism spectrum disorder is a complex and lifelong neurological and developmental problem that appears during childhood. It affects the sufferer in a number of ways including impairing their ability to socially interact with others as well as their ability to communicate through verbal and nonverbal communication. It is often noticed by parents as the child reaches 3yr of age and begins to display odd, repetitive behaviours, or has problems interacting with them.

The causes of autism are not known; but it is thought that there is a complex interplay between genetic, environmental and neurological factors that affect brain development. In the UK it is believed that 1 in 100 of people has autism or autistic traits amounting to almost 700,000 sufferers.

**HISTORY**
Approach the topic sensitively in a non-threatening non-judgemental manner. Adopt a relaxed open posture that is calm and inviting. Try not to appear patronising nor paternalistic towards the parent(s). Do not be dismissive but try and engage with and explore the patient's ideas and concerns.

**Open questions**     How can I help you today? Can you tell me more about your child's behaviour?

**Focused questions**
*Autism*     When did you notice the change in your child?
  Communication     How does your child communicate? Do they speak? Did this start on time? Do they repeat themselves or a phrase a lot? Do they understand if you are joking with them?
  Social Interact.     Does your child have many friends? Do they enjoy playing with others or are more happy being alone? Do they avoid eye-contact with you or others?
  Playing     Does your child play with different toys or concentrate on one? Do they play with the whole toy or just with a small part of it?
  Routine     Do they have to have a clear routine such as when dressing or eating?
  Skills     Does your child have any exceptional talents? (memorising lists, drawing, musical)

*Behaviour*     How is your child's usual mood or demeanour? Has there been any change? Do they have temper tantrums or challenging behaviour? Do they hit themselves or carry out any repetitive behaviours such as rocking their body or flapping their hands?

**Associated history**
*Sleeping*     How is your child's sleep? Do they have any problems?
*Feeding*     How is their appetite? Do they eat well? Do they refuse any foods? Why do they refuse?
*Gastrointestinal*     Do they have any problems with their bowels? (constipation, diarrhoea, pain)
*Development*     Have there been any problems with the child's development or achieving milestones? (walking, eating, speaking, potty training)

**RED FLAGS**     If <3yr regresses on language or developmental milestones, suspicion of child abuse

**PAST HISTORY**
*Medical*     Enquire whether the child suffers from any medical condition (Downs, tuberous sclerosis, epilepsy, ADHD)? Do they have a learning disability?

| Immunisations | Check if they are up-to-date with their childhood immunisations? Have they taken any travel vaccines? |
|---|---|

## BIRTH HISTORY

| Pregnancy | Enquire whether the mother had any problems during pregnancy? Did you take any medications (sodium valproate)? |
|---|---|
| Gestation | Was the child born prematurely (<35wks)? |

## DRUG HISTORY

| Medication | Are they taking any medications? |
|---|---|

## FAMILY HISTORY

| Autism | Are there any illnesses that run in your family? (autism) |
|---|---|
| Schizophrenia | Did any of the parents have a psychosis or severe mood disorder? |

## SOCIAL HISTORY

| Home | Who lives with them at home? How are things at home? |
|---|---|
| Siblings | Do they have brothers or sisters? How is the relationship between them? Do they have any illnesses? |
| School | Do they go to nursery or school? How are they performing? |

## IDEA, CONCERNS, EXPECTATIONS

| Ideas | Tell me what do you think may have caused your child's problem? (MMR) |
|---|---|
| Concerns | What are your main worries regarding it? |
| Expectations | How did you want me to help your child? (single vaccines) |

---

### MMR & Autism

The MMR vaccine is a three-in-one vaccine that is administered as a subcutaneous injection and contains live attenuated viruses or measles, mumps and rubella. Immunisation of children nationwide was introduced in 1988 to help protect against measles, mumps and German measles (Rubella). It is given to children at 12–13 months of age with a further booster given between the ages of 3 and 5 years just prior to starting school.

Worries and concerns were first raised over the vaccine directly as a result of a paper that was written by Dr Andrew Wakefield et al. that was published in The Lancet in 1998. In the paper, they reported that 12 children had developed bowel symptoms as well as autistic features soon after being inoculated with the MMR vaccine suggesting a possible link between the three-in-one vaccine and autism. The author then suggested that it was safer to vaccinate with single vaccines instead of the triple vaccine. Following the article, many parents from all ethnicities and walks of life, were dissuaded from taking the MMR vaccine with take-up rates falling to 79.9% in 2003/4. However, more recently rates have reached 89.1%, which is still below the 95% required to make the programme effective.

The consensus of the medical and scientific community state that there is no scientific evidence for a credible link between the MMR vaccine and autism and that the lack of confidence in MMR has damaged public health. Single separate vaccines instead of the MMR vaccine would not reduce the chance of adverse effects but would rather increase the risk of children catching the disease due to the increased time waiting for full immunisation cover. In 2010, all the authors bar Dr Wakefield as well as the Lancet published a public retraction around the findings and conclusions of the paper.

---

**CSA TIPS**

Given the likely age of presentation, it is unlikely that you will be dealing with a child in the consultation. It is more likely, as the RCGP are using actors 7 years old or above, that you will be consulting with a parent worried about the behaviour of their child. They also may present with concerns that the child's change in behaviour is due to the MMR vaccine they had at 12-13 months of age, or following the pre-school MMR booster between the age of 3 and 5 years. It is important that you are receptive and empathetic to the plight and worries of the parent. However, you should try and educate and advise the parent about the lack of evidence of a link between MMR and autism.

**PHYSICAL EXAMINATION**

| | |
|---|---|
| *Vitals* | Not routinely required unless worries about autism |

**INVESTIGATIONS**

| | |
|---|---|
| *Bloods* | Not routinely required |

**MANAGEMENT PLAN**

| | |
|---|---|
| *Explaining* | When explaining the condition to the family; incorporate vocabulary that the parent used to describe their child's problems. Explain the likely diagnosis and what will happen next |
| *Referral* | Refer to a local autism clinic, or child psychiatrist to make the diagnosis |
| Social Services | Consider referral to social services for assessment for benefits or an assignment of a key worker. Consider referral for a carer's assessment |
| Education | Consider extra help or educational needs assessment for school performance |

**SAFETY NETTING**

| | |
|---|---|
| *Follow up* | Offer the patient a convenient follow-up appointment as relevant to their needs |

**EXPLANATIONS**

| | |
|---|---|
| *Autism* | This is a lifelong condition that affects how a child relates to, and communicates with other people and how they make sense of the world around them. We do not know what causes it, but it is thought that there may be a family or genetic component that interacts with certain factors in the brain and the environment and triggers the problem. |
| *Immunisations* | Immunisations are vital to help the body protect against specific diseases when we come into contact with them. Usually, this is done by injecting a small part of the virus into the body and training it to recognise it and fight against the diseases if exposed to them in the future. |
| MMR | The MMR vaccine protects against the viruses measles, mumps and rubella. Although each of these disease may be mild and self-limiting, they can have rare but quite serious complications. For example, measles can lead to death, mumps can lead to infection of the brain and infertility and rubella can lead to blindness and birth abnormalities to the unborn child if caught during pregnancy. |
| *MMR & Autism* | In the past there was only one medical article that suggested a possible link between MMR and autism. This article has been totally discredited by the medical profession and since then thorough research has been undertaken that dismisses any possible |

link between MMR and autism. In 2010, most of the authors of the original article, and the medical journal itself, published a public retraction of the paper rejecting it and its findings outright.

Single Vaccines   Under the NHS you cannot get the MMR as separate vaccines. The medical profession in the UK advises against taking these as there would be a time gap in giving the three vaccines separately. This could potentially put your child at risk of catching these diseases and being exposed to the life threatening complications that they may cause.

Attention deficit hyperactivity disorder is a behavioural disorder which is characterised with inattention, hyperactivity or acting impulsively which are not appropriate for their age. It often presents in childhood (3-7yr) with impairment to their daily function (home, social activities, school) and is seen more often in boys than girls. Often the child can be easily distracted, forget things and have difficulty to follow instructions or complete tasks. They also can get bored after only a few minutes of doing an activity before switching swifty to another. For a formal diagnosis, symptoms must be present for 6mths with other causes such as learning difficulties excluded with impact upon two settings i.e. their home, school or social situations. Diagnosis should be made by a specialist.

## HISTORY
Approach the topic sensitively in a non-threatening non-judgemental manner. Adopt a relaxed open posture that is calm and inviting. Try not to appear patronising nor paternalistic towards the parent(s). Do not be dismissive but try and engage with and explore the patient's ideas and concerns.

**Open questions**   How can I help you today? Can you tell me more about your child's behaviour?

**Focused questions**

*ADHD*   When did you first notice a change in your child's behaviour?
 Inattention
  Concentration  Have they had difficulty concentrating on a task or play activity? Do they make careless mistakes in their school work or other activities?
  Distracted  Are they easily distracted? Do they struggle to complete tasks or follow instructions?

 Hyperactivity
  Restless  Are they more restless than other children? Can they remain seated through a class lesson? Are they always fidgeting?
  Overactive  Do they run or climb during times which is not appropriate?

 Impulsive
  Inpatient  Is your child generally impatient (waiting turn in games)? Do they blurt out things without thinking or worrying about the consequences?
  Interrupt  Do they interrupt others a lot? (conversation, playing)

**Associated history**
*School*   Have there been any problems with school? How are they performing? How is their relationship is with their friends?
 Adolescent  Any problems with the police? Do they use drugs?
 *Development delay*  Have there been any problems with the child's development or achieving milestones? (walking, eating, speaking, potty training)

## DIFFERENTIALS
*Autism*
 Social Interaction  Do they enjoy playing with others or are more happy being alone? Do they avoid eye-contact with you or others?
 Playing  Does your child play with different toys or concentrate on one?

| Communication | Did your child start speaking on time? Do they repeat themselves or a phrase a lot? Are they able to understand if you are joking with them? |
| Anxiety/depression | How is their mood recently? Any stress at school? Any bullying? |

## RED FLAGS

Child protections, abnormal development

## PAST HISTORY

| Medical | Enquire whether the child suffers from any medical condition (Downs, tuberous sclerosis, epilepsy, ADHD)? Do they have a learning disability? |
| Immunisations | Check if they are up-to-date with their childhood immunisations? Any travel vaccines? |

## BIRTH HISTORY

| Pregnancy | Enquire whether the mother had any problems during pregnancy or delivery? (low birth weight, premature) |

## DRUG HISTORY

| Medication | Are they taking any medications? |

## FAMILY HISTORY

| Medical | Are there any illnesses that run in your family? (autism, ADHD) |

## SOCIAL HISTORY

| Home | Who lives with them at home? How are things at home? |
| Siblings | Do they have brothers or sisters? How is the relationship between them? |
| Social services | Are they known to social services? |

## IDEA, CONCERNS, EXPECTATIONS

| Ideas | Did you have any thoughts what is causing your child's behavioural problems? |
| Concerns | Did you have any concerns about their behaviour? (school, concentration) |
| Expectations | How did you want me to help your child? (single vaccines) |
| Impact on life | How has their behaviour affected your family? |

## PHYSICAL EXAMINATION

| Vitals | Height, weight, growth charts |

## INVESTIGATIONS

| Bloods | Not routinely required |

## MANAGEMENT PLAN

| Explaining | When explaining the condition to the family. incorporate vocabulary that the parent used to describe their child's problems. Try to involve whole family in the management |

### Lifestyle

| Diet | Recommend diary of food and drink if parents suggest particular link with foods. Refer dietician if a link with food and behaviour has been identified |
| Fatty acids | Do not recommend fatty acid supplements to treat ADHD |

### Talking therapies

| | |
|---|---|
| Family therapy | Can be offered to the family |
| Group CBT | Can be offered to children or individual psychological treatment for older children |
| Education prog. | Teaches parents behaviour therapy techniques to use with their child such as offering structure to child's daily routine/day, rewarding positive interactions, implement clear rules for behaviour |

### Referral

| | |
|---|---|
| Moderate | Consider watchful waiting for upto 10wks. Refer for educational programmes |
| Severe | Refer to a the community Adolescent Mental Health Service (CAMHS) or specialist paediatrician |

### Specialists

Medication may be initiated (e.g. methylphenidate) if talking therapies fail. Side-effects include abdominal pain, nausea, indigestion. Growth is not usually affected but recommended to monitor growth during treatment

### SAFETY NETTING

| | |
|---|---|
| Follow up | Offer the patient a convenient follow-up appointment as relevant to their needs |

### EXPLANATIONS

| | |
|---|---|
| ADHD | ADHD, otherwise known as attention deficit hyperactive disorder, is a common condition that affects your child's behaviour. It often presents with your child being alway restless or fidgeting, easily distracted and having a short attention span. However, in ADHD, these symptoms are so severe it affects their ability to function on a day to day basis (i.e school, social function, home). |
| Diagnosis | Unfortunately there is no single test to diagnose ADHD. We can refer your child to the specialist for a formal assessment. This may involve a chat with both the child and parent as well as an observation of your child performing certain tasks. They may also request for a report from the school to get the whole picture before making a diagnosis. |
| Treatment | Whilst there is no cure for ADHD, there is lots of support for the parents and child. These include education programmes and talking therapies. If this does not work we can also consider medication that can help control some of the symptoms. |
| Methylphenidate | Ritalin is believed to work by stimulating part of the brain that helps control and manage your child's mental and behavioural reactions. |

# *13.5 Meningitis*

Meningitis relates to the infection or inflammation of the protective surface layer of the brain and spinal cord known as the meninges. It can become infected via bacterial, viral or even due to TB. The most common cause is viral meningitis which usually presents as a mild disease, however, all suspected meningitis cases should be considered bacterial unless proven otherwise. Since bacterial meningitis is a life-threatening condition that is particularly serious in children and young people. Due to the introduction of child immunisation with MenC and HiB, the demographics of the causes of meningitis is changing with streptococcus pneumoniae (pneumococcal disease) and neisseria meningitidis (meningococcus) being the most common causes.

## HISTORY
### *Principles*

| | |
|---|---|
| *Listen to mum* | If the child is of a young age and attends with a parent, i.e. the mother, listen carefully and acknowledge what they the mother is saying. Acknowledge the level of concern of the parent / carer in making your diagnosis |
| **Open questions** | Can you tell me more about your child's problems? Could you tell me about what has been troubling them? |

## Focused questions

| | |
|---|---|
| *Meningitis* | When did it all begin? How long has it been going on for? Is it getting worse or better? |
| Rash | Do they have a rash? When you press on it does it go away? |
| Neck Stiffness | Do they have any pain on their neck? Is it stiff? |
| Mental State | Is your child irritable or drowsy? Did they become confused or even semi-conscious? Do they only wake up if you shake or shout at them for a while? |
| Photophobia | Does your child have problems with the light? Do they get pain when they look directly at it? |
| Seizures | Have they fitted or had a seizure? |
| | |
| *Septicaemia* | When did it all begin? How long has it been going on for? Is it getting worse or better? |
| Joint pain | Do they have any arm, leg or joint pains? |
| Cold limbs | Despite having a fever, were their arms and feet still cold? |
| Rigors | Are they suffering with shivers or shakes? |

## Associated history

| | |
|---|---|
| *Nausea & vomiting* | Did your child feel sick or vomited? |
| *Fever* | Have they had a temperature? How high did it get to? |
| *Lethargy* | Are they active and awake or sleepy and tired? |
| *Headache* | Have they complained of a headache? Whereabouts is it? |
| *Feeding* | How is their appetite and eating? Are they eating less? |
| *Fluids* | Are they passing urine alright? How many wet nappies? |

## RED FLAGS

Evolving non-blanching rash, delirium, focal neurological signs, rapidly deteriorating

## PAST HISTORY

| | |
|---|---|
| *Premature* | Was your child born premature? |

| Shunt | Were they diagnosed with hydrocephalus? Do they have a shunt? |
| Immunisations | Check if they are up-to-date with their childhood immunisations? Any travel vaccines? |

**DRUG HISTORY**

| Medication | Is your child taking any medications? |

**SOCIAL HISTORY**

| Gatherings | Is your child studying? Did they attend any crowded events? (boarding school, youth camps) |
| Travel | Did your child go abroad and return recently? |
| Home | Who lives with them at home? |
| Siblings | Do they have brothers or sisters? Do they have any illnesses? |

**FAMILY HISTORY**

| Medical | Do any medical conditions affect other family members? |

**IDEA, CONCERNS, EXPECTATIONS**

| Idea | What do you think may be causing your child's illness? |
| Concerns | Is there anything that is worrying you specifically? |

**CSA TIPS**

Meningitis is a serious condition that is life-threatening. Parents attending with an unwell child who are overtly worried should be taken seriously and their concerns should not be dismissed. In such cases, it is important to take a history and assess the child for features of meningitis or septicaemia. If you do suspect then urgently referral to hospital via 999 is warranted with stat benzylpenicillin if there is a rash. Consider how you would take a history of a parent worried about meningitis over the telephone. Consider suggesting to the parents to do check the child's temperature and to do the glass test if at home.

**PHYSICAL EXAMINATION**

| Vitals | BP, pulse, temp, RR, CPT (>3 sec), O2 Sats |

**Normal Heart and Breath Rates for Healthy Children**

| Age | Normal (Beats per minute) | Normal (Breaths per minute) |
| --- | --- | --- |
| birth–1 yrs | 100-160 | 30-60 |
| 1–3 yrs | 90-150 | 24-40 |
| 3–6 yrs | 80-140 | 22-34 |
| 6–12 yrs | 70-120 | 18-30 |
| 12–18 yrs | 60-100 | 12-16 |

| General | Inspect the child generally - are they tired, withdraw, limp or confused? Do they look pale? Do they have a high-pitched cry? Do they look dehydrated (sunken eyes, reduced skin turgor)? |
| Rash | Observe for rash anywhere on the body. Does it blanch? Is it >2mm in diameter? |
| Palpate | Feel the peripheries for evidence of cold. In infants is the fontanelle bulging? |
| Neurological | Perform a general screening using AVPU - are they Alert? Do they respond to Voice, or Pain or are they totally Unresponsive? Perform a generalised CN examination (abnormal pupils) and neurological assessment. Do they flinch when a bright light is shone into their eyes? |

**Special tests**

| | |
|---|---|
| Kernig's sign | Does the child complain of pain when the knee is passively extended keeping the hips flexed? |
| Brudzinski's sign | Do the hips flex when the head is bent forward |

## INVESTIGATIONS — *Secondary care initiated*

| | |
|---|---|
| *Bloods* | FBC (infection), CRP, glucose, U&Es, Coagulation screen (DIC) |
| Cultures | Blood cultures for bacterial infection |
| *Urine* | Exclude alternative causes |
| *CXR* | Exclude alternative causes of fever |
| *Lumbar Puncture* | CSF sent for gram stain, TB, cytology, glucose protectin and culture |
| *CT / MRI* | Brain abscess, herniation |

## MANAGEMENT

### Conservative

| | |
|---|---|
| *General* | Wash you hands and have good hygiene. Do not share drinks, straws or utensils. Stay healthy and cover your mouth when your cough or sneeze |
| *Travel* | If travelling to Hajj or sub-Saharan Africa consider taking Meningococcal (ACWY) injection |
| *Gatherings* | Avoid large social gatherings |
| *Immunisations* | Ensure they are immunised with the DoH schedule (Men. C, Haem. B, Pneumococcal) |
| *HPA* | Inform the Health Protection Agency / CCDC about the diagnosis |

### Medical

| | |
|---|---|
| *Admit* | Call 999 and request an urgent ambulance |
| Bacterial (rash) | If suspect bacterial meningitis then give stat IM benzylpenicillin. <1yr 300mg, 1-9yr 600mg and >10yr 1200mg |
| Allergy | If penicillin allergy withhold. Consider cefotaxime as an alternative |
| Viral | Refer to hospital for supportive therapy and possible initiation of aciclovir |
| *Prophylaxis* | Identify possible close contacts in the week before onset of illness (pupils in dormitory, all household contacts, partners). Offer prophylaxis for meningococcal disease ciprofloxacin stat (azithromycin stat in pregnancy) |

## SAFETY NETTING

| | |
|---|---|
| *Red flags* | Ensure that explain to the parents red flags symptoms (rash, photophobia, Tumbler test) to look out for and to seek medical advice if they encounter them |
| *Follow up* | Review after discharge from hospital |
| *Audiology* | Ensure that they are booked for an audiological assessment 4 weeks after discharge |

## EXPLANATIONS

| | |
|---|---|
| *Meningitis* | This is a serious condition where the surface cover of the brain becomes infected or inflamed because of a bacterial or viral infection. If left alone, it may cause serious brain damage and that is why we have to send your child urgently to hospital. |
| *Septicaemia* | This is a condition that is when the infection passes from the brain into the blood and begins to spread and grow. This can cause serious damage to the body and needs to be treated urgently in hospital. |

Tumbler Test
This is a test that helps to see whether the rash your child has is because of blood poisoning. What you do is get a clear glass and press it against the spots. If the spots go away then this is good. However, if the spots do not change, then you should see a doctor urgently.

Lumbar puncture
This is a medical procedure that is when a needle is inserted into the lower spine to take some liquid from the fluid that bathes the brain and spinal cord. This fluids is called the CSF and we can send it to the lab to check for any signs of infection.

Upper respiratory tract infections are illnesses that are caused by an infection affecting the throat (pharyngitis, tonsillitis), sinuses (sinusitis), nose (rhinitis), ears (otitis), trachea (tracheitis) and larynx (laryngitis). They all usually present as self-limiting conditions most commonly triggered by viruses and give symptoms such as lethargy, myalgia, fever. Symptoms worsen for the first three days before gradually clearing on their own. Occasionally, bacteria may be implicated in the infection process and may require clearing with a course of antibiotics.

## HISTORY
### Principles

| | |
|---|---|
| *Listen to mum* | If the child is of a young age and attends with a parent, i.e. the mother, listen carefully and acknowledge what they the mother is saying. Acknowledge the level of concern of the parent / carer in making your diagnosis. |
| **Open questions** | Can you tell me more about your child's problems? Could you tell me about what has been troubling them? |

### Focused questions
*Otitis media*

| | |
|---|---|
| Otalgia | Do they have any ear pain? Does it throb? Does your child rub or pull their ears a lot? Does it make a popping sound? |
| Otorrhoea | Any discharge from the ear? What colour is it (blood stain, yellow)? Did the ear pain settle after you noticed the discharge? |
| With effusion | |
| Hearing | How is their hearing? Do they have the TV on loud? Do they often ask things to be repeated? |
| Learning | Has there been a delay in their speech or language development? Do they lack concentration at school? |

*Tonsillitis*

| | |
|---|---|
| Sore throat | Do you have a sore throat? How long has it being going on for? |
| Dysphagia | Is it affecting you to swallow? |
| Otalgia | Are you experiencing any ear pain? |
| Other | Do you have any difficulty or any noisy breathing? (stridor) |

*Croup*

| | |
|---|---|
| Cough | Do they have a cough? How long for? Is it a barking cough? Is it worse at night? |
| Hoarseness | Did the child's voice become hoarse? |
| Stridor | Any breathing problems or noise particularly when breathing in? |
| Trigger | Do the symptoms get worse when the child cries or gets upset? |

*Sinusitis*

| | |
|---|---|
| Nasal | Have they had a blocked nose or discharge from the nose? What colour is it? |
| Facial pain | Any headaches or pain over their face? Is it worsened when bending forward? |
| Cough | Any coughs? |

## Associated history

| | |
|---|---|
| *Fever* | Have they had a temperature? How high did it get to? When did it start? |
| *Nausea & vomiting* | Did your child feel sick or vomited? |
| *Lethargy* | Are they active and awake or sleepy and tired? |
| *Headache* | Have they complained of a headache? Whereabouts is the headache? |
| *Feeding* | How is their appetite and eating? Are they eating less? |
| *Fluids* | Are they passing urine ok? How many wet nappies? |
| *Previous* | Has this illness happened before? |

## RED FLAGS

Evolving non-blanching rash, delirium, focal neurological signs, rapidly deteriorating child, stridor or breathing difficulty

## DIFFERENTIALS

| | |
|---|---|
| *Meningitis* | Have you noticed a rash? When you press on it does it go away? Any neck stiffness, drowsiness or problems with the light? |
| *Otitis externa* | Do you swim? Does your ears itch a lot? |
| *Scarlet fever* | Any bright red spot or rashes over the body (neck, upper chest)? When did it start (2nd day)? Any colour change to the tongue (strawberry)? |

## PAST HISTORY

| | |
|---|---|
| *Otitis media* | Does your child suffer from Down's syndrome or have a cleft palate? |
| *Immunisations* | Check if they are up-to-date with their childhood immunisations? |

## BIRTH HISTORY

| | |
|---|---|
| *Premature* | Was your child born premature? (OM) |
| *Feeding* | Did the child breast or bottle feed? When did they stop breast feeding? |
| *Dummy* | Did the child use a dummy or pacifier after 11 months of age? |

## DRUG HISTORY

| | |
|---|---|
| *Medication* | Is your child taking any medications? Are they allergic to any antibiotics? |

## SOCIAL HISTORY

| | |
|---|---|
| *Passive smoking* | Does any family members smoke? |
| *Home* | Who lives with them at home? Any brothers or sisters? Does anyone at home have any illnesses or symptoms? |
| *Nursery* | Did the child recently start at nursery or daycare? |

## FAMILY HISTORY

| | |
|---|---|
| *Medical* | Do any medical conditions affect other family members? |

## IDEA, CONCERNS, EXPECTATIONS

| | |
|---|---|
| *Idea* | What do you think may be causing your child's illness? |
| *Concerns* | Is there anything that is worrying you specifically? |
| *Expectations* | How did you think I could help? (antibiotics) |

## CSA TIPS

Despite being extremely common, URTIs still cause much angst and worry for parents and carers alike. Looking after a hot, feverish and miserable child is not an easy task and parents frequently attend the GP for a magical panacea that will make everything better overnight; and It is still incorrectly believed that this is in the form of antibiotics. When dealing with a tired and stressed carer, it is important to remain empathetic and show your concern and worry about the child's health. You will have to educate and explain the natural course of the illness before safety netting and advising if and when, they may have to return.

**PHYSICAL EXAMINATION** *perform focused examination based on clinical findings*

| | |
|---|---|
| *Vitals* | Pulse (tachycardia), temp, RR, CPT (>3 sec), O2 Sats |
| *General* | Inspect the child generally (tired, withdrawn, pale). Look for signs of dehydration (sunken eyes, decreased skin turgor) |
| Rash | Observe for rash on the body. Check for blanching and size. Check texture (sandpaper - scarlet fever) and peeling of skin |
| *Throat* | Use a tongue depressor. Inspect for red, enlarged tonsils or exudates. Inspect tongue for colour (strawberry). Check for halitosis |
| *Ears* | Inspect the ears (not displaced). Look for the colour of the TM (red, cloudy, blue), shape (bulging, retracted) and presence of fluid level. Check for any perforations or discharge and loss of light reflex |
| Mastoiditis | Check for any redness, tenderness of the mastoids |
| *Sinuses* | Palpate frontal, maxillary, ethmoid sinuses |
| *Chest* | Inspect for tachypnoea, intercostal recession, stridor. Listen for wheeze or crepitations |
| *Lymph nodes* | Consider palpating the cervical lymph nodes (tonsils, anterior, posterior, pre and post auricular, occipital) |
| *Other* | Palpate for splenomegaly if glandular fever suspected |

**INVESTIGATIONS** *investigate underlying cause*

| | |
|---|---|
| *Bloods* | *Not routinely required:* FBC, CRP, Antistreptolysin O (ASO) titres |
| Other | LFTs, Blood film (mononuclear leucocytosis), monospot test for glandular fever |
| *Swab* | *Not routinely required:* ear discharge swab, throat swabs |
| *Specialist* | Audiometry (persistent hearing loss) or pneumatic otoscope for OM with effusion |

**MANAGEMENT** *treat underlying cause*

***Otitis media (OM)***

| | |
|---|---|
| *Advice* | Reassure, often resolves within 4d without abx. Advise parents not to smoke, Avoid dummies (>6mths old), consider breast feeding |
| *Analgesia* | Offer paracetamol or NSAIDs in all cases |
| *Antibiotics* | Avoid antibiotic unless severe. Recommend 5d oral (not drops) amoxicillin or erythromycin |
| *Refer* | Admit if <3mths, mastoiditis or systemically very unwell. Refer to ENT if persisting symptoms unresponsive to abx, discharge or perforation >2-3wks, impaired hearing |

---

**Guidelines for antibiotics in otitis media -** *Ref: Adapted NICE (2008) Respiratory tract infections*

- Bilateral acute otitis media in <2yr
- If systemically very unwell
- High risk of comorbidity (immunosuppressed, CF, premature, organ disease)
- Acute otitis media in children with otorrhoea
- Has signs of complications (mastoiditis)

---

***OM with effusion***

| | |
|---|---|
| *Advice* | Reassure, often resolves 6-12wks (90%) with monitoring. Advise parents not to smoke |
| Hearing loss | Promote learning by speaking face to face with slower rate of speech, switch off distractions (TV, music), daily reading, move seat near the front of class |

| | |
|---|---|
| *Antibiotics* | Antibiotic or antihistamines not recommended |
| *Refer* | If hearing loss, refer for audiology. If significant hearing loss (including bilateral), Down's or development delay refer ENT |
| *Surgery* | Considered if persistent bilateral OM with effusion >3mths with hearing loss. Treatment with grommets or adenoidectomy. Alternatively hearing aids or autoinflation may be offered |

### Tonsillitis/sore throat

| | |
|---|---|
| *Advice* | Reassure, sore throat, pharyngitis and acute tonsillitis often resolves by 1wk. Avoid hot drinks, drink adequate fluid intake. For older children recommend salted gargles, lozenges, hard boiled sweets, ice cream for symptomatic treatment |
| *Analgesia* | Offer paracetamol or NSAIDs in all cases |
| *Antibiotics* | Use centor criteria to support decision. If antibiotics indicated give 10d of Penicillin V or if allergy, Erythromycin for 5d. Avoid broad spectrum abx (Amoxicillin - maculopapular rashes). Give delayed prescription if worsening or not improved >3d |
| *Refer* | Admit if signs of peritonsillar abscess, refer if sore throat or painful swallowing >3wks |
| Tonsillectomy | Refer for operation if >=5/yr, severe enough to impact daily function, sleep apnoea |
| *Follow up* | Review as soon as possible if has SOB, stridor, drooling, dysphagia, severe pain, cannot keep fluid down, becomes systemically very unwell |

---

**Centor Criteria to Diagnose Group A beta-haemolytic streptococcus**

A patient with a sore throat and >=3 features would benefit from antibiotic use

- Tonsillar exudate
- Tender anterior cervical lymph nodes
- Absence of cough
- Fever

---

### Croup

| | |
|---|---|
| *Advice* | Reassure, often self limiting illness, often resolves within 2d but can persist for 1wk. Have upright if crying or has stridor. Ensure adequate fluid intake. Do not recommend steam inhalation rather cool air by stroll outside |
| *Antipyrexia* | Offer paracetamol or NSAIDs for high fever |
| *Antibiotics* | Antibiotic and cough medication not recommended |
| *Steroids* | Give stat oral dexamethasone (0.15mg/kg) or prednisolone (1mg/kg) |
| *Refer* | Admit if severe croup, persistent stridor at rest, respiratory distress, intercostal recession or cyanosis. Hospital may consider nebulised epinephrine (adrenaline) |
| *Follow up* | Review as soon as possible if has worsening SOB, restless, high fever or pale. Call 999 if becomes cyanosed, drowsy/unusually sleepy, struggles to breath or drooling. |

### Acute sinusitis

| | |
|---|---|
| *Advice* | Reassure, self limiting illness often lasts for 2.5wk. Have adequate fluid intake. Apply warm face packs |
| *Analgesia* | Offer paracetamol or NSAIDs for pain. Sodium chloride nasal drops can be considered |
| *Nasal steroids* | Considered in adults only for prolonged symptoms |
| *Antibiotics* | Antibiotic if evidence of bacterial infection such as purulent discharge (often unilateral), severe local pain (often unilateral), high fever >38°, marked worsening symptoms). Prescribe high dose amoxicillin, penicillin V or, if allergic, doxycycline (if >12yr) or erythromycin |
| *Refer* | Admit if systemically unwell or intracranial (meningitis) or orbital spread (cellulitis). Refer to ENT if recurrent (>3 requiring abx in yr) |
| *Follow up* | If symptoms worsen, high fever, or severe pain which is mainly unilateral |

# DIFFERENTIAL DIAGNOSIS

| Condition | Characteristic exam feature |
|---|---|
| Otitis media | Common condition, peak age 6-15mth, rare in school age. Risk factors include passive smoking, nursery, bottle feeding, craniofacial abnormalities, winter, dummy use. Can be viral (RSV, rhinovirus) or bacterial (strep. pneumoniae, H.influenzae). Children report ear pain (older child), pulling or rubbing ears, cough, poor feeding and high fever (>40°). OE: red, cloudy, bulging tympanic membrane +/- fluid level. Occasional perforation with discharge seen |
| Otitis media with effusion | Known as 'glue ear', collection of fluid within middle ear without signs of with inflammation. Seen in 1-6yr olds. Can cause hearing loss (resolves wks to mths) that can sometimes cause language delays. Similar risk factors to otitis media. OE: Often no signs of inflammation of TM, effusion (blood, mucoid, purulent) with loss of light reflex, yellow or blue retracted drum and fluid level with air bubbles |
| Tonsillitis | Common illness in children. May present with sore throat, painful swallowing, headache and loss of voice. Pain may radiate to ears. O/E red tonsils with exudate, tender anterior cervical lymph nodes |
| Sinusitis | Bacterial or viral infection of the sinuses (frontal, maxillary or ethmoid). Presents with cold or flu-like illness and symptoms include fever, tenderness over the sinus, halitosis nasal congestion with rhinitis, pressure/throbbing over the head which is worsened when bending forward |
| Croup | Viral infection (e.g. parainfluenza) affected infants from 6-36mth particularly in autumn/spring season. Starts with coryzal symptoms, sore throat, mild fever progressing to barking cough, hoarseness or inspiratory stridor with high fever (>40°). Cough often at night or when child agitated |
| Bronchiolitis | Caused by RSV. Often seen in winter months. Typically affects <1yr and presents with fever with runny nose. Worsening symptoms include irritable cough, worsening SOB and feeding difficulties. O/E widespread fine creps with high pitched wheeze |
| Scarlet fever | Produces characteristic red blush blanching rash that starts on day 2 that slowly fades over 3wks. Can start from upper chest or neck spreading to abdomen and extremities, skin creases that can peel off (toes, fingers). Has sandpaper texture. Associated with exudative tonsillitis, (red spots on palate, flushing face, and strawberry tongue |
| Glandular fever | Infectious disease spread by saliva caused by EBV. Presents with fever and acute fatigue with worsening sore throat, lymphadenopathy and macular rash. Can last for 2-3wks. Check for splenomegaly. Complication include splenic rupture |

# EXPLANATIONS

**Otitis media**

The ear is separated into different zones with the ear canal being the outer ear and the small space behind the eardrum, the middle ear. Otitis media means that your child has an infection of the middle ear. This often affects the ear drum making it red and angry and can cause an ear ache.

**OM with effusion**

This is a condition where there is a build-up of fluid behind the eardrum instead of air. This can cause dulled hearing or hearing loss.

**Grommet**

A grommet is a tiny tube or pipe that helps drain out fluid that may build up behind the eardrum. A tiny cut is made to the eardrum and the grommet is placed across it. It should improve hearing quite quickly.

**Adenoidectomy**

Adenoids are small lumps of tissue that are found in the back of the throat (upper part of the back of the nasal cavity) that are part of the immune system which help fight infections. If your child catches lots of colds then these can be inflamed and press on the entrance of the Eustachian tubes (tube connects middle ear to back of the nose) that can block fluid from draining from the middle ear and increase the air pressure there.

**Autoinflation**

This is when your child inflates a special balloon using their nose. it helps keep the eustachian tube open and therefore help drain out fluid from the middle ear.

**Croup**

Croup is a viral infection that affects the voice box (larynx) and windpipe (trachea). As it a result it can give you the harsh breathing sound (stridor) when you breath in and barking cough.

**Tonsillitis**

Tonsillitis is when your tonsils become infected. Tonsils are two small lumps of tissue that are found on either side of the back of the throat that are part of the immune system which help fight infections.

**Tonsillectomy**

This is the name of the operation that is used to remove the tonsils. It is considered only if your child has recurrent signs of infection (5 episodes in a year). It is undertaken under a general anaesthetic where they will be made to sleep and the tonsillar tissue will be removed using either a surgical knife or by a heat probe.

**Sinusitis**

This is an infection or inflammation of the linings of the sinuses. Sinuses are small, air-filled spaces found in the skull around the cheekbone and forehead. They can get infected after you catch a cold or may be from tooth infection that spreads into it.

**Antibiotics**

Most of the time URTIs are caused by viral infections. Antibiotics are only good at killing bacteria and do not not viruses. Often your immune system is strong enough to kill most infections including both virus and bacteria. Also antibiotics, if prescribed, can cause side effects such diarrhoea, stomach upset or rashes.

# 13.7 Urinary Tract Infection (UTI)

A urinary tract infection (UTI) is defined as any infection that affects the urinary tract from the kidney to the urethra. It is fairly rare in children with girls being more prone than boys. Structural abnormalities such as abnormal kidneys, vesicoureteric reflux or genital malformations may increase the risk of developing a UTI, however, in most cases there is no evidence of any problem. More commonly, functional problems such as holding the urine or constipation may be found and should be corrected. The most common bug implicated is Escherichia coli (>75%) then Klebsiella.

## HISTORY
**Open questions**    Can you tell me more about your child's problems? Could you tell me about what has been troubling them?

## Focused questions
*Urinary*    When did all the problems begin? How long has it been going on for? Is it getting worse or better?

Pain    Is there any pain when your child passes wee? What does it feel like (burn, stinging)? Is there any tummy pain? Or pain in the kidney area?

Frequency    Are they going more often? How many times a day? How many wet nappies?

Nocturia    Does your child pass urine at night? How many times? Do they wet the bed?

Blood    Is there any blood in the urine?

*Functional*

Constipation    Does your child open their bowels regularly? how often do they go?

Holding    Does your child voluntarily hold their wee not to go toilet?

## Associated history
*Nausea & vomiting*    Did your child feel sick or vomited?

*Fever*    Have they had a temperature? How high did it get to?

*Lethargy*    Are they active and awake or sleepy and tired?

*Feeding*    How is their appetite and eating? Are they eating less?

*Fluids*    Are they passing urine ok? How many wet nappies?

## Differentials
*Diabetes*    Do they feel thirsty all the time? Have you lost any weight?

## RED FLAGS    Dehydrated, lethargic, child abuse

## PAST HISTORY
*Premature*    Was your child born premature?

*Abnormalities*    Did your child have any kidney or spine problems from birth?

*UTI*    Have they had a UTI before?

## BIRTH HISTORY
*Pregnancy*    Enquire whether the child had any problems shown on the scan during pregnancy? (renal malformation)

## DRUG HISTORY

| | |
|---|---|
| *Medication* | Is your child taking any medications? |
| *Immunisations* | Check if they are up-to-date with their childhood immunisations? |

## SOCIAL HISTORY

| | |
|---|---|
| *Home* | Who is at home with them? |

## FAMILY HISTORY

| | |
|---|---|
| *Medical* | Do any medical conditions affect other family members? (renal disorders) |

## IDEA, CONCERNS, EXPECTATIONS

| | |
|---|---|
| *Idea* | What do you think may be causing your child's illness? |
| *Concerns* | Is there anything that is worrying you specifically? |
| *Expectations* | How were you hoping we could address this problem? |
| *Impact on life* | How has the illness affected the family? Any embarrassment at school? |

## CSA TIPS

UTI's affecting children are more serious the younger the child and may indicate underlying renal malformations. In the CSA it is unlikely that you will get a child <3 years appearing however, an anxious parent may present wanting to discuss the management plan following an abnormal MC+S. It is more likely that you will be faced with a young child (and parent) who has urinary incontinence or new onset bedwetting. A clear history from the patient and a collateral from the parent, along with an examination should help you discern a working diagnosis. Consider the presence of child abuse in a child who presents with recurrent UTI symptoms in absence of a medical cause or in the presence of other factors (excess genital itching or bruising, inappropriate sexual play).

## PHYSICAL EXAMINATION

| | |
|---|---|
| *Vitals* | BP, pulse, temp, height, weight (growth charts) |
| *General* | Inspect the child generally are they tired, withdrawn or limp? Do they look pale or dehydrated? (sunken eyes, decreased skin turgor) |
| *ENT* | Examine the ears and throat to exclude other causes of fever. Examine for cervical chain LN |
| *Abdomen* | Examine the abdomen for swelling (bladder), masses (kidney) or pain. Palpate for constipation and loin pain |
| *Genitals* | Examine for any evidence of vulval adhesions or phimosis in boys. Is there any evidence of superficial irritation? |

---

### Distinguishing between Lower and Upper UTIs

| | |
|---|---|
| *Upper* | Affects the kidney (and ureter) - signs of loin pain, high swinging fever, rigors |
| *Lower* | Affects the bladder (and urethra) - signs of dysuria, frequency and urgency |

---

## INVESTIGATIONS

| | |
|---|---|
| *Bloods* | *Not routinely indicated.* FBC (infection), CRP, glucose, U&Es |
| *Urine* | Dipstick (leucocytes, nitrates, blood, glu) and send for MC+S (even if -ve) to confirm diagnosis |
| *US* | If recurrent UTIs looking for structural deformity, thickening bladder |

| Specialist | Micturating cystography (urethral defects) if suspect UTI in <3mths. DMSA scintigraphy (renal defects) if suspect UTI in <3yrs or recurrent UTI in >3yrs |
|---|---|

## MANAGEMENT
### Conservative

| Fluids | Ensure children drink plenty of water in small amounts regularly |
|---|---|
| Hygiene | Wash hands after going to the toilet. Avoid bubble baths |
| Toileting | Advise parents on correct techniques such as wiping from front to back for girls and not to repeat using the same tissue. Ensure the child has good access to a potty or toilet and encourage to go when they feel the need |
| Clothing | Avoid tight fitting clothes and wear cotton underwear |
| Constipation | Increase fibre intake (brown bread, cereal, fruit and vegetable) and exercise regularly |

### Medical
UTI

| Aged <3mth | If UTI suspected then admit under paediatrician |
|---|---|
| Aged 3mths + | If first UTI treat with trimethoprim (lower UTI) or augmentin (upper UTI) |
| Urgent | If any high risk factors (poor urine output, dilated bladder, poor growth, genetic abnormality) then refer urgently to hospital |
| Recurrent UTI | If the child has 3 lower UTIs, 2 upper UTIs or 1 lower and 1 upper UTIs, then refer to paediatrician for assessment |
| Prophylaxis | *Secondary care initiated.* Consider long term antibiotics in patients with severe recurrent UTIs or structural abnormalities |

## SAFETY NETTING

| Follow up | Ensure parents have appropriate follow up to return 2-4 weeks if no improvement. To return as an emergency if child dehydrated or lethargic |
|---|---|

## EXPLANATIONS

| Urinary Tract | A UTI is an infection of the urinary tract. The urinary tract are the organs that make urine and help pass it out of the body. The tract starts at the two kidneys that lie in the loin area. The kidney washes out the toxins (poison) from the blood and passes out as urine. These pass down 2 tubes called the ureters than then enter the bladder. The bladder is like a reservoir and holds the urine until it is stretched enough to make you want to go. The urine then passes from the bladder outside through a tube called the urethra. |
|---|---|
| UTI | A UTI is when a germ (typically a bacteria) gets into the urine and affects the urinary tract. This normally comes from the bowel and happens if we do not clean or wash properly after going to pass a stool motion. The bug can grow quickly in the bladder and cause an infection there, or it may even travel upwards to affect the kidney as well. |
| Collecting Urine | It is important that we get a urine sample from your child so that we can check if they have an infection in their urine. This can sometimes be difficult. However, with some tips this can be done easily but requires patience. |
| Clean Catch | For young children, wash their genitals and place them on your lap. Put a sterile bowl underneath them and give them fluids and encourage them to pass urine. Once the |

sample is collected we can transfer it to a universal container and send to the lab for checking.

Mid-Stream  In older children you can take a mid-stream urine sample. Before doing the sample, it is important that you clean your child's genital area well. Do not allow their skin or body to touch the bottle when passing urine and try not to touch the top of the bottle with your fingers as well. When they begin to wee, try not to collect this sample, but when they are mid-flow catch this in the container.

# 13.8 Limping child

Children are often active mobile beings who are difficult to keep still. When a child presents with a limp it can be quite a worrying sight for the parents. Often a limp is caused by a simple sprain, minor injury or even a splinter in the foot. However, if there is no obvious cause to the limp then further evaluation is required. The most common cause of a limp is an irritable hip triggered by an URTI but other more serious causes such as septic arthritis or perthes should be excluded.

## HISTORY

**Open questions**      How can I help you today? Tell me more about the limp your child has been experiencing

## Focused questions

| | |
|---|---|
| *Limp* | When did you first notice the limp? How long has it been going on for? |
| Site | Does it affect one or both legs? |
| Onset | Did it come on quickly or gradually? |
| Trauma | Have they had a fall or injury recently? |
| Pains | Do they have any pain anywhere (hip, knee, bone)? When is the pain worse? (night) |
| Swelling | Have you noticed any swelling of any of their joints? |
| Movements | How does it affect their movement? (difficulty walking, refusal to stand) |

**RED FLAGS**      Fever or sweats (septic arthritis), trauma (fracture), weight loss or night pain (malignancy)

## Associated history

| | |
|---|---|
| *Fever* | Have they noticed any fever or sweats? Have they felt any shivers? |
| *Viral infection* | Have you had any coughs or colds recently? Any viral illness? |
| *Weight loss* | Have they lost any weight? |
| *Rashes* | An skin or nail changes? |

## PAST HISTORY

*Medical*      Have you ever suffered from any medical conditions? (Sickle cell, rickets, SLE, anorexia nervosa)

## FAMILY HISTORY

*Medical*      Does anyone in the family suffer from any hip problems? (RA)

## DRUG HISTORY

*Medication*      Are you taking any medications? (steroids)

## SOCIAL HISTORY

| | |
|---|---|
| *Home* | Who lives with them at home? How are things at home? |
| *School* | Do they go to nursery or school? Have they had any days off because of their symptoms? |

## IDEA, CONCERNS, EXPECTATIONS

*Ideas*      Have you had any thoughts what may be causing your limp?

| | |
|---|---|
| *Concerns* | Do you have any worries about it? |
| *Expectations* | How did you think I could help you today? |
| *Impact on life* | How have the symptoms affected your life? |

**PHYSICAL EXAMINATION** *Refer to hip pain chapter*

| | |
|---|---|
| **INVESTIGATIONS** | *depend on cause* |
| *Infection screen* | |
| Bloods | Hb, WCC, CRP, ESR |
| Other | MSU, throat swab, aspiration of synovial fluid (septic arthritis), blood c/s |
| *Hip / Pelvic Xray* | To exclude fracture or avascular necrosis of femoral head (Perthes). Consider AP/lateral hip xray for slipped upper femoral epiphysis |
| *Specialist* | US (irritable hip), MRI, Bone scan |

| | |
|---|---|
| **MANAGEMENT** | *treat underlying cause* |
| **Irritable hip** | Reassure as often resolves within 2wks. Recommend rest and analgesia. Keep leg flexed and externally rotated. If effusion consider aspiration. Once pain settles recommend mobilisation i.e. swimming |
| **Perthes'** | Advise rest. Refer to orthopaedics for bracing or surgery. Heals over 2-3yrs |
| **SUFE** | For slipped upper femoral epiphysis, advise rest and avoid walking. Offer analgesia and refer to orthopaedics for screw insertion or reconstructive surgery |
| **Septic arthritis** | If suspects admit into hospital for surgical drainage and antibiotics |
| **Juvenile arthritis** | Refer rheumatologist. Treatment similar to RA i.e. NSAIDs, steroids (intra-articular, oral), methotrexate |

| | |
|---|---|
| **SAFETY NETTING** | |
| *Follow up* | Review in 1-2wks to ensure limp is improving |

**DIFFERENTIAL DIAGNOSIS**

| Conditions | Characteristic exam feature |
|---|---|
| **Irritable hip** | Common in boys between 2-12yr (mean 6yr), associated with viral infection (mild fever) or mild trauma. Presents with acute hip pain with gradually improving limp over 10d. Both hips often affected. Child is systemically well. O/E Hip held in flexion, abduction and moderate external rotation. Limited ROM particularly adduction & extension (increases intracapsular pressure). Often diagnosis of exclusion |
| **Perthes disease** | Avascular necrosis to the femoral head resulting in abnormal growth. Seen in 3-11yr (peak 4-7yr), more common in boys. 10% bilateral. Presents with insidious onset (over 1mth) hip pain or knee pain (synovitis) causing a limp. O/E short stature, reduced abduction and internal rotation with leg length inequality, +ve thomas test |
| **Malignancy** | E.g. neuroblastomas, leukemias (ALL), osteosarcomas. Present with pain at night and/or |

| | bone pain distant from the joint |
|---|---|
| **Juvenile idiopathic arthritis** | Arthritis developing in <16yrs for >3mths. Vary in presentation but often affects large joints. May present with painless limp. Associated features include fever (swinging), maculopapular rash, arthralgia. Similar features to RA |
| **Septic arthritis / osteomyelitis** | Bacterial infection of the joint space often from spread from blood, penetrating wound or local infection (chronic osteomyelitis). Often seen in immunosuppressed, DM, RA, steroid use, recent joint surgery. Presents with high fever and unwell child with redness, swollen, tender hip joint. Often absent movements due to pain with point tenderness. Signs of tachycardia and swinging pyrexia |
| **Slipped upper femoral epiphysis** | Upper femoral epiphysis slips across the femur displaced postero-inferiorly. Rare cause of limp. More common in boys than girls with peak age in early adolescent (10-15yr). Left hip > right but can be bilateral. Child often overweight with hypothyroidism. Presents with pain in hip, groin medial thigh or referred to knee. Worse with walking or running. O/E reduced ROM hip (resists internal rotation), leg is externally rotated and shortened |

**EXPLANATIONS**

*Irritable hip*      This is when a there is an inflammation to the lining of the joint often as a reaction to a common cold or viral infection.

*Perthes disease*      This is a condition where there is reduced blood supply to the head of the thigh-bone causing portions of it to die and soften and breaks down. With time new blood vessels regrow with blood supply is returned to normal, however, there can be some distortion to the shape of the bone.

*SUFE*      Slipped capital femoral epiphysis is when the surface of the thighbone (head of femur) slips or slides across the underlying growth plate or growing part of the bone (epiphysis). As a result the thigh-bone may not fit inside the hip socket properly.

*Septic arthritis*      This is where the joint becomes infected with germs (bacteria) causing pain and swelling of the joint. Treatment is required urgently to stop permanent joint damage.

*Juvenile arthritis*      Often arthritis is assumed to affect older people but sometimes they can affect children. when this happens it is called juvenile arthritis.

# 13.9 Nocturnal enuresis

Nocturnal enuresis relates to the problem of bedwetting in a child of an age where control is expected. is defined as involuntary wetting during sleep in the absence of congenital or acquired defects. It occurs more commonly in boys and in those of lower social classes. It can be quite a distressing and embarrassing disorder for parent and child alike and it is important to broach the subject in an emphatic and non-judgemental way. Underlying illness or side-effects of medication need to be reliably excluded if the child had been previously dry at night for more than 6 months.

Most children with enuresis do not suffer from psychological disorders or other illnesses and conditions associated with urinary symptoms (e.g. urinary tract infection, diabetes) rarely present with enuresis. Daytime enuresis is more common in girls and is usually due to urge incontinence as a result of bladder instability.

Medical management for nocturnal enuresis is often considered after the child is >5 years old. Most children are continent during night and day by age of 3-4 years of age. However, approximately 20% of 5 year olds wet the bed twice a week falling to 9% of 9 year olds. Primary nocturnal enuresis is when child has never stopped bed wetting whilst secondary is when the child had been dry for the previous 6 months.

**HISTORY**

**Open questions**          Can you tell me more about your child's symptoms?

**Focused questions**

| | |
|---|---|
| *Enuresis* | When did you first notice the bed wetting? |
| Onset | Did it come on suddenly or over a period of time? |
| Pattern | How long has the bedwetting been going on for? How many nights a week? How many times a night? |
| Volume | Do they pass a large amount of urine? |
| *Primary / secondary* | Are they wet during the day? Have they ever been dry? |
| *Daytime* | How often do they pass urine during the day? Any accidents or feeling of urgency? |

**Associated history**

| | |
|---|---|
| *Development* | Have there been any problems with the child's development or achieving milestones? (walking, eating, speaking, potty training) |

**Differentials**

| | |
|---|---|
| *Constipation* | Any problems with their bowels? How often do they go? |
| *UTI* | Any pain passing urine? Do they go toilet often? Do they rush to the toilet? |
| *Diabetes* | Do they feel thirsty all the time? Have they lost any weight? |
| *Distress* | Are they being bullied at school? Any family problems (maltreatment)? Are they starting new school? |
| *Excess fluid* | How is their diet? Do they drink just before going to sleep? Any fizzy drinks? Do they drink tea or coffee? |

**RED FLAGS**          Painless jaundice, weight loss

**PAST HISTORY**

| | |
|---|---|
| *Medical* | Have you ever suffered from any medical conditions? (Diabetes, ADHD) |

## FAMILY HISTORY

*Enuresis*                    Did anyone else in your family suffer from bedwetting?

*Diabetes*                    Are there any illnesses that run in your family such as diabetes?

## DRUG HISTORY

*Medication*              Are you taking any medications?

## SOCIAL HISTORY

*Home*                      Who lives with them at home? How are things at home?

    Siblings              Do they have brothers or sisters? How is the relationship between them? Do they have any illnesses?

    Social services    Are they known to social services?

*School*                  Do they go to nursery or school? How are they performing? Any unauthorised days off?

## IDEA, CONCERNS, EXPECTATIONS

*Ideas*                     Have you had any thoughts what may be causing your child's symptoms?

*Concerns*              Do you have any worries about it?

*Expectations*         How did you think I could help your child today?

*Impact on life*       How have the symptoms affected your life? (avoid sleep overs, school trips, stress to parents)

## CSA TIPS

Children presenting with bedwetting, particularly those in their elder years, may feel acutely embarrassed by it. They may have faced social isolation and bullying that has affected their self-esteem and led them to truant from school. Attending the surgery with a parent in presence, may have required many days of mental preparation and thought about how to explain their problem. It is important that you are sensitive and empathetic when engaging with them and exclude any possible underlying medical condition.

## PHYSICAL EXAMINATION

*Vitals*                    Temp (fever), BMI, monitor growth

*Abdominal exam*     Examining the abdomen (constipation) and genitalia if appropriate

*Neurological*

    Spine                Inspect the back for sacral dimple, naevus or hair (meningomyelocele)

    Lower limb         Perform lower limb neurological assessment including ankle reflexes

## INVESTIGATIONS

*Urine*                     urine dipstick / MCS (DM, UTI)

*Specialist*             US scan (bladder, kidney)

## MANAGEMENT

### Conservative

*Reassure*

    <5yr                 Reassure that nocturnal enuresis is common (5% of 10yr olds) and often resolves spontaneously without treatment. Consider potty by bed

    >5yr                 If <2/wk consider monitoring only. If more consider treatments (alarms)

*Diary*                     Offer bladder diary including daytime fluid intake and urine output over 1wk

| | |
|---|---|
| *Toilet* | Encourage toilet training. Take to toilet if wakes up in night. Trial of nights (>=2) in a row without nappies/start pants. Empty child's bladder before going to sleep |
| *Void* | During day, void every 2-3hrs and avoid holding when they have the urge to urinate |
| *Mattress* | Waterproof cover for mattress, absorbent quilted sheets or pads |
| *Excess fluid* | Avoid excessive fluid intake particularly 1 hour before bed or abnormal toileting patterns. Daily intake for 4-8yr olds 1-1.4L, 9-13yr olds 1.2-2.3L |
| *Behaviour* | |
| Rewards | Suggest star charts for agreed behaviour rather than simply dry nights, i.e. drinking correct volume of fluid, going to toilet before sleeping, clean sheets |
| Avoid | Stress not the child's fault. Do not use penalty systems if patient fails (taking stars away). Punitive measures or blame should be avoided |

**Medical**

| | |
|---|---|
| *Enuresis alarm* | Enuresis alarm if not responded to lifestyle advice (often in >=7yr old). It wakes the child when they start urinating. They can be worn in the trouser or be a sensor pad that is placed under the child. Conditions the child to wake up and go to the toilet once they start passing urine. Eventually the child learns to wake up and hold their bladder before wetting the bed. Can be trialled for 4mth until 2wks of continuous dry nights achieved. Treatment may last 3-5 months. Alarms not recommended for <5yr as requires co-operation |
| *Desmopressin* | Offer desmopressin (200mcg po or 120mcg sublingual) >7yrs old if rapid or short-term improvement sought i.e. social occasion or alarm is unsuccessful or inappropriate. Taken at night as a tablet. Only sips allowed 1hr before taking medicine and up to 8hrs after. Effective for short term use or one off measures (short holiday trips). Review within 3mths |
| Side effects | Risk of fluid overload (hyponatremic convulsions), headache, nausea, abdominal pain. |
| *TCAs* | (imipramine) Have antimuscarinic effects, prescribed by specialists. Considered when all other options explored |

**Follow up**

| | |
|---|---|
| *Enuresis* | Review 4wks after recommending an enuresis alarm or starting on desmopressin |
| *Information* | Patients can get information from ERIC (Education and Resources for Improving Childhood Continence) |

**Refer**

| | |
|---|---|
| *Primary* | Refer to enuresis clinic if primary cause identified or daytime symptoms. Refer if has failed despite 2 courses of treatment (alarm, desmopressin, both) |

**DIFFERENTIAL DIAGNOSIS**

| Condition | Characteristic exam feature |
|---|---|
| **Nocturnal Enuresis** | Common (15% of 5yr, 5% of 10yr, 2% of 15yr). Associated with FH or ADHD. Often caused by sleep arousal difficulties (sensation of full bladder), polyuria or bladder dysfunction (overactive). Exclude other causes such as UTI, constipation, psychological |

| UTI | Common (8% of girls at 5yr). Nocturia, frequency, urgency. May have smelly and dark urine. OE: suprapublic pain, dipstick: protein, nitrates. If 2x +ve MSU <5yrs need referral |
|------|------|
| DM Type 1 | Rare. Causes weight loss, severe thirst, hunger, tiredness, frequency and nocturia. If very high may lead to ketoacidosis. O/E: thin, unwell child. Raised BM's. Dipstick: ketones, glu. Needs urgent referral to hospital. |

**EXPLANATIONS**

*Nocturnal enuresis*    Nocturnal enuresis is the medical way of saying bedwetting. It is a very common condition that affects 5% of 10 year old children. It happens when there is too much urine in the bladder at night, but your child is unable to feel it and awake to go to the toilet. In most cases the child is completely well and there is no serious cause. However, sometimes if the child is stressed from school, exams or bullying that may trigger it. There are also certain drinks that can make it worse and these contain caffeine like coffee, tea or coke. Stopping or cutting down these may help.

*Desmopressin*    Desmopressin works by copying the actions of a naturally produced hormone or messenger (ADH) therefore reducing the volume of urine produced by the kidneys so less collects in the bladder and therefore past at night. It usually works quickly and well and is useful particularly if your child is going away on holiday or for a sleepover at a friend's house.

*Alarms*    We normally use a pad and alarm that works very well to awake the child and prevent bedwetting. It is basically a simple device that is placed in the child's trousers when they sleep at night. As soon as the wetting starts, the alarm sounds and awakes the child to help prompt them to go to the toilet. Over time, the child learns to feel when their bladder is full and awakes themselves before having an accident.

# 13.10 Functional Constipation

Constipation is a common problem in children with some estimates claiming that up to 30% of children suffer from it. In both the primary and secondary care settings it is one of the most common attendances with around one quarter of a paediatric gastroenterologist workload being due to it. It is defined as the decrease in the frequency of bowel movements with the passage of hard stools that may give rise to pain.

The vast majority of sufferers are due to functional problems with only 5% being due to an underlying medical condition. There is no single agreed definition as to when a patient is constipated. However, Rome III have created some diagnostic criteria for functional constipation. Chronic constipation is defined when the problem persists for >2mths and is found in around one third of cases.

---

**Rome III Diagnostic criteria for functional constipation** - *Ref: Rome III Diagnostic Criteria for FGIDs*
Must include one month of at least two or more of the following (children >4yrs)
- Two or fewer defecations per week
- At least one episode/week of incontinence after the acquisition of toileting skills
- History of retentive posturing or excessive volitional stool retention
- History of painful or hard bowel movements
- Presence of a large fecal mass in the rectum
- History of large diameter stools which may obstruct the toilet

---

## HISTORY

**Open questions**     Can you tell me more about your child's problems? Could you tell me about what has been troubling them?

**Focused questions**

*Constipation*     When did all the problems begin? How long has it been going on for? Is it getting worse or better?

Frequency     Does your child open their bowels regularly? How often do they go?

Straining     Do they struggle to pass a motion?

Appearance     Do the stools look like rabbit droppings? Are they often so large that they block the toilet? *Use the Bristol Stool chart to identify the stool type*

Pain     Is there any pain when they go to the toilet for a poo?

Incontinence     Do they soil their undergarments?

Posture     How does the child sit when they have to go toilet? Do they stand on tiptoes, straight-legged with an arched back?

Triggers     Did it start after moving house? Starting school? After potty training? Any new stress in the family? (new additions, parental arguing)

**Associated history**

*Nausea & vomiting*     Did your child feel sick or vomited?

*Feeding*     How is their appetite and eating? Is it worse when they have not gone and better after going? What milk are your using? Did the constipation start when you tried to wean the child onto solids?

*Fluids*     Are they passing urine alright, at least 2x day? How many wet nappies?

*Blood*     Is there any blood on the toilet paper or pan when they have finished?

**Differentials**

| | |
|---|---|
| *Intest. obstruction* | Are they passing any wind or flatus? Are they vomiting? |
| *Hypothyroid* | Are they tired all the time? Are they not putting on weight? Do they feel cold? |
| *Fissure* | Is there blood on the toilet paper? Is it very painful when they go? |

**RED FLAGS**          Constipation from birth, Abdominal distention, vomiting, child abuse

**PAST HISTORY**

| | |
|---|---|
| *Premature* | Was your child born premature? |
| *Disability* | Is your child suffering from Down's syndrome or cerebral palsy? |
| *UTI* | Have they had a UTI before? |

**BIRTH HISTORY**

| | |
|---|---|
| *Pregnancy* | Enquire whether the child had any problems shown on the scan during pregnancy? |
| *Birth* | Did the child pass stools within 48 hours? |

**DRUG HISTORY**

| | |
|---|---|
| *Medication* | Is your child taking any medications? |
| *Immunisations* | Check if they are up-to-date with their childhood immunisations? |

**SOCIAL HISTORY**

| | |
|---|---|
| *Home* | Who is at home with them? Have you move house recently? |
| *Siblings* | Do they have brothers or sisters? How is the relationship between them? Any new arrivals? |
| *School* | Do they go to nursery or school? How are they performing? Any days off? Any bullying? |

**FAMILY HISTORY**

| | |
|---|---|
| *Medical* | Are there any medical conditions that affect other family members? |

**IDEA, CONCERNS, EXPECTATIONS**

| | |
|---|---|
| *Idea* | What do you think may be causing your child's illness? |
| *Concerns* | Is there anything that is worrying you specifically? |
| *Expectations* | How were you hoping we could address this problem? |
| *Impact on life* | How has the illness affected the family? Any embarrassment at school? |

**CSA TIPS**

Constipation is an embarrassing problem that sufferers may feel shy to talk about. Parents too may delay presenting worried that they may be castigated for having poor parenting skills. When broaching the subject you should be receptive and empathetic, whilst remaining supportive and encouraging. It is an extremely common problem and once any red flags or medical causes have been excluded, it can be managed fairly straightforwardly.

**PHYSICAL EXAMINATION**

| | |
|---|---|
| *Vitals* | BP, pulse, temp, height, weight (growth charts) |
| *General* | Inspect the child generally are they well or silent and listless? |
| *Abdomen* | Inspect for distention. Palpate for swelling (impacted faeces), pain and for constipation Auscultate for bowel sounds |

| PR | Not routinely required. However, if you suspect congenital abnormalities inspect the anus Look for anal fissures |
|---|---|

## INVESTIGATIONS

| | |
|---|---|
| Bloods | Not routinely indicated. FBC (infection), U&Es (dehydration), TFTs (hypothyroid), tTGA antibodies (coeliac) |
| AXR / US | Not needed in primary care |
| Specialist | Transit studies |

## MANAGEMENT
### Conservative

| | |
|---|---|
| Reassure | Reassure of the diagnosis of functional constipation and no underlying serious medical condition has been found. Explain it is very common (30% of children) and treatable |
| Diary | Offer bowel diary including daytime fluid intake and dietary intake |
| Fluids | Ensure children drink plenty of water in small amounts regularly |
| Toileting | Advise parents on correct techniques. Use warm water or vaseline around the anus to soothe it and help pass the stools. Consider simple massage of the abdomen prior to going to the toilet starting from the rIght hip area (RIF) up and across, down towards the left hip (LIF) |
| Diet | |
| Fruit | Increase fruit and vegetable – apple, pear prune, apricot. Dry fruits have higher concentration of sorbitol. Can be via fresh fruit juice |
| Fibre | Increase fibre consumption by eating coarse bran, whole grain bread, flour, brown rice and wholemeal spaghetti |
| Exercise | Encourage exercise 30-60 minutes daily |
| Behaviour | |
| Rewards | Star charts for agreed behaviour i.e. drinking correct volume of fluid, going to toilet at regular intervals |
| Avoid | Stress not the child's fault. Do not use penalty systems if patient fails (taking stars away). Punitive measures or blame should be avoided |

### Medical

| Constipation | |
|---|---|
| Oral | Use Movicol Paed plain as first line. If after 2wks no improvement then add stimulant laxative (bisacodyl, senna). Consider lactulose instead of Movicol if patient intolerant |
| PR | Do not use unless PO failed. Consider sodium citrate enema. Do not use phosphate enemas except in hospital setting |
| Maintenance | Commence maintenance treatment until several weeks after regular bowel motion is established. Titrate down the doses over a period of months depending on stool consistency and frequency |

## SAFETY NETTING

| | |
|---|---|
| Follow up | Ensure parents have appropriate follow up to return 1-2 weeks to adjust response |
| Referral | Consider referral if any red flags or poor response to treatment |

**DIFFERENTIAL DIAGNOSIS**

| Condition | Characteristic exam feature |
|---|---|
| **Anal fissures** | Tear to anal mucosa often posterior to anal canal. Pain on defecation with blood on toilet paper. Associated with constipation. On examination fissure visible. PR exam very tender |
| **Obstruction** | Colicky abdominal pain, distension, absolute constipation including wind. Bowels not opened. 'Tinkling' bowel sounds |

**EXPLANATIONS**

*Constipation*      Constipation simply means that stools are not being passed as frequently as they should. It may also mean that sufferers pass painful and hard stools. Sometimes it can cause crampy tummy pain and give rise to symptoms like bloating or even vomiting.

*Laxatives*      Laxatives are medications that help relieve constipation. Some of them work by making the stools more bulky and therefore encouraging you to go (bulk forming). Others work by increasing the amount of water in your bowels therefore making the stools pass more smoothly (osmotic). The last type works by encouraging the muscles in the bowel to increase the movement of the stools through your bowels.

*Impaction*      Occasionally the stool can become very hard that it gets stuck in the back passage. This can cause very alarming symptoms such as abdominal pain and swelling of your tummy. Occasionally the faeces may leak around the blockage, causing soiling of the underwear.

Dementia is an irreversible and progressive condition that usually affects the elderly causing impairment of cognitive function and personality without affecting consciousness. Patients may suffer with amnesia (memory loss), anomia (inability to recall names), apraxia (inability to co-ordinate), aphasia and agnosia (loss of ability to recognize objects, persons). The diagnosis is made once the symptoms have been present for more than 6 months. As symptoms progress, patients may wander, suffer hallucinations, become doubly incontinent and eventually need 24 hour care.

Over 50% of dementias are caused by alzheimer's, 25% are due to vascular dementia and 15% due to Lewy bodies. Although there are no treatments to cure dementia, there are medications that might delay cognitive deterioration.

**HISTORY**

Approach the topic sensitively in a non-threatening, non-judgemental manner. It may be difficult to broach the subject as the patient may lack insight, so begin by making your first few questions designed to put the patient at ease. If any carers are present, seek permission from the patient to take a collateral history.

| | |
|---|---|
| **Open questions** | Can you tell me more about your memory difficulties? History can be from a relative, carer or neighbour |

**Focused questions**

*Cognitive Symptoms*

| | |
|---|---|
| Memory | When did you first notice problems with your memory? How long has it been going on for? |
| Pattern | Did it develop suddenly (delirium), over a period of time (Alzheimer's) or in a step like fashion (vascular)? |
| Types | Do you forget immediate things (appointments, names, keys), recent memories (telephone no, cooking) or past things (birth/important dates, recognising family and friends)? |
| Orientation | Have you ever been disorientated with what day it is or the time? |
| Communication | Have you had problems with speaking or writing? Have you misunderstood people at times? Are you finding yourself repeating your questions more often than before? |
| Tasks | Do you feel it more difficult to make decisions? Are you making more decisions now that you regret later on? Are you finding it difficult to complete everyday tasks that you could do previously? (paying bills, following recipes) |

*Behaviour / Emotional Symptoms*

| | |
|---|---|
| Low mood | Have you been feeling low recently? Which came first, low mood or forgetfulness? (pseudodementia) |
| Anhedonia | Have you lost interest in doing things you used to do? |
| Withdrawal | Are you no longer interacting with people? Do you feel withdrawn from life? |
| Sleep | How has your sleep been recently? |
| Delusions | Have you felt that someone was out to harm you in anyway? |
| Hallucinations | Have you seen or heard anything that others have not noticed? |
| Disinhibition | Have you ever done an action that your felt embarrassed? (going outside undressed) |

*Neurological Symptoms*

| | |
|---|---|
| Walking | Have you had problems with mobility? When you walk do you shuffle? Have you been falling more recently? |
| Apraxia | Are you having problems with dressing, grooming or cooking? |

## Associated Questions

| | |
|---|---|
| *ADLs* | Are you having problems with looking after yourself? Are you able to cook? Can you feed yourself? Are you washing yourself regularly? |
| *Suicide* | Have you ever felt so low that you wanted to end it all? Have you ever acted upon these thoughts? How do you feel today? |

## Differentials

| | |
|---|---|
| *Depression* | Have you been feeling low recently? Do you feel disinterested in life or worthless inside? |
| *Delirium* | Did your symptoms come on quickly? Does your forgetfulness come and go? Are they worse at night? Do you feel that people are against you or do you see things that are not there? Have you had a temperature? |
| *Parkinson's disease* | Do you have a tremor in your hands? Have you noticed it takes longer to do things like get up from a chair or walk? Do you have difficulty writing? |
| *Bereavement* | Did someone close to you died recently? |
| *Hearing* | How is your hearing? |

## RED FLAGS

| | |
|---|---|
| | Suicidal ideation, severe memory loss, risky or aggressive behaviour, abuse or neglect |
| *Risk to self* | Have you left the gas cooker on? |
| *Wandering* | Have you ever got lost when you went out that you could not find your way back home? |

## PAST HISTORY

| | |
|---|---|
| *Psychiatric* | Have you ever had these symptoms before? Have you ever been treated for depression, anxiety or psychosis? Have you ever been admitted to a mental health ward? |
| *Medical* | Do you have any medical conditions such as a CVA, DM, IHD, Cholesterol? Have you ever had a head injury? Have you had a recent infection? (UTI, chest infection) |

## FAMILY HISTORY

| | |
|---|---|
| *Psychiatric* | Does anyone in your family suffer from Alzheimer's or any other mental illnesses? |

## DRUG HISTORY

| | |
|---|---|
| *Medication* | Are you taking any medications? (anticholinergics, TCAs, opiates, BDZ's) |

## SOCIAL HISTORY

| | |
|---|---|
| *Support network* | Who lives with you at home? Do you have any close friends or family? |
| Carers | Do you have any carers? Are they helping you doing day to day tasks? |
| *Occupation* | Are you currently working at the moment? How has your symptoms affected you at work? Are you making more mistakes? |
| *Drive* | Do you drive? |
| *Smoker* | Do you smoke? How many cigarettes do you smoke per day? |
| *Alcohol* | Do you drink alcohol? How much do you drink and how often? |

## IDEA, CONCERNS, EXPECTATIONS

| | |
|---|---|
| *Idea* | Do you have any idea about what may be causing your symptoms? |
| *Concerns* | Do you have any worries about your forgetfulness? |
| *Expectations* | How were you hoping I could help you? |
| *Impact* | How have your symptoms affected your life? |
| *Insight* | Do you believe you have any problems with forgetfulness? |

## CSA TIPS

Dementia becomes more common as a person ages. When presenting for assessment in the early stages, a patient may have insight and be acutely aware that they are suffering with increasing forgetfulness due to its impact on them. In such cases it is important to make a full assessment and exclude other possible more common causes such as depression and stress. Patients in the latter stages of dementia may lack insight about their illness and may require collateral history from carers or family members to make the diagnosis.

## PHYSICAL EXAMINATION

| | |
|---|---|
| *Vitals* | BMI, BP, temperature |
| *Examination* | Examine for signs of increased CVD risk factors, carotid bruit, reduced peripheral pulses |
| *Screening* | In 2013 the DoH commissioned a Dementia DES to screen all at-risk patients for memory loss. At-risk patients included, patients >60yrs with CVD, CVA, PVD or DM, >40yrs with Down's, patients >50yrs with LD or neurodegenerative conditions (PD) |
| *Questionnaire* | |
| 6-CIT | 6 memory questions. Total of 8 or more suggestive of dementia |

---

### 6 Cognitive Impairment Test (CIT)

| | |
|---|---|
| *Year* | What year is it? (score 4 if incorrect) |
| *Month* | What month is it? (scores 3 if incorrect) |
| *Recall* | Repeat after me: John / Smith / 41 / West Street / Manchester |
| *Time* | What time is it? (scores 3 if >1hr incorrect) |
| *Count* | Count backwards from 20-1 (scores 2 for a mistake, scores 4 if >1) |
| *Backwards* | Say the months of the year in reverse (scores 2 for a mistake, 4 if >1) |
| *Repeat recall* | Repeat the address stated previously (score 2 for each mistake, max 10 for 5 mistakes) |

---

| | |
|---|---|
| Mini-COG | 3 steps including recall and drawing of a clock. GPCOG more detailed |

---

### 6 Cognitive Impairment Test (CIT)

| | |
|---|---|
| *Memorise* | Ask to recall 3 unrelated words and repeat to ensure learning i.e. Banana, Sunrise, Chair |
| *Clock* | Request to draw a clock (circle, hour hands, numbers) and show 11:10 |
| *Recall* | Ask to recall the 3 words used previously |
| *Interpretation* | 0 recalled words or 1-2 recalled but abnormal clock suggest impairment |

---

| | |
|---|---|
| MMSE | Detailed memory test checking orientation (time & place), registration (name 3 objects), recall (address), calculation (count backwards from 7), language (reading & writing), drawing (pentagons). Scored out of 30 |
| Other | Mini-MTS, Screen for depression (PHQ-9) |

## INVESTIGATIONS

| | |
|---|---|
| *Bloods* | FBC, serum B12 & folate, ESR, CRP, glucose, U&Es, LFTs, TFT, calcium |
| *Not routine* | |
|     Bloods | Syphilis, HIV requested if risk factors present |
|     Urine | MSU for infection to exclude delirium |
|     CXR | Exclude chest infection, bronchial carcinoma (brain mets) |
|     ECG | If CVD is suspected |
|     CT/MRI | For evidence of vascular dementia (subcortical vascular changes) |

## MANAGEMENT

### Conservative

| | |
|---|---|
| *Advice* | Discuss with patient and family/carer sensitively the possibility of dementia |
| *Lifestyle* | |
|     Diet | Cut down alcohol (exacerbates forgetfulness). Eat well and regularly. Stop any recreational drugs and stop smoking |
|     Exercise | Take regular exercise to reduce weight. Recommend structured exercise programmes (over 6mths improves cognition) or dancing |
|     Mind | Offer cognitive stimulation programmes (problem solving, memory provoking), multisensory stimulation (exposed to light effects, tactile, sound), music or art therapy, massage, aromatherapy, animal assisted therapy (interacting with trained pet or animal) |
| *Memory* | Develop a routine to help compensate for poor memory (fixed place for leaving keys). Use memory aids such as writing things down, populating to-do lists (daily planner), diary for important dates or events |
| *Disorientation* | Fit higher door handles or locks to prevent wandering and getting lost. Fit alarms to the door to contact carers when main door opened. Consider pendant alarms |
| *Hazards* | Declutter the house removing excess clothes, pots and pans. Remove tripping hazards and label drawers with its contents |

| | |
|---|---|
| *Support for Carers* | |
|     Peer group | Give details about peer-support group for carers of dementia sufferers (Alzheimer's Society, Carers UK, Dementia support Group) |
|     CBT | Consider cognitive behavioural therapy or group psycho-education |
|     Respite | Offer short-break care (day care, adult replacement, short term or overnight residential care) to allows carer some respite |

### Refer

| | |
|---|---|
| *Memory clinic* | Refer to memory clinic for the diagnosis of dementia or known suffer with significant depression/psychosis, risky behaviour or medico-legal issues (capacity, driving) |
| *MDT* | Refer to multidisciplinary team (OT, physio, neuropsychiatry, social services) to assess functional capacity (continence, safety at home, self care etc) |
| *OT* | Evaluate performance and need. Help environmental modification to help complete tasks such as cooking, cleaning and washing independently |
| *Social Services* | Consider a referral to the social services to assess need at home. Other services such as Meals on Wheels or benefits advice |

### Medical

| | |
|---|---|
| *Medication* | Initiated by specialist (psychiatrist, neurologist), e.g. acetylcholinesterase inhibitors (donepezil, galantamine) often in moderate Alzheimer's disease (MMSE 10-20) or lewy |

body dementia (rivastigmine). Not for vascular dementia or mild cognitive impairment. Memantine given in severe Alzheimer's disease

| | |
|---|---|
| Antipsychotics | Should not be prescribed routinely e.g. haloperidol, olanzapine, risperidone. Increased risk of CVA and mortality rates. Considered only in severe symptoms (psychosis, anxiety causing distress) as last resort |
| Antidepressants | Can be offered in major depressive disorder. Care with interaction with anticholinergics (affect cognition), often specialist led. Consider CBT |

Safety
| | |
|---|---|
| Housing | Consider sheltered accommodation or change in residence |
| Driving | Should inform DVLA. Licence to review annually and a formal driving assessment may be necessary (group 1). Group 2 licence will be refused or revoked |

| | |
|---|---|
| Capacity | Assess capacity to make decisions (Mental Capacity Act 2005) |
| Power of Attorney | Whilst having capacity, patient's can nominate (written document) an individual to act on their behalf to make healthcare decisions if they were to lose capacity in the future (Lasting Power of Attorney) |
| Advance decisions | Similar to living wills and legally binding. Permits decision to refuse treatment even if it results in their death i.e. antibiotics for pneumonia |
| Adv.statements | Can recommend treatment, and respect their belief. Must be considered by doctors but not legally binding |
| Place of care plan | Patients can recommend their preferred place of care ie. where they would like to die |
| Will | Can write a will to determine their financial matter after their death |
| IMCA | The Independent Mental Capacity Advocate is for patients who lack capacity and do not have an advocate (friends/family/carer). Can challenge serious medical treatment, change of residence or support in vulnerable adult cases (abuse) |

---

**Mental Capacity - Mental Capacity Act (2005)**

| | |
|---|---|
| Principles | Patients assumed to have capacity. People have right to have support when making decision and permitted to make unwise ones. If a patients lacks capacity then the decision should be made in their best interests and least restrictive intervention to their rights and freedom |
| Lacks capacity | Patients lack capacity if they have an impairment to mental function *and* if they do not understand information related to the decision, unable to retain it, unable to utilise it to make a decision, or unable to communicate their decision to others |

---

| | |
|---|---|
| End of life | Discuss with patient, when they have capacity, end of life strategies including place of care plan to enable them to die with dignity. Consider palliative care measures including Liverpool care pathway or Gold standards framework |
| DNR | Discuss with the patient their resuscitation decisions (DNR) |

**SAFETY NETTING**

| | |
|---|---|
| Suicide risk | Review the patient frequently in primary care. Consider contacting Crisis Resolution & Home Treatment team for urgent assessment |
| Sectioning | Try voluntarily, if not, consider compulsory admission (if risk to self or others) |
| Safeguarding | Follow local safeguarding pathways for child protection or vulnerable adults |
| Follow up | Offer a series of appointments in primary care, with short gaps in more serious cases |

# DIFFERENTIAL DIAGNOSIS

| Condition | Characteristic exam feature |
|---|---|
| Alzheimer's | Progressive memory loss (often short term). Behavioural changes such as wandering and withdrawal. Dyspraxia (difficulty dressing) and problems communicating (dysphasia). Care result in personality changes. FHx present |
| Vascular Dementia | Stepwise deterioration with evidence of vascular disease (IHD, PVD, BP). Often starts more acutely, with gait problems, personality changes with insight intact until late |
| Lewy Body | Fluctuant with parkinsonian symptoms (rigidity, gait problems and tremor). May have delirium-like periods and visual hallucinations |
| Frontotemporal degeneration | Found in younger patients <65yrs. Mainly suffer from disinhibitions, early loss of insight, personality changes with preservation of memory |
| Delirium | Clinical diagnosis. Sudden onset and fluctuating consciousness usually worse at night. May have confusion, disorientation with fear and aggression. Delusions & hallucinations may be present. Common causes include infections (UTI/chest), drugs (sedative, analgesic), constipation, poor nutrition |

## EXPLANATIONS

*Dementia*

Dementia is a condition that causes a progressive decline of the brain's functionality. It causes gradual memory loss, slowing down of thinking speed and can affect one's understanding, judgement and language. It can worsen and affect your ability to remain independent and look after yourself.

*Alzheimer's*

Alzheimer's disease is a type of dementia which causes the brain to shrink (atrophy) with the amount of brain chemicals (neurotransmitters), that allow parts of the brain to talk to one another, reduced. Over time there is gradual death of brain cells with worsening of the condition.

*Vascular dementia*

This is where the patient suffers from several tiny strokes that affects the thinking areas of the brain. The blood vessels supplying the brain can become blocked and as a result blood cannot reach that area causing damage.

*Lewy body dementia*

This is a type of dementia that shares similarities to both Alzheimer's disease and Parkinson's disease. Lewy bodies are a type of abnormal proteins that build up in the nerve cells of the brain and can result in lower levels of brain chemicals (neurotransmitters) which can interfere with how the brain works normally.

*Delirium*

Delirium is a mental state that may present suddenly and cause symptoms similar to dementia. A person may display signs of confusion, forgetfulness and disorientation. Although patients with delirium may appear quite unwell, the condition is usually reversible once the reason has been identified; which is commonly because of a chest or urine infection, or may even be due to side-effects of common medications.

Falls are unintentional loss of balance resulting in the individual coming to a rest on the ground. They are very common in the elderly with 30% of >65yr having a fall in the last 1yr and 1 in 2 people having falls have had a history of previous falls of 2 or more in the last yr. Falls predisposes patients for having serious injury such as fractures (wrist, femur) particularly in patients with osteoporosis. They can have a significant impact upon the patient creating a fear of having another fall resulting in the patient failing to mobilise or exercise. As a result in muscle weakness which puts them at risk of further falls.

## HISTORY

**Open questions**   Can you tell me more about the falls you have been experiencing? Could you tell me about what has been troubling you?

## Focused questions

| | |
|---|---|
| *Falls* | When did you last have a fall? What exactly happened? (trip) |
| Frequency | How often has it happened? |
| Witness | Did anyone see you fall? What did they say happened? |
| Injuries | Did you sustain any injuries? (fracture, head) |
| Previous episodes | Has it happened before? When exactly? |
| Dizziness | Did you feel light headed before you fell? Did the room spin around? Did it happen after looking up? (BPPV) |
| LOC | Did you lose consciousness or blackout when you fell? |

## Associated history

| | |
|---|---|
| *Hazards* | Do you have any loose rugs anywhere? Did you trip over anything (cable)? How is your footwear? when did you last change them? |
| *Arthritis* | Do you have any joint pains? Do you get enough exercise? |
| *Vision* | How is your vision? (cataracts, partial sighted, macular degeneration) |
| *Incontinence* | How is your bladder control? Do you ever leak? |
| UTI | Any burning feeling when you pass urine? Do you pass urine often? |
| *Dementia* | Have you had any memory problems? |

## DIFFERENTIALS

| | |
|---|---|
| *Cardiac* | Did you have any chest pain or palpitations? (arrhythmia) |
| *Epilepsy* | Do you get warning signs before hand (prodromal - taste, smell)? Did your body go stiff and then fit? Did you bite your tongue or wet yourself? |
| *TIA* | Did you have slurred speech? Any weakness of your arms or legs? |
| *Postural hypotension* | Do you feel lightheaded when you stood up? Do you take any BP tablets? |
| *Situational syncope* | Where you shaving at the time (carotid sinus)? Where you passing urine? |

## RED FLAGS

Sudden onset, recent head injury, exercise induced LoC, focal neurology

## PAST HISTORY

| | |
|---|---|
| *Ischaemic* | Do you suffer from any medical conditions? (AF, DM, HTN, CVD) |
| *Osteoporosis* | Do you suffer from thinning of the bone? |
| *CNS* | Do you suffer from dementia, strokes, epilepsy or Parkinson's disease? |

## DRUG HISTORY

| | |
|---|---|
| *Medication* | Are you taking any medications? (polypharmacy, antihypertensives - postural hypotension, hypoglycaemics, antiarrhythmics, psychoactive - BDZ anticonvulsants) |

## FAMILY HISTORY

| | |
|---|---|
| *Osteoporosis* | Does anyone in the family suffer from thinning of the bones? |

## SOCIAL HISTORY

| | |
|---|---|
| *Mobility* | How is your mobility? Has it changed recently? Do you exercise often? |
| Stairs | Do you have stairs where you live? |
| *Support network* | Who lives with you at home? Do you have any close friends or family? |
| Carers | Do you have any carers? Are they helping you doing day to day tasks? |
| Coping | Are you coping currently? |
| *Occupation* | Are you currently working or retired? |
| *Alcohol* | Do you drink alcohol? How much do you drink and how often? |
| *Smoker* | Do you smoke? How many cigarettes do you smoke per day? |

## IDEA, CONCERNS, EXPECTATIONS

| | |
|---|---|
| *Idea* | Do you have any idea about what may be causing your falls? |
| *Concerns* | Do you have any worries about it? (fear of falling) |
| *Expectations* | How were you hoping I could help you? |
| *Impact* | How have your symptoms affected your life? |

## PHYSICAL EXAMINATION

| | |
|---|---|
| *Vitals* | Lying and standing BP (hypotension), pulse (AF, bradycardic), BMI |
| *Inspect* | Look at general appearance (anxious, pale), muscle wasting, tremor |
| *Cardiovascular* | Listen for heart murmurs (AS), enlarged heart (HOCM), carotid bruits |
| *Neurological* | *Perform focused examination based on clinical findings:* |
| Gait | Check for broad-based, ataxic, scissoring gait |
| Turn 180° test | Ask to stand up, turn around 180°. If requires >4 steps further assessment required |
| Get up & go | 'Timed up & Go' test: Time patient getting up from a chair without using arms, walk 3m then turn around, return and sit down in chair. Can use their own walking aid |
| Tone | Check for hypertonia |
| Power | Check power of limbs compared to normal side |
| Reflexes | Consider biceps, tricep, supinator, knee or ankle |
| Cranial nerves | CN examination (e.g. visual fields, V, VII) |

## INVESTIGATIONS — *depends on clinical findings*

| | |
|---|---|
| *Urine* | MSU or dipstick to exclude UTI |
| *Bloods* | Hb (anaemia), glucose (DM), U&Es (dehydration), LFT, TFT, B12 |
| *Imaging* | CXR (Enlarged heart), DEXA (osteoporosis) |
| *Cardiac* | ECG (Arrhythmia, bradycardia), 24 ECG - If ECG normal and cardiac sounding, Echo (Heart murmurs), 24hr BP |
| *Specialist* | CT/MRI (subdural, subarachnoid), carotid doppler (TIA), tilt-table, carotid sinus massage |

## MANAGEMENT

### Conservative

| | |
|---|---|
| Polypharmacy | Rationalise drugs if on multiple medications |
| Exercise | Recommend muscle strengthening and balance training. Recommend exercises (Tai Chi) |
| Support groups | Suggest Age Concern, Help the Age, Age UK |
| Adaptation | Recommend non-slip mats in bathroom, mopping up wet floors, decluttering house (moving furniture, wires), insert bright bulbs |
| Feet | Wear well-fitted shoes, trim toenails |
| Housing | Consider wearing pendant alarm, sheltered accommodation/warden controlled flat |
| Alcohol | Advice to cut down or avoid alcohol |

### Medical

| | |
|---|---|
| Osteoporosis | Consider Vit D and calcium including bisphosphonates if history of fractures or osteoporosis |

### Refer

| | |
|---|---|
| Physiotherapy | Structured exercise programmes |
| OT | Home hazards assessment (loose rugs, cable, furniture, wet surfaces, dim light) or if equipment needs to be installed (handholds). May require walking aids (stick, ZF) |
| Chiropodist | If requires foot care |
| Vision | Optician for vision assessment or ophthalmologist for cataracts |
| Endocrinologist | Refer to an endocrinologist if you suspect autonomic neuropathy |
| Falls clinic | If multifactorial, complex case requiring MDT or unknown cause refer to falls clinic |

## SAFETY NETTING

| | |
|---|---|
| Follow up | Review annually to check risk factors or sooner if has recurrent falls |

## EXPLANATIONS

| | |
|---|---|
| Falls | Falls can happen to anyone but as we get older they become more serious as it puts you at risk of fracture to your bones. Falls can happen for many reasons, most are due to a simple trip or wearing poor shoes, other causes included having health problems such as poor vision, dizzy spells, arthritis etc. |

# 15.1 Depression

Depression is the most common mental health disorder that GPs encounter with over 1 in 20 adults experiencing an episode of depression a year. It can vary in intensity ranging from a single mild episode to a severe recurrent lifelong disorder. The average length of a depressive episode is just over 6 months with a risk of recurrence of at least 50% after a first episode and rising to 70% after a second episode. Patients may present predominantly with biological symptoms known as 'somatic depression'. Patients with severe depression may even harbour delusions or auditory hallucinations. In approximately 4% of cases the depression will be severe enough to lead them to take their own life and hence it is important to always screen for suicidal ideation.

### HISTORY
Approach the topic sensitively in a non-threatening, non-judgemental manner. It can be quite difficult to broach the subject initially, so begin by making your first few questions designed to put the patient at ease.

| | |
|---|---|
| **Open questions** | Can you tell me more about how you are feeling? |
| *Cues* | If the patient is reluctant to talk or appears withdrawn, displaying little eye contact, reflect this non-verbal cue to them by saying; You look upset? Is anything bothering you? |

**Focused questions**

| | |
|---|---|
| *Depression* | When did you first start feeling like this? How long has it been going on for? |
| *Core Symptoms* | |
| Low mood | Have you been feeling low recently? |
| Anhedonia | Do you find it difficult to in enjoy the activities that you usually would get pleasure in doing? Have you lost interest in doing things you used to do? |
| Fatigue | How would you describe your energy levels? Do you tire easily? |

| | |
|---|---|
| *Cognitive Symptoms* | |
| Concentrate | Are you able to concentrate on things (tv/paper)? Do you find that you are easily distracted? |
| Self-esteem | How do you perceive yourselves? Do you lack self esteem or self belief? |
| Beck's triad | Do you feel you have no worth (worthless)? Do you feel that someone can help you (helpless)? How you see the future (hopeless)? |

| | |
|---|---|
| *Biological Symptoms* | |
| Sleep | How is your sleep? Do you find that you wake up early and struggle to go to sleep again (early morning waking) or do find it hard to go to sleep in the first place? |
| Food | How has your appetite been? Have you lost or gain weight recently? |
| Libido | Are you in a relationship? Are you still interested or enjoy sexual relations? |

| | |
|---|---|
| **Associated Questions** | |
| *Delusions* | Have you felt that someone was out to harm you in anyway? (persecutory) |
| *Hallucinations* | Did you see or hear anything that others have not noticed? Were the voices about you? |
| *Suicide* | Have you ever felt so low that you wanted to end it all? Have you ever acted upon these thoughts? Have you ever harmed yourself? How do you feel today? |

## Differentials

| | |
|---|---|
| Mania | Have you ever so high that you felt really energetic and excited? Have you been spending more than you had anticipated? |
| Bereavement | Did someone close die recently? |
| Postnatal Depres. | Did you give birth recently? When did your symptoms start? (<6wk of birth) |

## RED FLAGS

Suicidal ideation, persecutory delusions or hallucinations (risk to others), children

## PAST HISTORY

| | |
|---|---|
| Psychiatric | Have you ever had these symptoms before? Have you ever been treated for low mood, anxiety or psychosis? Have you ever been admitted to a mental health ward? |
| Medical | Do you have any medical conditions such as an underactive thyroid? (CVA, DM, IHD) |

## FAMILY HISTORY

| | |
|---|---|
| Psychiatric | Does anyone in your family suffer from depression or any other mental illnesses? |

## DRUG HISTORY

| | |
|---|---|
| Medication | Are you taking any medications? (steroids, COCP, indomethacin, ranitidine, beta-blockers, opioids) |

## SOCIAL HISTORY

| | |
|---|---|
| Relationships | Are you currently in a relationship? How are things? Do you have any children? |
| Support network | Who lives with you at home? Do you have any close friends or family? |
| Occupation | Are you working or studying at the moment? Do you have any financial worries? |
| Smoker | Do you smoke? How many cigarettes do you smoke per day? |
| Alcohol | Do you drink alcohol? How much do you drink and how often? |
| Recreational drugs | Have you ever used any recreational drugs? Have you used heroin or cannabis? |

---

**Diagnosing Depression** - *Ref: NICE (2009) Depression, the tx and mx of depression in adults*
Diagnosis of depression requires 1 or 2 core symptoms with =>5 associated symptom
- During the past month have you been feeling, down, depressed or hopeless?
- During the past month have you had little interest or pleasure in doing things?

| | |
|---|---|
| Associated symptoms | Disturbed sleep (more/less), changes to appetite and/or weight, fatigue, agitation or slowing of movements, poor concentration, feeling worthless or guilt, suicidal thoughts |
| Sub-threshold | 2-5 associated symptoms with 1 core |
| Mild depression | >5 associated symptoms with mild impairment to function |
| Mod depression | Symptoms or functional impairment are between 'mild' and 'severe' |
| Severe depression | Most symptoms with markedly interference to daily function +/- psychotic symptoms |

---

## IDEA, CONCERNS, EXPECTATIONS

| | |
|---|---|
| Idea | Do you have any idea about what may be causing your symptoms? |
| Concerns | Do you have any worries about it? |
| Expectations | How were you hoping I could help you? |
| Impact | How have your symptoms affected your life? |

## CSA TIPS

Given that depression is so common, it is likely that you will face a case in the exams. Patients may attend with symptoms of low mood and unhappiness for which they are seeking help from you, their GP regarding diagnosis and management. Others may attend with similar symptoms but may have more pressing concerns around an inability to cope at work and require assistance in this regard.

## PHYSICAL EXAMINATION

| | |
|---|---|
| *Vitals* | BMI |
| *Questionnaire* | |
| PHQ-9 | 9 questions, 3 points each, total score of 21, >11 requires intervention |
| Severity | 0-4 none, 5-9 mild, 10-14 moderate, 15-19 moderately severe, 20-27 severe |
| HADS | 14 questions (7 on depression, 7 on anxiety), total score of 21, >9 requires intervention |
| Severity | 0-7 normal, 8–10 borderline, 11+ case |

## INVESTIGATIONS

| | |
|---|---|
| *Bloods* | Often not indicated. FBC, ESR, glucose, U&Es, LFTs, TFT, calcium |

## MANAGEMENT

### Conservative

*Lifestyle*

| | |
|---|---|
| Exercise | Take regular exercise and try and get out even for a walk |
| Diet | Cut down alcohol. Eat well and regularly. Stop any recreational drugs e.g. cannabis |
| Sleep | Relax in a dark room with minimal distraction. Go to sleep at the same time every night and have a light snack |

| | |
|---|---|
| *Sick Certificate* | Offer short fit-note. Consider amended duties or altered hours if finding it difficult to carry out certain tasks or attend in the morning |

*Self Help*

| | |
|---|---|
| Material | Can prescribe books or leaflets to help guide patients with their symptoms. RCPsych recommends the 'Overcoming' series |
| On-line | Computer programmes or internet guided treatments like NICE recommended, 'Beating the Blues' or 'FearFighter' |

*Talking therapies*

| | |
|---|---|
| Counselling | Refer to counsellor or therapist for mild depression |
| CBT | Consider cognitive behavioural therapy for mild / moderate depression |
| Others | Consider referring for specific therapies such as couple therapy, bereavement counselling, interpersonal psychotherapy, computerised CBT or group therapy |

### Medical

| | |
|---|---|
| *Titration* | Consider medications with moderate to severe depression. May take 2-4wk before they feel any improvement. Must use for 6mth following remission of symptoms to reduce relapse risk |

| | |
|---|---|
| *SSRIs* | 1st episode use selective serotonin reuptake inhibitor e.g. citalopram, fluoxetine or paroxetine. 2nd line SSRIs include escitalopram, mirtazapine |
| Side effects | GI symptoms, GI bleed, increased anxiety and agitation for first 2-4wks |

| | |
|---|---|
| Interactions | NSAIDs (add PPI), warfarin (avoid, consider mirtazapine), aspirin, triptans |
| Discontinue | Gradually taper over 4wks (not required for fluoxetine). If stops suddenly may experience discontinuation symptoms (restlessness, difficulty sleeping, mood change, sweaty, GI- N&V, diarrhoea, paresthesia) |
| *SNRI* | Consider venlafaxine or duloxetine if poor response to SSRIs or in severe depression. 2nd line treatment. Check BP after initiating |
| Side effects | Nausea, dizziness, dry mouth |
| CI | Uncontrolled hypertension, CVD |
| *TCA* | Not to be used if risk of overdose nor as first line. Consider if severe depression or failure to respond to SSRIs e.g. amitriptyline, clomipramine, lofepramine |
| Side effects | Dry mouth, drowsiness, blurred vision, constipation, urinary retention |
| CI | Immediate after MI, arrhythmia (block) |
| *ECT* | Consider only as last resort in severe, treatment resistant depression |
| *Pregnancy* | Consider if benefits > risks. Fluoxetine only SSRI licenced in pregnancy. Small risk of congenital heart disease in early pregnancy and neonatal withdrawal symptoms in third trimester |

**Switching Antidepressants**

| | |
|---|---|
| SSRI → SSRI | Initial SSRI should be reduced then stopped before another SSRI started |
| SSRI → TCA | Cross taper i.e. reduce one and increase other (exception fluoxetine) |
| SSRI → Venlafaxine | Cross taper but start venlafaxine 37.5mg od, increase slowly |
| Fluoxetine → Venla. | Withdraw then start venlafaxine 37.5mg od, increase slowly |
| Fluoxetine → SSRI | Withdraw gradually, leave 7d gap before starting SSRI |
| Fluoxetine → TCA | Withdraw gradually, leave 7d gap before starting TCA |

**SAFETY NETTING**

| | |
|---|---|
| *Suicide risk* | Review the patient frequently in primary care. Consider contacting Crisis Resolution & Home Treatment team for urgent assessment |
| Sectioning | Try persuading voluntarily, if not compliant consider compulsory admission (if risk to self, or to others) |
| Safeguarding | Follow local safeguarding pathways for child protection or vulnerable adults |
| *Follow up* | Offer a series of appointments in primary care, with short gaps in more serious cases |

**DIFFERENTIAL DIAGNOSIS**

| Condition | Characteristic exam feature |
|---|---|
| **Subthreshold depression** | Few symptoms of depression but able to cope with everyday life. Dysthymia when symptoms go on for 2yrs |
| **Seasonal affective disorder** | Symptoms of depression occur annually each year often in winter and resolving in spring |
| **Abn.Bereavement** | Abnormal reaction to a bereavement (>2mth). Feelings of guilt, preoccupation of |

| Reaction | worthlessness with psychomotor retardation. Can have thoughts of death |
|---|---|
| Bipolar | 2 contrasting emotional states i.e. depression/mania. In elevation phase patient is overactive, irritable, distracted, disinhibited, suffers from insomnia, has flights of idea or pressure of speech. Can also have grandiose ideas |
| Anorexia | Affects young girls after the age of 16. Low BMI <17.5. Missing meals, vomiting or using laxatives. Obsessed with body image and looking in the mirror. OE: Thin, yellow skin, pale conjunctiva, calluses on knuckles, pallor, low bp and bradycardia. |

## EXPLANATIONS

*Depression*

Depression is a common mental illness that makes people have a low mood, and lack of interest in doing things. Patients may also have feelings of guilt, tiredness, poor sleep and poor concentration. Although people feel unhappy from time to time, when it is persistent and begins to affect your life then it is known as depression.

*Cause*

Depression may happy for many reasons. It could be because of a life-changing illness you have been diagnosed with or it could be because of a specific situation like a loss of job or a death of a loved one. However, on many occasions we may never know what triggered the depression.

*CBT*

This is known as cognitive behaviour therapy and is a powerful psychological treatment that is often used in patients with mild or moderate depression. It works by making you appreciate yourself, others and the environment and how you relate to it with your thoughts and feelings. It involves fairly intensive work with a therapist over a number of sessions to identify the deep rooted issues affecting you and helps you to deal with them using your own thoughts, behaviours and positive emotions.

*SSRI*

Research has shown that in patients who suffer from depression or low mood, they often have low amounts of a chemical messenger or hormone called Serotonin. This is a special chemical in the brain that is believed to influence and improve mood, sleep and feelings. SSRIs work to stop the breakdown of this hormone and hence increases its levels.

Sleep disorders affect 1 in 3 people at some time in their life. It is characterised by an inability to fall asleep or stay asleep for a sufficient enough time to feel refreshed in the morning. Having a lack of sleep may present with symptoms such as forgetfulness, daytime tiredness, irritability or anxiety. It may present itself as a primary disorder, or more usually, as a symptom of another mental health illness such as mania, depression, anxiety or PTSD. It is more common in women and with increasing age.

## HISTORY
Approach the topic sensitively in a non-threatening, non-judgemental manner. It can be quite difficult to broach the subject initially, so begin by making your first few questions designed to put the patient at ease.

**Open questions** — Can you tell me more about the symptoms you have been experiencing? What problems have you had with your sleep?

*Cues* — If the patient is reluctant to talk or appears appear withdrawn, displaying little eye contact or spontaneity, reflect this non-verbal cue to them by saying; You look upset? Is anything bothering you?

*Screening* — *Ask patients who suffer from anxiety or depression:* Do you experience difficulty sleeping? Do you have problems falling or staying asleep?

**Focused questions**

*Sleep* — When did your sleep problem first start? How long has it been going on for? Does it affect you every day or just occasionally?

Quality — How would you rate the quality of your sleep between 1 (poor) - 5 (very good)?

Sleep routine — Talk me through how you go to sleep? When do you go to sleep? What time do you wake up? Do you wake up in the middle of the night? Do you nap during the day? How many hours of sleep do you get?

*Triggers (ideas)* — Have you noticed anything that could be causing your poor sleep?

Occupation — Are you currently working or studying at the moment? Do you have any stress at work? Do you work a shifting pattern (nights)? Are you studying late at night?

Financial — Do you have any financial worries? (loss of job, mortgages, debt)

Relationships — Are you currently in a relationship? How are things? Do you have any children? Do they sleep well at night?

Environmental — Has there been any changes to your environment (noisy neighbour)? Have you been abroad recently (jet lag)?

Diet — Do you drink tea or coffee? Do you use energy drinks or cola?

**Associated Questions**

*Depression* — Have you been feeling low recently? Do you feel disinterested in life or worthless inside? How is your eating habit?

*Anxiety* — Do you feel anxious or worried a lot? How often do you feel this way? Do you suffer from panic attacks?

*Psychosis* — Have you seen things or heard things that you could not explain? Do you feel someone is out to harm you in anyway?

*Suicide* — Have you ever felt so low that you wanted to end it all?

| Other | Do you get any symptoms such as a cough, pain, shortness of breath or passing urine a lot at night that is affecting you to sleep? |
|---|---|

## Differentials

| Sleep apnoea | Do you snore when you sleep? Has your partner noticed you can stop breathing for a few seconds/minutes? Do you feel sleepy and unrefreshed in the morning? |
|---|---|
| Heart Failure | Do you have problems breathing when sleeping? How many pillows do you use at night? Do you have any pink phlegm? Do you have any ankle swelling? |
| Panic disorder | Do you suffer from unexpected panic attacks often for no reason? Do they last for a few seconds or minutes? Do you get palpitations? |

## RED FLAGS

Depression, alcohol, recreational drugs

## PAST HISTORY

| Psychiatric | Have you ever had these symptoms before? Have you ever been treated for depression, mania, anxiety or panic attacks? Have you ever been diagnosed with ADHD? |
|---|---|
| Medical | Do you have any medical conditions? Have you ever been diagnosed with restless legs syndromes or an overactive thyroid? |

## FAMILY HISTORY

| Psychiatric | Does anyone in your family suffer from mental illnesses? Has anyone close like your parents or siblings been previously diagnosed with anxiety disorder or panic attacks? |
|---|---|

## DRUG HISTORY

| Medication | Are you taking any medications (ritalin, nicotine replacement, alpha and beta-blockers, oral steroids)? Have you ever taken diazepam (rebound insomnia)? |
|---|---|

## SOCIAL HISTORY

| Stress | Is there anything in your life that has caused you much stress and anxiety? |
|---|---|
| Smoker | Do you smoke? How many cigarettes do you smoke per day? |
| Alcohol | Do you drink alcohol? How much do you drink and how often? |
| Recreational drugs | Have you ever used any recreational drugs? (crack, amphetamines, ecstasy) |

## IDEA, CONCERNS, EXPECTATIONS

| Concerns | Do you have any worries about it? |
|---|---|
| Expectations | How were you hoping I could help you? |
| Impact | How have your symptoms affected your life? |

## PHYSICAL EXAMINATION

| Vitals | BMI, BP, pulse |
|---|---|
| Examination | Perform cardiac or thyroid examination if indicated |
| Questionnaire | |
|    Epworth | Offer the Epworth sleepiness questionnaire to assess severity of OSA |

## INVESTIGATIONS

| Bloods | *Not routinely performed.* Consider TFT, pro-BNP |
|---|---|
| Diary | Offer a 2 week sleep diary |

| | |
|---|---|
| *Sleep Studies* | Secondary care may refer for polysomnogram and the multiple sleep latency test to check for presence of insomnia or sleep apnoea |

## MANAGEMENT
### *Conservative*
Lifestyle

| | |
|---|---|
| Diet | Avoid caffeine <6hrs before bedtime, consider stopping all caffeine. Do not eat a heavy meal before sleeping nor sleep on an empty stomach |
| Alcohol / smoking | Advise to stop or cut down alcohol and smoking |
| Drugs | Stop any recreational drugs |
| Exercise | Regular daytime exercise (jogging, swimming, cycling) helps reduce stress and make you feel tired. However avoid exercise 4hrs prior to bedtime |
| Relaxation tech. | Recommend relaxation techniques e.g. deep breathing exercises, take a warm bath before sleeping or listen to calming music |
| Driving | Advise the patient not to drive if feels drowsy/sleepy |

*Sleep hygiene*

| | |
|---|---|
| Environment | Ensure you lie in a dark room, use thick blinds or curtains or an eye mask. Ensure the room is quiet with ambient temperature. If it is noisy around you, wear ear plugs to minimise this Switch off any tv, smartphones or tablet devices and close any books. Turn away any clocks to avoid clock-watching |
| Routine | Advised to go to wake up and go to sleep a fixed times every day. Avoid napping during the day. Relax prior to sleeping |
| *Self Help* | Offer leaflets on understanding sleep disorders and managing it (Overcoming series) |

*Talking therapies*

| | |
|---|---|
| CBT | Consider referral for cognitive behavioural therapy (individual or group) |
| Others | Consider stimulus control or sleep restriction therapy, biofeedback, paradoxical intention |

### *Medical*

| | |
|---|---|
| *Hypnotics* | Consider in short term insomnia where daytime sleepiness is severe. Offer a maximum of 2wks medication. Consider short acting BDZ (temazepam, lorazepam) or non-BDZ (zopiclone, zolpidem). Do not recommend diazepam (daytime anxiety) |
| Side effects | Warn patient about risk of drug tolerance and dependency. Avoid against driving or operating machinery. Causes drowsiness, confusion |
| *Melatonin* | Consider in >55yr with persistent insomnia. Initiate for 3wks and continue for 13wks in total if respond |
| *Antidepressants* | Some have sedative effects such as amitriptyline, mirtazapine. Consider if has concurrent depression or anxiety only |
| *Referral* | Consider if symptoms persist for >4wks refer to psychiatrist |

## SAFETY NETTING

| | |
|---|---|
| *Follow up* | If on hypnotics review face to face prior to offering a repeat prescription in 2wk |

# 15.3 Psychosis

Psychosis in a mental health disorder whereby the sufferer is unable to distinguish between real life and their imagination. It usually affects adults and young people from 16-30 years of age. It is characterised by holding fixed unshakeable beliefs also known as delusions or vivid hallucinations invariable auditory but may also present as tactile or visual. Psychosis can be caused by a wide range of disorders including bipolar disease, head tumour, substance abuse, but is most commonly due to schizophrenia.

## HISTORY
Approach the topic sensitively in a non-threatening, non-judgemental manner. It can be quite difficult to broach the subject initially, so begin by making your first few questions designed to put the patient at ease.

| | |
|---|---|
| **Open questions** | Can you tell me more about how you are feeling? |
| *Cues* | If the patient is reluctant to talk or appears suspicious or fidgety reflect this non-verbal cue to them by saying; You look preoccupied? Is there something on your mind? |

**Focused questions**

| | |
|---|---|
| *Psychosis* | When did you first start feeling like this? How long has it been going on for? What do you think caused it? How has it affected you? |
| *Delusions* | |
| Persecutory | Do you think that someone is plotting against you? Is it a specific person or agency? |
| Grandiosity | Do you believe that you have special powers that others do not possess? |
| Reference | Have you ever felt that the TV/radio was communicating directly to you? |
| Perception | Do you interpret things differently compared to other people? |
| Control | Do you believe that you are being controlled by an outside force? |
| Nihilistic | Do you believe the world is in a state of destruction? How do you view yourself? |
| Cotard's | Do you believe you insides are rotten? |
| Ekbom's | Or do you believe you have been infested by an organism? |
| Fixed | How certain are you about these thoughts? |

| | |
|---|---|
| *Hallucinations* | |
| Auditory | Do you ever hear voices when someone is not there? Tell me about the voices? How many people are there? |
| 3rd person | Do they speak about you? (third person, running commentary) |
| 2nd person | Do they speak to you directly? (second person, depression) |
| 1st person | Do you ever hear your own thoughts being repeated like an echo? (echo de pense) |
| Location | Do you hear the voices from inside (pseudo) or outside (real) your head? |
| Content | What do you hear? What do they say? (derogatory/praiseworthy) |
| | Do they tell you to harm yourself? (severe depression) |
| Visual/olfactory | Have you seen or smelt things that others have said were not there? (head injury, organic, temporal lobe epilepsy) |
| Formication | Have you felt something walking on your skin like a bug? (alcohol, cocaine) |

| | |
|---|---|
| *Thought Disorder* | |
| Insert/withdrawal | Have you felt that someone is putting thoughts into your head or taking them out? |
| Broadcasting | Do you think that others can hear what you are thinking? |

## Negative Symptoms

| | |
|---|---|
| *Lack of motivation* | Do you feel that you no longer have any motivation to do things? |
| *Asocial* | Do you still mix with friends or family? |
| *Self neglect* | Are you still washing yourself or cleaning the house? |

## Differentials

| | |
|---|---|
| *Mania* | Have you ever felt so high or really excited? Do you have difficulty controlling your spending? Have you notice yourself becoming more promiscuous? |
| *Depression* | How is your mood? Do you still enjoy your past-times? |
| *PTSD* | Have you ever experienced a life threatening event? Do you get nightmares? |
| *Puerperal Psychosis* | Did you give birth recently? When did your symptoms start? (shortly after birth) |

## RED FLAGS

Suicidal ideation, persecutory delusions or hallucinations (risk to others), children

## PAST HISTORY

| | |
|---|---|
| *Psychiatric* | Have you ever had these symptoms before? Have you ever been treated for schizophrenia or depression? Have you ever been admitted to a mental health ward? |
| *Medical* | Do you have any medical conditions? Do you suffer with any chronic conditions like HIV, TB, dementia? Have you ever had a brain tumour? |

## FAMILY HISTORY

| | |
|---|---|
| *Psychiatric* | Does anyone in your family suffer from schizophrenia or any other mental illnesses? |

## DRUG HISTORY

| | |
|---|---|
| *Medication* | Are you taking any medications? (steroids, levodopa, opioids) |

## SOCIAL HISTORY

| | |
|---|---|
| *Relationships* | Are you currently in a relationship? How are things? Do you have any children? Who looks after them? |
| *Support network* | Who lives with you at home? Do you have any close friends or family? |
| *Occupation* | Are you currently working or studying at the moment? Do you have any financial worries? |
| *Smoker* | Do you smoke? How many cigarettes do you smoke per day? |
| *Alcohol* | Do you drink alcohol? How much do you drink and how often? |
| *Recreational drugs* | Have you ever used any recreational drugs? (LSD, cocaine, amphetamines, ketamine) For each enquire about the quantity, frequency, pattern of use and how they take it |

---

### Diagnosing Schizophrenia

Schneider's first rank symptoms used to diagnosed schizophrenia include:

- Auditory hallucination (3rd person, running commentary, echo de la pense)
- Thought disorder (insertion, withdrawal, broadcasting)
- Delusions of perception   • Delusions of control   • Somatic hallucinations

---

## IDEA, CONCERNS, EXPECTATIONS

| | |
|---|---|
| *Idea* | Do you have any idea about what may be causing your symptoms? |
| *Concerns* | Are you worried about some of the thoughts you are having? |
| *Expectations* | Do you think I can help you? How? |
| *Insight* | Do you believe you are unwell? |

## CSA TIPS

Patient suffering with psychosis usually lack insight and are unable to recognise they are unwell. When assessing the patient's symptoms it is important to challenge their perception to test for insight. If this is not done in a non-judgemental way they may get angry and disengage in the consultation particularly if they think you consider that they are mentally unwell. You should practice how you would explain to a patient that they need to see a psychiatrist without causing undue angst or anxiety in the patient.

## PHYSICAL EXAMINATION

| | |
|---|---|
| *Vitals* | BMI, weight, BP |

## INVESTIGATIONS

| | |
|---|---|
| *Bloods* | FBC, Fasting glucose, lipid profile, LFT |
| *Specialist* | |
| MRI scan, EEG | Exclude organic psychosis i.e. temporal lobe epilepsy |
| Urine drug screen | Exclude drug induced psychosis i.e. LSD, amphetamines |

## MANAGEMENT

### Conservative

*Lifestyle*

| | |
|---|---|
| Smoking | Offer cessation advice. Consider NRT (bupropion or varenicline increase risk of neuropsychiatric symptoms) |
| Alcohol | Advise to cut down alcohol intake |
| Exercise | Give exercise advice. Refer to healthy eating or physical exercise programme (obesity SE of medication) |
| Co-morbidities | Offer interventions for abnormal glucose and cholesterol levels (higher incidence of diabetes and CVD) |
| Diet | Advise to eat well and regularly |

| | |
|---|---|
| *Work* | Offer supported employment programmes if wishes to return to work |

*Talking therapies*

| | |
|---|---|
| CBT | Consider cognitive behavioural therapy for all patients |
| Family intervent. | Offered to families with members suffering from schizophrenia who live with them |
| Art therapies | Offered to patients with negative symptoms |

### Medical

| | |
|---|---|
| *Antipsychotics* | Do not initiate medication unless you have experience in doing so |
| | 2nd generation drugs (e.g. amisulpride, clozapine, olanzapine, quetiapine, risperidone, aripiprazole) are better treating negative symptoms |
| Side effects | Antimuscarinic (dry mouth, blurred vision, urinary retention, constipation), drowsiness, weight gain, sexual dysfunction |
| Extrapyr. | Parkinsonism (tremor), dystonia (torticollis, oculogyric crisis), akathisia (severe restlessness), tardive dyskinesia (e.g. rhythmic involuntary movement e.g. chewing and pouting of jaw) |
| Blood tests | FBC, U&E, LFT measured at start of therapy then yrly. Request prolactin (hyperprolactinaema) |
| ECG | Before initiating perform ECG if PMH of CVD |
| BP | Check at initiating and upon dose titration |

| | |
|---|---|
| *Depot* | Consider if patients prefer after acute episodes or patients attempts covertly to avoid adherence to medication which is clinically essential |

**Referral**

| | |
|---|---|
| *Early referral* | Refer urgently to community team if first presentation of psychotic symptoms |
| *Re-Referral* | Re-refer if poor response to treatment, poor compliance, intolerable SE, substance misuse, or risk to self or others. |

**SAFETY NETTING**

| | |
|---|---|
| *Suicide risk* | Contact Crisis Resolution & Home Treatment team for urgent assessment |
| Sectioning | Try persuading voluntarily, if not compliant consider compulsory admission (if risk to self, or to others) |
| Safeguarding | Follow local safeguarding pathways for child protection or vulnerable adults |
| *Follow up* | Offer a series of appointments in primary care, with short gaps in more serious cases |

**DIFFERENTIAL DIAGNOSIS**

| Condition | Characteristic exam feature |
|---|---|
| **Schizophrenia** | Schneider's 1st rank symptoms (auditory hallucination, Thought disorder, delusions of perception & control). Negative symptoms include asocial behaviour, lack of motivation, poor concentration, lack of self care |
| **Depression** | Low mood and effect with cognitive and biological symptoms, delusions (worthless), hallucinations (derogatory auditory) |
| **Puerperal Psychosis** | Onset 2-4d after delivery, clouding of consciousness, delusions (paranoid), hallucinations associated with affect (depressed/hypomania). Risk of infanticide |
| **Bipolar** | Contrasting emotional states (depression/mania). In elevation phase patient is overactive, irritable, distracted, disinhibited, suffers from insomnia, has flights of idea or pressure of speech. Can also have grandiose ideas |
| **PTSD** | Exposure to traumatic life event. Flashbacks & nightmares, avoidance behaviour and numbing, hypervigilance state |

**EXPLANATIONS**

| | |
|---|---|
| *Schizophrenia* | Schizophrenia is a mental illness that can cause people to have disorganised thoughts, beliefs and experiences. It can cause people to lose touch with reality making it hard for them to tell the difference between real thoughts from false ones. |
| Treatment | Antipsychotics are often used to treat schizophrenia. They works by affecting the balance of brain chemicals (neurotransmitters). |

# 15.4 Suicidal ideation

Patients suffering from mental health illnesses are at an increased risk of self harming and attempting suicide. In the UK it is believed that over 4000 people die from suicide every year with many more self-harming and attempting suicide. It is important to screen for suicidal ideation in all patients who present with low mood, anxiety, schizophrenia or self-harm as evidence shows that almost 50% of patients who go on to die from suicide have visited their primary care physician within a month of their death; and of those who have attempted suicide over 90% have had suicidal thoughts or ideation in the past year.

---

**Risk Factors for Suicide** - *Ref: Self-harm, suicide & risk: helping people who self-harm, RCPsych College 2010*

| | |
|---|---|
| *Gender* | Men are 3x than more likely than Female |
| *Age* | >40 yrs |
| *Depression* | 70% of suicides suffered from a form of depression |
| *Previous attempt* | 30-40x increased risk of death in those who have attempted before |
| *Alcohol abuse* | Alcoholics have a lifetime risk of suicide of 3-4% |
| *Loss rational thinking* | Schizophrenics have a 10% lifetime risk of suicide |
| *Loss of support* | Divorcees or widowed women |
| *Organised plan* | Patients who have planned their suicide or left a note or will |
| *Unemployed* | Low socioeconomic status 2-3x increased risk |
| *Chronic illness* | Patients with chronic diseases (MS, epilepsy, pain, disability & cancer) |
| *Professions* | Doctors, veterans |

---

## HISTORY

Approach the topic sensitively in a non-threatening, non-judgemental manner. It can be quite difficult to broach the subject initially, so begin by making your first few questions designed to put the patient at ease.

| | |
|---|---|
| **Open questions** | Can you tell me more about what happened? |
| *Cues* | If the patient appears withdrawn, displaying little eye contact, reflect this non-verbal cue to them by saying; You look upset? Is anything bothering you? |
| *Confidentiality* | Reassure that everything they say will is in confidence unless others are at risk |

### Focused questions

*Pre-Attempt*

| | |
|---|---|
| Trigger | Did anything trigger or make you try and take your life? (bereavement, significant life event) |
| Mood | How was your mood at the time? |
| Premeditated | Did you plan it or was it spontaneous? |
| Inform | Did you tell anyone that you wanted to harm / take your own life? |
| Precautions | Did you make sure no one was around when you tried to end it? |
| Note | Did you write a final will or note? Or close your bank accounts? |

*Attempt*

| | |
|---|---|
| When | When did you try and take your life? Where were you at the time? |
| Method | How did you try and end it all? Did you use a weapon? Or take an overdose? Did you try and jump from a height or hang yourself? |

| | |
|---|---|
| Overdose | Do you remember what medications you took? Did you mix different medicines? Do you know how many of each tablets you took? |
| Intention | Did you think the amount of tablets you took would be enough to end your life? |
| Alcohol / drugs | Before you tried it, did you drink a lot of alcohol or use recreational drugs? |
| Found | How were you found? Did anyone help you? Did you go and seek help? |

*Post-Attempt*

| | |
|---|---|
| Thoughts | How do you feel now that you are still alive? Are you happy that you are with us? Or are you angry that you were not successful? |
| Intent | Did you really want to die? Was it more of a cry for help? |
| Ideation | Do you still have any thoughts or desire not to be alive? |

**RED FLAGS**    On going suicidal ideation, meticulous planning, violent method. Risk to others

**PAST HISTORY**

| | |
|---|---|
| *Psychiatric* | Have you ever had these symptoms before? Have you ever been treated for depression, anxiety or psychosis? Have you ever been admitted to a mental health ward? Have you been diagnosed with a personality disorder or anorexia? |
| *Self-Harm* | Have you ever tried to commit suicide in the past or self-harmed before? |
| *Medical* | Do you have any medical conditions? Do you suffer with any chronic conditions like CVA, DM, HIV, IHD, MS, epilepsy, chronic pain? |

**FAMILY HISTORY**

| | |
|---|---|
| *Psychiatric* | Does anyone in your family suffer from depression or any other mental illnesses? Has anyone attempted suicide in your close family (first-degree relatives)? |

**DRUG HISTORY**

| | |
|---|---|
| *Medication* | Are you taking any medications? (SSRI, champix, sibutramine, amitriptyline) |

**SOCIAL HISTORY**

| | |
|---|---|
| *Relationships* | Are you currently in a relationship? How are things? Do you have any children? |
| *Support network* | Who lives with you at home? Do you have any close friends or family? |
| *Occupation* | Are you currently working or studying at the moment? Do you have any financial worries? Did you recently lose your job? |
| *Abuse* | Has there been a history of abuse? (physical, sexual or emotional) |
| *Smoker* | Do you smoke? How many cigarettes do you smoke per day? |
| *Alcohol* | Do you drink alcohol? How much do you drink and how often? |
| *Recreational drugs* | Have you ever used any recreational drugs? |

---

**Protective factors in Suicide**

There are factors that may decrease the risk for a patient to commit suicide some of these include having strong social support, being a religious person, having children in the home or being pregnant, access to clinical interventions for mental and substance disorders

---

**IDEA, CONCERNS, EXPECTATIONS**

| | |
|---|---|
| *Expectations* | Were you hoping for anything in particular from me today? (sick note, referral, support group, emotional support) |
| *Impact on life* | How has it affected your life? (job, relationships) |

## CSA TIPS

Assessing suicidal risk is a key skill that doctors need to be able to perform in a non-judgemental way. Patients may attend with common mental health problems but actually be harbouring suicidal ideations. In such situations it would be key for you to pick up on the cues and assess their suicidal risk. If you are unable to establish rapport, or make the patient feel at ease, they may not be so forthcoming as to the real reason for their attendance and the consultation may not be resolved in the ensuing time.

## PHYSICAL EXAMINATION

| | |
|---|---|
| *Vitals* | BMI, BP, Pulse |
| *Injuries* | Assess and document any physical injuries |
| *Risk Assessment* | Is the patient at low, medium or high risk to themselves or to others? |

## INVESTIGATIONS *Not routinely indicated in primary care*

| | |
|---|---|
| *Bloods* | FBC, ESR, glucose, U&Es, LFTs, TFT, calcium, paracetamol & salicylate levels |
| *Urine* | For common recreational drugs (opiates, BDZs, barbiturates, amphetamine, methadone) |
| *ECG* | Looking for co-morbidities or cardiac arrhythmias post OD |

## MANAGEMENT

| | |
|---|---|
| **Emergency** | In the case of acute injuries (glue, stitches), overdose it is important to stabilise the patient and call 999 to take to A&E |

### Prevention

| | |
|---|---|
| *Medication review* | Offer regular medication reviews. Drugs such as aspirin, paracetamol, codeine, BDZs, sleeping tablets and amitriptyline are rationalised |
| *Weekly scripts* | Consider giving weekly scripts for patients at higher risk of suicide |
| *Carer* | Advise having a carer or relative administer the medications from a locked cupboard or directly observed therapy (DOT) |

### Conservative

*Lifestyle*

| | |
|---|---|
| Alcohol | Cut down alcohol. Refer to local detox programmes or alcohol advisors |
| Drugs | Stop any recreational drugs e.g. cannabis and refer to drugs advisor. Consider dual diagnosis teams if concurrent mental health illness |

| | |
|---|---|
| *Benefits / Job* | Consider fit-note if unable to work. Refer to benefits advisor, social services or job centre if needs advice around housing and employment |
| *Carers* | Refer to social services for a care package if unable to cope (disability) |

### Conditions

| | |
|---|---|
| *Depression* | If patient depressed then treat via self help, CBT or SSRIs |
| *Bereavement* | If recent death, treat via CBT or SSRIs. Refer to bereavement counsellor |
| *Chronic Disease* | Tighter control, refer to appropriate secondary care specialist, rationalise pain treatment or refer to pain teams |

### Suicide

| | |
|---|---|
| *Low Risk* | Consider telephone assessments or frequent follow up in primary care. Refer to local psychotherapy services for treatment of any anxiety or depression. Consider referral |

| | to local PCMHT services. Give telephone no for Samaritans, 24hr emergency psychiatric services |
|---|---|
| *High Risk* | Refer to Crisis Resolution & Home Treatment team for urgent assessment. Refer for CPN or mental health key-worker |
| Sectioning | Try persuading voluntarily, if not compliant consider compulsory admission (if risk to self, or to others) |
| Safeguarding | Follow local safeguarding pathways for child protection or vulnerable adults |

---

## Mental Health Act 2007

Patients can be compulsorily admitted to hospital if they have a mental disorder that warrants treatment at hospital and it is in the interest of their health & safety or others

| | |
|---|---|
| *Section 2* | Admitted for 28d for assessment. Application from an AMHP (approved mental health professional) or relative, supported by 2 Drs, one who is approved by section 12 (psychiatrist) |
| *Section 3* | Admitted for 6mth for treatments. Application as above. Must be assessed on Section 2 first |
| *Section 4* | Admitted for 72hrs (emergencies only if delay to get section 2). Require an application from AMHP and a doctor (GP). Permits emergency assessment |
| *Section 135* | Court permits forced entry into a house for a person believed to suffer from mental disorder |
| *Section 136* | Transfer patient from public place to safety by the police. Permits examination by a Dr and AMHP |

---

## SAFETY NETTING

| | |
|---|---|
| *Follow up* | Offer a series of appointments in primary care, with short gaps in more serious cases. Give emergency details to patient (i.e. crisis team) if they feel the need to self harm again. |

## EXPLANATIONS

| | |
|---|---|
| *Self harm* | Self harm is when someone hurt themselves in order to deal with or forget about a difficult experience or emotions that causes them pain. Some hurt themselves physically by cutting themselves, burning their skin, overdosing or hitting the wall. However, whilst it may make you feel better for a short time it does not often cure the problem and sometimes make you feel worse. |

# *15.5 Anxiety disorder*

Anxiety disorders refer to the mental health disorders that lead to patients suffering from symptoms including fear, anxiety, restlessness, irritability and may lead to physical symptoms including palpitations, sweating and tremor. There are a number of different conditions that come underneath the anxiety umbrella including PTSD, social anxiety, generalised anxiety disorders, panic and phobias. Although a specific trigger may be present it is not always necessary for the diagnosis to be made.

## HISTORY
Approach the topic sensitively in a non-threatening, non-judgemental manner. It can be quite difficult to broach the subject initially, so begin by making your first few questions designed to put the patient at ease.

| | |
|---|---|
| **Open questions** | Can you tell me more about the symptoms you have been experiencing? |
| | Could you tell me about what has been troubling you? |
| *Cues* | If the patient appears withdrawn, displaying little eye contact, reflect this non-verbal cue to them by saying; You look upset? Is anything bothering you? |

**Focused questions**

| | |
|---|---|
| *Anxiety* | When did you first start feeling like this? How long has it been going on for? Is it always there (continuous) or does it come come and go (episodic)? |
| Triggers | Have you noticed anything that brings it on? (panic disorder, phobia) |
| Avoidance | Do you ever avoid certain situations due to fear or anxiety? |
| Palpitations | Have you felt that your heart thumping rapidly in your chest? |
| SOB | Do you get short of breath when it occurs? |
| Sleep | Does it affect your sleep? |
| Other | Do you ever experience at the same time hot flushes, sweats, dizzy spells, pins and needles, tiredness, muscle aches or have a sense of impending doom? |

**Associated Questions**

| | |
|---|---|
| *Depression* | Have you been feeling low recently? Do you feel disinterested in life or worthless inside? How is your eating habit? |
| *Suicide* | Have you ever felt so low that you wanted to end it all? |

**Differentials**

| | |
|---|---|
| *GAD* | Do you feel anxious or worried everyday without reason? Do you find it hard to concentrate? Do you feel restless or irritable all the time? |
| *Panic disorder* | Do you suffer from unexpected panic attacks often for no reason? Do they last for a few seconds or minutes? Do you get palpitations? |
| *Phobia* | Do you feel anxious when faced with a specific situation (heights, open spaces, flying)? Do you try and avoid it (public speaking, meeting people)? Do you get similar symptoms when encountering animals (snakes, spiders)? |
| *PTSD* | Have you experienced a traumatic event in the past? Do you suffer from nightmares or flashbacks? Do you constantly feel on edge? See PTSD chapter |
| *OCD* | Are you overwhelmed with unpleasant ideas that occur repeatedly? Do you feel as if you must complete them? Do you feel some relief if you do? See OCD chapter |
| *Hyperthyroidism* | Have you noticed that you cannot tolerate warm weather? Have you had any recent weight loss, increased appetite or tremor of your hands? |

| **RED FLAGS** | Risk to self or others |
|---|---|

**PAST HISTORY**

| *Psychiatric* | Have you ever had these symptoms before? Have you ever been treated for depression, anxiety or panic attacks? |
|---|---|
| *Medical* | Do you have any medical conditions such as an overactive thyroid? |

**FAMILY HISTORY**

| *Psychiatric* | Does anyone in your family suffer from mental illnesses? Has anyone close like your parents or siblings been previously diagnosed with anxiety disorder or panic attacks? |
|---|---|

**DRUG HISTORY**

| *Medication* | Are you taking any medications (salbutamol, ritalin, thyroxine)? Have you ever taken diazepam? |
|---|---|

**SOCIAL HISTORY**

| *Occupation* | Are you currently working at the moment? Do you have any stress at work? Do you have any financial worries (loss of job, mortgages, debt)? |
|---|---|
| *Smoker* | Do you smoke? How many cigarettes do you smoke per day? |
| *Alcohol* | Do you drink alcohol? How much do you drink and how often? |
| *Diet* | Do you drink tea or coffee? Do you use energy drinks or cola? |
| *Recreational drugs* | Have you ever used any recreational drugs? (crack, amphetamines) |
| *Relationships* | Are you currently in a relationship? How are things? |
| *Support network* | Who lives with you at home? Do you have any close friends or family? |

**IDEA, CONCERNS, EXPECTATIONS**

| *Idea* | Do you have any idea about what may be causing your symptoms? |
|---|---|
| *Concerns* | Do you have any worries about it? |
| *Expectations* | How were you hoping I could help you? |
| *Impact* | How have your symptoms affected your life? |

**CSA TIPS**

Anxiety disorder is an extremely common problem with women mainly suffering from the condition. Patients may simply attend requesting general advice about minimal symptoms they are experiencing and may simply require lifestyle interventions. However, anxiety can be extremely debilitating and in other cases you may be faced with a patient who is fearful of going outside or mixing with people due to a severe social anxiety disorder.

**PHYSICAL EXAMINATION**

| *Vitals* | BMI, BP, pulse |
|---|---|
| *Examination* | Perform cardiac or thyroid examination if indicated |
| *Questionnaire* | |
| HAD | Hospital Anxiety and Depression scale consists of 7 questions for each condition and is categorised as normal, mild, moderate and severe depending on responses |
| GAD-7 | Generalised Anxiety Disorder Questionnaire has 7 questions to be completed with each being scored out of three depending on severity. Answers are categorised as minimal (0-4), mild (5-9), moderate (10-14) and severe (15-21) depending on responses |

## INVESTIGATIONS

| | |
|---|---|
| *Bloods* | *Not routinely required.* FBC, ferritin, B12 & folate (deficiencies), TFT |
| *ECGs* | Consider with chest pain or palpitations to exclude arrhythmia |

## MANAGEMENT
### Conservative
*Lifestyle*

| | |
|---|---|
| Reassure | Explain condition to patient and attempt to reassure by informing them their symptoms are not due to a physical illness rather anxiety related |
| Exercise | Regular exercise such as jogging, swimming, cycling helps reduce stress and release tension. Recommended to do 2.5hrs weekly |
| Relaxation tech. | Recommend relaxation techniques e.g. deep breathing exercises, yoga |
| Diet | Avoid caffeine |
| Alcohol | Advise to stop or cut down alcohol to safe limits (14u or 21u/wk) |
| Drugs | Stop any recreational drugs e.g. cannabis. |

*Self Help*

| | |
|---|---|
| Material | Offer books, CDs or leaflets on understanding anxiety and managing it (overcoming series) |
| Group therapy | Suggest to join group therapy |
| Online | Try online resources (FearFighter, Anxiety UK, Mind) |

*Talking therapies*

| | |
|---|---|
| CBT | Consider referral for cognitive behavioural therapy (individual or group) |
| CCBT | Refer to computered or web-based CBT supported by practitioner |
| ERP | Exposure and Response Prevention is a type of CBT used to confront repetitive thoughts and to reduce compulsive behaviour. Consider in OCD |
| Group therapy | Recommend psychoeducational group-based therapy that encourages observational learning. 12 patients per therapist |
| Applied relaxation | CBT trained practitioner offers training on series of relaxation techniques (muscle, cue controlled) applied in situations that trigger anxiety. Consider in GAD |
| Desensitisation | Systematic desensitisation is useful to treat phobias. Exposes to phobia until anxiety settles |
| Hypnotherapy | Little evidence around effectiveness. Some suggest helps in social disorders & phobias |

### Medical

| | |
|---|---|
| *Antidepressants* | Initiate an SSRI Advise patients it may take 2-4wk before they feel any improvement. Can experience worsening of anxiety in first 2-4 wks as medication is started. If no improvement >2mth consider increasing dose or changing to alternative SSRI or SNRI (venlafaxine). |
| GAD | Sertraline is first line, alternative SSRI include escitalopram or paroxetine. If not tolerated consider SNRI or pregabalin (third line) |
| *Benzodiazepines* | Diazepam can be consider for short term (2-4wks) in severe anxiety and irritability. Warn patient about risk of drug tolerance and dependency |
| *Beta Blockers* | Propranolol useful in reducing the physical symptoms (sweating, palpitations) |
| *Insomnia* | Advise on sleep hygiene. Consider short course of hypnotics or sedative antidepressants (mirtazapine) |
| *Referral* | Consider if symptoms persist for >4wks refer to psychiatrist |

## SAFETY NETTING

| | |
|---|---|
| *Suicide risk* | Review the patient frequently in primary care. Consider contacting Crisis Resolution & Home Treatment team for urgent assessment. Give Samaritans number for emergency |
| Sectioning | Try persuading voluntarily, if not consider compulsory admission (if risk to self, or to others) |
| Safeguarding | Follow local safeguarding pathways for child protection or vulnerable adults |
| *Follow up* | Offer a series of appointments in primary care, with short gaps in more serious cases |

## DIFFERENTIAL DIAGNOSIS

| Condition | Characteristic exam feature |
|---|---|
| **Generalised Anxiety Disorder** | Generalised anxiety that impacts of day to day activities on most days. Symptoms include tension, restlessness, fatigability, insomnia. Present for 6mths for diagnosis to be made |
| **PTSD** | Exposure to traumatic event (e.g. rape, natural disaster), flashbacks (vivid), nightmares, avoidance behaviour, emotional numbing, hyperarousal |
| **Acute Stress Reaction** | Acute symptoms of anxiety, low mood, irritability, poor sleep from a stressful event. Lasts minutes to hours. Physical symptoms include palpitations, headaches, SOB and nausea |
| **Adjustment Disorder** | Due to a change in a person's life or after a major life event (moving house/divorce). Symptoms similar to acute stress reaction or depression. Resolves once stressor removed |
| **Panic Disorder** | Unpredictable, recurrent, panic attacks with severe anxiety, palpitations, tremor, SOB, chest pain or paresthesia. Often lasts 5-10 minutes but can last for few hours |
| **Obsessive-compulsive disorder (OCD)** | Recurrent obsessions (unpleasant ideas, urges) and compulsions (desire to complete). Experiences anxiety if attempts to resist and temporary relief if does e.g. cleaning, counting, hoarding |
| **Phobia** | Specific anxiety or fear to a particular thing (animals, travel) or situation (social anxiety disorder, agoraphobia). Results in avoidance behaviour with impact on daily function |

## EXPLANATIONS

| | |
|---|---|
| *Anxiety* | Anxiety is something all people will experience from time to time. Most people feel tense when sitting an exam or attending a job interview and this is quite normal. However, an anxiety disorder is when these symptoms continue and become overwhelming such that they begin to interfere with your day to day activities. |
| *Panic disorder* | Panic disorder is where patients experience repeated, often unpredictable, panic attacks. You can have, without warning and suddenly, palpitations, hot flushes, chest pains and tremors. This can happen when the brain gets over-excited and sends |

several nervous impulse to the rest of the body which can lead to the release of a hormone called adrenaline. Whilst this is normal reaction when someone is in danger, in panic attacks the body unfortunately produces the same response for situations that are not dangerous or life threatening.

*Phobia*

A phobia is a type of anxiety disorder that is caused by a persistent and enduring fear about an object or situation such that the sufferer goes to great lengths to avoid. The symptoms may be debilitating and may interfere with your life such that you are fearful even to go out.

*OCD*

OCD, or obsessive-compulsive disorder, is a condition where a patient experiences quite unpleasant thoughts (obsessions) that repeatedly enter into their mind that make them feel really anxious e.g. feeling dirty, worried about unlocked doors, needing to organise things. They often are overwhelmed with a compulsive desire to do things that can help deal with their obsession and relieve their anxiety e.g. wash hands, lock doors, counting. However, whilst they may feel better for a few moments their symptoms come back repeatedly.

# 15.6  Post traumatic stress disorder (PTSD)

Post traumatic stress disorder is a mental health condition that develops following a person being exposed to an extremely stressful, distressing or frightening event. Common events that may induce PTSD include rape, robbery, military combat, severe natural disasters and serious road traffic incidents. Sufferers usually present with recurrent memories, severe anxiety and flashbacks whereby the patient may relive the event. It is thought that 1 in 3 people develop the symptoms of PTSD following an adverse event, however, the symptoms may not necessarily start immediately following it, rather in most patients symptoms develop many months afterwards.

## HISTORY
Approach the topic sensitively in a non-threatening, non-judgemental manner. It can be quite difficult to broach the subject initially, so begin by making your first few questions designed to put the patient at ease.

| | |
|---|---|
| **Open questions** | Can you tell me more about the symptoms you have been experiencing? How long have they been going on for? |
| *Cues* | If the patient appears appear withdrawn, displaying little eye contact, reflect this non-verbal cue to them by saying; You look upset? Is anything bothering you? |
| *Screening* | In asylum seekers / refugees or any patients 1 month post severe disaster, patients should be asked about PTSD symptoms |

**Focused questions**

| | |
|---|---|
| *Traumatic event* | Have you ever experienced a major traumatic event? (abuse, torture, military combat, natural disaster, serious RTA) |
| *Re-experiencing* | |
|   Flashbacks | Do you get repeated distressing memories or emotions of the event? Do you have a sense that you are reliving it as if the event was happening again? |
|   Nightmare | Do you see the events in your dreams as nightmares? |
| *Avoidance* | Do you tend to avoid people or situations that remind you of the event? |
| *Emotional Numbing* | Do you feel that you struggle to experience feelings or feel detached? |
| *Hyperarousal* | Do you find yourself get very irritable often for no reason? Do you feel that you are alway on edge? (hypervigilance) |

**Associated Questions**

| | |
|---|---|
| *Anxiety* | Have you been recently been feeling anxious? |
| *Depression* | Have you been feeling low recently? Do you feel disinterested in life or worthless inside? How is your sleep or eating habits? |
| *Suicide* | Have you ever felt so low that you wanted to end it all? |

**Differentials**

| | |
|---|---|
| *GAD* | Do you feel anxious or worried everyday without reason? |
| *Panic disorder* | Do you suffer from panic attacks often for no reason? |

| | |
|---|---|
| **RED FLAGS** | Suicidal ideation, delusions or hallucinations, risk to others |

## PAST HISTORY

*Psychiatric*       Have you ever had these symptoms before? Have you ever been treated for depression, anxiety or panic attacks?

*Medical*           Do you have any medical conditions such as a thyroid disorder? Do you suffer with any chronic debilitating conditions like cancer, HIV?

## FAMILY HISTORY

*Psychiatric*       Does anyone in your family suffer from mental illnesses?

## DRUG HISTORY

*Medication*        Are you taking any medications (salbutamol, ritalin, thyroxine)? Have you taken any L-dopa, beta-blockers or donepezil (nightmares)?

## SOCIAL HISTORY

*Occupation*        Are you currently working at the moment? (military, emergency services - e.g. firefighters, ambulance drivers)

*Smoker*            Do you smoke? How many cigarettes do you smoke per day?

*Alcohol*           Do you drink alcohol? How much do you drink and how often?

*Recreational drugs* Have you ever used any recreational drugs? (crack, amphetamines)

*Relationships*     Are you currently in a relationship? How are things? Do you have any children?

*Support network*   Who lives with you at home? Do you have any close friends or family?

## IDEA, CONCERNS, EXPECTATIONS

*Idea*              Do you have any idea about what may be causing your symptoms?

*Concerns*          Do you have any worries about it?

*Expectations*      How were you hoping I could help you?

*Impact*            How have your symptoms affected your life?

## CSA TIPS

Patients suffering with symptoms of PTSD may not necessarily be aware that they are due to a previous adverse incident that took place in their life. Consequently, patients may only be attending to see you complaining of insomnia or nightmares many months after the event. It is also important to screen for symptoms in patients who are asylum seekers or refugees as they are highly likely to have either seen or experienced violence and emotional turmoil.

## PHYSICAL EXAMINATION

*Vitals*            BMI

*Questionnaire*

   TSQ        Offer Trauma Screening-Questionnaire (TSQ). Consists of 10 questions given >1mth after exposed to trauma. Asks which symptoms they have experienced >1 in past week. >5 consider intervention

## MANAGEMENT

### Conservative

*Lifestyle*

   Alcohol    Known risk factor. Advise to stop or refer to alcohol programme

   Drugs      Stop any recreational drugs e.g. cannabis

   Sleep      Relax in a dark room with minimal distraction. Go to sleep at the same time every night and have a light snack

| Watchful waiting | Consider in mild symptoms <4wks to monitor if resolve without treatment |
|---|---|

**Self Help**

| Material | Offer books or leaflets on understanding PTSD and how to manage it |
|---|---|
| Group therapy | Suggest to join group therapy (combat stress, rape crisis, victim support, CRUSE). Consider signposting members of family to support group |
| Online | Try online resources (UK psychological trauma society, veterans UK, Anxiety UK) |

**Talking therapies**

| CBT | Consider trauma focused cognitive behavioural therapy (8-12 sessions) |
|---|---|
| EMDR | Consider referring for eye movement desensitisation and reprocessing |

**Medical**

| Antidepressants | Consider medications with such as paroxetine or mirtazapine if patient declines referral to specialist services. Remain on medication SSRI for 6mths and upto 12-15mths if severe or chronic PTSD. If responds well titrate down dose after 1yr |
|---|---|
| Anxiety | Diazepam can be consider for short time to improve anxiety and irritability. Propranolol may be helpful in panic attack like symptoms |
| Insomnia | Consider short course of hypnotics or sedative antidepressants (mirtazapine) |
| Referral | Consider if symptoms persist for >4wks refer to PTSD clinic |

**SAFETY NETTING**

| Suicide risk | Review the patient frequently in primary care. Consider contacting Crisis Resolution & Home Treatment team for urgent assessment |
|---|---|
| Sectioning | Try persuading voluntarily, if not, consider compulsory admission (if risk to self, or to others) |
| Safeguarding | Follow local safeguarding pathways for child protection or vulnerable adults |
| Follow up | Offer a series of appointments in primary care, with short gaps in more serious cases |

**DIFFERENTIAL DIAGNOSIS**

| Condition | Characteristic exam feature |
|---|---|
| **PTSD** | Exposure to traumatic event (e.g. rape, natural disaster), flashbacks (vivid), nightmares, avoidance behaviour, emotional numbing, hyperarousal. Risk factors include occupation (firefighters, army - prisoners of war), rape victims, RTAs, refugees |
| **Depression** | Low mood and effect with cognitive and biological symptoms, delusions (worthless), hallucinations (derogatory auditory) |
| **Abnormal Bereavement Reaction** | Abnormal reaction to a bereavement (>2mths). Feelings of guilt, preoccupation of worthlessness with psychomotor retardation. Can have thoughts of death. May have dreams about partner |
| **Acute Stress Reaction** | Acute symptoms of anxiety, low mood, irritability, flashbacks and avoidance. Physical symptoms like palpitations, headaches, shortness of breath and nausea may be present. Starts suddenly almost immediately after a stressful event and usually does |

| | not last more than a few months |
|---|---|
| **Adjustment Disorder** | Due to a change in a person's life or after a major life event. Symptoms include anhedonia, hopelessness, anxiety and crying. The condition usually resolves once the stressor is removed |
| **Generalised Anxiety Disorder** | Increased generalised anxiety that impacts of day to day activities. Symptoms include tension, restlessness, fatigability, insomnia and must be present for 6 months for diagnosis to be made |

## EXPLANATIONS

*PTSD*

Post Traumatic Stress disorder is a condition that some people develop after being exposed to significant amounts of stress from a very traumatic event such as a serious road traffic accident, natural disaster or due to military combat.

*Trauma focused CBT*

Trauma focused cognitive behaviour therapy is a type of psychological treatment where a trained therapist may challenge your traumatic memories and make you confront them. They will then help empower you to cope and gain control over the distress and anxiety that has arisen from it. They will help change the way the brain negatively links the traumatic experience to the fear that you feel or guilt that you are some how to blame for what happened.

*EMDR*

Eye movement desensitisation and reprocessing has been shown to work well in treating PTSD. It works by following the therapist's finger whilst they ask you to recall aspects of the traumatic event. It is unclear how it works but it appears to desensitise the brain's abnormal thought patterns about the event.

*SSRI*

Whilst SSRI have commonly been used to treat depression, they have been found to help patients with PTSD by altering the balance of the chemical messenger or brain hormone called serotonin. SSRIs work to stop the breakdown of this hormone and hence increases its levels.

# 15.7 Obsessional-Compulsive Disorder (OCD)

OCD is an anxiety disorder that is characterised by repetitive, unpleasant, intrusive thoughts that create feelings of fear, and unease in the sufferer that are subsided by undertaking repetitive behaviours. Sufferers usually recognise actions as being excessive or irrational, but are compelled to repeat them to reduce anxiety levels. They often recognises that the thoughts originate from themselves and not someone else. Common symptoms include excessive hand washing, repeated checking whether doors are locked, being obsessively meticulous, making sure that everything is in a specific order.

## HISTORY

Approach the topic sensitively in a non-threatening, non-judgemental manner. It can be quite difficult to broach the subject initially, so begin by making your first few questions designed to put the patient at ease.

| | |
|---|---|
| **Open questions** | Can you tell me more about the symptoms you have been experiencing? |
| | Could you tell me about what has been troubling you? |
| *Cues* | If the patient appears withdrawn, displaying little eye contact, reflect this non-verbal cue to them by saying; You look upset? Is anything bothering you? |

**Focused questions**

| | |
|---|---|
| *OCD* | When did you first start feeling like this? How long has it been going on for? (>2wks) |
| | Has anything made it worse or triggered off your symptoms? (life events, stressors) |

| | |
|---|---|
| *Obsessions* | Do you get unpleasant thoughts or ideas that enter into your mind? |
| Feel | How do these thoughts make you feel? (disgusted, anxious) |
| Repetitive | Do they happen all the time? |
| Intrusive | Do they enter your mind against your will? Are they your own thoughts? Do you think these thoughts are unreasonable? |
| Content | What thoughts do you get? (fear of dirt or germs, worried of unlocked door or fire left on, wanting perfection, hoarding) |
| Resist | What happens when you try and resist or ignore them? (anxiety) |

| | |
|---|---|
| *Compulsions* | |
| Type | Do you get a burning desire on compulsion to do things? What things do you do? |
| Cleaning | Do you find that you are always cleaning your hands or the house? Do your daily activities take a long time to finish? |
| Checking | Do you find that you have to have to keep checking things repeatedly such as the gas taps, light switched off, door locked? |
| Order | Do you feel that you have to have things in an exact order? |
| Hoarding | Do you find that you collect things that have little sentimental value to you? |
| Relief | What happens when you give into your compulsions? Do you get some relief? |

**Associated Questions**

| | |
|---|---|
| *Suicide* | Have you ever felt so low that you wanted to end it all? |

**Differentials**

| | |
|---|---|
| *Depression* | Have you been feeling low recently? Do you feel disinterested in life or worthless inside? How is your eating habit? |

| | |
|---|---|
| Schizophrenia | Have you seen or heard things that you cannot explain? Do you feel that someone may be out to harm you in anyway? Do you feel that someone can insert thoughts into your head? |

**RED FLAGS**   Risk to self or others

**PAST HISTORY**

| | |
|---|---|
| Psychiatric | Have you ever had these symptoms before? Have you ever been treated for depression, anxiety or panic attacks? |
| Medical | Do you have any medical conditions? |

**FAMILY HISTORY**

| | |
|---|---|
| Psychiatric | Does anyone in your family suffer from mental illnesses? Has anyone been diagnosed with anxiety disorder, panic attacks or OCD? |

**DRUG HISTORY**

| | |
|---|---|
| Medication | Are you taking any medications? (ritalin) |

**SOCIAL HISTORY**

| | |
|---|---|
| Occupation | Are you currently working at the moment? Does your symptoms make it hard or impossible to go to work? Has anyone commented about your behaviour? |
| Smoker | Do you smoke? How many cigarettes do you smoke per day? |
| Alcohol | Do you drink alcohol? How much do you drink and how often? |
| Recreational drugs | Have you ever used any recreational drugs? |
| Relationships | Are you currently in a relationship? Has it affected it? |
| Support network | Who lives with you at home? Have you spoken about it to your close friends or family? |

**IDEA, CONCERNS, EXPECTATIONS**

| | |
|---|---|
| Idea | Do you have any idea about why you are having these repetitive thoughts? |
| Concerns | Do you have any worries about it? |
| Expectations | How were you hoping I could help you? |
| Impact | How have your symptoms affected your life? |

**CSA TIPS**

OCD are characterised my intrusive thoughts and repetitive behaviours that can interfere with a sufferer's life causing them to lose their job or affect on their family situation. Most patients may delay presentation to the GPs due to embarrassment and present later on with more intrusive thoughts and ruminations. Although patients will realise their behaviours are irrational, they may not know how to control them and will attend to discuss the different management options available to them.

**PHYSICAL EXAMINATION**

| | |
|---|---|
| Vitals | BMI, BP, pulse |
| Examination | Perform cardiac or thyroid examination if indicated |
| Questionnaire | |
| OCI | Obsessive-Compulsive Inventory consists of 42 questions for a range of repetitive behaviours and thoughts that has distressed or bothered a patient over the past month. Each question is rated from 0 (never) to 4 (almost always) on a frequency score and similar 0-4 score for a distress scale. it is scored out of 168 with an OCI inventory of >40 suggesting OCD |

| Y-BOCS | Yale–Brown Obsessive-Compulsive Scale is an alternative tool consisting of 10 items, each question scored from 0-4 with a maximum score of 40 |
|---|---|

## INVESTIGATIONS
*Bloods*  Not routinely required

## MANAGEMENT
### Conservative
*Lifestyle*

| Reassure | Explain condition to patient and attempt to reassure by informing them their symptoms are not due to a physical illness rather anxiety related |
|---|---|

*Self Help*

| Material | Offer books, CD, leaflets on understanding OCD and managing it (Overcoming series) |
|---|---|
| Group therapy | Suggest to join group therapy |

*Talking therapies*

| CBT | Consider referral for cognitive behavioural therapy (individual or group) |
|---|---|
| CT | Cognitive therapy can be used in addition to ERP. Helpful for patients who suffer from obsessions but no compulsions. Can be individual or group |
| ERP | Exposure and Response Prevention is a type of CBT used to confront repetitive thoughts and to reduce compulsive behaviour |
| Hypnotherapy | Little good evidence around effectiveness. Some suggest short term help in OCD |

### Medical

| Antidepressants | Consider initiating an SSRI (citalopram). Advise it may take 12wk before they feel any improvement. Can experience worsening of anxiety in first 2-4wk as medication is started |
|---|---|
| TCA | If poor response to SSRI may consider clomipramine 25mg od increasing to 100-150mg od after 2wks. Continue treatment for 12mths |
| Baseline | Check BP and perform ECG if CVD |
| Side effects | Dry mouth, drowsiness, blurred vision, constipation, urinary retention |
| CI | Immediate after MI, arrhythmia (block) |
| Antipsychotics | In addition to SSRI to augment response |

| *Referral* | Consider if symptoms persist for >4wks refer to psychiatrist |
|---|---|
| National Service | Consider referral to the National Service for Refractory OCD for patients with severe refractory OCD that has failed response to 2 different SSRIs and CBT |
| Neurosurgery | Ablation neurosurgery only considered for the most severe end of the spectrum |

## SAFETY NETTING

| *Suicide risk* | Review the patient frequently in primary care. Consider contacting Crisis Resolution & Home Treatment team for urgent assessment. Give Samaritans number for emergency |
|---|---|
| Sectioning | Try persuading voluntarily, if not, consider compulsory admission (if risk to self, or to others) |
| Safeguarding | Follow local safeguarding pathways for child protection or vulnerable adults |
| *Follow up* | Offer a series of appointments in primary care, with short gaps in more serious cases |

# EXPLANATIONS

*OCD*  OCD, or obsessive-compulsive disorder, is a condition where a patient experiences quite unpleasant thoughts (obsessions) that repeatedly enters into their mind that makes them feel really anxious e.g. feeling dirty, worried about unlocked doors, needing to organise things. They often are overwhelmed with a compulsive desire to do things that can help deal with their obsession and relieve their anxiety e.g. wash hands, lock doors, counting. However, whilst they may feel better for a few moments their symptoms come back repeatedly.

*ERP*  This is a type of cognitive behaviour therapy known as exposure and response prevention. Essentially it is an exposure based treatment that works on your obsessions and tries to help you face them in a controlled way. It involves facing your fears or anxieties and prevents you from acting upon your impulsive behaviours. Initially you may feel quite anxious and distressed, but over time your body adapts the anxiety response gradually reduces and becomes more bearable. If done properly, around 75% of patients get some sort of relief from their OCD symptoms.

# *15.8 Alcoholism*

Alcohol dependency syndrome is a fairly common condition afflicting western societies. It is due to excessive consumption of alcohol such that one finds it difficult to cut down despite being at risk of significant mental or physical harm. It is thought that 9% of men and 4% of women suffer from alcohol dependency syndrome at some point in their lifetimes. Excessive alcohol consumption can cause a number of physical ailments including gastritis, hepatitis, cirrhosis, erectile dysfunction and pancreatitis, as well as mental problems such as depression, insomnia and anxiety.

Alcohol also causes numerous social problems including, relationship breakdown, loss of employment and criminality. The DoH recommends that men should drink no more than 3u daily (total 21u weekly) and females no more than 2u daily (14u a week) to minimise the harmful consequences.

## HISTORY
Approach the topic sensitively in a non-threatening, non-judgemental manner. It can be quite difficult to broach the subject initially, so begin by making your first few questions designed to put the patient at ease.

| | |
|---|---|
| **Open questions** | Can you tell me more about the symptoms you have been experiencing? Could you tell me about what has been troubling you? |
| *Cues* | If the patient appears embarrassed, displaying little eye contact, reflect this non-verbal cue to them by saying; You look upset? Is anything bothering you? |

**Focused questions**

| | |
|---|---|
| *Alcohol* | How long have you been drinking for? How much do you drink in a typical day? (convert to units per day) |
| Pattern | Can you describe a typical drinking day? |
| Types | What types of alcohol do you drink? (whisky, beer, wine) |
| Binge | Are there times where you drink more than you would normally? |
| Reason (ideas) | Is there any reason why you are drinking this much? |

**Units and measure of alcohol**

| | |
|---|---|
| *Beer* | Half pint (1u), half pint strong beer (2u). Large bottle or strong beer 440ml can (3units) |
| *Wine* | Small (125ml) glass (1.5unit), medium (175ml) glass (2units), large (250ml) glass (3units) Bottle (750ml) of wine (9units) |
| *Spirits* | Single short (25ml) of spirits (1 unit), bottle (750ml) of spirits (30 units) |

*CAGE questionnaire*

| | |
|---|---|
| Cut down | Have you tried to cut down how much alcohol you drink? |
| Angry | Have you felt angry if people comment on your drinking? |
| Guilty | Have you felt guilty about how much you drink? |
| Eye Opener | Do you ever drink first thing in the morning? |

*Dependence syndrome*

| | |
|---|---|
| Cravings | Do you have a strong desire to drink? |
| Primacy | Would you say alcohol was a priority over other aspects of your life? |
| Control | Do you have difficulty controlling how much you drink? |

| Tolerance | Are you drinking more alcohol to get the same effect? |
| Neglect | Do you find that you neglect other responsibilities because of your drinking? |
| Withdrawal | Do you experience any symptoms (tremors, shakes, nausea, fits, hallucinations) when you go without alcohol for a period of time? |
| Relieved | Are these symptoms relieved by drinking more alcohol? |

## Associated Questions

| *Neurology* | Have you ever lost consciousness, had dizzy spells or poor coordination? Do you suffer from any pin and needles in your limbs? |
| *Liver* | Have you noticed your skin or your eyes going yellow? Any abdominal pain? |
| *Depression* | Have you been feeling low recently? Do you feel disinterested in life or worthless? |
| *Self-harm/Suicide* | Have you ever harmed yourself to feel better inside? Have you ever felt so low that you wanted to end it all? |
| *Psychosis* | Have you ever felt insects crawling on your skin (formication) or seen things you could not explain? |
| *Injuries* | Have you sustained any injuries from your alcohol drinking? |

## RED FLAGS

Depression, Liver disease (jaundice), encephalopathy, neuropathy

## PAST HISTORY

| *Psychiatric* | Have you ever had these symptoms before? Have you ever been treated for depression, anxiety or panic attacks? |
| *Drinking* | Have you ever tried giving up or reducing your drinking in the past? Did you attend alcohol anonymous or any local groups? |
| *Medical* | Do you have any medical conditions? Have you ever suffered with peptic ulcer disease, pancreatitis, liver disease or raised BP? |

## FAMILY HISTORY

| *Psychiatric* | Does anyone in your family suffer from mental illnesses? Has anyone been diagnosed with alcohol or substance misuse? |

## DRUG HISTORY

| *Medication* | Are you taking any medications or OTC preparations? (warfarin, COCP, anti-epileptics) |

## SOCIAL HISTORY

| *Stress* | Is there anything in your life that has caused you much stress and anxiety? How was your childhood (abuse, neglect, parental alcoholism)? |
| *Occupation* | Are you working at the moment? (publican, sailor, manual labourer- roofer, painter, builder) |
| *Smoker* | Do you smoke? How many cigarettes do you smoke per day? |
| *Drive* | Do you drive a vehicle? |
| *Recreational drugs* | Have you ever used any recreational drugs? |
| *Relationships* | Are you currently in a relationship? Does your partner drink? Has it affected it? |
| *Children* | Do you have any children? Did you ever have a social worker? |
| *Criminality* | Have you ever had a brush with the law because of your drinking? |

## IDEA, CONCERNS, EXPECTATIONS

| *Idea* | Do you think the levels of alcohol you are drinking is damaging for you? |
| *Concerns* | Do you have any worries about how much you are drinking? |

| Expectations | How did you want me to help you? |
|---|---|
| Impact | How has your drinking affected your life? |

## CSA TIPS

In the examination it is unlikely that you will be faced with a patient suffering with acute alcoholic withdrawal symptoms or delirium tremens requiring admission. Most cases of alcoholism will be picked up from asking screening questions as part of your routine health promotion questioning when taking a social history. If a patient drinks excessively, this may be a cue that the case revolves around this issue and it is essential that your undertake a more validated assessment of the patient's drinking habits and attempt to provide a brief intervention.

## PHYSICAL EXAMINATION

| Vitals | BMI, BP, pulse (AF) |
|---|---|
| Inspection | Inspect for signs of liver disease (ascites, spider naevi), tremor, jaundice |
| Examination | |
| Abdomen | Enlarged liver, ascites, signs of chronic liver disease |
| Neurology | Wide based gait (ataxia), confusion, peripheral neuropathy |

## INVESTIGATIONS

| Bloods | FBC (macrocytosis), B12, LFT, GGT |
|---|---|
| Others | ALT, AST, Albumin, clotting, or lipid (raised) |

| Questionnaires | Offer brief alcohol screening to all newly registered patients >16yr (DES). Screened using FAST or AUDIT-C. If positive, offer full AUDIT questionnaire |
|---|---|
| AUDIT-C | Scores =>5 is positive - higher risk drinking |
| Often | How often do you have a drink containing alcohol? |
| Units | How many units of alcohol do you drink on a typical day when you are drinking? |
| Excess | How often have you had 6 or more units (if female), or 8 or more (if male), on a single occasion in the last year? |
| | |
| FAST | If scores =>3 is positive - higher risk drinking |
| Excess | How often have you had =>6 units (female), or =>8 (male), on a single occasion? |
| Forget | How often during the last year have you been unable to remember what happened the night before because you had been drinking? |
| Impact | How often during the last year have you failed to do what was normally expected of you because of drinking? |
| Concern | In the last year has a relative or friend, or a doctor or other health worker been concerned about your drinking or suggested you cut down? |

## MANAGEMENT

### Conservative

| Brief Intervention | Provide a brief, 5 minute intervention. Discuss the patient's drinking habits and the cost vs benefits of drinking. Explore the health risks and impact it is having on their life. Advise about the DOH recommended weekly units for men (21u) & women (14u) |
|---|---|

### Lifestyle

| Avoid | Try and avoid places that have alcohol readily available such as pubs, clubs and supermarkets. Throw out reminders of alcohol from the the house (alcoholic beverages, empty bottles) |
|---|---|

| | |
|---|---|
| Going out | If going out with friends offer to buy others a round whilst missing yourself out. If you are drinking in a group ensure that you are the slowest drinker and sip your drink instead of gulping it down. Buy less concentrated forms of alcohol as you attempt to wean yourself off |
| Drinking | Try and have alcohol days off when you do not drink any alcohol. This will help reduce tolerance. Purchase small glasses or mugs to reduce the overall amount you drink. Replace alcohol with soft drinks |
| Driving | Alcohol dependence must inform DVLA. Cannot drive for 1yr until free of alcohol problem and 6mths for alcohol misuse. May require licence revocation and normalisation of blood tests |

*Self Help*

| | |
|---|---|
| Material | Offer books, leaflets on understanding alcoholism and managing it (Overcoming series) |
| Group therapy | Suggest to join Alcoholics Anonymous |

*Talking therapies*

| | |
|---|---|
| CBT | Consider referral for cognitive behavioural therapy (individual or group) to help alter unrealistic thoughts and beliefs |

**Detoxification**

| | |
|---|---|
| Community | Daily monitoring and treatment to ensure compliance for patients who drink >15u/day |
| Inpatient | Consider in patients who drink more than 30u of alcohol a day, have delirium tremens or epilepsy, or drink 15-20u daily but have severe depression, psychosis. Patients who are homeless or increased risk of suicide should be considered for inpatient detox |

**Medical**

*Acute Withdrawal*

| | |
|---|---|
| BDZ | Chlordiazepoxide is classically used to help reduce tremor and agitation. Alternative may be diazepam. Short courses to restrict chances of dependency |
| Vitamin B | Oral vitamin B complex or as multivitamins to reduce neurological symptoms |

*Relapse Prevention (specialist led)*

| | |
|---|---|
| Acamprosate | Usually used with counselling. Start as soon as you beginning alcohol withdrawal and continue for 6mths. Helps maintain abstinence as reduces cravings. Usual dose of 666mg tds |
| Naltrexone | Opioid antagonist that reduces the pleasure derived from drinking alcohol and helps to prevent relapse. Usually taken as a maintenance dose of 50mg tablet per day once detoxification is completed and treatment may last up to 6 months |
| Disulfiram | Works by causing physical side effects when drinking alcohol such as nausea, vomiting, flushing, palpitations and dizziness. Once started taken at a dose of 200mg daily for 12 weeks. Advise to avoid alcohol in food, perfumes and sprays as may get side effects |

**SAFETY NETTING**

| | |
|---|---|
| *Follow up* | Offer a series of appointments in primary care, with short gaps in more serious cases. Advise if symptoms of delirium tremens to review as soon as possible. Equally advise if signs of jaundice, haematemesis, abdominal pain (pancreatitis) or drowsiness for urgent review |

**DIFFERENTIAL DIAGNOSIS**

| Condition | Characteristic exam feature |
|---|---|
| **Alcohol dependence** | Patients experience cravings, preoccupation of drinking alcohol (despite knowing harmful). Alcohol is drunk to reduce withdrawal symptoms (tremor, insomnia, sweating, hallucinations), overtakes life to the point of neglect and tolerance (volume drunk would cause LOC for normal drinkers). Can use SADQ (questionnaire) |
| **Delirium tremens** | Often develops 2-3d after cessation of heavy alcohol consumption. Experiences delirium (disorientation of time & place), drowsiness, agitation), tremor of hands, sweating, hallucinations (formication) |
| **Pancreatitis** | Inflammation of pancreas presenting with acute upper abdominal pain, radiating to back and N&V. Can cause peritonitis (shoulder-tip pain, abdo tenderness) |
| **Wernicke encephalopathy** | Caused by thiamine deficiency, reversible. Wernicke symptoms include acute confusion, ataxia (broad based gait), ophthalmoplegia (fixed pupil, nystagmus, bilateral lateral rectus palsies), & peripheral neuropathies (legs) |
| **Korsakoff Psychosis** | Lack of thiamine causes irreversible damage. Presents with retrograde amnesia (before onset of condition) and anterograde amnesia (inability to memorise new information), confabulation (invented memories for gaps in memory), lack of insight |
| **Liver cirrhosis** | End stage liver disease. Presents with lethargy, pruritus, fever, weight loss, swelling of abdomen (ascites). Signs include jaundice, clubbing, palmar erythema, leukonychia, spider naevi, gynecomastia |

**EXPLANATIONS**

*Alcoholism*

Alcoholism is when a person has developed physical and psychological dependence on drinking alcohol such that if they were not to drink they would suffer with uncomfortable symptoms and feel generally unwell. This dependence drives further drinking so much so that even if the patient realises they should stop drinking, they find it extremely difficult to do so.

*Ill-Effects*

Drinking alcohol over a long period of time can cause health problems. The alcohol can affect a number of different vital organs in your body including the brain (depression, encephalopathy), heart (BP, irregular beats), liver (hepatitis, cirrhosis) and pancreas (inflammation). It can also cause erectile dysfunction, obesity and diabetes. Excessive alcohol can even put you are an increased risk of getting different cancers including, throat, liver and breast cancer.

*Cirrhosis*

Cirrhosis is where the liver slowly gets replaced by scar tissue (fibrosis). As a result the liver loses its ability to function properly. This can affect the liver's ability to purify the blood and clearing toxins and poisons and making proteins that are important for the blood to clot. It can also affect the blood flow to the liver causing back pressure called portal hypertension.

# 15.9 Drug Dependency

Substance misuse or drug dependency is an increasingly common phenomenon whereby a person has a compulsive need to use drugs in order to function. Failure to obtain drugs leads to uncomfortable withdrawal symptoms such as anxiety, shaking, excessive sweating and lack of concentration. A person can become addicted to a large number of substances including glue, nicotine, alcohol and caffeine, however in this chapter we will be focusing on illegal substances such as heroin, cocaine, MDMA, LSD and cocaine.

## HISTORY

Approach the topic sensitively in a non-threatening, non-judgemental manner. It can be quite difficult to broach the subject initially, so begin by making your first few questions designed to put the patient at ease.

| | |
|---|---|
| **Open questions** | Could you tell me about what has been troubling you? |
| *Expectations* | How were you hoping I could help you today? (detoxification or maintenance therapy, methadone for withdrawal symptoms, letter for court, housing) |
| *Cues* | If the patient appears embarrassed, displaying little eye contact, reflect this non-verbal cue to them by saying; You look upset? Is anything bothering you? |
| *Confidentiality* | Reassure that everything they say will be in confidence unless others are at risk |
| *Screening* | Screen for substance abuse if they have suffer from mental health disorders, alcoholism or in prison |

| **Focused questions** | |
|---|---|
| *Drugs* | What drugs are you currently taking? How long have you been taking them? When did you start? How much are you using? Has the amount changed recently? |
| Method | How do you take them? (orally, injection, snorting, smoking) |
| Needles | Do you inject the drugs? Do you share needles or equipment? (syringes) |
| Costs | How much are you spending to support your habit? |
| Overdose | Have you ever had an overdose recently? What happened? |
| Detoxification | Assess the patients motivation to change: Is there any reason why you want to stop now? Have you tried stopping before? |

| *Dependence syndrome* | |
|---|---|
| Cravings | Does your body have a strong desire to take drugs? |
| Control | Do you have difficulty controlling how much you drugs you take? |
| Tolerance | Are you finding that you need to take more drugs to get the same effect? |
| Withdrawal | Do you experience any withdrawal symptoms (muscle aches, restlessness, anxiety, cravings, sweating, insomnia) when you stop taking drugs? |
| Neglect | Do you find that you neglect other responsibilities because of your drug habit? |

| **Associated Questions** | |
|---|---|
| *Liver* | Have you noticed your skin or your going yellow? Any abdominal pain? |
| *Depression* | Have you been feeling low recently? Do you feel disinterested in life? |
| *Suicide* | Have you ever felt so low that you wanted to end it all? |

| **RED FLAGS** | Risk to self, vulnerable children/adults (pregnancy), liver disease |
|---|---|

## PAST HISTORY

| | |
|---|---|
| *Hepatitis B or C* | Has anyone informed you that you suffer from hepatitis B or C? |
| *HIV* | Have you ever been checked for HIV? |
| *Psychiatric* | Have you ever been treated for depression, anxiety or panic attacks? Have you ever had a psychotic episode or been diagnosed with schizophrenia? |
| *Medical* | Do you have any medical conditions? |

## FAMILY HISTORY

| | |
|---|---|
| *Psychiatric* | Does anyone in your family suffer from mental illnesses? Has anyone had problems with alcohol or substance misuse? |

## DRUG HISTORY

| | |
|---|---|
| *Medication* | Are you taking any medications or OTC preparations? |

## SOCIAL HISTORY

| | |
|---|---|
| *Smoker* | Do you smoke? How many cigarettes do you smoke per day? |
| *Alcohol* | Do you drink alcohol? How often and how much do you drink? |
| *Housing* | Where do you live currently? Are you homeless? |
| *Occupation* | Are you working at the moment or unemployed? Are you on benefits? |
| *Criminality* | Have you ever had a brush with the law because of your drug use? |
| *Finance* | How do you finance your drug habits? (sex workers, stealing) |
| *Support network* | Who lives with you at home? Do you have any close friends or family? |
| *Relationships* | Are you currently in a relationship? Does your partner use drugs? |
| *Children* | Do you have any children? Did you ever have a social worker? |

## IDEA, CONCERNS, EXPECTATIONS

| | |
|---|---|
| *Idea* | Do you think the drugs you are using are harmful for you? |
| *Concerns* | Do you have any worries about how much you are using? |
| *Impact* | How has your recreational drug use affected your life? |

## CSA TIPS

Patients presenting with drug dependence or substance abuse may not disclose their behaviour unless you provide them with reassurances that everything they tell you will be confidential and will not be shared with any outside agencies unless there was a risk of harm to others or to themselves. Patients who use drugs may also be engaging in other high-risk activities such as unsafe sex, sharing needles, criminality or sex work. It is important that you attempt to broach these topics and advise on the risk of catching a blood borne virus such as Hep A, B or HIV.

## PHYSICAL EXAMINATION

| | |
|---|---|
| *Vitals* | BP, pulse (bradycardia), temperature (hypothermic) |
| *Inspection* | Inspect for signs of liver disease if indicated. Inspect poor dental caries and poor nutrition |
| *Examination* | |
| Skin | Look for any injection or puncture marks on the elbow or legs. Look for signs of infections (sepsis, thrombophlebitis, cellulitis, abscess) |
| Other | if clinically indicated, listen to chest to exclude chest infections or TB. Feel the liver for an enlarged liver (hepatitis) |

## INVESTIGATIONS

| | |
|---|---|
| *Bloods* | LFT, GGT, Hepatitis B & C, HIV |
| Other | FBC (anaemia, infections) |
| *Urine* | Perform a urine drug screen. Screen prior to initiating opioid substitution treatment |
| *ECG* | Check for bradycardia (opiates) or arrhythmias. Methadone can cause long QT syndrome |

## MANAGEMENT
### Conservative

| | |
|---|---|
| *Brief Intervention* | Discuss their drug habits and the cost vs benefits of using drugs. Explore the health risks as well and impact it is having on their life. Do not recommend to go 'cold turkey' |
| *Harm reduction* | |
| Sharing needles | Inform of the risks of sharing needles (Hep B, HIV) and recommend testing. Offer needle exchange programme for safe disposal |
| Immunisation | Recommend immunisation for tetanus, hepatitis A and B |

| | |
|---|---|
| *Self Help* | |
| CAB | Refer to Citizens Advice Bureau for financial problems |
| Social services | Refer to social services to assist in housing or social issues |
| Group therapy | Suggest to join Narcotics Anonymous, Cocaine Anonymous or SMART |

| | |
|---|---|
| *Other* | |
| Social | Support the patients access to welfare benefits, housing (letter) |
| Driving | It is illegal to drive whilst under the influence of drugs. Drug users must inform DVLA if they used in the past 3 years. Licence considered if drug free for 1yr (group 1) or less (consultant led maintenance programme) |

### Medical

| | |
|---|---|
| *Refer* | Do not prescribe beyond your competence. Refer to a local drug dependency unit. Involve drug/key worker to support the patient |
| *Methadone* | Often first choice. If alcohol intake is significant methadone may not be appropriate. Often initiated on low doses. Liquids only licenced |
| Side effects | 'Clouding' effect, GI (N&V, constipation), dry mouth, headaches, reduced libido, amenorrhoea |
| *Buprenorphine* | Consider if suffered SE of methadone (drowsiness), wishes detoxification from heroin, on liver enzyme inducer/inhibitor drugs (rifampicin anticonvulsants). More likely to develop withdrawal symptoms |
| Side effects | Bitter taste, constipation, insomnia, nausea, sweating, headaches |

| | |
|---|---|
| *Supervised* | Both can be offered under supervised consumption i.e. pharmacist |
| *Withdrawal sympt.* | Observe for restlessness, irritability, insomnia, headaches, sweating, aches and pains, yawning, rhinorrhoea, dilated pupils, GI symptoms (abdo pain, nausea, vomiting, diarrhoea) |
| Treatment | Treat symptomatically i.e. loperamide (diarrhoea), metoclopramide (N&V), hyoscine or mebeverine (stomach cramps), paracetamol or NSAIDs (aches and pain), anxiety (propranolol) |
| *Other* | |
| Traveling abroad | Requires letter from prescribing doctor. Keep in hand luggage. If traveling >3mths requires special licence to travel with controlled drug |

| | |
|---|---|
| Pregnancy | Involve social services and CP if appropriate. Maintenance therapy of methadone recommended. Higher dose in 3rd trimester considered due to slowed gut mobility. Vomiting from morning sickness can reduce methadone intake. Offer antiemetics or quick prescription replacement |
| Pain | For acute pain continue maintenance dose of opioid medication. Offer paracetamol or NSAIDs. If severe and on methadone, offer morphine sulphate with dose titrated for pain. Monitor respiration |

## SAFETY NETTING

| | |
|---|---|
| *Child protection (CP)* | If any concerns for welfare of child refer as per local guidance |
| *Follow up* | Offer appointment within the week to establish if they are coping, achieving shared targets or tied with the local services. Offer daily appointments if initiating detoxification or maintenance treatment |

## DIFFERENTIAL DIAGNOSIS

| Condition | Characteristic exam feature |
|---|---|
| **Drug dependence** | Patients experience cravings, preoccupation for the drug (despite knowing harmful). Drugs are taken to reduce withdrawal symptoms (tremor, insomnia, sweating, hallucinations), overtakes life to the point of neglect and tolerance |
| **Cocaine** | Excessive use presents with dilated pupils, increased energy levels and excitability, insomnia, hallucinations, paranoia and palpitations. |
| **Heroin** | Overdose presents with depressed breathing, dry mouth, pinpoint pupils, low BP and constipation. May cause drowsiness, delirium and eventual coma. |
| **Ecstasy** | Excess use may present with headache, chest pain, blurred vision, nausea and vomiting, faint, raised BP, hyperthermia. OD may cause loss of consciousness, seizures and paranoia. |
| **LSD** | Overuse may lead to hallucinations, panic attacks, despair, feeling of death, fear and synesthesia (sensory crossover) |

# 15.10 Eating disorders

Eating disorders refers to the group of conditions that as a result of a person's altered eating habits puts their health and wellbeing at risk; usually out of a morbid fear that they will become obese or fat. The most common disorders are anorexia nervosa and bulimia, with bulimia being 5x more common than anorexia. It is thought that well over 1.5 million people are affected by an eating disorder in the UK with around 2% of women being affected at some point in their life. Although women are 10x more likely to be diagnosed with an eating disorder than their male counterparts, its prevalence is beginning to increase in the male population as well.

## HISTORY

Approach the topic sensitively in a non-threatening, non-judgemental manner. It can be quite difficult to broach the subject initially, so begin by making your first few questions designed to put the patient at ease.

| | |
|---|---|
| **Open questions** | Can you tell me more about the symptoms you have been experiencing? Could you tell me about what has been troubling you? |
| *Cues* | If the patient appears embarrassed, displaying little eye contact, reflect this non-verbal cue to them by saying; You look upset? Is anything bothering you? |
| *Screening* | In high risk patients (young women with low BMI), ask screening questions such as: Do you think you have an eating problem? Do you worry excessively about your weight? |

---

### The SCOFF Questionnaire

Screen for eating disorders. ≥2 positive questions suggests diagnosis of anorexia nervosa or bulimia

- Do you make yourself **S**ick because you feel uncomfortably full?
- Do you worry you have lost **C**ontrol over how much you eat?
- Have you recently lost more than **O**ne stone in a 3 month period?
- Do you believe yourself to be **F**at when others say you are too thin?
- Would you say that **F**ood dominates your life?

---

### Focused questions

*Eating disorders*

| | |
|---|---|
| Weight | Have you had any problems with your weight? How much weight have you lost? Over what time period? Did you mean to lose the weight? (intentional) |
| Diet | What do you eat in a typical day? Has your eating pattern changed recently? Do you avoid certain foods? Do you ever binge eat? |
| | Are you eating more healthily at the present time (fruit and veg)? Do you find yourself wanting to cook for others and not want to eat yourself? |

*Prevent weight gain*

| | |
|---|---|
| Purge | Do you ever make yourself throw up? (self induce, excess laxatives) |
| Medication | Do you use any medications to lose weight? (diuretic, appetite suppress.) |
| Exercise | Do you exercise? How much exercise do you do? |

*Psychological sympt.*

| | |
|---|---|
| Fear of fatness | Do you worry about your weight alot? Are you scared of putting it on? Do you enjoy losing it? |

| Body image | Are you happy with your body? (Desire to be thin) |
| Denial | Do you believe that you may have a weight problem? |

## Associated Questions

| Depression | Have you been feeling low recently? Do you feel disinterested in life or worthless inside? |
| Self-harm/Suicide | Have you ever harmed yourself to feel better inside? Have you ever felt so low that you wanted to end it all? |

## Differentials

*Anorexia nervosa*

| Hair growth | Have you noticed any abnormal hair growth anywhere on your body? |
| Menstrual history | When was your last period? Are they irregular? (amenorrhoea) |
| Hypothyroidism | Do you feel tired all the time? Do you have an intolerance to the cold? Do you suffer from constipation? |

*Bulimia nervosa*

| Eating | Are you finding that you raid the fridge for fattening foods like biscuits, chocolates or cakes? And then you make yourself sick to get rid of the food? |
| Guilt | Do you ever regret your behaviour of trying to lose weight? (by vomiting) |
| Other sympt. | Do you ever feel bloated, suffer from indigestion or a sore throat (from vomiting)? Have you had any problems with your teeth? |

**RED FLAGS**  Suicidal ideation, BMI < 14, electrolyte imbalance, bradycardia (<40bpm)

## PAST HISTORY

| Psychiatric | Have you ever had these symptoms before? Have you ever been treated for depression, anxiety or panic attacks? |
| Medical | Do you have any medical conditions? |

## FAMILY HISTORY

| Psychiatric | Does anyone in your family suffer from mental illnesses? Has anyone been diagnosed with eating disorders, depression or substance misuse? |

## DRUG HISTORY

| Medication | Are you taking any medications or OTC preparations? (laxatives, slimming pills, thyroxine) |

## SOCIAL HISTORY

| Stress | Is there anything in your life that has caused you much stress and anxiety? How was your childhood? (abuse, neglect) |
| Occupation | Are you currently working at the moment? Do you do dancing, modelling or acting? |
| Smoker | Do you smoke? How many cigarettes do you smoke per day? |
| Alcohol | Do you drink alcohol? How much do you drink and how often? |
| Recreational drugs | Have you ever used any recreational drugs? |
| Relationships | Are you currently in a relationship? Has it affected it? |
| Support network | Who lives with you at home? Have your close friends or family mentioned that they are worried about your weight? |

## IDEA, CONCERNS, EXPECTATIONS

| | |
|---|---|
| *Idea* | Do you have any idea about why you want to lose weight? |
| *Concerns* | Do you have any worries about it? |
| *Expectations* | How were you hoping I could help you? |
| *Impact* | How have your symptoms affected your life? |

## CSA TIPS

Most doctors consider eating disorders to be the domain of the consultant psychiatrist. However, given their widespread prevalence amongst young women (and increasing prevalence in men), a competent GP would be expected to screen for and diagnose relevant cases. In patients who attend with a morbid obsession about their weight or incessantly looking at themselves in the mirror, you should broach the subject about an eating disorder sensitively and work to take a clearer history.

## PHYSICAL EXAMINATION

| | |
|---|---|
| *Vitals* | Temp, height & weight, BMI, BP, pulse (arrhythmia - hypokalaemia) |
| *Inspection* | Inspect the teeth for erosion of tooth enamel, knuckles for calluses (Russell's sign - induced vomiting) |
| *Examination* | |
| Inspection | Pale, emaciated, bowed appearance, delayed puberty |
| Muscle power | Test muscle power by asking them to to sit up without using their hands (sit up test). Ask them to stand from a squatting position without using their hands (squat test) |

## INVESTIGATIONS

| | |
|---|---|
| *Bloods* | U&E's (hypokalaemia) |
| Others | FBCs, Ferritin, LFT's, CK, bone profile (PO4), TFT's or ESR if indicated |
| *ECG* | Patient may get bradycardia or arrhythmias, prolonged QT |
| *X-ray* | Only if concerned about fractures |
| *DEXA* | When admitted as inpatient |

## MANAGEMENT

### Conservative

*Lifestyle*

| | |
|---|---|
| Diary | Keep a food diary about what you eat and when you eat it. Record your emotions at the time and see if there is any link |
| Eating | Eating food at the regular mealtimes and do not snack |
| Dietician | Referral to an eating disorder trained dietician to discuss with the patient around calories, food intake and a healthy diet |
| Weight | Do not weigh yourself more than once a week. Try and avoid looking at yourself in the mirror |
| Dental | If the patient is vomiting, advice avoid brushing after vomiting, rinsing with mouthwash and reducing any acidic food intake. Refer to a dentist for assessment of dentition |

*Self Help*

| | |
|---|---|
| Material | Offer leaflets on understanding eating disorders and managing it (Overcoming series) |
| Group therapy | Suggest to join group therapy |
| *Talking therapies* | |
| CBT | Consider referral for cognitive behavioural therapy (individual or group) |

| Family | Consider for children or adolescents. Helps the family implement a healthy diet and also helps resolve any family based conflicts |

| Specialists | |
| CAT | Cognitive analytic therapy to help resolve unhealthy past events that impact on current behaviours |
| IPT | Interpersonal psychotherapy to help concentrate on your interactions with others and to deal with your emotional needs (reduced self-esteem, self-doubt) |

## Medical

| Laxatives | Stop or reduce any laxatives the patient is taking |
| Vitamins | May need oral multivitamins |
| Referral | Refer patient to specialist eating disorder clinic. Consider inpatient admission if risk to self, very low BMI or patient has deranged electrolytes |

## Specialists-led

| Antidepressants | Consider SSRI (fluoxetine 60mg) in bulimia to reduce the binges. Advise patients it may take 2-3 weeks before they feel any improvement. Can experience worsening of anxiety in first few weeks as medication is started |
| Energy drinks | Fortisip / Complan may be prescribed by dietician to aid weight gain |
| Antipsychotics | Olanzapine may be used in anorexia to reduce the anxiety and ruminations caused by the disorder. Often initiated by hospital |

## SAFETY NETTING

| Suicide risk | Review the patient frequently. Consider contacting Crisis Resolution & Home Treatment team for urgent assessment. Give Samaritans number for emergency |
| Sectioning | Try voluntarily, if not, consider compulsory admission (if risk to self, or to others) |
| Safeguarding | Follow local safeguarding pathways for child protection or vulnerable adults |
| Follow up | Offer a series of appointments in primary care, with short gaps in more serious cases |

## EXPLANATIONS

| Anorexia | Anorexia is an eating disorder that mainly affects young women. Although there a number of different factors that may trigger it such as genes, recent stress event, a large component is social pressures and the need to confirm to a certain body size. Sufferers usually worry about increasing weight and incorrectly think that they are overweight despite not being clinically so. As a result, they miss food or eat low calorie food to lose weight and try and achieve what they think is the right body weight for them. By doing this, they may restrict their body from vital vitamins and minerals that are required to function leaving them feeling tired, weak, dizzy and may even lead to quite serious illnesses and ultimately death. |

| Bulimia | This is an eating disorder in which the sufferer is worried about their body image but has episodes of uncontrollable binging on fatty foods and then forcefully expelling their stomach contents by vomiting or taking laxatives to prevent weight increase. |

csa exam
breaking bad news
ethical
negotiating
challenging
genetics
angry patient
claudication
focused history
complaints

MRCGP

anxiety
time keeping

consultations
abdominal pains  depression

CSA cases

summarising  psychosocial
ideas concerns expectations
diabetes  hypertension
heart failure

# MRCGP CSA Cases

Practice cases for the
MRCGP CSA exam

*by Muhammad and Nazmul Akunjee*
*MRCGP CSA course GP facilitators*

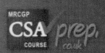

# 16.1 Genetic case

## Candidate's brief

### Patient medical records

| | |
|---|---|
| **Name:** | Margaret Kennie (31 years) |
| **Past medical history:** | Asthma (2000) |
| **Drug history:** | Folic acid 400 mcg |

### Letter from Genetic clinic (1 week ago)

*Letter from Genetic Screening to GP:* I am writing to summarise the results of the genetic screening tests. The couple had performed the initial tests but unfortunately they did not attend the follow-up appointment for the explanation of the results. Of note, the partner was tested previously and had been told he was a carrier.

Cystic Fibrosis occurs when a child inherits a defective copy of the CF gene from both parents. A defect in the gene is not the same in all cases. However, in the couples' case both partners have inherited the commonest type of defect called delta F508 gene and they are therefore both carriers. This means that there is a 1 in 4 risk of any child being born from the two partners being affected with CF.

*Dr Michael Shumer - Consultant Geneticist*

### Consultation (4 weeks ago)

*Dr Andrews:* Patient reports she is pregnant. LMP 1 week late - approximately 5 weeks gestation. Commenced on folic acid. Advice given in pregnancy regarding healthy eating, diet and alcohol - Emma's diary given. Non-smoker but drinks a glass of wine on occasions. Has agreed to stop for pregnancy. No cats in the house. Family history of CF. Organised referral to genetic clinic due to anxieties.

# Actor's brief

*Background:* You are Margaret Kennie, a 31 year old, IT columnist for an online technology magazine.
*Approach:* You are well dressed and are softly spoken. You are a confident middle-class lady.
*Opening statement:* 'Doctor, I guess you know I'm pregnant, but I am a little worried.'

## History

*Open history*

- You have been trying for a baby for a while with your partner and have just got pregnant. You are obviously very happy but also very anxious to make sure your baby is born healthy (verbal cue).
- *Verbal cue:* You missed your outpatient appointment, as you had been *'overwhelmed with everything'.*

### Reveal history if asked

*DNA*

- You have been quite anxious about whether your child will be born healthy. After you and your partner had the blood test you were *'overcome by nerves'* and could not face the results. You already know that your partner is a carrier of the CF gene.
- You missed the appointment but now having done some research on the web are more confused than ever. You managed to pluck the courage and book the appointment today with the doctor to know, *'once and for all'.*

*Cystic Fibrosis*

- You have a cousin called, Daniel, who was diagnosed with Cystic Fibrosis. He is the son of your aunt (Martha) on your dad's side.
- Your aunt and her partner, Tom, had a very difficult time bringing up Daniel. They were told that he would die before he passed his teenage years but instead he is still alive and is currently 22 years old. However, when he was younger he had lots of chest infections and was quite unwell needing constant 1-2-1 lung physiotherapy. He was *'always in and out of hospital'* and had a few close brushes with death due to pneumonia. However, he is more stable now and he is keen to be a physiotherapist and help others with the same condition.
- After seeing how Daniel grew up, you know enough about CF and its treatment. However, now that you are pregnant - *'It's hitting home, I need to know if my child has it or not!'*
- You do not want an explanation about the condition.

- *Ideas:* You want to know the blood results: whether your child has cystic fibrosis or not.
- *Concerns:* You are worried that your child has cystic fibrosis.
- *Expectations:* You want the results of the genetic tests as you want to know if your baby has CF definitively or not.

*Past medical history*

- You have suffered with Asthma for over 10 years but are well controlled with inhalers. For the last 1-year you have not needed to use your inhalers at all.

*Past obstetric history*

- You have no previous pregnancies, children or terminations.

- You have been previously reluctant to get pregnant with your knowledge that something was wrong with the genes in your family. However, you are overtly aware that *'time is running out and nature does not wait for anyone'*.
- You are really excited with your pregnancy but you are finding it hard to celebrate with this hanging over you.

*Family history*

- As above regarding CF.
- You have no other medical problems in your family.

*Drug history*

- You no longer need your inhalers. You take folic acid 400mcg as prescribed.
- You have no drug allergies.

*Social history*

- You do not smoke but drink the occasional glass of wine at least 3 times a week; usually at social events.
- Your mood is stable and you sleep and eat well.
- *Relationship:* You have been with your partner for 3 years and decided to try for a child this year, as things between yourselves have never been better. You are happy with him and he is very supportive. He will support any decision you make about the baby.
- *Occupation:* You live in a 2 bedroom flat with a minimal mortgage. You have no financial worries and have a good job in the city as an IT journalist with a regular column for an online magazine.
- *Diet:* You are conscious of what you eat after Dr Andrews informed you what is good for your baby. You have read all the books and avoid all the foods that you are meant to. You do not want either antenatal or booking advice today.

---

### *Nub of the case*

- You are a middle class lady who is pregnant and worried about her baby having Cystic Fibrosis.
- You missed your genetic clinic appointment, as you were too nervous of the results. Both you and your partner have already had your DNA/swab taken.
- You have a cousin who has CF and has struggled with his health from it (recurrent chest infections).
- You believe that the doctor is going to inform you whether your baby has CF or not. You are surprised it is only a probability score.
- You want to know how to test for sure whether your baby has it or not.

---

**How to respond**
- *Results:* If the doctor informs that you and your partners are carriers of CF gene act surprised and worried. Ask to clarify what that means for your baby: *'Does that mean my baby has it?'*
  - If the doctor informs you that there is a 1 in 4 chance that your baby has CF appear surprised and confused and suggest, *'I thought I will be finding out today definitely whether my child had it or not. What does 1 in 4 mean?'*
  - Accept an explanation of the chance of inheriting CF if explained accurately.
    - Remain puzzled if performed poorly.
  - After explanation, demand to know how you can be tested to be 100% sure your baby has CF or not.

- **Investigations:** If the doctor suggests that there are tests that can be done in the womb, seek clarification what tests and when they can be done. Also ask how it is performed.
  - If the doctor suggests it is done by a needle, act alarmed and quite surprised (non-verbal cue).
    - Your concern, if asked, is whether the needle will hit your baby and cause bleeding to your child inside your womb: *'What if you insert the needle and hit my baby?'* Be reassured if they explain that it is ultrasound guided.
  - Enquire about the risks of the test i.e. miscarriage, harm to the fetus.
  - If the doctor suggests that you can wait until your child is born and then perform a sweat test reply that you must know now *'to put your mind at ease'.*
    - You believe that you will have an *'awful 7 months'* of pregnancy if you did not know.

- **Implications:** If the doctor asks you the question about what you would do if you learnt that your baby had CF then reply, *'I really want this baby and I will do everything to keep it.'*
  - Explain further that you want to be fully prepared for any eventuality and you learnt lessons from Daniel's experience and you believe that there are good treatments and support for children with CF.
  - Already you have seen Daniel live longer than expected with current treatments and you have been reading alot about viral gene technology and believe that by the time your baby is older, medical advancements will mean your baby is almost cured of CF.

## Examination findings

|  | Vitals | Examination |
|---|---|---|
| BP | 110 / 68 | Declines as has appointment in 3 days time with own midwife |
| Pulse | 81 bpm | |
| BMI | 29 | |
| Temp | 37.1˚C | |

## CSA Case points

This scenario is testing your ability to discuss genetics testing with a pregnant mother. The mother is already quite well informed about the condition at hand, Cystic Fibrosis, and is keen to find out definitively as to whether her current pregnancy may be suffering with the condition. The case centers around taking a good history as well as the concurrent psycho-social problems surrounding the mother and ultimately exploring how exactly she wants to proceed if she were to learn the definitive results from further testing.

### CANDIDATE BRIEF

The candidate's brief offers a key insight into the possibility that this case will focus on a genetic topic. It is revealed that the mother is currently pregnant and that she has a family history of Cystic Fibrosis. As a result she has been referred to speak to the geneticist. However, as per the Consultant's letter, she missed the follow-up appointment to discuss the results in detail. The geneticist has informed you that both partners were found to be carriers. Prior to the patient entering the room, you should plot out a genetic tree and calculate the risks of being a carrier and suffering the full-blown disease. Consider ways of how to communicate the different risk to the mother if she is attending today to discuss these.

Given the mother's anxiety about Cystic Fibrosis warranting a genetics referral, and the clear family history, it would be prudent to consider exploring these two issues further in the consultation. It is likely that she is attending today due to missing her appointment and perhaps, given that you are her GP, she is more likely to trust your explanation and be comfortable to ask questions.

The patient is currently only on folic acid that was commenced a few weeks prior. However, there is a note that they have suffered from asthma. It may be useful to establish how well controlled the patient's asthma is and whether they are currently taking any treatment for this. It is a well-known fact that in about a third of pregnancies patients with asthma may get a worsening of symptoms.

From the candidate's brief you can approximate that she is 9 weeks pregnant, however, there is very little antenatal history recorded in the notes. It may well be worth asking more history surrounding the mother's obstetric background. Has she been pregnant before? Had she had any terminations (if so, particularly was it due to a possible congenital deformity)? Does she have any children now? If so, are they healthy?

## INTERPERSONAL SKILLS
Genetic cases are quite sensitive consultations since they broach subjects that may affect whether a pregnancy will be continued or not. The advice given during the consultation may alter the plans a mother, or the parents have for their child. Hence, one has to be quite conscious of the issues and broach the topic with the delicateness it deserves.

As the patient begins, she starts with an opening statement that expresses her anxieties surrounding the pregnancy. It is important to use open questions to help allow the patient to offer her true feelings and the surrounding history as freely as possible without interruption. Ensure that you always act empathically if the patient reveals any anxieties, or concerns. Make sure that you do not over complicate any explanation or use excessive medical jargon particularly when speaking about genes and inheritance. This will only serve to confuse and confound the patient and is likely to make them feel even more anxious than they already are.

*Negative indicators:*
- Fails to listen to the patient and obtain a detailed understanding of the issues.
- Fails to identify or respond to cues.
- Fails to use open questions and appears abrupt.
- Uses excessive medical jargon when communicating the risk.

## DATA GATHERING
Although the patient describes her anxieties about the pregnancy and the possibility of cystic fibrosis it is important to try and establish what she already knows. It may be an idea to quickly summarise the previous consultation back to her, to check she agrees with what was said and then to request whether she received a copy of the letter from the genetics clinic. It would be relevant as well to establish why she missed the follow-up appointment with the hospital.

*DNA*
- Try and find out why the patient missed the follow-up appointment? Did she do this willingly or was the appointment forgotten? If she missed it intentionally, what was the reason? What was she afraid of finding out? Does she want you to communicate the risk of CF today to her?

*Cystic Fibrosis*

- Why is the patient so worried about the risk of Cystic Fibrosis? Has she or her partner been tested before? Does she know anyone with CF and what was their experience with it? What does she understand about CF?
- Does she want you to explain the condition today? Or was she expecting something else from the consultation.

*Psycho-social context*

- Establish the impact the symptoms have had on the patient's cousin i.e. attendance to numerous hospital appointments, number of admissions and near-death experiences (ITU admissions).
- Determine the patient's current living arrangements and who they live with. What does their partner know about CF? What would the partner want to do if the child had CF?
- Check if they smoke or drink and signpost to health promotion initiatives as appropriate.

*Negative indicators:*

- Takes only a superficial history about the presenting complaint and fails to elicit subtle signs of anxiety about the pregnancy.
- Makes superficial assumptions about the patient's health and does not elicit relevant psycho-social context i.e. impact on life-expectancy.

## CLINICAL MANAGEMENT SKILLS

When a patient attends for their first appointment after finding out they are pregnant, it is important to ascertain their intentions with regards to keeping the baby or having a termination (TOP). This becomes more evident when dealing with sensitive topics such as genetic scenarios. If one were to assume that the patient intended to have a TOP, this may be taken as being judgmental and dramatically change the tone of the consultation. Often a good question to ask early on would be:

**'If you found out that your baby had this condition, how would it change things? Would it change whether you wanted to keep this pregnancy or not?'**

*Inheritance*

- **Explanation:** Explain to the patient the mode of inheritance: *'Genes come in pairs with one from each pair coming from both parents. A person suffering from CF inherits one copy of the sleeping defective gene from each parent who are the recessive carrier.'*
  - Explain other possible outcomes: *'If a person inherits a single defective gene than this means that they do not have the disease but are a carrier. This means they can pass on the gene to their children, but will not be affected with the disease themselves.'*
  - Explain to the patient the risk to their child: *'In your case, since both your partner and yourself are carriers there is a 1 in 4 (25%) chance that your baby will have Cystic Fibrosis. In other words if you were to have 4 children with your partner we would expect 1 child completely well without any defective gene, 2 children who are well and healthy but are carriers of the defective gene, and 1 child who will have CF.'*

*Definitive tests*

- Discuss with the patient options to conduct more accurate tests in-utero to determine whether the fetus has CF: *'Chorionic villus sampling or amniocentesis are techniques that allow us to take a sample from the womb of the baby's cells. We will pass a fine needle through the wall of your tummy. It is performed in early pregnancy (11-14 CVS, 16wk - amniocentesis) and we will use ultrasound to guide us to ensure the baby is safe.'*

- Explain the risks associated with Chorionic villus sampling or amniocentesis: *'However, the test is not 100 percent accurate and there is a slight risk of causing a miscarriage (1/100).'*

*Post delivery/diagnosis*

- Offer the patient alternative methods to diagnose Cystic Fibrosis including the heel prick test or sweat test. Emphasise that these tests can only be conducted once the baby has been delivered.

- **Referral:** Support the mother in her decision to keep the baby. Suggest that you can organise an early obstetric and paediatric referral. Offer patient organizational details or charity information for patients with CF.

- **Follow-up:** Consider reviewing the patient in a few weeks after they have had time to discuss with their partner or the midwife. Consider seeing the patient with their partner to further explore the issues.

*Negative indicators:*

- Uses inappropriate (e.g. technical) language.
- Fails to offer suitable options for investigating CF i.e. CVS or amniocentesis.
- Fails to incorporate patient's ideas and expectations into the management plan i.e. patient wants to keep the child regardless of diagnosis and would like in-utero testing to be prepared.

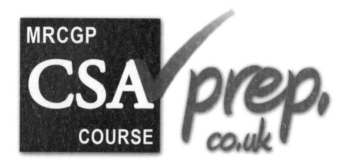